THE HISTORY OF MEDICATIONS FOR WOMEN

Materia medica woman

THE HISTORY OF MEDICATIONS FOR WOMEN

Materia medica woman

Michael J. O'Dowd

Consultant Obstetrician Gynaecologist
Portiuncula Hospital, Ballinasloe, Co. Galway, Ireland

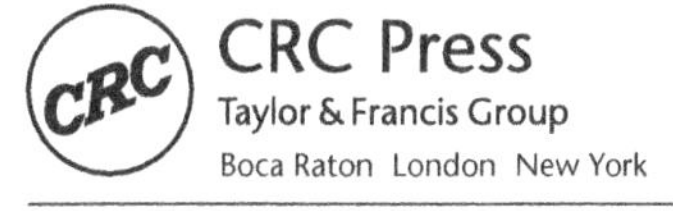

CRC Press is an imprint of the
Taylor & Francis Group, an informa business

Library of Congress Cataloging-in-Publication Data
O'Dowd, Michael J.
The history of medications for women / by M.J. O'Dowd.
p. ; cm.
Includes bibliographical references and index.
ISBN 1-85070-002-8 (alk. paper)
1. Materia medica--History. 2. Women--Medical care--History. I. Title.
[DNLM: 1. Drug Therapy--history. 2. Genital Diseases, Female--history. 3. Alternative Medicine. 4. Genital Diseases, Female--drug therapy. 5. Obstetrics--history. 6. Women's Health. WP 11.1 O26h 2000]
RS62. O36 2000
615'.1'082--dc21s 00-038506

British Library Cataloguing in Publication Data
O'Dowd, Michael J.
The history of medications for women
1. Women – Health and hygiene – History 2. Drugs – History
3. Women – Diseases – Treatment – History
I. Title
615.1'082

CRC Press
Taylor & Francis Group
6000 Broken Sound Parkway NW, Suite 300
Boca Raton, FL 33487-2742

First issued in paperback 2019

ISBN-13: 978-1-85070-002-9 (hbk)
ISBN-13: 978-0-367-39756-2 (pbk)

Typeset by Siva Math Setters, Chennai, India

Visit the Taylor & Francis Web site at
http://www.taylorandfrancis.com

and the CRC Press Web site at
http://www.crcpress.com

Contents

Dedication

To Christine, wife, partner, lover, mother of our children,
best friend, and my personal Materia Medica Woman.

Acknowledgments

My special thanks to David Bloomer for accepting *The History of Medications for Women* for publication, and for his patience while awaiting the final manuscript. To Helen Lee, Scientific Editor, and to all at Parthenon Publishing.

Christine, organised my personal and professional life to allow time for research and writing, and helped with advice, formatting and typing. Margaret Mannion for data processing and typing. Florence Grenham for data processing. Mike O'Reilly for computer programming and software support. Katy O'Dowd for research on Thomas Cross and Nicholas Culpeper. Clare O'Dowd for work on complementary medicine. Michael and David O'Dowd for computer support. Judy and Joe Lieberman for medicinal plants of Philadelphia. Ulrika Grubner, Schloss Arnskaug, Neustadt an der Orla, Germany, translated portions of *Der Schwangern Frauen und Hebammen Rosengarten* of 1513.

Robert Mills, Librarian, Royal College of Physicians, Dublin. Helen Rivett, The Librarian and staff, The Royal Society of Medicine, London. The Librarian, The British Lending Library. Patricia Want, Librarian, Royal College of Obstetricians and Gynaecologists, London. The Librarian, Wellcome Library, London. Susan Rishworth, Archivist, American College of Obstetricians and Gynecologists, Washington, for her gift of *The Philadelphia Practice of Midwifery* by Charles Meigs (1842) during my visit in 1997. Ballinasloe Community Information Society.

Some of the older documents were obtained on microfiche from: Inter Documentation Company bv, PO Box 11205, 2301 EE Leiden, The Netherlands. Other older sources were a number of facsimile obstetric books from: The Classics of Obstetrics and Gynecology Library, Gryphon Editions, 3000 Cindel Drive, PO Box 6003, Delran, New Jersey 08075, USA.

The booksellers, Patrick Pollack, Nigel Phillips and Victor Daniels, England; Stokes Books, Dublin; Vanessa Parker and Roger Grimes, Rare Ould Times, Westport; Patrick Rowan, Belfast; Robert Campbell, Montreal, and others.

To Elliot Philipp who started it all. To my family for their support and understanding of many absences.

Section 1

Introduction 1

THE EVOLUTION OF MATERIA MEDICA WOMAN

At the beginning of 1994 I sat in the library of the College of Physicians, Dublin, and read Ireland's oldest text on midwifery, the *Speculum Matricis*, written by the Cork-based physician and accoucheur, James Wolveridge, and published in 1671. My motive at the time was to glean some information for a book to be entitled 'The History of Obstetrics and Gynecology In Ireland', an epic as yet unborn. It occurred to me that most of the text of the *Speculum Matricis* consisted of recipes for exotic-sounding nostrums for the problems encountered with fertility, pregnancy and childbirth. Drug names such as asafetida, bezoardic medicine, castoreum, diamargariton and styrax jumped from the pages but found no connections in my twentieth century brain. The seeds of motivation were sown and it became a priority to research the history of materia medica for women.

THE SCOPE OF MATERIA MEDICA WOMAN

Materia Medica Woman is a book that contains lists of medications used by, or prescribed for, women from earliest times to the present, a form of historical catalog. The histories of many remedies are described in detail in the form of monographs while others, though listed, are ignored. Some botanical, chemical, pharmacological and therapeutic details are included, as are extensive quotations from old and rare books, and from modern texts. Some of the history of obstetrics and gynecology, and of general medicine, complements the text, as do a number of short biographies and illustrations.

The 'Materia Medica Woman Project' set out to discover what medications were prescribed for women, but not whether they all had demonstrable therapeutic benefits for the illnesses for which they were prescribed. Except in the monographs or special subject areas, no great attempt was made to discover whether the medications were subjected to modern laboratory or therapeutic analysis: that is work for a different project. *Materia Medica Woman* is a primer for further study on the historical aspects of medications for women. *Materia Medica Woman* is not a textbook of botany, pharmacology, pharmacognosy or therapeutics. The medications in the book are included purely for their historical interest and are neither debunked nor recommended for dispensing. Drugs should not be taken except under the care and guidance of a skilled professional.

RESEARCH: PROBLEMS AND SOLUTIONS

The research involved identifying source material suitable for the historical periods, civilizations and the special subjects as outlined in the Contents. All of the medications in each of the specific source books were cataloged, as were the indications for their use. The information was placed in a specially designed analytical computer program. Partial or complete lists of the cataloged medications are scattered throughout the text of *Materia Medica Woman*. Many problems were encountered during the research, the compilation of facts, and the eventual writing of the book. Some of the difficulties had a number of solutions and the choices made were entirely my own. The following problems and solutions are examples.

Theory of medicine

Historically, the main theory of medicine evolved from the cultures of ancient Greece and Rome and was handed down as humoral medicine, a form of diagnostics, prognostics and therapeutics quite different from the twentieth century view. Medications were prescribed using completely different logic but, in spite of this, many were effective. Humoral medicine (and its adaptations) existed for millennia and carried its own authority. No attempt was made to change its diagnostic categories in this book although modern terminology is often used to replace the ancient. Examples are the use of 'hemorrhage' for 'flooding' and 'menorrhagia' for 'great excess of the courses, or flowers'.

Drug names

The problems

Drug names, whether animal, vegetable or mineral, varied over the centuries. A plant, for instance, most often had an original name in Greek or Latin, but had alternative names in both languages. From an etymological point of view the English name for the plant was often quite unrelated to the Greek or Latin versions and to compound the problem a single plant could have a number of synonyms. The parts of the plant, whether fresh or stored, which were used as medication could vary, as could the dosage. Throughout the ages almost all prescriptions were compound in nature, and the plant in question could be mixed with a large number of other animal, mineral, or plant components to form the final medication. The medication could then be administered in a number of different ways – by fumigation, my mouth, as a plaster, or per rectum, for example.

The solutions

Plants and other medications have been identified where possible by their modern English names, but not always by their official Latin names. There were some remedies that could not be identified but they were, however, cataloged by their original name and listed in the text. In most instances, the *Materia Medica Woman* listing did not retain information on whether the herb was fresh or dried, or whether flower, leaf, stem, root or seed was used. Many authors' works were quoted in the text of *Materia Medica Woman* and on those occasions specific plant parts were mentioned as in the original author's text. The specific plant was allocated to its 'category of use' without indicating what other medications were in the compound and without relating how it was administered. This method of recording reduced the number of variables per medication and simplified matters, but led to instances such as that of water (a vehicle) being classified as a treatment. As some remedies consisted of over fifty components the simple approach was the most appealing.

Translations of source material

The content of translated older works varied according to whether the work was rendered into English from Greek, Latin, Arabic, French or German and from what source the translation was made. The translators did not necessarily agree on the names of all the medications mentioned in a text and some speculative terminology occurred. My choice of a particular translation was based on who the translator was, the clarity of the translated English, or sometimes simply by what translation was available to me. A case in point was the work of Aetius of Amida: James Ricci made a translation that was logical and easy to read and I chose his text as the source for cataloging medications from the Aetius era.

Indications for therapy

Indications for therapy did not always fall into clear-cut groups, particularly in texts before the eighteenth century. For example, many drugs were used 'to help labor'. Did that mean that the medications were oxytocics, analgesic/sedatives, or that they were just offered as a 'pick-me-up', or tonic, in a nourishing broth? The solution to this problem was to put remedies into diagnostic categories according to the historical sources, although this system did lead to some duplication. Labor drugs in older texts could therefore be assigned to groups such as 'to start labor', 'to help labor', 'to relieve labor', etc., although the expected action of the drug was not always obvious in a modern context.

PRESENTATION

Catalogs are not much fun to read so an historically-based text was written to complement drug lists in the Chapters on different eras, civilizations and/or special subjects. Chapters in the Chronology section comprise a brief dip into the history and, where appropriate, the mythology of the era. General medical theories were summarized in the early chapters but as humoral medicine became the norm from the time of ancient Greece and Rome until the eighteenth century the humoral concepts, once outlined, were not repeated in depth. The historical aspects of obstetrics and gynecology were explored and enlivened by quoting verbatim from books of the period. The old forms of English spelling were retained to add 'texture' to the script.

Most chapters contain a 'Selection of Materia Medica for Women' chosen from the drug lists of the era in question. The drugs were usually chosen because they were the most frequently mentioned medications in the group. The chapter on the late Middle Ages, for example, has monographs highlighting aetites, eagle-stone, dragon's blood, iris, savin, shepherd's purse and wax, while the twentieth century selection includes drugs such as aspirin, folic acid, thalidomide and many more. 'Lists of Medications', and/or 'Medications and their Uses', accompany most chapters but their sum falls short of the entire Materia Medica Woman catalog. A number of pertinent biographies are included. Appropriate references accompany all chapters and for many of the older texts the subject matter and the page numbers are mentioned.

HIGHLIGHTS OF MATERIA MEDICA WOMAN

Remarkable treatments

- Much of the materia medica of ancient Assyria (c. 4000 BC) is still in use today in herbal medicine.
- Malachite and kohl were used by the ancient Egyptians to prevent bacterial eye infection and became fashionable as make-up.
- Mummy medicine was used as a uterine expulsive.
- Arab physicians treated skin lesions with mercury, which was introduced into Europe by the Crusaders. Initially a treatment for syphilitic skin sores, mercury became the usual treatment for generalized syphilis from the fifteenth to the twentieth century.
- Dragon's blood was prescribed for a variety of female complaints during the Middle Ages.
- Penicillin was derived from a fungus found on decaying blue hyssop.
- Cephalosporins were developed from sewage outlet effluent.
- Opium came from meconium.
- Castoreum, the dried secretion of the preputial glands of the beaver, was used as an oxytocic and for a number of female complaints.
- Quinine, from cinchona bark, was used to treat the pyrexia of puerperal fever.
- Estrogens were discovered in the American pussy-willow.
- Epsom salts beat the scourge of eclampsia.
- Mexican yam was found to contain diosgenin which allowed large-scale production of progesterone.
- Anticoagulants were discovered in sweet clover when castrated bullocks bled to death.
- Anti-D (RhoGam) was developed in male prisoners at Sing Sing Penitentiary.
- The ovaries of 2500 pigs were used to yield 1 mg of progesterone.
- Aspirin was obtained from willow tree bark and meadowsweet.
- Lanolin was discovered by the Greeks and Romans in the sweaty wool of skin-folds close to sheep udders.
- Mothers' milk was a common ingredient of 'powerful' Egyptian medications.
- Human placenta is used as a medication in China and was used in the West for cosmetics and for extracting hormones until recently.
- Ergot was obtained from smutted rye.
- Ether, the first anesthetic used in midwifery, was obtained by the action of acid of sulfur on plant-derived alcohol.
- Leeches were used for a variety of conditions, including breast engorgement, and for many years physicians were known as 'leeches'.

- Lydia Pinkham's pills, an American nostrum for female complaints in the nineteenth and twentieth centuries, were commemorated in song in both centuries.
- Intra-uterine electrical therapy was an early twentieth century remedy for menorrhagia.

Remarkable authors

The most notable aspect of many of the works featured in *Materia Medica Woman*, and one that must gain admiration and respect, was that the authors cared passionately about their chosen subject, whether it was botany, herbal medicine, obstetrics, pharmacology, pharmacognosy or therapeutics. The ancient authors managed to compile vast amounts of readable data filling many hundreds of pages per book and one wonders how they tackled the problems of research, compilation of materials, writing, correcting and eventual publication.

- Dioscorides' herbal of the first century AD was the basis of all herbals for almost 2000 years.
- Soranus of Ephesus (second century AD), the author of *Gynecology*, wrote the most important book on midwifery of all time.
- Almost 1500 years later, Eucharius Rösslin ushered in the renaissance of midwifery with his *Der Schwangern Frauwen und Hebammen Rosengarten*, translated as *The Byrth of Mankynde*.
- Nicholas Culpeper, 'Divine and Gent', beloved of the poor and reviled by physicians, changed forever the practice of therapeutics and is one of the unsung 'greats' of medical history.
- The trials and tribulations of being a man-midwife are explored in the biography of Fielding Ould.
- Samuel Bard wrote the first American textbook published there and his well organized materia medica was the best in any obstetric book of the nineteenth century.
- Carl Linnaeus was mainly responsible for the binominal classification of species used today but he was ridiculed for his sexual classification of plants.

The most remarkable discoveries

- Mercury, the main treatment for syphilis for almost 600 years.
- Ergot, used to prevent postpartum hemorrhage by midwives from the Middle Ages, was introduced into medical practice by John Stearns in 1807.
- Anesthesia, developed by James Young Simpson in 1847, paved the way for the relief of the 'Curse of Eve', the pain of labor.
- Blood transfusion, first used therapeutically by James Blundell 1818.
- Chemotherapy of puerperal sepsis with prontosil by Leonard Colebrook and Maeve Kenny in 1936.
- Penicillin, discovered in 1928 by Alexander Fleming and developed by Florey, Chain and colleagues in the 1940s.
- Hormonal contraception, which became a reality after the discovery of diosgenin and clinical trials partially funded by women and championed by a devout Roman Catholic.
- Epsom salts (magnesium sulfate), for eclampsia, used since the nineteenth century but established as the best treatment in the late twentieth century.
- Hormone replacement therapy: 'We stand at the threshold. Like Moses glimpsing the Promised land' (see Chapter 17).
- Taxol, from the bark of Pacific yew, used in chemotherapy of female cancers.

CONCLUSION

From early 1994 until the manuscript was completed some five years later, I learned about asafetida, bezoardic medicine, castoreum, diamargariton and styrax, and my mind savored those once alien-sounding names, and hundreds more, as I tracked down the many strange and wonderful medications that comprised the materia medica of women from ancient Assyria to the end of the twentieth century. Now I look around me with a modulated twentieth-century brain and wonder where the new Taxol or similar 'wonder drug' for women will be found. Will it be synthesized *de novo* in a laboratory or obtained from mares' urine, from a plant or frog skin, from a chicken-run or from the effluent of a sewage pipe discharging into the sea? And will I forget that some illnesses require the patient to hitch their boat to a mooring-post and listen to the soothing sounds of the water as they wait for time and 'inner healing' to provide the remedy? Will modern medicine rediscover its roots in herbal medicine and become an all-encompassing whole of allopathic and complementary medicine? Whatever the future holds the Materia Medica Woman Project was a source of fascination, inspiration and fun, allied with plenty of problem-solving and seat polishing. I hope you enjoy it as much as I did.

Section 2

Origins

The prescription 2

THE ORIGIN OF THE PRESCRIPTION

The word 'prescription' is derived from the Latin (*prae*, before + *scribo*, I write) and is a formula which lays down, in advance, rules or directions for the preparation and administration of the ingredients of a medical remedy.

Nowadays medical prescriptions are simple in format because standard drug formulations were introduced into therapeutics during the twentieth century. Contrast this with the 1920s when 80% of prescriptions filled in American pharmacies required a knowledge of preparation and compounding (Cowen and Helfand, 1990 p. 219). The classic prescription, written in Latin or English (and often in the form of standard abbreviations) was complex to write and to prepare. Each prescription contained a number of parts.

1. Name of the patient: the address might also be included.
2. Superscription: a heading in the form of an instruction to the dispenser. The symbol Rx was used and was an abbreviation of the Latin (*recipe*, take).
3. The instruction: a list of ingredients, together with the amount of each. Contained in this was:
   (a) a basis, which was the principal ingredient;
   (b) an adjuvant, which could enhance or hasten the action of the basis;
   (c) a corrective, to counteract any undesirable effects of the drug(s) used; and
   (d) a vehicle, usually flavoring or coloring material.
4. The subscription: this stated the form the preparation had to take and the amount to be dispensed, e.g. *fiat mistura* (FM) meant 'let a mixture be made', while *mitte* would mean 'send'.
5. The signature: this referred to the directions to be given to the patient. The term *signeture* or *sign* meant 'let it be labeled' and the subsequent instructions were written in Latin, in abbreviated form, or in English, e.g. 'one tablespoonful to be taken at night'.

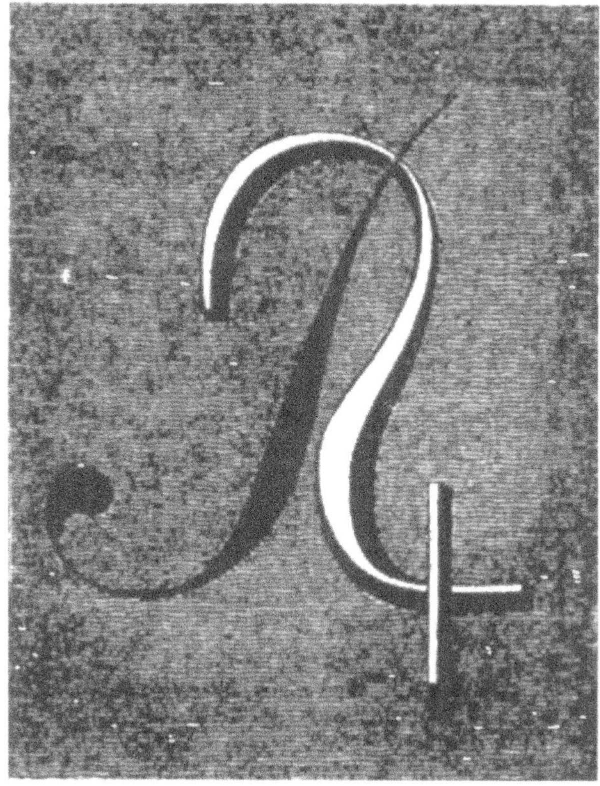

Figure 1 The Rx symbol for a prescription

The prescription was complete when signed and dated by the prescribing doctor.

THE ORIGIN OF THE Rx SYMBOL

The Eye of Horus

It is believed that the abbreviated Rx sign may be derived from ancient Egyptian mythology and that it signifies the 'Eye of Horus' (Lyons and Petrucelli, 1987 p. 77). Horus was one of the principal gods of ancient Egypt. He was represented as a hawk or falcon, or shown in human form with a falcon's head. He had two main identities, that of the sun god Horus, or as the son of Isis and Osiris. Isis was the Egyptian goddess of motherhood and fertility, and Osiris, who was the God of fertility and vegetation, later became Lord of the Underworld. Horus was often depicted as a child being breastfed by his goddess mother.

Osiris and Isis were brother and sister but also man and wife. Osiris was the heir to all the Egyptian gods. He introduced the cultivation of food and plants and brought civilization to his people. His brother, the wicked god Seth, was jealous of his power and popularity and determined to kill Osiris. In a pretense of friendship, Seth invited Osiris to a banquet. After his arrival, the evil brother imprisoned Osiris in a lead-lined chest which was thrown into the river Nile. The casket became entwined in the branches of a sapling which grew into a fragrant tamarisk tree. Isis found the body of her dead husband and hid it in the marshes of the Nile delta. While out hunting, Seth discovered the body. He cut it into 14 pieces which he scattered throughout the lands of Egypt. With the help of her sister, Isis collected 13 of the body parts and reassembled them in an embalming process so creating the first mummy (Patrick and Croft, 1987 p. 39). Despite her magical powers Isis could not bring Osiris back to life. However, she fashioned a golden phallus to replace the dead god's missing body-part and by mystical means she infused Osiris with the life of her loins, warming him enough to awaken his sexual energy and make her pregnant (Cotterell, 1989 p. 102). Thus was Horus conceived and from that time on Osiris became Lord of the Underworld.

When Horus reached maturity he aspired to the role and responsibilities previously held by his father, and which were held in trust for him by his mother. Seth opposed this move and their conflict lead to many adventures. During one bitter encounter Seth gouged out the eye of Horus. Temporarily blinded and in pain, Horus sought refuge with Isis. By magical means she replaced the eye and bathed it with healing milk. The eye was completely restored and from then it was known as the udjat, the 'whole (or sound) eye'. This miraculous event signified that the 'Eye of Horus' was all-powerful. It became a symbol of soundness, strength and danger, but also of protection (Clayton, 1990 p. 103). Horus became ever more potent and through a

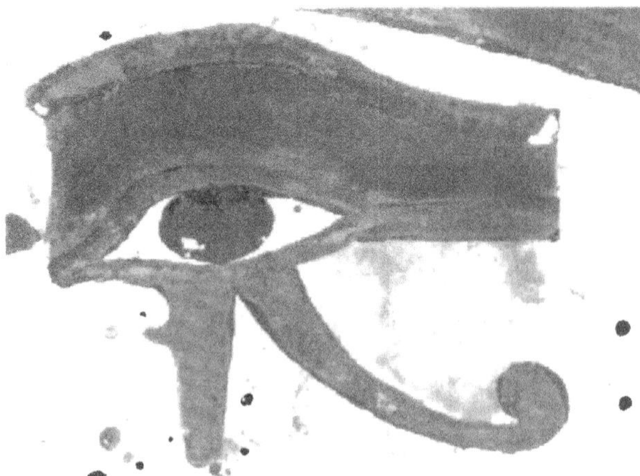

Figure 2 The eye of Horus (Courtesy of the Louvre, Paris)

series of events overcame his uncle Seth to assume his father's earlier role as god of fertility and vegetation. Thereafter each Pharaoh or King of ancient Egypt was regarded as Horus incarnate (David, 1987 p. 96).

The typical appearance of the 'Eye of Horus', etched in dark eye make-up, was due to the Egyptian custom of applying green and black eye paint. Green pigment which symbolized fertility was obtained from malachite, a copper ore. A gray-black eyeliner, used as protection against eye infection, contained the pigment kohl, which was made from galena, a lead ore.

So, the Eye of Horus became a design for an amulet which was second only to the scarab or sacred beetle as a mascot of Ancient Egypt. Of elaborate design, the sign became simplified to resemble an Rx, and was placed on all objects associated with danger, such as ships, chariots – and prescriptions (Guthrie, 1945 p. 20).

As time went by the Eye of Horus became used as a practical shorthand to quantify the ingredients of a prescription. The udjat eye contained 64 parts and each area of the eye formed a fraction of the total. Each division could represent a proportional volume or fraction of the total ingredients (Estes, 1989 p. 95).

Jupiter and astrology

Paris, in his *Pharmacologia* (1882 p. 17), asserted that the Rx sign represented the Roman astrological symbol for the planet Jupiter. Up to the Middle Ages, physicians believed that the planets influenced a

PHARMACOLOGIA:

COMPREHENDING

The Art of Prescribing

UPON

FIXED AND SCIENTIFIC PRINCIPLES;

TOGETHER WITH THE

HISTORY OF MEDICINAL SUBSTANCES.

BY

J. A. PARIS, M.D. F.R.S. F.L.S.

Fellow of the Royal College of Physicians of London;
Honorary Member of the Board of Agriculture;
Fellow of the Philosophical Society of Cambridge; and of the Royal Medical Society of Edinburgh;
and late Senior Physician to the Westminster Hospital.
&c. &c. &c.

IN TWO VOLUMES.

VOLUME THE FIRST.

Quis Pharmacopœo dabit leges, ignarus ipse agendorum?---Vix profecto dici potest, quantum hæc ignorantia rei medicæ inferat detrimentum.

GAUB: METHOD: CONCINN: FORMUL.

Fifth Edition, enlarged.

LONDON:

PRINTED AND PUBLISHED BY W. PHILLIPS,
George Yard, Lombard Street;
SOLD ALSO BY T. & G. UNDERWOOD, FLEET STREET.

1822.

Figure 3 Frontispiece from J. A. Paris, *Pharmacologia: Comprehending The Art of Prescribing* (1822)

person's health and Jupiter was thought to be the most powerful of all the heavenly bodies in the curing of disease. Jupiter, the largest planet in the solar system, was named after the king of the Roman gods.

Beryl Rowland, in her *A Medieval Woman's Guide To Health* (1981 p. 12), stressed the importance of astrology in medicine. She wrote that 'the professionally trained doctor often carried prognosticatory tables and equipment necessary for accurate zodiacal calculations' and that the Abbess Hildegard of Bingen (1098–1179) had 'urged parents to note the time of conception in order to facilitate astrological calculations'. An illustration by Amman for Jacob Rueff's second edition of his *De Conceptu et Generatione Hominis* (1580) shows the birth scene of a pregnant noblewoman with midwives in attendance and astrologers debating the alignment of planets and constellations while casting a horoscope to foretell the infant's future.

Douglas Guthrie, in his *A History of Medicine* (1945 p. 129), wrote that '[a] very common illustration [of the time] was the "zodiac man" showing the relation of the various heavenly bodies to the human frame, a belief widely held in the Middle Ages and still further developed during the sixteenth century'. Johannes de Ketham provided such an illustration in his *Fasiculus Medicine* of 1491 in which the zodiac sign Scorpio, for example, was related to the genital organs. Astrological symbols were of importance because 'the best time for giving medicines or for drawing blood was ascertained by a study of [those] constellations and of the moon' (Guthrie, 1945 p. 129).

According to Paris (1882 p. 17), the planetary influence pervaded the botanical history of the Middle Ages 'there was not a plant of medicinal use … that was not placed under the dominion of some planet'. In conclusion, Paris wrote that 'the character which we at this day place at the head of our prescriptions, and which is understood, and supposed to mean recipe, is a product of the astrological symbol of Jupiter disguised by the addition of the down stroke, which converts it into the letter R*x*.'

Although astrology remained popular with the sixteenth and seventeenth century herbalists Turner, Culpeper and Lovel, the art gradually disappeared from orthodox medicine at about that time. However, some romantics believe that the sign for Jupiter still adorns our prescription sheets to this day.

Recipe

Pragmatists realize that *recipe*, Latin for take, is a direction for making a prescription and may reason that the *x* is merely an abbreviation replacing the 'ecipe', thus giving rise to the rather less charming version of the derivation of the R*x* symbol.

References

Clayton, P. (1990). *Great Figures in Mythology*, p. 103. (Leicester: Magna Books)

Cotterell, A. (1989). *The Illustrated Encyclopoedia of Myths and Legends*, p. 102. (London: Cassell Publishers Ltd.)

Cowen, D. L. and Helfand, W. H. (1990). *Pharmacy. An Illustrated History*, p. 219. (New York: Harry N. Abrams Inc.)

David, R. (1987). Egypt. In Cavendish, R. (ed.) *Mythology. An Illustrated Encyclopoedia*, p. 96. (London: Macdonald Ltd.)

Estes, J. W. (1989). *The Medical Skills of Ancient Egypt*, p. 95. (USA: Science History Publications)

Guthrie, D. (1945). *A History of Medicine*, pp. 20, 129. (London: Thomas Nelson and Sons Ltd.)

Lyons, A. S. and Petrucelli, R. J. (1987). *Medicine. An Illustrated History*, p. 77. (New York: Abradale Press, Harry N. Abrams)

Paris, J. A. (1822). *Pharmacologia; Comprehending The Art of Prescribing upon Fixed and Scientific Principles; Together with The History of Medicinal Substances*, p. 17. (London: W. Phillips)

Patrick, R. and Croft, P. (1987). *Classic Ancient Mythology*, p. 39. (London: Galley Press)

Rowland, B. (1981). *A Medieval Woman's Guide To Health*, p. 12. (London: Croom Helm)

Rueff, J. (1580). *De Conceptu et generatione Hominis*. (Frankfurt am Main: Sigismund Feyerabend)

Ergot 3

INTRODUCTION

The technique of induction of labor by artificial means began around 1756 and, although there were many uterine stimulants in vogue, no single remedy could be relied upon. Meanwhile, prolonged or 'tedious' labor was a major source of maternal distress and of maternal and fetal mortality. The introduction of ergot in 1807, and of pituitary extract about one hundred years later, radically transformed the perception and the process of labor (read more on the topic of prolonged labor in the chapter on Anesthesia and Analgesia).

Ergot was one of the most important drugs ever introduced to obstetric and gynecological practice. When used to control the third stage of labor, this uterine stimulant reduced the maternal death rate due to postpartum hemorrhage from about 0.3 per 1000 live and stillbirths in the pre-1940s, to a record low of 0.06 per 1000 in 1952 (Moir, 1955).

Ergot is a fungus and is the winter resting stage of *Claviceps purpurea*, a parasite on rye (*Secale cereale*, L.) but sometimes also found on wheat and other grasses. The fungus grows from the infected plant to form a long, black, slightly curved body, known as the sclerotium, which stands out conspicuously from the ears of the rye. The word 'ergot' is derived from old French *argot*, 'a cock's spur', to which ergot has a marked similarity of form. A related fungus, *Ustilago maydis*, causes corn smut, and appears as a brown–black powder containing innumerable spores. Also known as corn ergot, the substance was formerly used as an emmenagogue and parturient (Grieve, 1992).

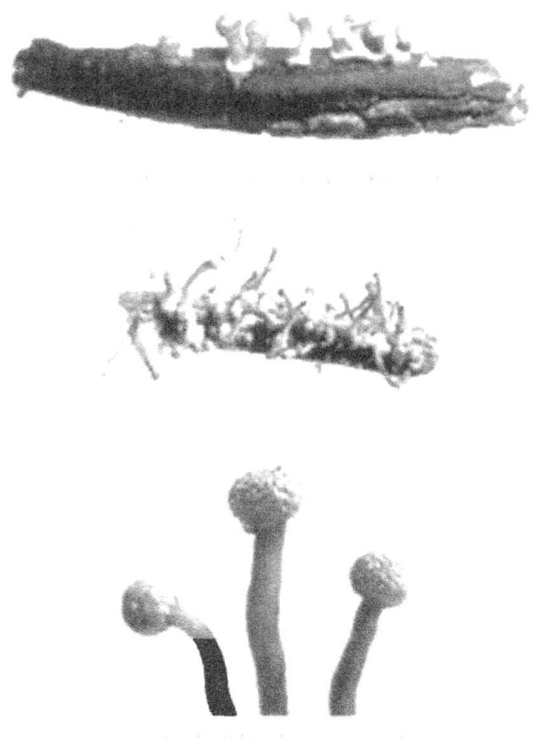

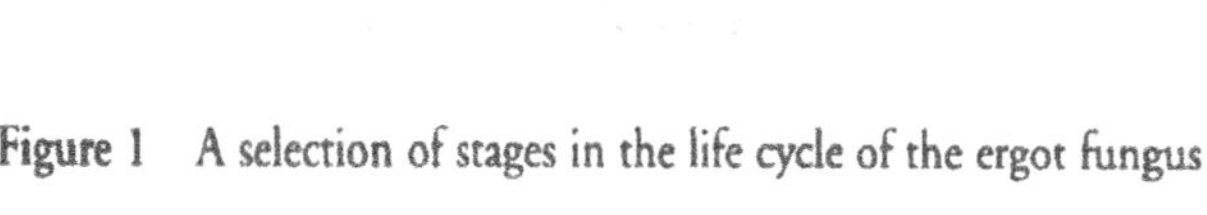

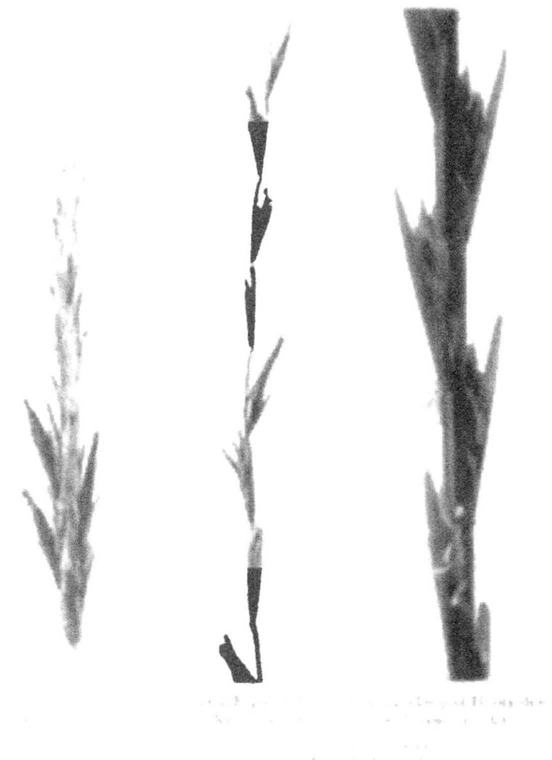

Figure 1 A selection of stages in the life cycle of the ergot fungus

Earliest references

In his *Historical Account of Pharmacology*, Chauncey D. Leake of the University of California in San Francisco, states that ergot was mentioned by the eminent Arab medical writer, Gerber, in his book on poisons, *Kitab as-sumum*, in AD 750. A translation by the German, Alfred Siggel, in 1958 served as Leake's source. Many of the drugs mentioned by Gerber are similar to those in the old Egyptian medical papyri and, 'most of them seem to have been taken chiefly from Dioscorides. New, however, are ergot (*Secale cornutum*)' and some others (Leake, 1975).

There is no mention of ergot, that I can find, in translations of the ancient Egyptian medical papyri, nor in translations of the great works of Theophrastus (c. 370–287 BC), Pliny (AD 23–79), Dioscorides (c. AD 40–80), Soranus (AD 98–177) or Paul of Aegina (AD 625–690). However, Theodore Rall and Leonard Schleifer (1985) in an essay on *Drugs Affecting Uterine Motility* related that, as early as 600 BC, an Assyrian tablet alluded to a 'noxious pustule in the ear of grain', and that in one of the sacred books of the Parsees (descendants of emigrants from Persia to India in the eighth century BC) the following pertinent passage occurs, 'Among the evil things created, are noxious grasses that cause pregnant women to drop the womb and die in childbed'. The early Greeks and Romans did not cultivate rye and Rall and Schleifer concluded that there was 'no undisputed reference to ergot poisoning in the early Greek and Roman literature'. The rye grain was introduced to Europe soon after the Christian era and written descriptions of ergotism did not appear until much later.

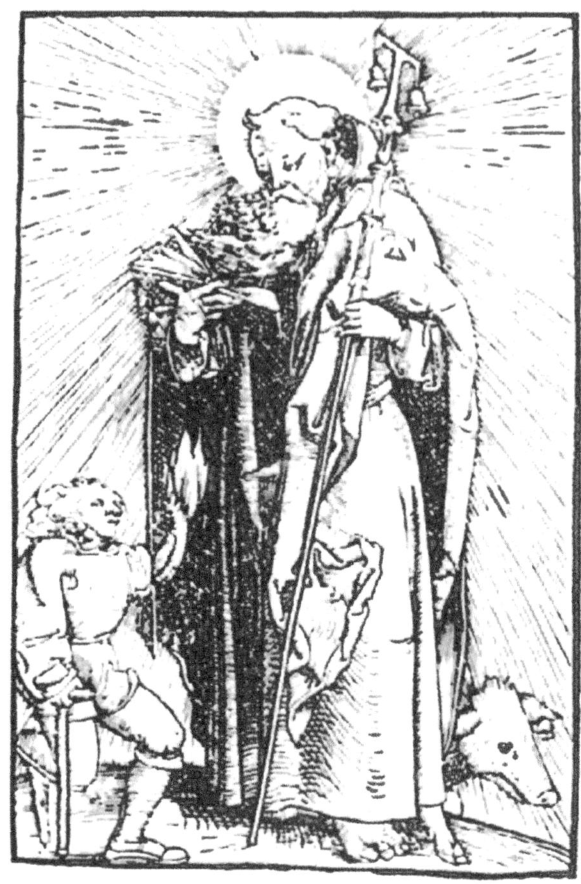
Von dem kalten Brandt.
O Anthoni heiliger Man/
Warumb nimbst dich der Arzney an?
Sie Gott dem Herrn gebürt die Ehr/
Und keinem Menschen sonst nit mehr.

Figure 2 St Anthony

Ergot and St Anthony's fire

Throughout the Middle Ages a number of disease epidemics ravaged the population of Europe. One such epidemic was Saint Anthony's fire, or ergotism, which was caused by ingestion of bread made from rye contaminated with ergot. Rye was commonly used for breadmaking in France and Germany so that those areas were most affected. The disease only appeared in wet seasons when weather conditions promoted growth of the fungus. Affected individuals developed tingling of the skin and burning pain in their extremities. Gangrene of the limbs followed and was often accompanied by hallucinations and convulsions before the individual died. Animals also suffered from ergotism and it is related that it caused pregnant sows to litter before their time. The earliest reference to ergotism is to be found in the *Annales Xantenses* (from the church in Xanten in the lower Rhine region) and dates from AD 836.

A plague of 'the fire' occurred in and around Paris in AD 945. Sufferers flocked to the church of St Mary where they were tended and fed with bread which was ergot-free. In many instances, their symptoms abated but on their return home 'the fire' was rekindled. At a later date, a brotherhood of monks devoted to

St Anthony set up hostels in areas affected by ergotism and nursed the sick. The monk's bread was fungus-free and many sufferers were cured. Thus, in the thirteenth century, St Anthony became associated with 'the fire' which subsequently bore his name (Barger, 1931). In 1597 the medical faculty at Marburg investigated the likely causes of St Anthony's fire and concluded that it was due to eating bread made from by rye blighted with ergot (Haggard, 1929). As a result, rye bread became unpopular and, from that time, epidemics of ergotism were infrequent. However, an outbreak of possible St Anthony's fire occurred in southern France in 1951. Toxic symptoms were 'officially' reported as being due to contamination with an agricultural fungicide, but John Fuller (1968) investigated the affair and was convinced that ergotism was responsible.

Early obstetric use of ergot

In his historical and exhaustively researched monograph on *Ergot and Ergotism*, George Barger, professor of medical chemistry in the University of Edinburgh, wrote that the first unmistakable mention of the drug itself, as distinct from its toxic effects in epidemics, was in a German book, the 1582 edition of Adam Lonicer's *Kreuterbuch*. The following descriptive segment was quoted from Lonicer: 'long, black, hard, narrow corn pegs, internally white, often protruding like long nails from between the grains in the ear'. Their use by women to induce uterine contractions was mentioned and the dose of three sclerotia or about 0.5 g accorded with modern practice in the nineteenth century (Barger, 1931). Camerius, in 1668, wrote of its use to accelerate childbirth in certain parts of Germany. The first French publication on ergot was by Dodart in 1676 and preceded its first mention in England by a year. Munchausen of Germany first recognized that ergot was a fungus in 1764.

Although Lonicer and others had mentioned the use of ergot by pregnant women, it was not until 1787 that Paulizky reported in the *Neus Magazin für Aerzte* that powdered ergot had been introduced to The Netherlands (some 30 years previously). The powder was called 'pulvis ad partum' and was administered by midwives or, on occasion, by some physicians. This was the first recognition of the oxytocic action of ergot in a medical journal.

The Paris naturalist and apothecary, Antoine-Augustin Parmentier (1737–1813), recorded in 1764 that a midwife at Chaumont, a Madame Depille, used ergot to treat prolonged labor (Radcliffe, 1967), although the year is given as 1770 by Barger (1931). Desgranges, a physician at Lyons, reported in 1818 that ergot, which he called 'poudre obstetricale', was (ground up in a coffee mill and) offered as a decoction to laboring women by a local midwife since 1777. He also commented that, in the neighborhood of Lyons, ergot had been used from time immemorial – and that it was also dispensed to cattle.

INTRODUCTION OF ERGOT INTO OFFICIAL MEDICINE

John Stearns (1770–1848), a doctor in Saratoga county, New York gains the credit for introducing ergot to modern obstetric practice. He wrote a letter at Waterford, NY dated 25th January 1807 to a Dr Samuel Akerly, physician to the New York City Dispensary, in which he gave an account of the therapeutic use of ergot. His letter, entitled Account of the Pulvis Parturiens, a Remedy for quickening Childbirth, was later published in the *Medical Repository of New York* (Stearns, 1808). Stearns wrote as follows: 'in compliance with your request I herewith transmit you a sample of the "pulvis parturiens" which I have been in the habit of using for several years, with the most complete success. It expedites lingering parturition without producing any bad effects on the patient.... I have generally found this powder to be useful when the pains are lingering, have wholly subsided, or are in any way incompetent to exclude the fetus'. He then advised that the fetal presentation should be ascertained and that there should be no obstruction to delivery as, 'the violent and almost incessant action which it [ergot] produces in the uterus precludes the possibility of turning'. He advised a dose of powder equivalent to 5 to 10 grains, but found that nausea and vomiting were induced when the dose was large. He also commented that 'with the suddenness of its operation; it is, therefore, necessary to be completely ready before you give the medicine'.

Soon afterwards, Oliver Prescott, a Fellow of the Massachusetts Medical Society read his *Dissertation on the Natural History and Medicinal Effects of the Secale*

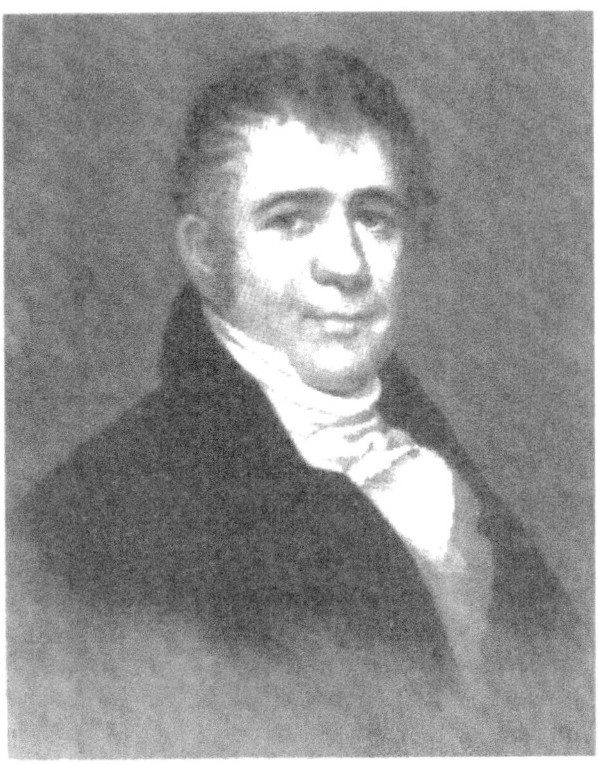

Figure 3 John Stearns (1770–1848)

cornutum, or Ergot at the annual meeting of the society at Boston on 2nd June 1813. He pointed out the great value of the drug in uterine hemorrhage but cautioned against its use by the inexperienced accoucheur. Published later in the same year (Prescott, 1813), his paper was reprinted and translated into French and German and aroused the interest of European physicians to the medicinal use of ergot. However, soon afterwards, Jacob Bigelow, a medical botanist in Boston, discussed the contraindications to its use and hinted at the harm done by the new drug.

Ergot soon became an essential drug in the obstetric materia medica but, despite the early warnings of dramatic side effects, the remedy was used inappropriately in early labor and soon led to deaths of mothers and infants due to the almost incessant action it induced in the uterus. In 1822, Hossack wrote that 'the number of still-born children had increased so much that an inquiry was instituted by the Medical Society of New York' and that 'the pulvis ad partum … may with almost equal truth be denominated the "pulvis ad mortem"', but he did approve of its use for postpartum hemorrhage. It was as a drug for that indication that ergot became indispensable and by its correct use the rye fungus was responsible for saving countless mother's lives.

Stearns (1822), relying on his experience of ergot, wrote his masterly dissertation *Observations on the Secale cornutum, or Ergot, with Directions for its Use in Parturition*, in which he enlarged his indications for use of ergot to include miscarriage, retained placenta, postpartum hemorrhage or where hemorrhage or lochial discharges were too profuse immediately after delivery. He related that his early knowledge of ergot was obtained from a Scottish immigrant woman whom he had met in Washington. As the risks of using ergot in labor became more apparent, it was no longer prescribed to hasten the birth process and the indications as outlined in Stearn's 1822 paper hold through to the present day.

Ergot was first mentioned in a textbook of materia medica by Chapman of Philadelphia in 1817 and was included in the original edition of the *United States Pharmacopoeia* of 1820, the same year that the drug was introduced to English midwifery by a doctor Merriman (Radcliffe, 1967). In 1828, Adam Neale of Scotland reviewed 720 reported cases in which ergot was used by practitioners in Europe and North America, either to hasten labor and placental delivery or to control hemorrhage (Dunn, 1993). Ergot was admitted to the Pharmacopoeia of the London College of Physicians in 1836 and thus, within 30 years of John Stearns original report, ergot became firmly established in Europe and was included in the various materiae medica throughout the continent.

Early chemical analysis

The earliest chemical investigations of ergot took place in the eighteenth century but, following Stearns report of 1807, a plethora of papers recording chemical and medical investigations on the fungus appeared in the scientific press. It was during this same time that chemistry developed into a modern science and pharmacology followed suit – an early achievement, for instance, was the isolation of morphine from opium. Regarding ergot, a major breakthrough occurred in

1842 when a crude pharmaceutical extract of ergot called 'ergotine' was prepared by Bonjean. However, it was not until 1875 that Tanret obtained a pure crystalline alkaloid which he called 'ergotinine', but unfortunately this particular extract was (later) found to be devoid of activity. By 1906, Barger and Carr of London had isolated another alkaloid, 'ergotoxine', which was found to stimulate the uterus and, if administered in large enough doses, caused all the side effects of ergot. Further interest was aroused with Stoll's discovery of 'ergotamine' in 1918 and this product was widely used in obstetric practice under the trade names Femergin and Gynergen.

As other ergot alkaloids were discovered, it became apparent that the rye fungus was a rich chemical storehouse of the most unexpected substances. Histamine, tyramine and acetylcholine were first discovered in ergot. Ergosterol, another ergot alkaloid, was found to be related to vitamin D. Much later, it was discovered that the ergot alkaloids all derived from a complex molecule named lysergic acid, a modification of which produced the drug lysergic acid diethylamide (LSD, a much abused 'mind bending' drug of the 1960s) which was originally introduced in 1954 in the assessment of certain psychiatric conditions.

Another by-product was di-hydroergotamine, evolved by Stoll through hydrogenation of the lysergic acid portion of ergot alkaloids, and this drug became popular in the treatment of migraine. Bromoergocrypytine, used to treat hyperprolactinemia and Parkinsonism, is a more recent isolate.

The discovery of ergometrine

The first announcement of ergometrine, the new and definitive ergot alkaloid for use in obstetric practice, appeared in the *British Medical Journal* (Dudley and Moir, 1935). The discovery and subsequent investigations of the drug owes much to the research of John Chassar Moir who later became Nuffield professor of obstetrics and gynaecology at Oxford University, England. Invited to take part in research on the rival merits of ergotoxine and ergotamine, Moir decided to record the effects of those drugs on the puerperal uterus, using a method of recording intrauterine pressure which had been described in 1927 by Bourne and Burn. During what was then the routine 7th-day postnatal check, a vaginal examination was carried out and a small pressure transducer was inserted into the still open uterine cavity. The puerperal uterus was found to be an ideal test organ. Results showed that although ergotoxine and ergotamine stimulated the uterus, their action was slow with a 20 minute delay after intramuscular injection or up to 2 hours delay if administered by mouth. Moir noted that this did not accord with Stearns' observation of 'the suddenness of its [ergot's] action' and reasoned that ergot contained some other active substance which was as yet undiscovered.

Moir turned his attention to the aqueous extract of ergot which contained neither ergotoxine or ergotamine, but was then official in the *British Pharmacopoeia* and appeared clinically effective. Moir (1955) related that 'the first recording ... was indeed memorable and [my] lasting impression was one of sheer astonishment' as he observed the effect of liquid extract of ergot on the uterus of a puerperal woman. He subsequently reported this 'new active principle' which contained the 'John Stearns effect' in the *British Medical Journal* (Moir, 1932).

In collaboration with H.W. Dudley, a research chemist in the National Institute of Medical Research, Moir further researched the aqueous extract of ergot. On February 9th 1935, an active preparation, soon to be called ergometrine, was evaluated and found to produce a perfect 'John Stearns effect'. The announcement of this new alkaloid wonder drug appeared in the *British Medical Journal* of March 1935 (Dudley and Moir, 1935) and thus ergometrine replaced the other ergot extracts which were in use, although liquid extract of ergot was still available in the 1950s.

Soon after Dudley and Moir's report, Thompson of Baltimore, Kharasch and Legault of Chicago, and Stoll and Burckhardt from Basel almost simultaneously announced their isolation of new water-soluble ergot principles, all of which were found to be identical to ergometrine. However, the official name for ergometrine varied, and in the USA the title was ergonovine with a proprietary name of ergotrate. The Sandoz firm in Switzerland used Stoll's term 'ergobasine' and then went on to market Stoll's semi-synthetic methylergometrine product as methergin (Moir, 1970).

THE MODERN USE OF ERGOT

Ergometrine became the drug of choice to prevent or arrest postpartum or postmiscarriage hemorrhage due to uterine relaxation, and to aid placental detachment, its delivery and thus to shorten the 3rd stage of labor. The routine administration of ergometrine with the appearance of the fetal shoulder was first proposed by Davis of Chicago and the studies which followed proved the efficacy of this form of management (Moir, 1970).

One disadvantage of the use of ergometrine was an increased incidence of retained placentae due to spasm of the uterus. This problem was overcome by combining with the drug a modified Brandt–Andrews technique of controlled cord traction, which was evaluated by Rowe of Australia in 1962 and by Spencer of London in the same year (Spencer, 1962). There was also the problem of retention of a second twin or third triplet if the drug was administered after the birth of the first infant. The putative use of ergometrine to promote involution of the postpartum uterus was discounted in a study by Moir and Russell (1943).

Clinical research showed that the effects of ergometrine become apparent within 5 to 7 minutes after oral administration but the response time was shortened to about 60 seconds for intravenous injection. Ergometrine was found to induce uterine spasm which, after an elapse of 10 minutes, changed to strong contractions with decreasing force for a further 30 to 40 minutes. With the help of tocographic studies, Embrey and colleagues at Oxford demonstrated the advantages of combining oxytocin, with its speed of action, and ergometrine, with its duration of effect. The combination was called syntometrine, the intramuscular use of which became a substitute for intravenous ergometrine (Embrey, 1961; Embrey, Barber and Scudamore, 1963). Syntometrine contained ergometrine maleate 0.5 mg and synthetic oxytocin 5 units in a 1 ml ampoule.

The disagreeable side effects of nausea or vomiting and hypertension had been recognized for many years (Ringer, 1888) but it is only recently that synthetic oxytocin (syntocinon), with its lesser toxicity, has replaced syntometrine as the drug of choice to prevent postpartum hemorrhage.

Endpiece on ergot

Chasser Moir wrote extensively on the use of ergot and I can do no better than quote his concluding remarks in an essay on the history of ergot: 'when next you handle the ergometrine ampoule pause for a moment. Give a thought to the strange fungus that infests the head of the rye grass, to St Anthony and his monks, to the immense sum of learning that ergot research has added to medical science; and, not least, thank God for His provision of this strange and wonderful medicine' (Moir, 1955).

References

Barger, G. (1931). *Ergot and Ergotism*, pp. 12, 43, 7. (London: Gurney and Jackson)

Dudley, H. W. and Moir, J. C. (1935). The Substance Responsible, for the Traditional Clinical Effect of Ergot. *BMJ*, 1, 520–3

Dunn, P. M. (1993). Adam Neale (c.1780–1832) and Ergot of Rye. *Arch. Dis. Childhood*, 68, 617–18

Embrey, M. P. (1961). Simultaneous intramuscular injection of oxytocin and ergometrine: A tocographic study. *BMJ*, 1, 1737–38

Embrey, M. P., Barber, D. T. C. and Scudamore, J. H. (1963). Use of syntometrine in prevention of PPH. *BMJ*, 1, 1387–89

Fuller, J. G. (1968). *The Day of St. Anthony's Fire*. (London: Hutchinson)

Grieve, M. (1992). *A Modern Herbal*, pp. 338–9. (London: Tiger Books International)

Haggard, H. W. (1929). *Devils, Drugs and Doctors. The Story of the Science of Healing from Medicine-Man to Doctor*, pp. 216–19. (London: Heinemann)

Leake, C. D. (1975). *An Historical Account of Pharmacology to the 20th Century*, p. 75. (Springfield: Charles C. Thomas)

Moir, J. C. (1932). The action of ergot preparations on the puerperal uterus. *BMJ*, 1, 1119–22

Moir, J. C. (1955). The History and Present-day use of Ergot. *Can. Med. Assoc. J.*, 72, 727–34

Moir, J. C. (1964). The obstetrician bids, and the uterus contracts. *BMJ*, 2, 1025–29

Moir, J. C. (1968). Obituary. Sir Henry Dale. *J. Obstet. Gynecol. Br. Common.*, 75, 1076–78

Moir, J. C. (1970). The Use of Ergot in Obstetrics. In E. E. Philipp, J. Barnes, and M. Newton (eds) *Scientific*

Foundations of Obstetrics and Gynaecology, pp. 649–52. (London: Heinemann)

Prescott, O. (1813). *A Dissertation on the Natural History and Medicinal Effects of the Secale cornutum, or Ergot.* (Boston: Cummings and Hilliard)

Radcliffe, W. (1967). *Milestones in Midwifery*, p. 71. (Bristol: John Wright and Sons Ltd.)

Rall, T. W. and Schleifer, L. S. (1985). Drugs Affecting Uterine Motility. In Goodman Gillman, L. S. Goodman, T. W. Rall and F. Murad (eds) *The Pharmacological Basis of Therapeutics*, pp. 926–45. (New York: Macmillan Publishing Company)

Ringer, S. (1888). *A Handbook of Therapeutics*, p. 523. (London: H. K. Lewis)

Spencer, P. M. (1962). Controlled cord traction in management of the third stage of labour. *BMJ*, 1, 1728–32

Stearns, J. (1808). Account of Pulvis Parturiens, a Remedy for Quickening Child-birth. *The Medical Repository (New York)*, Second Hexade, 5, 308–9

Stearns, J. (1822). Observations on the Secale cornutum, or Ergot-with Directions for its use in Parturition. *Phil. J. Med. Physical Sci.*, 5, 36–45

Lettuce 4

THE LETTUCE PLANT

Common name: Lettuce
Botanical names: *Lactuca sativa, Lactuca virosa*
Synonyms: Wild lettuce, green endive

The word lettuce comes from the Old French, *laitue*, derived from the word for milk. The Latin version comes from *lac*, milk. Wild lettuce, from which all present-day varieties developed, secreted a large volume of milky sap, giving rise to its name.

Lettuce varieties

Lactuca virosa (Latin, *virosus*, meaning 'poisonous' and, *fetid*, 'the wild variety'), and *Lactuca sativa* (Latin, *sativus*, for 'sown' or 'planted') are the two types of lettuce alluded to by Gerard in his *Herball* (1636 p. 64): 'there be of lettuce two sorts, the one wild or of the field and the other tame or of the garden', and belong to a species of annual or perennial herb, most of which are edible (Hyam and Pankhurst, 1995 p. 271).

The constituents of lettuce

The fresh lettuce plant, when cut, exudes a latex known as 'lactucarium' which contains lactucone, lactucin and lactucic acid. In addition the leaves may contain traces of a mydriatic alkaloid. Also contained in the sap are gum, essential oils, and mannitol.

HISTORY OF LETTUCE

The remains of lettuce plants similar to cultivated lettuce, or *Lactuca sativa*, have been recovered from a Mesolithic (c. 5000 BC) site on the Isle of Wight (Godwin, 1956 p. 148). It is estimated that lettuce farming began in Persia before 550 BC and according to Herodotus, lettuce was used for salads and served to the Persian kings for more than four hundred years before the Christian era (Lindley and Moore, 1870 p. 655). In ancient times the plant had a bitter taste which has disappeared as a result of cross-pollination and selection.

Lettuce is mentioned in the Bible in Numbers 9, 11: 'together with unleavened bread and bitter herbs'. The plant was mentioned by many of the great writers of antiquity including Theophrastus, Pliny, Dioscorides and others. Gerard's *The Herbal or a General History of Plants* which was first published in 1597 described eight cultivated varieties of lettuce which were available in England.s

HISTORICAL USES OF LETTUCE

Galactagogue

It is known that lettuce grew wild in Ancient Egypt. The plant has a high fluid content and was thus very valuable as a thirst quencher in the hot climate. The plant, which secretes a large volume of milky juice, was fed to women after childbirth, to promote the flow of breast-milk. Culpeper in his herbal of 1652 and John K'Eogh (1735 p. 92) in his *Botanalogia Universalis Hibernica*, both recorded that lettuce 'increases milk in nurses'. Native Amerindian women drank lettuce tea to stimulate their milk flow (Lust, 1974 p. 254).

Aphrodisiac

The opalescent sap was also thought to have semen-like qualities and the tradition grew that lettuce was an effective aphrodisiac (Manniche, 1993 p. 112). Lettuce was the favorite food of Min, the Egyptian god of sexuality and fertility, who is depicted with an erect phallus in a relief carving at Thebes. He was also associated with rain and the growth of grain crops. The sacred white bulls of Min were fed lettuce during the harvest-time celebrations (Patrick and Croft, 1987 p. 53).

Lettuce was also the choice food of the evil Egyptian god Seth. On one occasion he attempted to rape his nephew Horus, as a show of power and to discredit the sun god. Horus caught the venomous seed in his hand and disposed of it in the marshes of the Nile delta. Being aware of Seth's liking for lettuce, Horus dressed some delicious leaves of the plant with his own semen. Unaware of what had happened, Seth ate the lettuce and later on the seed of Horus burst through the head of the evil one. Thus disgraced in the eyes of his peers, Seth retired from his battles with Horus (Clayton, 1990 p. 103). (See also Chapter 2.)

Anaphrodisiac

William Turner, the English physician famous for his three-volume *New Herball* published in London in 1568, remarked that lettuce was 'agaynst the rages of venery'. Culpeper wrote, in 1653, that lettuce was a cooling plant owned by the moon. Among its many properties he noted that 'it abateth bodily lust, [when] outwardly applied to the cods [testicles] with a little camphire'. His notions were in keeping with those of the Ancient Greeks and the puritan Pythagoreans who thought that lettuce (*L. sativa*) was an anaphrodisiac. Pythagoras claimed that the plant was the food of eunuchs. Nowadays, in contrast, a tincture of the whole lettuce plant is used by herbalists as a remedy for impotence (Ody, 1993 p. 164).

Analgesic, sedative and laxative

The sedative powers of lettuce were known since earliest times. In one fable from antiquity it is told that Venus, after the death of Adonis, threw herself on a bed of lettuces, to ease her grief, and repress her desires. The Greek physician Galen (c. AD 131–200) suffered from 'morbid vigilance' in later life which was cured by eating lettuce (Paris, 1822 p. 13).

Lettuce has been used since antiquity as an analgesic. Bellamy and Pfister (1992 p. 85) in their book on plant medicine wrote that lettuce seeds were contained in a mixture known as *spongia somnifera* or 'sleeping sponge'. The preparation, which contained opium, mandragora and other plant narcotics was used as an analgesic or anesthetic.

The dried sap of *L. virosa*, contains 'lactucarium', a mild opium-like narcotic (Grieve, 1992 p. 476). Lactucarium was introduced to European medicine either by a Dr Duncan of Edinburgh (Lindley and Moore, 1870 p. 655) or by Collin in 1771 and was later called 'lettuce opium' by Coxe in 1799 (Stuart, 1994 p. 210). From the Middle Ages, the dried sap of lettuce (*L. virosa*) was an ingredient in witches' ointments, and the North American Indians mixed lettuce into their magical smoking blends.

The use of 'well-buttered' lettuce as a laxative, by the childbearing woman was recorded by James Wolveridge (1671).

CURRENT USE OF LETTUCE

The lettuce plant, or its extracts, are now mainly used in complementary medicine. Known for its mild sedative and anodyne properties the sap may be used to treat restlessness, irritable cough, pain, priapism, nymphomania, and dysmenorrhoea (*British Herbal Pharmacopoeiae*, 1983 p. 126). Cultivation of the plant over time, however, has reduced the potency of its sap.

References

Bellamy, D. and Pfister, A. (1992). *World Medicine. Plants, Patients and People*, p. 85. (Oxford: Blackwell)

The British Herbal Medicine Association (1983). *British Herbal Pharmacopoeiae*, p. 126. (Bournemouth, UK)

Clayton, P. (1990). *Great Figures in Mythology*, p. 103. (London: Magna Books)

Culpeper, N. (1652). *Culpeper's Complete Herbal*, A Reprint of the 1826 version by Magna Books, Leicester (1981). p. 84. (London: Bloomsbury Books)

Godwin, H. (1956). *The History of the British Flora*, p. 148. (Cambridge: University Press Cambridge)

Grieve, M. (1992). *A Modern Herbal*, p. 476. (London: Tiger Books International)

Hyam, R. and Pankhurst, R. (1995). *Plants and their Names. A Concise Dictionary*, p. 271. (Oxford: Oxford University Press)

K'Eogh, J. (1735). *Botanalogia Universalis Hibernica*. An edited translation by Michael Scott (1986). p. 92. (Dublin: The Aquarian Press)

Lindley, J. and Moore, T. (1870). *The Treasury of Botany: A Popular Dictionary of the Vegetable Kingdom; with which is incorporated A Glossary of Botanical Terms*, p. 655. (London: Longmans, Green, and Co.)

Lust, J. B. (1974). *The Herb Book*, p. 254. (Toronto, London: Bantam Books)

Manniche, L. (1989). *An Ancient Egyptian Herbal*, pp. 61, 58. (London: British Museum Press)

Manniche, L. (1993). *An Ancient Egyptian Herbal* (Second Impression), p. 112. (London: British Museum Press)

Ody, P. (1993). *The Herb Society's Complete Medicinal Herbal*, p. 164. (London: Dorling Kindersley)

Paris, J. A. (1822). *Pharmacologia; Comprehending The Art of Prescribing upon Fixed and Scientific Principles; together with the History of Medicinal Substances*, p. 13. (London: W. Phillips)

Patrick, R. and Croft, P. (1987). *Classic Ancient Mythology*, p. 53. (London: Galley Press)

Stuart, M. (1994). *The Encyclopaedia of Herbs and Herbalism*, p. 210. (Cambridge: Edgerton International Ltd.)

Turner, W. (1568). *The Herball*. (London: Collen)

Wolveridge, J. (1669). *The Speculum Matricis*, p. 112. (London: E. Okes)

Woodward, M. (1927). *Gerard's Herball. The essence thereof distilled by Marcus Woodward from the editions of T. Johnson 1636*, p. 64. (London: Spring Books)

Mummy Medicine 5

WOLVERIDGE'S MUMMY MEDICINE

There is an intriguing prescription which includes the ingredient 'mummy' in James Wolveridge's book on midwifery care *The Speculum Matricis* (1671 p. 131).

Wolveridge's prescription was used 'to provoke the flowers, expel a dead child, and [expel] false conception' and contained the following ingredients: calamita, cassia lignea, cinnamon and styrax 'of each half an ounce; Mummy, two drachms; saffron, half a drachm, make all these into fine Powder: this may be taken in white-wine, a drachm at a time, for a week together, or more'. The ingredient that aroused my fascination was 'mummy'.

The word 'mummy' translates to Latin as *homo mortuus arte medicatus* thereby giving a clue to its derivation. Ernest A. Wallis Budge (1893 p. 173)

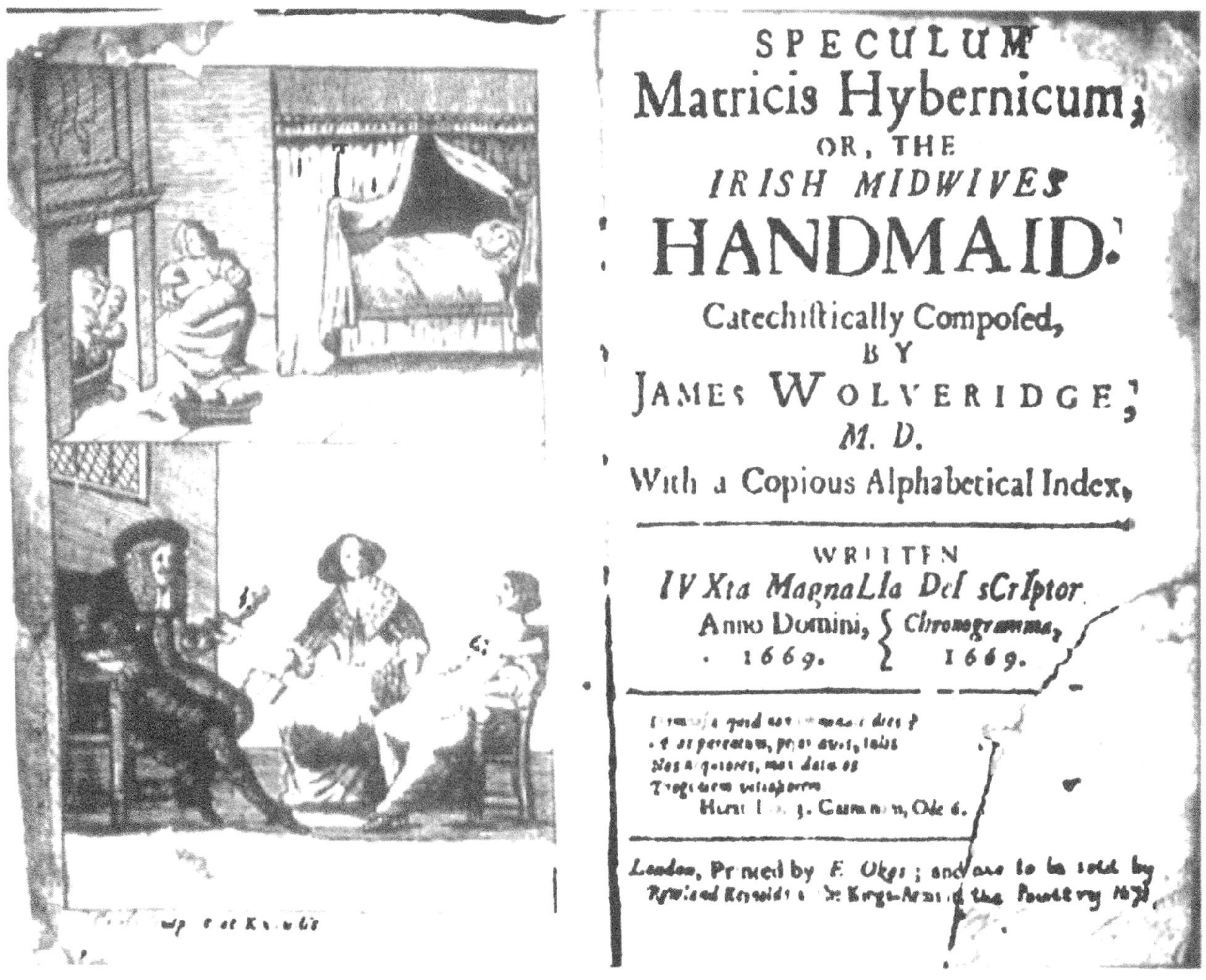

SPECULUM
Matricis Hybernicum;
OR, THE
IRISH MIDWIVES
HANDMAID:
Catechistically Composed,
BY
JAMES WOLVERIDGE,
M. D.
With a Copious Alphabetical Index,

WRITTEN
IVXta MagnaLIa DeI sCrIptor.
Anno Domini, { *Chronogramma,*
1669. 1669.

[illegible]

London, Printed by *E. Okes*; and are to be sold by [illegible]

Figure 1 Frontispiece from James Wolveridge's *Irish Midwives Handmaid*

relates that 'mummy' is a term applied to a body 'preserved by means of bitumen, spices, gums or natron'. He discovered that the word was found in Latin, Byzantine Greek and almost all European languages, derived in turn from the Arabic name for 'bitumen'. It was the word used by the Arabs for a body 'preserved by bitumen' and was also known to the Persians as 'a drug in medicine'. The Arabs mistook the dark (resin coated) mummy skin as being a result of preservation by bitumen but, in reality, bitumen was rarely used in the mummification process.

So, 'mummy', from the Arabic *mumiyah* (bitumen or asphalt), from the Persian *mum* (embalming wax), from the Latin *mumia*, from French *mumie*, entered the English language in the early seventeenth century and became defined as 'an embalmed or otherwise preserved dead body: the substance of such a body, formerly used medicinally: or, a bituminous drug or pigment' (Macdonald, 1972 p. 866).

MUMMIFICATION

Douglas Guthrie (1945 p. 27) contributed to the desiccation theory of the evolution of mummification. He wrote: 'The fact that dead bodies, buried in the dry hot sands of the desert, remained for many years in a remarkable state of preservation, may have suggested to the Egyptians that the natural preservation might be favored by artificial means'.

More recent observers claimed that the desiccation theory is 'an inadequate and flawed explanation [and that] the practice evolved simply to preserve the image of the body' (Shaw and Nicholson, 1995 p. 190). Whatever its origins, the process of embalming was practiced in Egypt from about 4000 BC to AD 600, and it is estimated that 500 to 700 million bodies were so treated.

The Greek historian Herodotus (c. 485–425 BC) provides a graphic account of the mummification process (Godley, 1921 p. 371). Soon after death the body was taken to the 'Place of Purification' and washed with a natron solution. Then, in a tent called the 'House of Beauty', the brain was removed with a bent iron through the nostrils and the skull was washed out with an infusion of drugs. Thereafter, a cut was made in the left flank with a sharp Ethiopian stone knife or 'obsidian' and the intestines, liver and

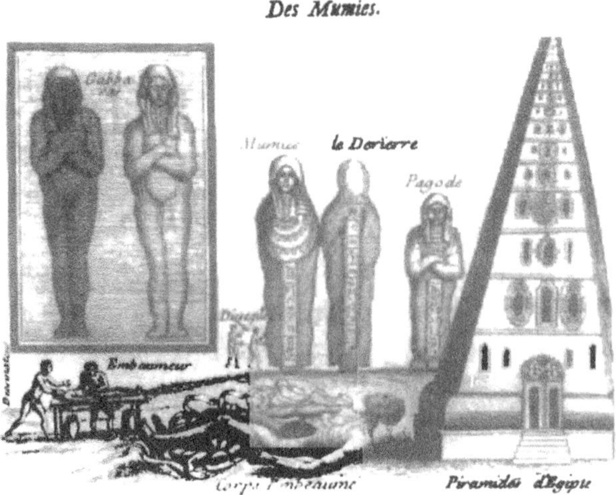

Figure 2 Egyptian mummies

lungs were removed. The abdominal incisions were made by the *paracentati* while other practitioners, the *taricheutai*, removed the organs. The heart was carefully preserved in the body and the kidneys, bladder and internal genitalia were also not removed.

The viscera were dried, cleansed, bandaged and placed in four capped canopic jars which were dedicated to the four sons of Horus: Amset (liver); Hapi (lungs); Duamutef (stomach); and Kebehsenuef (intestines). The abdominal cavity was packed with cassia, myrrh and other spices and the body was then placed in dry natron for 70 days. After that the body was washed and wrapped in fine cotton or linen bandages smeared with gum. The oils and creams applied to the body and bandages included caraway seed oil, cedar oil, incense, natron, raw rubber, turpentine, resins (sometimes replaced by honey) and wax. The mummy was then placed in a shaped wooden case and moved to a burial chamber. Less expensive methods were also available and Herodotus mentioned two cheaper forms of embalming.

MUMMIES AS MEDICINE

There is a compelling description of mummy as a medication in the first edition of the *Encyclopaedia Britannica* (1771 p. 315). There were, it appears:

> 'two different substances reserved for medicinal use under the name of mummy, though both in some

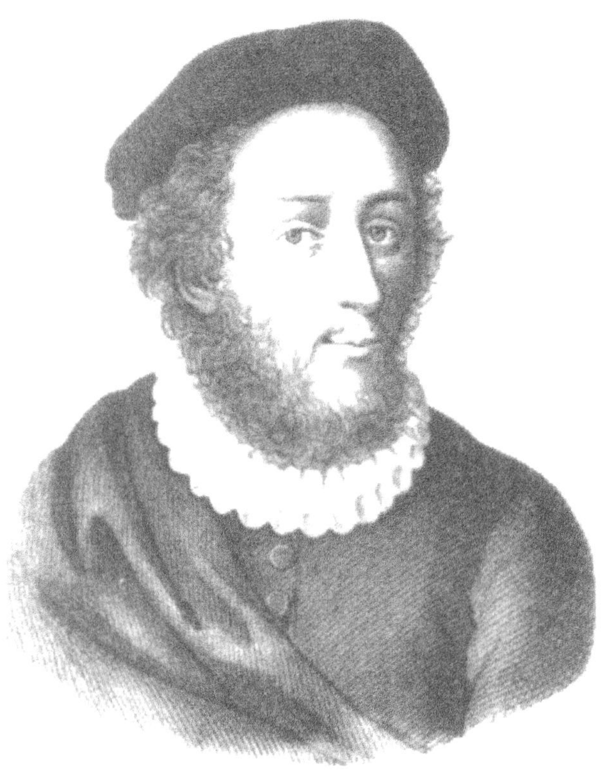

Figure 3 Guy de Chauliac (1300–1367)

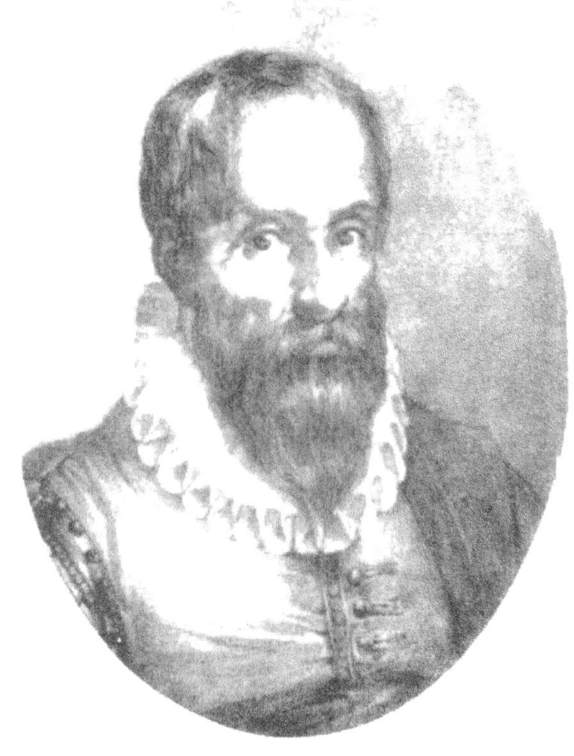

Figure 4 Ambroise Paré (1510–1590)

> degree of the same origin. The one is the dried and preserved flesh of human bodies, embalmed with myrrh and spices; the other is the liquor running from such mummies ... mummy has been esteemed resolvent and balsamic: but whatever virtues have been attributed to it, seem to be such as depend more upon the ingredients used in preparing the flesh than in the flesh itself; and it would surely be better to give those ingredients without so shocking an addition'.

Mummy produce could be ordered as balsams, extracts, ointments, powder or tinctures and these therapies formed part of the normal materia medica of apothecaries shops three to four centuries ago. One such therapy was *Aqua Divina* which derived from pulped mummy product. It is recounted that El-Magar, a Jewish physician from Alexandria, frequently prescribed mummy to his patients, for cuts, bruises and other ailments. He also used powdered mummy to treat both the injured Crusaders and their Saracen opponents. It is known that mummies were transported to Cairo and Alexandria and shipped from there by Portuguese and Venetian merchants to Lyon, in France, which was a commercial center for distribution of mummy medicines.

Guido Lanfranchi (better known as Lanfranc), who died c. 1315, is considered to be the founder of surgery in France and is best remembered for his practical contributions to the management of brain injuries. In his *Science of Surgery*, he prescribed mummy to be 'laid on the nucha' (the spinal cord) (Ayto, 1994 p. 358).

Another Frenchman, Guy de Chauliac, who was surgeon to Pope Clement VI in the fourteenth century, used ground up mummy as therapy. Guy, who was born in the late thirteenth century, wrote a huge seven-part work on surgery entitled *La Grande Chirurgie* (*Chirurgia Magna*), which contained 3299 quotations from previous medical authors. He was so influential that his methods dominated the surgical practice of France, and to a lesser extent that of England, for at least two centuries (Haeger, 1989 p. 89).

It is also reported that Francois I of France, mixed powdered mummy with rhubarb and carried it with him to apply to wounds or bruises, although he may also have taken the medication orally (Duin and Sutcliffe, 1992 p. 13).

An interesting tale is told of Ambroise Paré, the French surgeon and obstetrician, who in 1580 at the age of 70, attended a Monsieur Christophe des Ursins who had been thrown from a horse and knocked unconscious. When he recovered, the patient complained that mummy had not been applied to his wounds. Paré thereupon declared his disbelief in the remedy and expounded that mummy was 'sometimes made in France from the bodies of executed criminals' but that despite the deceit he believed the French mummy to be as good as the Egyptian preparation because 'neither were of any value'. His statements excited the violent opposition of the whole Paris Faculty of Medicine (Haggard, 1929 p. 324).

Despite the assertions of Paré and other illustrious medical men the use of mummy medicine continued right up to the eighteenth century. Indeed Becher's *Parnassus Medicalis Illustratus* of 1663 advocated mummy medicine for 'delayed women's time' – similar to James Wolveridge's indication – and also gave a recipe for artificial mummy (Stetter, 1993 p. 166).

In time, genuine mummy either became too expensive or ran into short supply, so that the bodies of slaves and executed criminals or those who had died 'of the most loathsome of diseases' were quickly mummified and sold as 'ancient' mummies. The trade in mummies suffered a reversal, however, in 1564 when a physician called Guy de la Fontaine discovered the deceitful practice and reported it to the Pasha (the Turkish/Egyptian Governor). Thereafter a heavy tax was imposed on mummy products and the trade died out slowly over the following two centuries (Wallis Budge, 1893 p. 175).

Mummy medicine was prescribed for various conditions, including epilepsy and gout; to inhibit or enhance blood clotting or as a panacea. The rationale for its use was based on a magical effect; mummies were 'tangible symbols of longevity' (Estes, 1989 p. 113). However it should be borne in mind that at least fourteen herbs and other agents were used during the mummification process (see below). Therefore, if genuine mummy was included in a prescription, it is possible that mummy products may have exerted a medicinal effect.

Products used in mummification

Balsam (resin)
Bitumen (rarely)
Cassia
Cedar oil
Cinnamon
Honey (rarely)
Myrrh
Natron
Palm wine
Syrmaea (purgative oil)

Ungents and products applied to the body after mummification

Caraway seed oil
Cedar oil
Incense
Natron
Rubber (raw)
Turpentine
Wax/Honey

It is of interest that at least five of the products used in mummification (balsam, cassia, myrrh, cinnamon and natron) were later used either to impede conception; to act as emmenagogues, or to expel an embryo or fetus. These five medications were mentioned for such uses in many influential medical texts right up to the Middle Ages (Riddle, 1992 p. 122).

So, James Wolveridge, in his intriguing recipe of 1671, which he used to 'provoke the flowers, expel a dead child, and [expel] false conception' not only prescribed mummy, which contained five expulsive agents but also advocated the use of calamita, styrax and saffron, which were in vogue as anti-fertility, abortive or expulsive drugs for many centuries. Whether his recipe was successful or not is a moot point but it appears that Wolveridge was well versed in the therapeutics of his time and that his medicines were based on the materiae medica of a long line of illustrious predecessors.

A SELECTION OF MUMMIFICATION AGENTS

Balsam a resinous product of various trees, with or without benzoic and/or cinnamic acid or esters, and still used in diseases of the urinary tract, for nasal catarrh, for leukorrhea and for bruises.

Bitumen asphalt, a dark brown or black substance, found wild and also as a residue of petroleum distillation.

Calaminta (possibly also known as calamint) related to thyme, and containing carvacrol (a phenol) and other mints, an antispasmodic. The ancients believed that it drove away serpents, particularly the dreaded Greek basilisk Kalos, the serpent king.

Caraway seed oil an aromatic carminative, containing carvene and carvol but little used now.

Cassia a coarse form of cinnamon, yielding purging cassia and senna was used as an emmenagogue, anti-galactagogue and for uterine bleeding.

Cedar oil contains substances which cause severe gastrointestinal irritation. Also stimulates menstruation and abortion.

Cinnamon aromatic astringent and carminative which was thought useful for uterine hemorrhage.

Honey nectar of flowers and secretion of *Apis mellifera*, antiseptic and antibacterial.

Incense gum or resin of frankincense (Fr. *franc encens*, pure incense), also known as olibanum. Aromatic, it was used for fumigation. Charred frankincense was powdered to produce kohl, a black powder used as an antiseptic eye paint. (Only applied to the body or bandages after mummification.)

Myrrh gum from the bark of *Commiphora*. Astringent and tonic, used in tooth powders/paste, for catarrh and formerly for amenorrhea.

Natron naturally occurring sodium carbonate and sodium bicarbonate, this is the chemists' Latin for 'sodium'. Collected from the shores and beds of ancient lakes in Egypt, and used for cleansing, purification, mummification, and in glass-making.

Palm wine the fermented sap from trees or shrubs of the Palmae family. Used as an antiseptic, palm extract is now known to contain the female hormone estrogen (as do apple seeds, pomegranate seeds, Scots pine, and willow flowers).

Rubber obtained in raw, or natural forms from at least 40 different plants by processing plant latex.

Saffron obtained from *Crocus sativus*, it contains colchicine, an alkaline diuretic which can cause intense purging.

Styrax a resin collected from *Liquidambar orientalis*, abounding in aromatic substances such as benzoin.

Syrmaea a purgative oil.

Turpentine originally a balsam of the terebinth tree (now from conifers), used as oil or spirit.

Wax obtained not only from bees but also from many plants, including the wax-myrtle and privet.

White wine the fermented juice of fruits, alcoholic and antibacterial.

References

Ayto, J. (1994). *Dictionary of Word Origins: The Histories of Over 8000 Words Explained*, p. 358. (UK: Columbia Marketing)

Duin, N. and Sutcliffe, J. (1992). *A History of Medicine: From Prehistory to the Year 2020*, p. 13. (London: Simon and Schuster)

Encyclopaedia Britannica (1771). *Encyclopaedia Britannica; or, a Dictionary of Arts and Sciences*, compiled upon a new plan By a Society of Gentlemen in Scotland. Vol. III, p. 315. (Edinburgh: A. Bell and C. Macfarquhar)

Estes, J. Worth (1989). *The Medical Skills of Ancient Egypt*, p. 113. (USA: Science History Publications)

Godley, A. D. (1921). *Herodotus. Translation for the Loeb Classical Library*, Four volumes. Vol. 1, Book 2, p. 371. (London: Heinemann Ltd.)

Guthrie, D. (1945). *A History of Medicine*, p. 27. (London: Thomas Nelson and Sons Ltd.)

Haeger, K. (1989). *The Illustrated History of Surgery*, p. 89. (London: Harold Starke)

Haggard, H. W. (1929). *Devils, Drugs, and Doctors. The Story of the Science of Healing from Medicine-Man to Doctor*, p. 324. (London: Heinemann)

Macdonald, A. M. ed. (1972). *Chambers Twentieth Century Dictionary*, p. 866. (Edinburgh: W. and R. Chambers Ltd.)

Riddle, J. M. (1992). *Contraception and Abortion from the Ancient World to the Renaissance*, p. 122. (London and Massachusetts: Harvard University Press)

Shaw, I. and Nicholson, P. (1995). *British Museum Dictionary of Ancient Egypt*, p. 190. (London: British Museum Press)

Stetter, C. (1993). *The Secret Medicine of the Pharaohs*, p. 166. (Chicago: Quintessence Co.)

Wallis Budge, E. A. (1893). *The Mummy*: (Chapters on Egyptian Funereal Archaeology), pp. 173, 175. (Cambridge: Cambridge University Press)

Wolveridge, J. (1671). *Speculum Matricis; or, The Expert Midwives Handmaid*, p. 131. (London: E. Okes)

Section 3

Chronology

Assyria 6

INTRODUCTION

The land between the eastern Mediterranean seaboard and the Persian Gulf has attracted several eponyms. The sector includes the modern territories of Lebanon, Iran, Iraq, Israel and Syria. This vast area, known as the 'Fertile Crescent' was so-called because the annual flooding of the great rivers in the region carried with it alluvial soil which remained behind to enrich the arid plains when the water levels subsided. The nomadic inhabitants settled down, became farmers, and tilled the fertile soil while gradually domesticating the wild animals and plants of the area. Villages were established at the beginning of the Neolithic period (c. 7000 BC) and then came the birth of the world's first cities in the fifth and fourth millennia BC with their amenities and complex economies. As this was man's original development from nomadic to rural, and then to urban lifestyle and the beginnings of agriculture and animal husbandry, the Fertile Crescent also became known as the 'Cradle of Civilization' (Caubet and Bernus-Taylor, 1991 p. 5).

THE ARCHEOLOGICAL STORY

Enclosed in the Cradle of Civilization was Mesopotamia, a country whose boundaries approximate to present-day Iraq. That ancient nation became known as 'The Land Between the Two Rivers' because of its geographical position between the mighty Euphrates and Tigris rivers. Mesopotamia had a turbulent history and was dominated in turn by the Ubaidians, Sumerians, Amorites, Babylonians (Akkadians), Kassites, Elamites, Assyrians, Chaldeans and Syrians. Their complex story is well told by Samuel Noah Kramer, one of the world's foremost authorities on Mesopotamian cultures and cuneiform writing (Kramer, 1969). It is from the colorful civilizations who dwelt in the region that we gain our earliest knowledge of ancient medicine. Impressed on clay tablets and stored in palace libraries, the ancient medical texts were lost for millennia and only rediscovered in the nineteenth century AD.

Babylon, established c. 2600 BC, was the mightiest city of Assyrian antiquity and was home to King Nebuchadnezzar. The site was discovered in 1899 by the German archaeologist Robert Koldawii. Directly after the First World War and the destruction of the Ottoman Empire, the newly-formed governments of the Near East established Departments of Antiquity and detailed scientific exploration of the Fertile Crescent began in earnest.

Archeologists over the centuries became aware of the importance of ancient Assyrian texts. The earliest writing was in the form of pictographs; symbols were impressed on mud tablets which retained the image when hardened in ovens, or in the heat of the sun. As time went by the pictographs were simplified and replaced by signs or symbols arranged in vertical, horizontal and oblique wedge-shaped lines inscribed with a wooden or bone pen which had a wedge shaped tip. The writing became known as 'cuneiform', from the Latin *cuneus*, a wedge. All attempts to decipher the Sumerian texts were, however, frustrated until 1765 when Carsten Niebuhr, a mathematician on a Danish expedition, identified three different types of writing inscribed together on the Assyrian clay tablets – old Persian, Elamite and Akkadian (Assyrian or Babylonian).

In the 1850s, a British archaeological team discovered over 25,000 hard-baked clay tablets and fragments inscribed with bilingual Sumerian–Akkadian texts at the site of the seventh century BC library of King Ashurbanipal at Nineveh. The collection included astronomical, medical, literary, and religious texts. Around 700 of the inscribed tablets were devoted to medical problems and it is estimated that the textual details were at least a thousand years old when the tablets were written.

THE BASIS OF THE ASSYRIAN MEDICAL SYSTEM

Most of our knowledge of disease and its treatment in ancient Assyria comes from a study of the Sumerian medical texts. Disease was regarded as a curse, thought to be a punishment by the gods on sinners or on those who unwittingly violated the moral code and was inflicted by evil demons. Although this was considered the chief cause of disease, a man could also fall ill as a result of black magic or sorcery. The Assyrians believed in contagion; the sick person was impure and contact with a bewitched woman or one with unclean hands could result in disease. Even worse was contact with the ghosts of children, of brides or of women who died in labor or while breastfeeding who, because they had died unfulfilled, were high among the list of spirits who caused disease. Assyrians could also fall prey to the 'Evil Seven', seven malign phantoms who were ever-ready to pounce on the unwary.

A diagnosis was reached when the doctor resorted to divination, usually by hepatoscopy. This involved a detailed examination of a sacrificed animal's liver. The Assyrians believed that the soul resided in the liver, the source of life and of emotion (the heart was considered the source of intellect and the uterus the site of compassion). A cheaper method of divination was to pour a drop of oil onto water and observe the outcome. Birth omens were also used as a method of divination for events of major consequence; abnormal births could indicate future tribulations. Astrology also played an important role.

Treatments included prayers, sacrifices and magico-religious ceremonies which were offered to the healing gods Marduk, the father of medicine, to Ninib, and to Ningishzida who had as his emblem a double-headed snake. Despite their spiritual belief system the Assyrians discovered that herbal remedies could be used to treat disease, so an extensive pharmacopoeia evolved. Remedies were variously: given by mouth; applied as salves and fomentations; inserted as suppositories and enemas; blown into body orifices or inhaled as vapors and fumigations (Lyons and Petrucelli, 1978 pp. 58–69).

The oldest known prescription from the era dates from c. 2100 BC and is inscribed in cuneiform script on a clay tablet which was discovered at Nippur in Iraq, about 60 miles south of present day Baghdad. The ingredients for seven internal medications and eight poultices are listed on the tablet (Estes, 1989 p. 94). A reading of the Assyrian prescriptions reveals that not all medications were quantified so it is likely that convention decreed certain measures. However the quantities of *gur, ka, mana*, and *shekel* are mentioned, the latter being the well-known Jewish equivalent of 14 grams.

The Babylonians were the first to regulate medicine using laws. King Hammurabi c. 1770 BC (see below) collected the ancient laws, codified them and had them recorded in cuneiform script. The Code of Hammurabi was engraved on a polished black diorite stele, a stone shaft of crystalline igneous rock over 2 m in height. The structure, which is on display in the Louvre, was uncovered in three large fragments during excavations at Susa in Iran in 1901. An engraving on the upper part of the shaft shows Hammurabi receiving the commission to write his code of laws from Shamash, the Babylonian sun god and god of justice. Below the carved picture are inscribed 282 laws dealing with issues as diverse as social structure and medical practice.

Hammurabi (1792–1708 BC)

King Hammurabi ascended the throne of Babylon c. 1770 BC and was one of the most celebrated rulers of the ancient Near East. He was renowned for his diplomatic ability and for his knowledge of military matters. Hammurabi inherited the small kingdom of Babylon which was less than 50 miles in radius. During his reign he developed and extended his realm to contain all the territory between the Syrian desert in the west and the Persian Gulf in the east. He is remembered most for his Code of Hammurabi, the earliest known legal system, a code which also contained laws to regulate the practice of medicine. Under his kingship, Babylon (named after a town 50 miles south of present day Baghdad) became the most civilized state of the era and in his own words was 'supreme in the world' (Kramer, 1969 p. 53).

FERTILITY AND CHILDBIRTH

The social unit, as in all societies, was the family. The customary age at marriage is not known, but the newly weds, whose union was bound by legal contract, frequently went to live with the husband's parents until they were old enough to be independent. The Code of Hammurabi contains details of the bride's dowry and how it should be dispersed in cases of divorce. Monogamy was usual but a man could take a second wife if the first failed to bear children. Divorce was available for failed marriage but adultery could be punished by death.

Women were held in high esteem by society and in many legal matters had equal rights with men, but were subject to the full rigors of the law when required. Should a woman '[crush] a man's testicle in an affray, one of her fingers shall be cut off' and if the second gland was affected then 'both her nipples shall be torn off'. Men's genital health was further considered in passages relating to venereal disease. Discharge of pus or blood, or urine like that of 'an ass ... like beer-yeast ... wine-yeast, or like gummy paint' pointed to a diagnosis of gonorrhea (Sigerist, 1951 pp. 429, 482).

The Code contains references to miscarriage: 'If a man strike a man's daughter and bring about a miscarriage, he shall pay ten shekels of silver for her miscarriage'. The text continues, 'if that woman die they shall put his daughter to death'. There are similar regulations which govern miscarriage in female slaves and in those who were free. The mythological demon of abortion was Dodib 'the strangler who kills the young in the womb' (Graham, 1951 p. 24).

Divination was used to predict the sex of the unborn: oil was dropped on water and if two rings developed, one large and one small, a boy could be expected. The pregnant Assyrian woman was protected against evil by amulets, magic rites and prayers. An incantation referring to pregnancy reveals the power of the evil spirits who could 'steal away desire and bring naught to seed; they tear out ... of the loins; they rend the [womb] of the nursing mother, and of the woman in travail. They stay the [offspring] and spread destruction' (Ricci, 1943 p. 29). The goddess Ishtar was invoked: 'May this woman gave birth happily. May she gave birth, may she stay alive and may the child in her fare well.... May she walk in health before thy divinity. May she give birth happily and worship thee' (Sigerist, 1951 pp. 399–40). Ishtar, the Assyrian goddess of love, was also known as 'The Mother of the Fruitful Breasts' and numerous figurines display her in typical 'breast-offering' pose. Later Christian writers belittled her holy sexual nature by calling her the 'Whore of Babylon'. Prayers were offered to avoid, at all costs, the wrath of the evil demon Labartu, a terrifying monster, who was thought to be responsible for causing the diseases of women, of fetal mortality and child-bed fever.

Little is known about the Assyrian customs of childbirth but it is likely that midwives were in attendance while the woman gave birth squatting on bricks or a delivery chair, as in the manner of their near-neighbors, the Egyptians. Children were breastfed for the first three years and wet-nurses were sometimes employed. Circumcision was not practiced and the custom appears to have originated in Africa where the Hebrews borrowed it from the Egyptians. The Code of Hammurabi sought to prevent abuse, and if an infant died and the wet-nurse substituted another child, her breasts were cut off. Adoption was allowed and the Code determined that such children should have the same rights as a child born to the adoptive parents. Not all children were well catered for, however, and unwanted offspring were allowed to die from exposure.

Assyrian deities relating to women

Dodib the abortion demon.
Labartu cause of disease, of preterm birth and child-bed fever.
Innana present at (loving) conception and at death in battle.
Ishtar love goddess and protector of pregnant women.
Gir an assistant to women in childbirth.
Ninhursag mother Earth, the source of all life, including plants.

THE ASSYRIAN HERBAL

The 42 drug names in this section are gleaned from a search through the text of Reginald Campbell

Thompson's *The Assyrian Herbal* (1924), a monograph on Assyrian vegetable drugs, based on a paper given to the Royal Society on 20 March, 1924. It appears that the author, who was a Fellow of Merton College, Oxford, had problems in finding a publisher and so wrote his text in longhand and produced stencil copies, some of which were printed by him at Boars Hill, Oxford and some by a Mr William Hunt, Broad St., Oxford. The book was distributed by Luzac and Co., London. Thompson, a renowned expert on Assyria, commented that 'difficulties in printing a monograph for which there is a limited public ... have rendered this form of production imperative'.

Thompson's study was based on approximately 120 fragments of plant lists in cuneiform script on a further 660 medical tablets, and on previous publications by other authors. He listed a total of 550 drugs of which 250 were vegetable, 120 mineral and 180 classified as 'other' or unidentified drugs. Also mentioned were alcohols, fats, honey, milk, oil, and wax which were used as vehicles or solvents for drug administration. Thompson found that many of the Assyrian plant names had found their way into Western languages. Examples include asafetida, saffron, myrrh, poppy (the Assyrian for which was *pa-pa*) and pine. The author's knowledge of ancient botany, languages and medicine is readily attested to by the contents of the text and also by the index with its addenda which are laid out in Assyrian, Arabic, Aramaic/Hebrew, English, Greek, Latin, Sumerian and Syriac.

Analysis of Thompson's text reveals that the 42 products mentioned by him for various 'female complaints' are readily categorized. They are placed here under nine main headings, and the text shown in quotes is taken directly from his script. The drugs, obtained from various parts of plants, were used either alone or in combinations, although referred to below as single agents.

Aphrodisiacs

Aphrodisiacs are common to peoples of all eras. It is likely that they were used as agents similar to our own fertility drugs as well as for increasing libido. The ancient Assyrians allowed a degree of sexual freedom, evidenced by the fact that venereal disease was known, and concubines and temple priestesses were available for sexual favors.

Among the five aphrodisiacs mentioned was **asafetida** (from the root of *Ferula foetida*). This vile-smelling gum resin was also obtained from *Narthex asafoetida* and other umbelliferae which grew near Babylon. Known to be an antispasmodic and carminative, and still used as such in herbal medicine (*British Herbal Pharmacopoeia*, or BHP, 1983 pp. 34–5) it was either taken alone or consumed in beer 'when a man goes to his wife and to another woman'. The drug became so popular that it attracted special taxation in second century AD Alexandria. Also known as 'evil's dung', low concentrations are used now to flavor Indian cooking and Worcestershire sauce (Wren, 1988 p. 18).

The **caper** (*Capparis spinosa*) was known in Assyria as 'the plant of the female pudenda perhaps suggested to the Babylonian mind by the [vulval] appearance of the flower' and was considered a 'drug for begetting and seed-setting'. The association between caper and vulva is probably the earliest example of what became referred to as the 'Doctrine of signatures', a system where like cures like, for example, heart-shaped plant leaves for heart conditions; red flowers for treating the blood; yellow flowers for jaundice. The caper contains capric acid which is responsible for its flavor. Never very popular as a medication, the plant has been used as a condiment and pickle for over 2000 years (Stuart, 1989 p. 165).

An unusual agent known as **lye** (strong alkaline solution) may have been used to stimulate passion (this is somewhat uncertain from Thompson's text), and could have been ingested or applied to the genitalia. Lye was obtained from saltmarsh plants (either *Salsola kali* or *Salicornia* sp.). The sun-dried plants were burnt in pits and the fused alkali collected at the bottom. The ashes were rich in iodine and other minerals. The juice of the salsola plant was also useful as a diuretic (Grieve, 1992 pp. 358–9).

The (stinging) **nettle** (*Urtica dioica*) may seem an unusual choice for an aphrodisiac but the seed was prized as an agent to stimulate sexual desire. The stinging leaves were used as a flagellator by some hardy enthusiasts at a later date – mainly as an antidote to consuming passion. Various parts of the nettle plant were prescribed for other less pressing

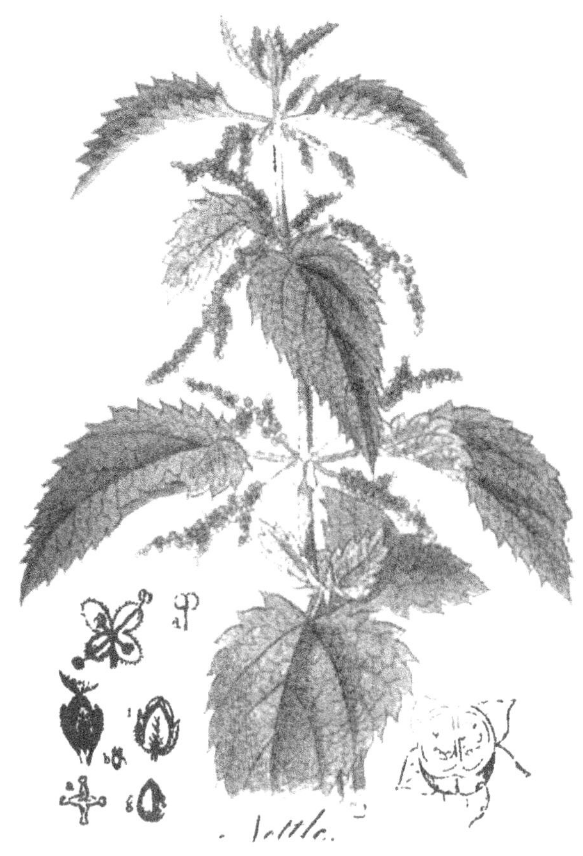

Figure 1 The nettle (*Urtica dioica*)

ailments and the nettle retains its place in the BHP (1983 pp. 224–5) as a therapy for uterine hemorrhage.

The **poppy** was called 'the plant of life' and the remedy was used 'when a man approaches his wife'. The plant in question was probably the red or corn poppy (*Papaver rhoeas*) as it appears that the red poppy was more popular or better known in pre-Roman times (Ellis, 1946 pp. 44–52). Much in vogue through the ages as a sedative, narcotic, hallucinogen and recreational drug, opium (from the white poppy, *Papaver somniferum*) is now banned except for strictly medicinal prescription.

Breast disease

Thompson included the remedies in this section 'for breast diseases/disorders' and did not enlarge further, but we can deduce that the drugs were used to promote lactation or were applied as remedies for breast engorgement, infection or cancer. Interestingly, each of the remedies in this section were still prescribed in the twentieth century. Of even greater interest is the fact that some of the Assyrian remedies were obtained from the bark or sap of trees. We now know that trees are a source of potent anti-cancer agents. Crude extract of the Pacific yew tree, *Taxus brevifolia*, was found to have cytotoxic activity against several tumors in 1971. The taxoids, docetaxel (Taxotere) and paclitaxel (Taxol), which are derived from the yew, are potent agents in the treatment of breast and ovarian cancers. What would the ancient Assyrians have thought, I wonder, of the research of Schiff and colleagues (1979 pp. 665–7) who highlighted the clinical potential of paclitaxel, a tree-bark extract?

The juice extract of the **chaste tree** (*Vitex agnus castus*) was applied alone, or in rosewater, as a poultice for breast disorders. The chaste tree has long been associated with women's diseases, and is currently available as a non-prescription drug in health food stores for the enhancement of lactation and for a variety of female ailments.

The **cypress tree** (*Cupressus* sp.) probably as a bark extract, was applied in a binding for diseases of the breast. Known to have astringent properties and to contain a volatile oil, cypress bark has antipyretic effects (Hocking, 1955 p. 64) and could have been beneficial.

Fenugreek (*Trigonella foenum-graecum*) was applied as a flour in a poultice for breast disease. An ingredient of curry powders, it is reported to have a number of medicinal effects. The *BHP* (1983 p. 216) includes fenugreek as a treatment for suppurating wounds, and in China it is applied in pessary form to treat cancer of the cervix.

Galbanum (from *Ferula galbaniflua*), a yellowish treacly liquid which forms a sticky mass, was applied directly to the breast. Galbanum retained its popularity as a remedy to the present century and was listed as 'a plaster [for use] in chronic inflammatory conditions' in Peter Wyatt Squire's *Companion to the British Pharmacopoeia* (1908 pp. 548–50).

Pine (*Pinus* sp.) is the remedy which is mentioned most frequently in the Assyrian pharmacopoeia

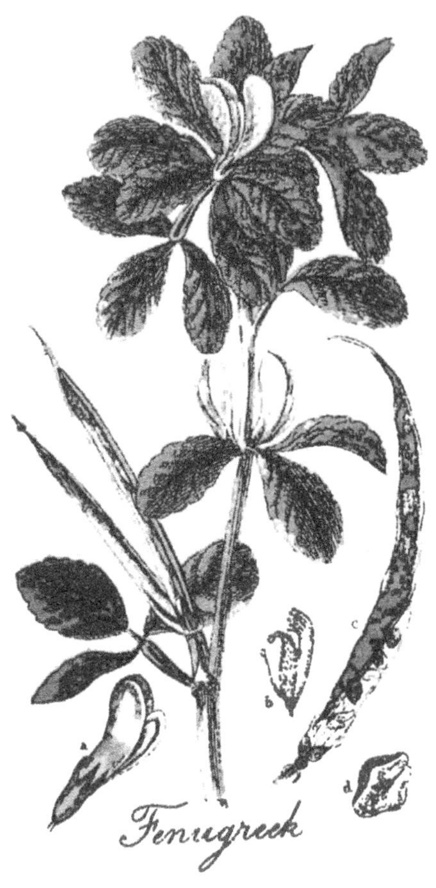

Figure 2 Fenugreek

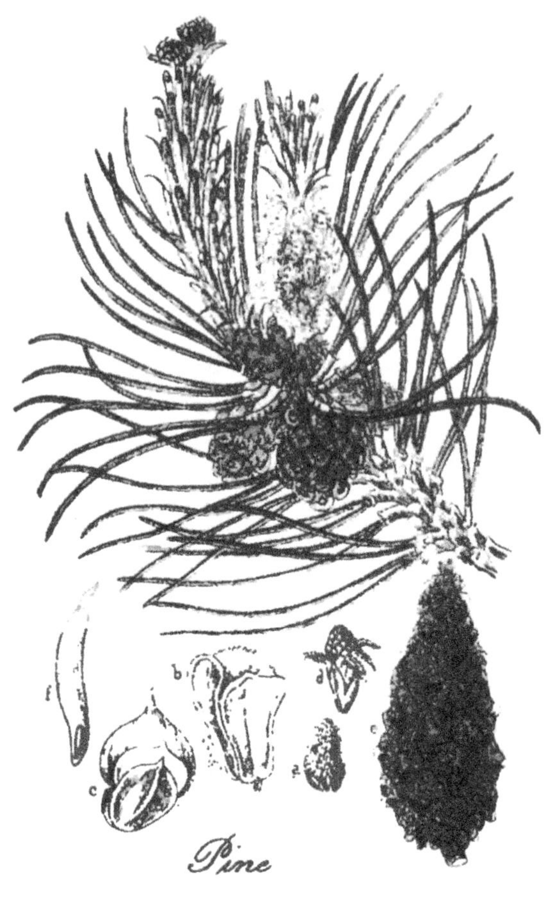

Figure 3 Pine (*Pinus* sp.)

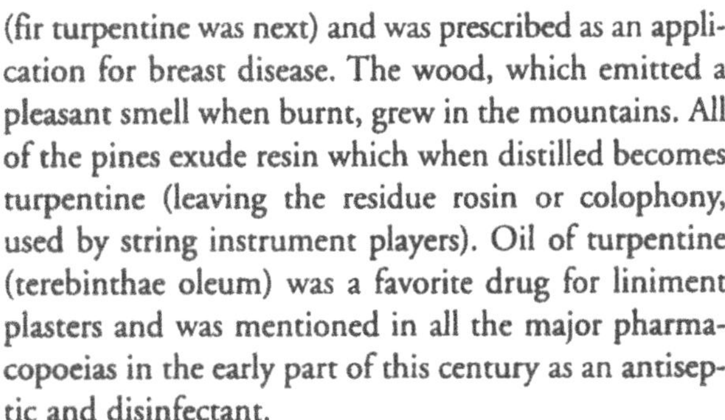

(fir turpentine was next) and was prescribed as an application for breast disease. The wood, which emitted a pleasant smell when burnt, grew in the mountains. All of the pines exude resin which when distilled becomes turpentine (leaving the residue rosin or colophony, used by string instrument players). Oil of turpentine (terebinthae oleum) was a favorite drug for liniment plasters and was mentioned in all the major pharmacopoeias in the early part of this century as an antiseptic and disinfectant.

Wild pea (*Lathyrus* sp.) was applied to the breast in a poultice, and George M. Hocking, professor of pharmacognosy and adviser to the *American National Formulary* noted its use in this form (1955 p. 123) in his book on natural medicinal and pharmaceutical materials and the plants and animals from which they are derived.

Labor

Analgesics

Each of the analgesics identified by Thompson in his *Assyrian Herbal* contained effective pain-relief in the form of hyoscine (scopolamine), one of the most widely used and potent anodynes and prescribed through the ages in some guise or other to the present day.

Thompson identified the **fox-grape** as a *Solanum* sp., which was used in Assyria as a potion for difficult labor. Both seed and sap were recognized to have analgesic effects. There is some confusion as the fox-grape is *Vitis labrusca*, the wild vine, and *Solanum* refers to a genus which includes the Nightshade plants, such as those which produce atropine and the narcotic hyoscine (scopolamine), all of which were still in use during this century. The author wrote that the

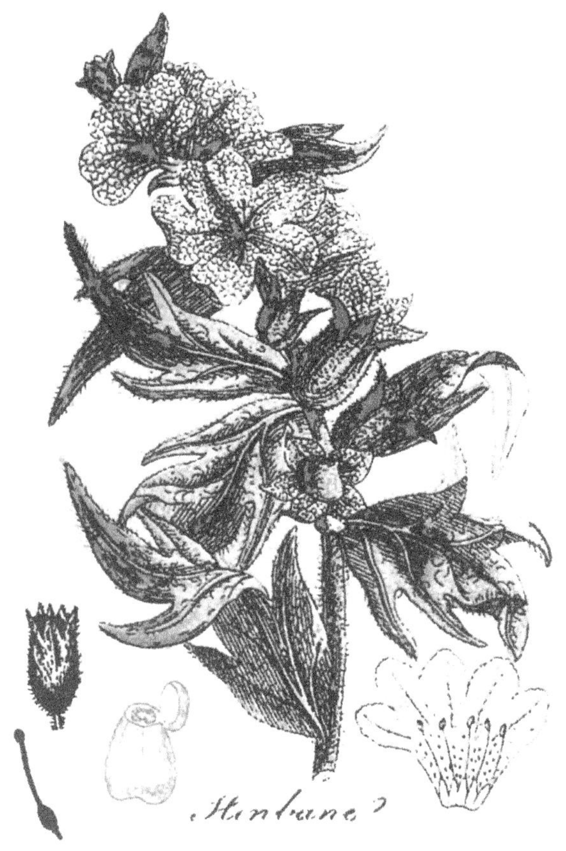

Figure 4 Henbane (*Hyoscyamus niger*)

fox-grape was also used to relieve penile pain or discomfort – if he was referring here to the vine, it is known that the seeds and leaves have astringent properties, helpful for skin lesions.

Henbane (*Hyoscyamus niger*) was taken alone, or in beer, for difficult labor and contains hyoscine and hyocyamine. Henbane was one of the drugs used in the 'soporific sponge' and was employed as an (unreliable) anesthetic in Greece and Rome. It was used world-wide until this century and was included in the major pharmacopoeias as a sedative and antispasmodic. It had less objectionable side-effects than Opium (Squire, 1908 pp. 644–5).

Extract of **Mandrake** (*Mandragora officinalis*), known as the 'devil plant' and the 'male namtar plant of the North', was used during difficult labor. It was advised that the stomach of a woman in difficult labor should be anointed seven times with root extract. Mandrake was known to many cultures and gained further fame when eulogized by Shakespeare in *Othello*, Act 3, Scene 3, line 331:

> Nor all the drowsy syrups of the world,
> not poppy nor mandragora.

The famous bard mentioned mandragora on six occasions and opium only once.

Oxytocics

The Assyrian remedies in this section had either purgative and spasmolytic, or analgesic, antiseptic and anti-inflammatory effects, all of which could benefit a woman in labor. All of the drugs are listed in Pharmacopoeias of this century. It would seem, however, that only those with purgative action could be thought of as oxytocics as it has long been held that aperients exert an ecbolic action on the uterus as a sympathetic response to irritation of the gut.

Thompson identified the Assyrian **ammi** plant as an umbellifer which he postulated may have been related to the mint plant. This herb has antiseptic and antispasmodic effects and should probably be categorized as an analgesic and spasmolytic rather than a uterine stimulant.

Another drug mentioned in this category was **asafetida**. The remedy, taken by mouth, stimulates the gut and acts as a mild purgative (Ringer, 1888 p. 380).

The seed or plant extract of the **castor oil plant** (*Ricinus communis*) was mixed with beer and applied directly to the uterus to aid contractions. Castor oil, a mild but speedy aperient became part of the 'OBE' ritual (oil, bath and enema), a much vaunted technique to hasten early labor and used world-wide in maternity care until the 1960s. The active principle of castor oil is ricinoleic acid. Direct application of oil to the abdomen can cause uterine activity. The technique is still used to this day when we 'rub-up' the uterus to make it contract.

Galbanum (the gum of *Ferula galbaniflua*) was used by fumigation 'to facilitate birth'. There were two principal varieties of the drug, one originating from the eastern Mediterranean seaboard and the other from Persia. Galbanum causes purgation if taken by mouth. As a fumigant its main actions are anti-inflammatory and antiseptic, useful qualities in the treatment a woman in prolonged labor.

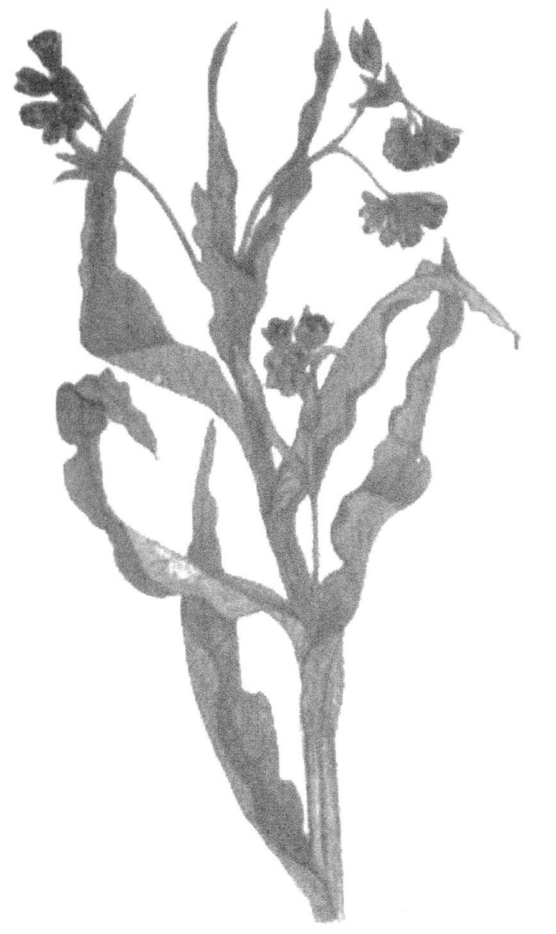

Figure 5 Hound's tongue

Hound's tongue (*Cynoglossum officinale*), or more probably **plantain** (*Plantago psyllium*), was taken as a drink 'for speedy accouchement' and could be accompanied by mint (antispasmodic) and a variety of *Solanum* (analgesic). The seed was also found useful. Thompson wrote that there was much confusion between hound's tongue and plantain and this made exact identification difficult. When cooked like a vegetable plantain could be applied locally to the uterus and may also have been used to treat venereal disease. Hound's tongue was a recognized anodyne over the centuries and was a constituent of ointment for painful hemorrhoids until recent times (Grieve, 1992 pp. 421–2). Plantain seeds yield a large amount of mucilage which is an effective laxative, and they are prescribed nowadays for irritable bowel syndrome (*BHP*, 1983 pp. 165–6).

Juniper (*Juniperus communis*) was taken alone or with plantain 'to speed accouchement'. Its action may have been to flavor the plantain (juniper gives gin its distinctive taste), its anti-colic or its anti-inflammatory effects. Oil of juniper was listed in all the major national pharmacopoeias in the early twentieth century, and remains as a spasmolytic and anti-inflammatory in the *BHP* (1983 p. 124).

Lye (strong alkaline solution) was noted as an ecbolic, used 'to deliver the dead child'. Various sodas, known as 'salts' were developed over the millennia for their purgative action, to stimulate labor and to treat postnatal breast engorgement .

Pistachio (*Pistacia terebinthus*), from which came the early true turpentine (Chian turpentine) was 'applied for speedy birth'. Alternatively, it could be administered with asafetida. Turpentine has antiseptic, diuretic and anti-inflammatory effects and could be given in enema form for obstinate constipation. Turpentine was listed in the pharmacopoeias for these medicinal uses until recent times.

Menstruation

Emmenagogues

With the exception of marigold and saffron this group of Assyrian remedies, are not acknowledged (in modern sources) to induce menstruation, although they all have active constituents.

The leaves and fruit of the **bay tree** (*Laurus nobilis*) are aromatic and stimulant and reputed to have narcotic effects. An oil made from the berries was used for colic and for amenorrhea. The tree was found extensively in Gilead (famous for its balm of Gilead, an oleoresin obtained from poplar buds, considered to have miraculous properties), and also grew in Palestine and Asia Minor.

The **caper** (*Capparis spinosa*) was said to 'stir the menses', and **cypress** (*Cupressus* sp.) wood shavings, taken in a drink, were also thought to be effective.

Marigold (*Calendula officinalis*) was useful as a diuretic and also as an emmenagogue and for pains 'in the loins'. The leaves were also applied for convulsions and the juice, with oil of roses, was much used to relieve headache. Marigold is noted as an emmenagogue in the *BHP* (1983 pp. 44–5).

Thompson identified the Assyrian urbatu plant as **papyrus** (*Cyperus papyrus*), later known as Egyptian papyrus. An extract was used to promote menstruation, as a diuretic, and as a treatment for snake bite or scorpion stings. Papyrus was of great economic importance in the ancient world and provided the first known form of paper. It was also used as fuel, for making baskets, sails and cordage, and for building punts or canoes. The plant was used in later times to ornament Egyptian temples and to crown the statues of Egyptian gods.

Saffron (*Crocus sativus*) was formerly used as an antispasmodic and emmenagogue (Grieve, 1992 p. 700) and appeared in recent pharmacopoeias as an ingredient to give coloring and flavor to medicines.

Storax (originally the solid resin from *Styrax officinale*), a balsam obtained from the trunk of *Liquidambar orientalis*, was used to promote menstruation but, as the centuries went by, it was usually prescribed as a stimulant and expectorant. The tree grew solitarily by rivers, or thickly in groves, throughout northern Mesopotamia and the inspissated juice of the bark had a vanilla-like odor.

Treatment for painful and heavy menstruation

All of the Assyrian drugs listed under this heading would have been useful medications for the indications specified. Most appear in the pharmacopoeias of recent times or are used in herbal medications for painful or heavy periods.

The evil-smelling **asafetida** (from *Ferula foetida* root), still in use as an antispasmodic, was prescribed as an emmenagogue until well into the nineteenth century (Graves, 1834 pp. 156–7). Both properties would have been helpful for the conditions for which they were prescribed.

Cassia (a coarse form of cinnamon) is still advocated as an antispasmodic (*BHP*, 1983 p. 69). The bark, which contains tannic acid and other chemicals, was also used for uterine hemorrhage.

The seeds of **hemp** (*Cannabis sativa*) were found to be good for their analgesic properties and were mixed and taken in beer for 'female ailments' and for heavy and painful periods. Hemp was much used through the ages as a sedative and analgesic. The plant was smoked or ingested as an hallucinogen in many cultures and is known by many slang names such as bhang, hashish and marijuana.

Marigold (*Calendula officinalis*) was applied externally, internally and as a fumigation for dysmenorrhea and excess menstrual loss and retains its place for these indications in herbal medicine (*BHP*, 1983 pp. 44–5; McIntyre, 1994 p. 95).

Another Assyrian remedy was **mint** (*Mentha* spp., *urnu* in Assyrian) which was useful for 'foul breath and to clean the mouth'. Mint was (and still is) used for colic and painful menstruation (*BHP*, 1983 p. 142; McIntyre, 1994 p. 143).

The **nettle** (*Urtica dioica*), a nutritious plant high in vitamins and minerals, contains formic acid and histamine in its stinging hairs. Nettles have an astringent action which led to their being applied to staunch bleeding and probably explains why the plant was advocated for reducing menstrual bleeding. The nettle still retains this indication in herbal medicine.

It appears that the Assyrian botanists knew the narcotic properties of both **poppy** and **mandragora**. Poppy juice was gathered by the children and women. Known as 'pa-pa', 'araru' or 'daughter of the field', the plant name translates easily to 'poppy' and also suggests an origin for the Latin *Papaver*. The plant in question was probably the red poppy, *Papaver rhoeas*. Of more importance is *Papaver somniferum* from which opium is obtained. Thompson included a long list of indications for the use of poppy and intimated that it may have been used for painful menses.

Dried **rose** (*Rosa* sp.), cooked in wine, was another Assyrian remedy for uterine pain. An important source of vitamin C and rose oil (attar), and famed for its fragrance, it was listed in the early twentieth century pharmacopoeias, and is prescribed to relieve dysmenorrhea and uterine congestion in herbal medicine (McIntyre, 1994 p. 253).

Treatment to stop menses

The leaves of the **marigold** (*Calendula officinalis*) were used 'to stay the menstrual discharge' and, according to McIntyre (1994 p. 62) the plant's astringent properties 'help reduce excessive [uterine] bleeding'.

The **windflower** (*Anemone pulsatilla*), either alone or with other plants, was placed in beer and drunk by a woman so that 'the menstruation shall be stayed'.

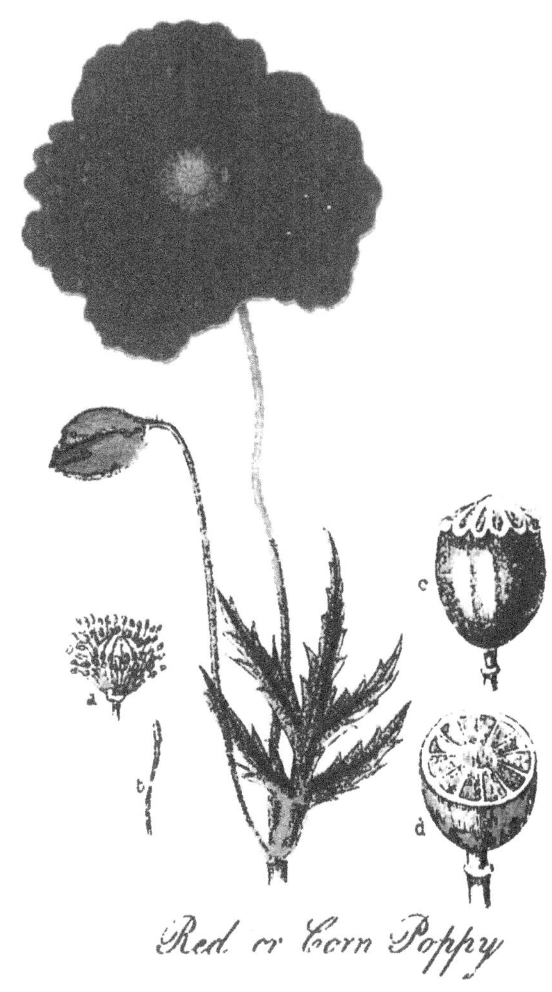

Figure 6 Poppy (*Papaver* sp.)

Modern books on herbalism suggest using the windflower for dysmenorrhea, scanty menses and premenstrual tension states (*BHP*, 1983 p. 174; McIntyre, 1994 p. 84; Wren, 1988 p. 227).

Penile problems

It is likely that the remedies for penile disorders were medications for venereal disease or skin ailments.

The seeds and leaves of **fox-grape** (*Vitis labrusca*) were used for their astringent properties. Maple (*Acer* sp.) extract, alone or in rosewater or milk, was also applied to the penis. As an astringent, it should have been helpful for skin inflammation or ulceration.

Thompson wrote that **rose** (*Rosa* sp.), often as rosewater, was mentioned extensively in the Assyrian medicinal tablets. The rose bush was rarely found in Mesopotamia so the dried flowers were probably imported from Persia. Oil of roses (Persian, 'attar', a very fragrant essential oil made chiefly from the damask rose) was used to disguise the unpleasant odor of some drug applications.

The red-blossomed **tamarisk** (*Tamarix* sp.), which grows along river beds and in marshes provides a fruit which the ancient Assyrians believed was a powerful amulet to ward off disease. The fruits (Manna) contain various sugars and are thought to be anti-inflammatory (Ratsch, 1992 p. 171).

Rupture of membranes

It is uncertain from Thompson's text if the remedies 'for too much fluid flowing' were used to treat rupture of the membranes with escape of liquor or for excess menstrual blood loss.

The root of the **cassia** plant (*Cinnamomum cassia*) was applied to the uterus 'with five other drugs' for the condition. The *BHP* (1983 p. 69) classifies *Cinnamomum cassia* as an antimicrobial. Could the Ancient Assyrians have understood that prolonged membrane rupture could lead to sepsis *in utero*?

Thompson wrote that the cassia known to the ancients should not be confused with senna which he believed could not be traced to Assyria earlier than the ninth century BC. He asserted that the cassia alluded to in the late cuneiform contracts was either cinnamon or a closely related plant. During Roman times Galen said that the finest cassia could be substituted for the lowest quality cinnamon. It is known that the medical properties of both are very similar.

Uterine disease

The *Assyrian Herbal* contains a number of remedies which the author classified as 'for [unspecified] uterine disease. The first such nostrum was **alamu**. Although not positively identified, this aromatic plant, possibly an umbellifer, was prescribed for external use in uterine disease and was sometimes administered with fennel (*Foeniculum vulgare*).

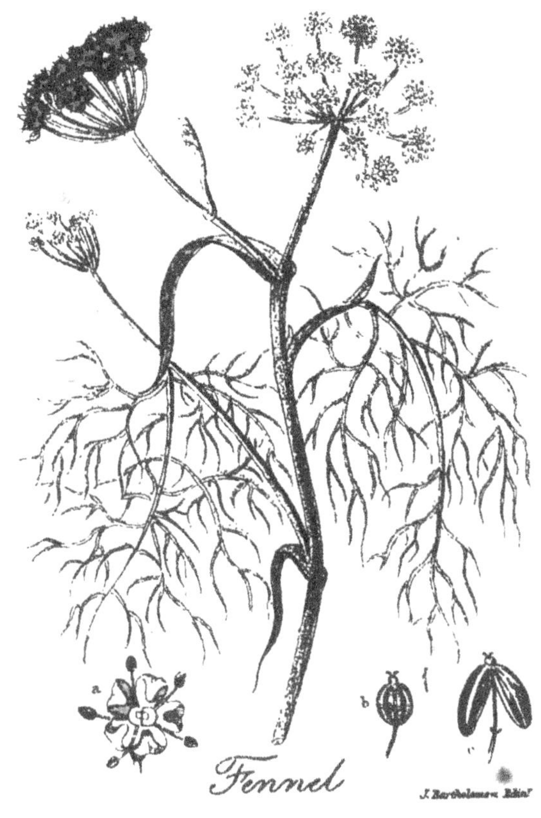

Figure 7 Fennel

Another plant remedy was **boxthorn** (*Lycium barbarum*) seed, which was taken in a potion and was thought to be helpful for uterine and menstrual disorders. The herb was identified as a thorny plant of Cappadocia and Lydia and as one of the Berberidaceae family.

Camomile or chamomile (*Anthemis nobilis*), which grew plentifully in the area, was prescribed when 'much water flows' and was also of general use for 'disease of the uterus'. Thought to be an anodyne, antispasmodic and anti-inflammatory it was listed in conventional medical pharmacopoeias to this century and is currently a favorite herbal and aromatherapeutic cure for women (Ody, 1993 p. 47; McIntyre, 1994 p. 41; *BHP*, 1983 pp. 60–1; Stuart, 1989 p. 170; Dye, 1992 p. 51). It was known in Germany as matricaria chamomile, an allusion to its beneficial effects in gynecology.

Extract of **cassia** bark (*Cinnamomum cassia*) was used externally for diseases of the uterus, possibly for its antispasmodic effects.

The **castor oil** plant (*Ricinus communis*) was applied 'with beer', possibly as a lubricant. Intriguingly, Thompson noted a similarity between the castor oil plant and savin (*Juniperus sabina*), a powerful uterine stimulant and emmenagogue (Stuart, 1989 pp. 209–10) which in large doses was said to cause abortion. Its use as such in ancient Assyria is purely conjecture. There are no references to abortion in Thompson's text and he did not state whether the emmenagogue drugs were used as abortifacients, although they may have been.

Fennel (*Foeniculum vulgare*), was used as a carminative and anti-colic agent in conventional medicine in this century (Squire, 1908 p. 540), and is still prescribed in herbal medicine as an antispasmodic and to reduce premenstrual bloating and fluid retention (Rogers, 1995 p. 28).

Kelp (*Laminaria* spp.) was known as the 'sprout of the sea' and as a drug 'from the middle of the sea'. It appears that most of the common seaweeds were used for making kelp. The weed was harvested from the rocks on the foreshore and was then partially dried and burned in pits. The ashes contained a form of soda mixed with many impurities which was applied directly to the uterus. It may have been useful as an astringent. The slender stems of *Laminaria* were in use in this century for cervical dilatation. The dried stem was placed in the cervical canal and could swell up to four times the size of its dry diameter by extracting water from the cervical stroma.

Opopanax (derived from *Opopanax chironium*), an umbellifer native to Asia Minor. When wounded a milky sap flows from the plant and hardens with time. The main constituents of opopanax are gum, resin, and a volatile oil. Also known as 'surgeon's opopanax', the drug was said to have antispasmodic and emmenagogue effects (Graves, 1834 p. 112; Grieve, 1992 p. 600).

Another agent 'for uterine disease' in the *Assyrian Herbal* was **storax** (from *Styrax officinalis*). Much used as incense during church ceremonies the plant contains benzoic acid and is in medical use as Benzoin Tincture Co., (*The British Pharmacopoeia*, 1932 pp. 438–9; Reynolds and Prasad, 1982 p. 314). An effective antifungal agent, it was combined with salicylic acid in Whitfield's ointment (Harvey, 1985 p. 973). It is

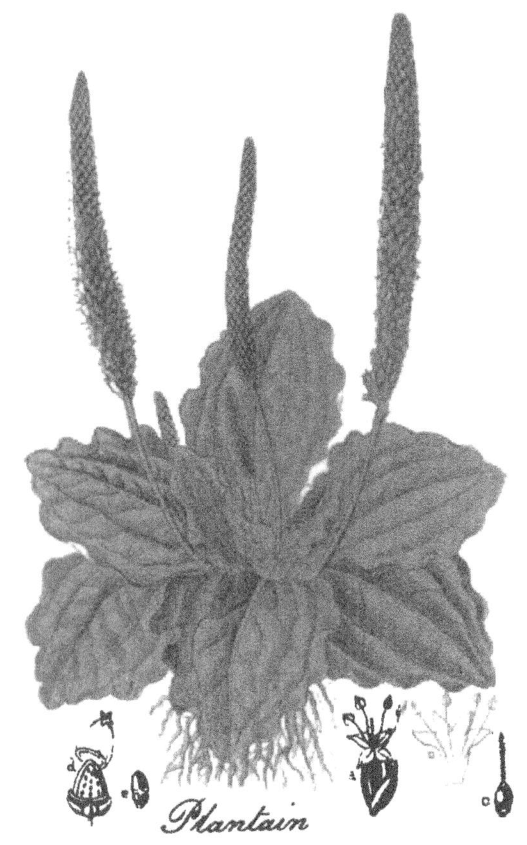

Figure 8 Plantain (*Plantago* sp.)

tempting to think that the Assyrians could have prescribed it for 'uterine' (possibly meaning uterus *and* genital tract) itch and discomfort. It is currently in vogue as treatment for 'cracked' nipples caused by breastfeeding.

Venereal disease

Evening primrose (*Oenothera biennis*) is 'similar in many ways to the water hemlock, a poisonous plant which could cause vomiting, convulsions and stupor, but if applied locally was known to have anodyne qualities and was used to treat pain in venereal disease'. In the seventeenth century, Nicholas Culpeper advised a salve of primrose leaves to help wounds to heal. Found in 1919 to contain gamma linolenic acid, evening primrose oil became a medical and commercial success in the management of premenstrual syndrome in the 1980s and 1990s.

Marigold (*Calendula officinalis*), used by the ancients for what was classified as venereal disease (presumably discomfort, discharge, irritation and itch) is favored by herbalists as an antifungal, anti-inflammatory and antiseptic (*BHP*, 1983 pp. 44–5; Ody, 1993 p. 43), particularly for infections of the female genital tract (McIntyre, 1994 p. 62).

Plantain (*Plantago* spp.), which contains glycosides, mucilage, and tannins has always had the reputation for being a healing herb, and Pliny advocated its use to heal wounds. It is still in vogue as a laxative and as a poultice for allergic or infected skin lesions (Ody, 1993 p. 86).

The resin from the **pistachio** tree (*Pistacia terebinthus*) was used in Assyria as a local application 'for gonorrhea'. Oil of **turpentine** has antiseptic, antispasmodic and hemostatic properties and was still included in *Martindale, The Extra Pharmacopoeia* in 1982 (Reynolds and Prasad, p. 670).

The **tamarisk** (*Tamarix* sp.) grows in copses and was probably the source of the biblical manna. The branches were the height of a camel rider and extract of the plant, which has astringent qualities, was applied to the penis to treat venereal disease. Plant extract or the seed of an unidentified plant, **tu-lal**, were also used.

Women's diseases

Some of the remedies mentioned by Thompson fall into the non-specific category of 'women's diseases'. The plants include **bay** (*Laurus nobilis*) and the **boxthorn** (*Lycium barbarum*). Also mentioned is the **chaste tree** (*Vitex agnus castus*) and its extract was applied with **asafetida** and **turpentine** for 'female complaints'. **Juniper** (*Juniperus communis*) was also added to remedies for some female complaints, probably for its antispasmodic effects.

Corn (*Triticum* sp.) is the only one of this group not previously dealt with. It was consumed in oil or beer. Apart from its nutritional value it could be used in the preparation of thick, viscous medicines. More specifically for women's diseases, it may have been, and still is, prescribed as herbal medicine, to treat gonorrhea and disorders of the urinary tract (Grieve, 1992 pp. 224–6; McIntyre, 1994 p. 148).

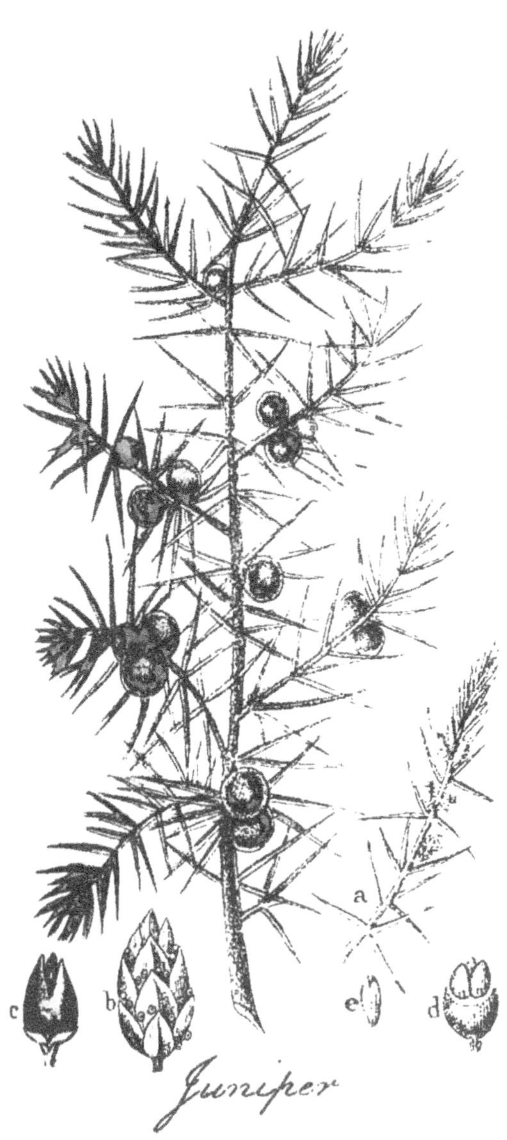

Figure 9 Juniper (*Juniperus* sp.)

MATERIA MEDICA IN ANCIENT ASSYRIA

Uses

Aphrodisiacs
Asafetida, caper, lye, nettle seed, poppy

Breast disease
Chaste tree, cypress, fenugreek, galbanum, pine, wild pea

Labor

Analgesics	Fox-grape, henbane, mandrake
Oxytocics	Ammi, asafetida, castor oil plant, galbanum, hound's tongue, juniper, lye, pistachio, plantain

Menstruation

Emmenagogues	Bay, caper, cypress, marigold, papyrus, saffron, storax
Painful/heavy menstruation	Asafetida, cassia, hemp, marigold, mint, nettle, poppy, rose
To stop menses	Marigold, windflower

Penile disorders
Fox-grape, maple, rose, tamarisk

Rupture of membranes
Cassia

Uterine disease
Alamu, boxthorn, camomile, cassia, castor oil plant, fennel, kelp, opopanax, storax

Venereal disease
Evening primrose, marigold, plantain, turpentine (fir), tamarisk, tu-lal

Women's diseases
Bay, boxthorn, chaste tree, corn, juniper

Selected remedies

Alamu, ammi, asafetida
Bay, boxthorn
Camomile, caper, cassia, castor oil plant, chaste tree, corn, cypress
Evening primrose
Fennel, fenugreek, fox-grape
Galbanum
Hemp, henbane, hound's tongue
Juniper
Kelp
Lye
Mandrake, maple, marigold, mint
Nettle
Opopanax
Poppy, papyrus, pine, pistachio, plantain
Rose
Saffron, storax
Tamarisk, turpentine (fir), tu-lal
Windflower, wild pea

References

The British Herbal Medicine Association (1983). *British Herbal Pharmacopoeia*, pp. 34–5, 44–5, 60–1, 69, 124, 142, 165–6, 174, 224–5, 216. (Bournemouth: UK)

Caubet, A. and Bernus-Taylor, M. (1991). *The Louvre. Near-Eastern Antiquities*, p. 5. (Paris: Scala Publications Ltd.)

Dye, J. (1992). *Aromatherapy for Women and Children*, p. 51. (UK: C. W. Daniel and Co.)

Ellis, E. S. (1946). *Ancient Anodynes*, pp. 44–52. (London: Heinemann)

Estes, J. Worth (1989). *The Medical Skills of Ancient Egypt*, p. 94. (USA: Science History Publications)

The General Medical Council (1932). *The British Pharmocopoeia*, pp. 438–9. (London: Constable and Co.)

Graham, H. (1951). *Eternal Eve*, p. 24. (New York: Doubleday and Co.)

Graves, G. (1834). *Hortus Medicus*, pp. 156–7, 112. (London: Longman). Reprinted as *Medicinal Plants*. (London: Bracken Books)

Grieve, M. (1992). *A Modern Herbal*, pp. 224–6, 358–9, 421–2, 600, 700. (London: Tiger Books)

Harvey, S. (1985). Antiseptics and Disinfectants; Fungicides: Ectoparasiticides. In Goodman and Gilman (eds) *The Pharmacological Basis of Therapeutics*, p. 973. (New York: Macmillan)

Hocking, G. M. (1955). *A Dictionary of Terms in Pharmacognosy*, pp. 64, 123. (Springfield, IL: Charles C. Thomas)

Kramer, S. N. (1969). *Cradle of Civilization. Great ages of man. A History of the World's Cultures*, pp. 53, 127–53. (The Netherlands: Time–Life International)

Lyons, A. S. and Pertrucelli, R. J. (1978). *Medicine. An Illustrated History*, pp. 58–69. (New York: Abrams)

McIntyre, A. (1994). *The Complete Woman's Herbal*, pp. 41, 62, 95, 143, 148, 253. (London: Gaia Books Ltd.)

Ody, P. (1993). *The Herb Society's Complete Medicinal Herbal*, pp. 43, 47, 86. (London: Dorling Kindersley)

Ratsch, C. (1992). *A Dictionary of Sacred and Magical Plants*, p. 171. (UK: Unity Press)

Reynolds, J. E. F. and Prasad, A. B. (1982). *Martindale. The Extra Pharmacopoeia*, pp. 314, 670. (London: The Pharmaceutical Press)

Ricci, J. V. (1943). *The Genealogy of Gynecology*, p. 29. (Philadelphia: Blakiston Co.)

Ringer, S. (1888). *A Handbook of Therapeutics*, p. 380. (London: H. K. Lewis)

Rogers, C. (1995). *The Women's Guide to Herbal Medicine*, p. 28. (London: Hamish Hamilton)

Schiff, P. B., Fant, J. and Horowitz, S. B. (1979). Promotion of microtubule assembly *in vitro* by taxol. *Nature*, 227, 665–7

Sigerist, H. E. (1951). *A History of Medicine*, Vol. 1, pp. 399–40, 429, 482. (Oxford: Oxford University Press)

Squire, P. W. (1908). *Squire's Companion to the Latest Edition of the British Pharmacopoeia*, pp. 540, 548–50, 644–5. (London: J. and A. Churchill)

Stuart, M. (ed.) (1989). *The Encyclopedia of Herbs and Herbalism*, pp. 165, 170, 209–10. (UK: Caxton)

Thompson, R. Campbell (1924). *The Assyrian Herbal*. (London: Luzac and Co.)

Wren, R. C. (1988). *Potter's New Cyclopedia of Botanical Drugs and Preparations*, pp. 18, 227. (UK: C. W. Daniel Co.)

Egypt 7

INTRODUCTION

The Ancient Egyptian civilization is the first great culture for which there are adequate records for the compilation of a materia medica of commonly used prescriptions in general and reproductive medicine. The physicians of the era used plant, animal and mineral compounds obtained locally but also imported from afar. We now know that many of their ingredients have definite pharmacological effects.

The ancient drug formularies were carefully recorded in papyral texts. A number of such compilations were discovered in the nineteenth century as was the method of their interpretation. The drugs were carefully measured and the physicians were aware of potential toxic side effects. The commonly used drug vehicles such as beer, honey and wine, also had medicinal effects. A mystical element, an input from the gods of medicine, was also important in treatment.

Although men did not attend at childbirth many formulations were evolved to assist with fertility, gynecology and the birth process. From Ancient Egypt came the first oral contraceptive and also the first urinary pregnancy test. The importance of breast changes in early pregnancy was also well known. Abortifacient, antiseptic, analgesic and other drug compounds were used. This chapter explores some of the concepts of Ancient Egyptian medicine and obstetrics and gynecology and also describes the materia medica for women's disorders in that era.

THE BASIS OF THE ANCIENT EGYPTIAN MEDICAL SYSTEM

According to myth, the human body was divided into many parts each of which came under the protection of a specific god or goddess. The penis, for instance, was watched over by Osiris (see Chapter 2). The heart was thought to be the principal organ of the body and the seat of all emotion and intellect. It was necessary not only for life but also in death. The deceased person's 'weighing of the heart' ceremony took place at the entrance to the Afterworld (the Duat). If the heart was so burdened with a guilty conscience that it weighed more than a feather, it was devoured by Ammut, a goddess demon, and the deceased could not enter the happy Kingdom of the Dead.

It was the Egyptian belief that air, water and blood were carried in afferent ducts or 'metu' to the body's organs, and that efferent *metu* transported organ products and waste material to the surface. Feces were thought to produce a noxious substance, *Whdw* (rotten stuff), rising levels of which could become dangerous to the heart and cause disease of the *metu*. The *Whdw* of flatulence was also found in the odor of infection and decay. *Whdw* could be controlled by washing, by emetics or purgatives, or by medications which cleansed wounds and septic areas. Disease was also attributed to worms, insects and supernatural causes.

THE ANCIENT HEALERS

There were three classes of healers – sorcerers, priests and lay physicians (*swnw*). Would-be physicians attended 'The House of Life', the equivalent of medical school, and collections of medical writings were kept for study in the temples. Galen, in the second century AD wrote that Greek physicians visited one such medical school and temple library at Memphis.

In his book *The Medical Skills of Ancient Egypt*, J. Worth Estes (1989 p. 20) recounts that c. 425 BC the Greek historian Herodotus wrote that 'all [of Egypt] is stuffed with physicians' and that 'the practice of medicine they split into separate parts, each doctor being responsible for the treatment of only one disease'. Thus it appears that medicine was well regulated and that some *swnw* were regarded as specialists in certain ailments and dubbed titles such as 'Physician of the Eyes', 'Shepherd of the Anus', and 'Chief of Dentists'. There were some female physicians and it is known that at one time during the Old Kingdom era a woman named Peseshet was the 'Overseer of Lady Physicians'.

ANCIENT EGYPTIAN TREATMENTS

Amulets, incantations and written or carved talismans were thought to have occult medical properties. Consequently they were widely used in healing and to ward off the demons responsible for disease. Votive offerings to the statues of healing gods were deemed helpful and water poured over such figurines was used for its curative properties. Temples were associated with healing and temple sleep and bathing in the holy temple waters were frequently-used remedies. Sometimes no treatment was offered and natural healing was awaited which was referred to as the patient being 'tied to his/her moorings'.

Many of the foods used in day to day cooking were also in use as medications. Cereals were the main crops grown in Ancient Egypt: emmer wheat was pounded to make flour for bread (as was the lotus plant fruit), and barley was brewed for beer. The vegetable crop included cucumber, garlic, leek, lettuce, onion and radish. The pulses, chickpeas, beans and lentils, were cultivated, and fruits, including dates, figs, grapes and melons, were also grown. Oil was obtained from sesame, and grapes, pomegranate and palm were fermented to make wine. Carob pods, dates, honey and raisins were used as sweeteners. Papyrus was used for making writing material and papyrus or flax were the basis for clothing, ropes and sails. Domesticated animals and wild game or fish were used as meats. Eggs, milk and cheese were available.

Although locally-available plant, animal and mineral products were used as medications many more were imported. Trading expeditions traveled by sea to 'the land of Punt' (possibly Zimbabwe) and returned with ebony, gold, incense, ivory, myrrh trees and also baboons and other animals. Many drug-containing plants were obtained and carried overland from neighboring countries.

Acacia, natron (desert salt), malachite and other local products were gathered and prescribed on an empiric basis. If they appeared to be effective, they were added to the ancient drug formularies and so became rational treatments. The medications (*phr.t*) of Ancient Egypt were prescribed with little alteration in their constituents over many centuries.

In her book, *An Ancient Egyptian Herbal* (1989), Lise Manniche has written a comprehensive account of the plant medications available in Ancient Egypt. For her source material she drew on the Ancient Egyptian papyri, texts from contemporary neighboring civilizations, treatises by classical authors, and the medical works of the Copts. She discovered that 'a surprisingly large amount [of the plants, trees and fruit mentioned in those sources] have medicinal properties recognized in modern herbal medicine' and that the ancients had 'certainly learned from experience that the treatment was efficient'.

It is known that the *swnw* prepared their own recipes, each component being accurately measured. Egyptian measures were based on the *ro*, or mouthful, equivalent to about 15 ml (Leake, 1975 p. 46). Other measures included the ***hekat*** (4.5 l) and the ***hin*** (about 0.5 l or 32 *ro*), or fractions of these measures. The protective 'Eye of Horus' (the ***udjat***) was placed on all prescriptions. Each area of the eye symbol represented a fraction of the 64 parts and could be used to indicate the proportion or fraction of medicinal products to be used in a prescription (see Chapter 2).

Liquid vehicles for drug delivery were used as solvents and diluents and included ale, honey, milk, oil, water and wine. Animal fat or beeswax formed the base for unguents and emollients. It is estimated that animal parts formed 42% of the ingredients mentioned in the Ebers Papyrus, the remainder being mainly of plant origin (Estes, 1989 p. 103). About 70% of prescriptions were designed for topical application and it appears that the *swnw* were aware of dose related side-effects and toxicity.

Many of the plant and mineral remedies of the time have been assessed and are now known to contain identifiable pharmacological properties. Although it is interesting to speculate on the action of drugs mentioned in the medical papyri it should be borne in mind that treatments were introduced on a magical or an empiric basis for symptom complexes which do not necessarily relate to modern diagnoses.

In a remarkable study by Pierre Rouyer, a French pharmacist who accompanied the Napoleonic invasion of 1798, it was found that 90% of the drugs commonly sold in Cairo at the end of the eighteenth century were in current use in France and the New World. At least a third of eighteenth century Egyptian drugs are also to be found in the Ebers Papyrus which dates from c. 1550 BC. Estes (1989 p. 114) opined that Greek and Roman medicine owed much to Ancient Egyptian practice. The Greco-Roman materia medica was preserved in the writings of the renowned Pedanius Dioscorides of Cilicia (now in Turkey), a physician to the Roman Legions in the first century AD. His text was translated into Arabic and eventually retranslated, reaching, in turn, Islamic Egypt and Renaissance Europe.

Ergot

There are a number of ingredients and recipes for women mentioned in Estes' definitive book. A surprising addition to the group is ergot, from the cereal and grass fungus, *Claviceps purpurea*, the cause of St Anthony's fire (contracted by eating bread made from smutty rye grain). Estes himself doubted if it was used in Ancient Egypt and quotes Chauncey Leake of the University of California in San Francisco as his reference (Leake, 1975 p. 75). Leake used as *his* source a translation of a book on poisons written c. AD 750 by Jabir ibn Hayyan, the earliest and highly respected Arab medical writer, but doubt remains whether ergot was used in Pharaonic times.

FERTILITY AND CHILDBIRTH

Fertility

The relationship between semen, intercourse and pregnancy was well recognized. According to Ancient Egyptian concepts, the semen (thought to originate in the spinal cord or in the heart) provided the seed which was nurtured in the womb to form the infant. Semen traveled by two *metu* to the testes where it awaited its future liberation. According to legend, the god Amun 'laid his heart' in Ahmes, a Pharaoh's wife, who became pregnant with the future Pharaoh Hatshesput.

In her book, *Magic In Ancient Egypt*, (1994 p. 120) Geraldine Pinch relates that human fertility was the domain of goddesses such as Isis, Hathor and Heket, the fertility of crops and animals being associated with the male deities Osiris and Min. Pregnancy was thought to be achievable by magico-religious means and the help of the powerful fertility gods was invoked. Fertility figurines were used to magically hasten the onset of conception. Human fertility could be threatened by spells cast by living persons or by the spirits of women who had died in childbirth, but adoption was sometimes possible for those unfortunate couples who remained childless (Robins, 1993 p. 77).

Among the many available treatments were herbal remedies such as honey and fenugreek which were ingested to 'loosen a child in the womb'. Animal testicles, suitably presented, or powdered placenta were included in fertility prescriptions. Milk or stallion's saliva were prescribed to increase women's libido and there were many remedies for male impotence and sterility including carob, juniper, oil, pine, salt and watermelon. The mandrake plant was introduced into Egypt during the New Kingdom era. The root contains a narcotic painkiller which was also used as an aphrodisiac. An unlikely but much-used aphrodisiac was lettuce (Tyldesley, 1994 p. 70), the favorite food of Min, the Egyptian god of sexuality. Wild lettuce contains small amounts of an opium-like chemical called lactucarium (see Chapter 4).

Menstruation

Menstruation, or lack of it, is mentioned on many occasions in the medical papyri and various prescriptions were offered as treatment. Stetter (1993 p. 105) quotes a magical spell to be intoned over a bunch of flax threads, bound and made into a tampon, which was inserted 'into her flesh' to arrest the flow of menstruation. Some translators have claimed that there is mention of sanitary protection in the laundry lists dating from the time of the New Kingdom, although this is disputed.

Marriage

Marriage was arranged in most instances and the average age of conjugal union was 12 to 13 years for females and 15 to 20 years for males. The couple regarded the loving relationship of Isis, with her undying love for Osiris, as their example of faithful marriage. Isis was seen as the ideal mother figure and portrayed with her infant son Horus on her lap.

Pregnancy

Pregnancy was diagnosed by examination of the breasts and skin and by testing the woman's urine (see below). The length of gestation was reckoned to be between nine and ten months. Sometimes magical knot amulets or 'Isis-knots' were worn to keep the womb shut, to prevent miscarriage. Swallow's liver 'dried, powdered and with liquid of fermented beverage' was applied to the abdomen of the woman who had miscarried. A special alabaster vessel, in the shape of a pregnant woman, was used to store oil. The oil was rubbed on the abdominal skin to prevent stretch marks and was also applied to the vulva during labor, especially at the anticipated time of delivery.

Childbirth

The birth of the gods was celebrated in specially constructed temples called *Mammesi* or birth houses. The delivery of Rudjedet, a pregnant priestess, is described in the Westcar papyrus and may reflect what happened in real life: four midwife goddess were present, Isis to the front, Nephthys at the rear and Heket to help conduct the delivery (Stetter, 1993 p. 89). The goddess Meskhenet, represented as birth brick with a female head, transformed herself into a birth stool for the delivery. Afterwards she foretold the fortunes and destiny of the newborn.

Mortal births took place in a part of the home separate from the rest of the household. Ostraca (tiles) which depict the birth bower show a plant which is similar to birthwort (*Aristolochia clematis*); extract of birthwort was once used to induce labor. Some commentators believe the plant to be bryony, which contains purgative juice. Birth amulets or magical ointments were placed on 'the head of the woman who is giving birth' (Barnes, 1956 p. 28). Midwives attended during the labor and offered remedies of honey and fenugreek for oral consumption or vaginal suppositories which could include beer and incense. Castoreum (musk, from the perineal sacs of the beaver) is mentioned by Ebbell in his 1937 translation of the papyri and the descendant midwives of the Ancient Egyptians used castoreum to expedite labor.

The woman gave birth while sitting or squatting on two (or four) birth bricks or on a birthing stool. The hieroglyphs meaning 'to give birth' show either a woman in squatting position or the use of a birthing stool or birthing bricks (Reeves, 1992 p. 19). The umbilical cord was cut with a flint (pesehkef) or an obsidian knife and spells were used to assist placental delivery and to curtail excess bleeding. Both the cord and the placenta were treated with respect and were buried in the home, as it was believed that this ensured the survival of the newborn. Some placenta was kept for use in fertility spells and a piece might even be offered to the infant – if refused, a poor outcome could be expected for the neonate.

The goddess Tauert, portrayed as a female hippopotamus with the limbs of a lion, the back and tail of a crocodile, pendulous breasts and a full belly, was particularly associated with the protection of women in childbirth. Bes, the dwarf god, was also linked with the birth process, especially at the time of placental delivery. After the delivery both mother and infant remained in the birth chamber for 14 days of 'purification'. The god Khnum bestowed the gift of good health to those newborn infants who met with his favor.

Not all births had a happy outcome. Some were complicated by prolonged labor with consequent formation of urinary fistulae, resulting in untreatable urinary incontinence. Such an obstetric complication is mentioned in the Kahun papyrus and physical evidence was documented by Professor Derry of Cairo in 1935 when he discovered an extensive vesico-vaginal fistula in the mummified remains of a woman called Henhenit, who was either a queen or dancer and who was one of the six ladies in the court of Mentuhotep c. 2000 BC (Mahfouz Bey, 1957 p. 23).

The puerperium

Infants were breastfed until the age of three years and lactation provided the best available means of fertility regulation. Mother's milk, particularly when feeding a male infant, was considered a powerful remedy. This belief was based on myths surrounding the goddess Isis who treated life threatening burns to the infant Horus by applying her own healing and nurturing breast-milk. On another occasion, she magically healed the left eye of Horus with milk, after it was gouged out by his evil uncle, Seth (see Chapter 2).

Wet-nurses were sometimes employed, particularly for royal children but also when a mother's own milk supply failed, or if a mother had died. Pottery vessels were used to hold excess mother's milk, probably for medicinal purposes. One prescription included finely ground papyrus plant and grain mixed with milk. A *hin* of this preparation was guaranteed to give the child a healthy sleep (Robins, 1993 p. 90).

FEMALE DISORDERS

Vesico-vaginal fistula, ovarian tumors, and calcified fibroids have been found in mummified remains but, as yet, no instance of female breast cancer has been discovered – this may be because this cancer usually occurs at an age to which survival was not then common. The average age of death was less than 40 years and many women died young due to difficulties encountered in childbearing. However, the Edwin Smith papyrus (c. 1600 BC), purchased at Luxor in 1862 and translated by James Breasted (1930), relates instructions concerning the treatment of a bulging tumor on the breast in a man (case 45). Some observers have suggested that the tumor was either gas gangrene, a tropical ulcer, or Kaposi sarcoma. A benign fibroadenoma of the left breast was discovered during examination of a female mummy, aged about 35, who died c. 835 BC.

The *swnw* believed that many female disorders related to malposition of the uterus. Consequently, they devised treatments for replacing the matrix into its normal pelvic position. Fumigations, medicated pessaries and even oral recipes were used but digital manipulation was not tried. The ghosts of the *swnw* influenced medical notions until recent times.

MALE DISORDERS

During the New Kingdom era (1570–1070 BC) images of Akhenaten (Amenhotep IV), Tutankhamun and other royal males reveal a family who had gynecomastia and a feminine body shape. It is unknown if this

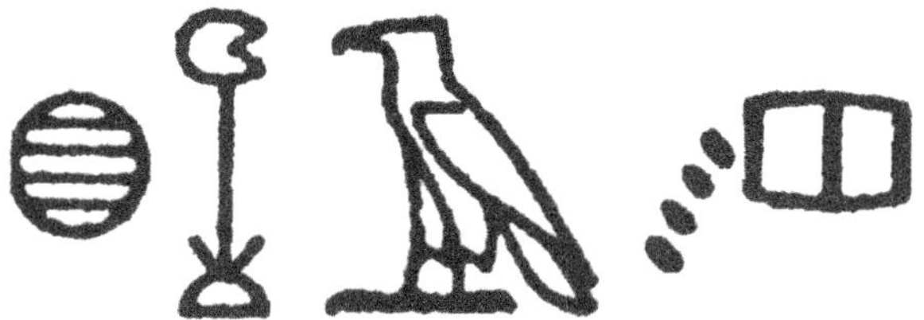

was a genetic defect or if it related to the effects of schistosomiasis or some other ailment. Schistosomiasis, caused by the bilharzia worm, results in cirrhosis of the liver. The visible manifestations of the disease include gynecomastia, umbilical hernia and enlargement of the scrotal sac due to increased abdominal pressure from ascites.

Circumcision

During the Old Kingdom era (2686–2181 BC) circumcision was performed on the nobility and priests, and honey was applied to the wounds to aid healing and avoid infection. While it may have had religious significance circumcision may also have been performed as a pubertal rite or in an effort to prevent balanitis. A circumcision scene from the mastaba (tomb) of Ank-ma-hor at Sakkara, which dates from the sixth dynasty, is the oldest-known image of any surgical technique.

THE MEDICAL PAPYRI

The medical papyri of Ancient Egypt are the oldest-known form of medical literature, containing the earliest writings on anatomy, surgery, gynecology and drug therapy. The papyri contain references to aphrodisiacs, sterility, impotence, contraception, miscarriage, labor, and remedies to protect the newborn and to promote the supply of breast milk.

The Ancient Egyptian scribes were experts in hieroglyphic writing, an elaborate form of picture-writing using about 700 signs. This form of writing was used on temples, monuments, tombs and religious papyri. Hieratic script, an abridged version of hieroglyphics, was developed for business contracts and other texts. Demotic script, which was a much simpler and faster version, was introduced at a later date.

Pages of the ancient papyri measured approximately 40 × 32 cm. Sheets of the papyrus were formed when the pith of papyrus reeds was cut into thin strips which were laid over each other in criss-cross fashion and pressed for about a week. The papyral texts were written in hieratic script with titles in red ink and the remainder of the text in black ink. The skill of reading hieroglyphs was lost about the six century AD when the Ancient Egyptian temples were closed down.

In 1799 a slab of basalt was discovered near Rosetta (Rashid) in the western delta. Hieroglyphic and demotic symbols and Greek inscriptions were engraved on the Rosetta Stone. Each script bore the same text, a message of gratitude to Ptolemy V, the Greek ruler of Egypt in the second century BC. Thomas Young deciphered the demotic script (published posthumously in 1831) and Jean-François Champollion began his translation of the hieroglyphic text in 1822. A vast storehouse of knowledge contained in the writings of the ancients was then opened up for research by Egyptologists.

The Kahun Papyrus

The Kahun Papyrus is the oldest of the surviving medical papyri and was compiled c. 1850 BC, during the Middle Kingdom era (2040–1782 BC). It is thought that the Kahun Papyrus was not an original but a copy of a much older text. The contents were first translated and published by Francis L. Griffith (1898). The papyrus (with other non-medical papyri) was discovered in 1889 by Sir William Flinders Petrie in a badly fragmented condition at Medinet el Faiyyum, some 60 miles south of Cairo. The document was reconstructed but many fragments are missing. A new translation was presented by John M. Stevens of Victoria in the *Medical Journal of Australia* (1975 p. 949).

The text of the Kahun Papyrus consists of 34 gynecological case histories which can be classified under the four main headings: disease, conception and contraception, fertility forecasting and pregnancy diagnosis, and miscellanea. The textual subdivisions of these headings are noted below by their number, in brackets, prefixed by the letter 'S'. Altogether, 29 medicinal products are mentioned in the Kahun text, of which 18 are plant in origin, five are of animal origin, four are of mineral origin and two are as yet unidentified.

Disease

This section contains 17 symptom-complexes thought to relate to diseases of the female genitalia. Seven of the medications mentioned could be given as a drink, and three could be eaten. Four were for local application. Three recipes were given as a douche, two as fumigants for the genitalia, and the last mentioned was a preparation for the woman to sit on.

A number of the assorted symptoms and signs were thought to be due to abnormal discharge of fluid from the uterus and birth canal (S.1, S.3, S.6, S.10.). One remedy for this was fumigation with frankincense (used for its fragrance) and new oil while eating raw asses' liver. A cool drink of almonds mixed with s's'-grain in cow's milk was an alternative recipe. Another drink, of finely ground beans and grass seeds, mixed with ale (made from barley, emmer wheat or dates, with an alcohol content of 6–8%) was cooked and drunk over four successive mornings. Smearing of the feet and calves with mud was also used. Soft wet earth often contains mold-producing fungi which have the ability to form antibacterial substances, so the application of mud could have been a more helpful remedy than it would at first glance appear.

Case history number S.2 related instructions 'for [a] woman whose womb has become diseased'. The woman declared that there was a smell of 'roast meat' from the genital area which was interpreted by Griffith as being characteristic of the odor of cancer of the uterus. Fumigation over 'anything that smelled of roast meat' was prescribed.

Instructions for a woman 'swollen after birth' declared that the woman should pour new oil into her vagina (S.4). A topical remedy for swelling of the genitalia was a mixture of finely-powdered green eye paint (malachite) and boiled cow's milk (S.15). Malachite (copper carbonate) and other copper salts were used as cosmetics during the Old Kingdom era. Research has shown that copper salts, of which malachite is the most useful, inhibit bacterial growth, so topical application of the substance to an infected pubic area could have been effective. Malachite was used both as an eye cosmetic and to combat eye infections. Malachite is also listed as an ingredient in 39 drug formulations in the Ebers Papyrus (Estes, 1989 p. 65).

Yet another prescription for a woman 'suffering in her vagina' was oil taken by mouth (S.9). This instruction appears to relate to a sexually abused woman, 'one who has been maltreated', and is probably the first recorded case of rape.

Womb pains (S.5) and spasms of the uterus (S.11) were treated by fumigation with frankincense and oil and application of ass urine to the vagina, or by drinking *h'wy*-food which would induce emesis. Strips of fine linen soaked in myrrh (an astringent and antiseptic) were applied to promote menstruation (S.12). If that failed, a vaginal douche of myrrh and new oil was prescribed.

Menorrhagia (and possibly miscarriage) was treated by sitting on lees of sweet ale. Date juice could be added to increase its efficacy. Lees (the sediment of alcoholic drinks) contains yeast, vitamins and antibacterial substances but it is unknown whether it would lessen menstrual flow.

Other instructions are detailed for 'want in her womb' (S.6), for 'disquiet' of the womb (S.8), and for further disorders (S.13 and S.14) thought to relate to the uterus.

Conception and contraception

There are eight entries in this portion, of which five are concerned with conception and three with contraception. Four of the agents used were applied by douche and in two instances the woman was advised to sit on the medication. Fumigation of the genitalia and insertion of a 'medicated' pessary were each mentioned once.

Milk was prescribed as an aphrodisiac (S.18). The naked woman, who was with her husband, was advised to pour half a dipper of milk (which had been set aside earlier) into her vagina. The next entry (S.19) is concerned with the diagnosis of pregnancy.

As a further aid to conception, the patient was advised to fumigate herself with the smoke of sweet ale, dates, frankincense, new oil, fermented mash and *hywy*-liquid, all placed in a basket and burnt on a fire (S.20). Then, for acute pains of the womb (and possibly to promote menstruation) the woman was advised to sit, with her thighs apart, on well pounded dried dates mixed with sweet ale (S.24). In the last segment on conception (S.25), the woman was advised to sit on canal water which contained *hprwr*-plants and *i'b* of *mst*.

To prevent conception (cases S.21, S.22, S.23), the vagina was irrigated with crocodile dung which was dispersed in sour milk. Alternatively honey and natron (alkaline sodium salts) were placed in the birth canal. Another suggestion was to pour sour milk into the vagina.

The use of crocodile dung to prevent conception may have developed as a result of its mechanical effect or its alteration of the vaginal pH level. Alternatively, the feces may have been used for their magical effect: the crocodile was associated with Seth, the malign Egyptian god who had attempted to injure his sister Isis during her pregnancy. Seth amulets could be used either to open the womb (to promote menstruation, conception or birth) or to close it (causing miscarriage or hemorrhage). Seth was frequently depicted on uterine amulets which were used for their magico-medicinal properties and to ward off evil. The dung of the Seth/crocodile figure may have been a replacement for an amulet. Of course the presence of crocodile feces was likely to decrease male libido and it may be that this is how the dung achieved its desired effect. Vaginal administration of crocodile dung, or 'residue of noxious matter', is also mentioned as a contraceptive in the Ramesseum Papyrus IV, c. 1700 BC (Barnes, 1956 p. 29).

The application of sour milk or natron as contraceptives could have had a spermicidal effect by increasing the vaginal pH. Honey was likely to act either as a mechanical barrier or as a spermicide due to its hypertonicity. Analysis of the ingredients contained in the medical papyri shows that honey was used in over 30% of prescriptions. It was used as a vehicle for oral, anal and vaginal medication but was also applied directly to wounds, e.g. after circumcision. Honey has an antibacterial effect because it is hypertonic, and it also contains propolis, an antiseptic. Glucose oxidase, an enzyme secreted by bee salivary glands reacts with plant glucose to form gluconic acid and hydrogen peroxide, both of which are antibacterial (Estes, 1989 p. 69).

Fertility forecasting and pregnancy diagnosis

Five direct methods of examination were described for determining fertility. Fumigation and sitting the patient on medication were each advised once.

To determine whether a woman would become pregnant it was advised to place an onion bulb 'in her belly' (in the vagina). If she could scent the onion's odor in her nostril on the following morning it was likely that she would give birth (S.28). This test, to check the patency of the birth canal, was also mentioned in the Carlsberg Papyrus and many centuries later (c. 450 BC) was advocated by the Greek 'father of medicine', Hippocrates. To predict the number of children she would have, the woman was asked to sit on a floor strewn with lees of sweet ale and mash of dates. If this caused vomiting, she was likely to give birth and the number of times she was sick determined the number of her future offspring (S.27).

The woman with hale and hearty complexion (S.31), whose breast blood vessels were distended (S.26), whose belly and *mnï* part were touched – and presumably found enlarged (S.29, S.32), or who had issue of blood from her nostril (S.30), was likely to have conceived and to deliver.

Miscellanea

There are two further notations at the conclusion of the papyrus: one prescribed ground beans to prevent toothache in the pregnant woman (S.30); the other described a woman with vesico-vaginal fistula and advised in doom laden prophesy that 'she will be like this forever' (S.34).

The Ebers Papyrus

Dating from c. 1550 BC, the Ebers Papyrus was bought by the German Egyptologist, Georg Ebers, from an Arab in Luxor in 1873. Ebers published a German translation of the text at Leipzig in 1875. The Norwegian, Bendix Ebbell, published another translation in 1937. The papyrus appears to be a collation of texts of diverse origin and is a valuable source of information on Ancient Egyptian drug lore.

The Ebers Papyrus contains 876 prescriptions and mentions 500 substances used in treatment. Altogether, about 6% of the medications listed in the papyrus were for ailments of the female genitalia. The papyrus records a number of ointments, salts and aromatic resins which could be used to hasten birth if inserted into the vagina (Estes, 1989 p. 59). There is a prescription for a perineal binding impregnated with cedar shavings and crushed onions for correcting menstrual irregularity (Eb.832). Cedar shavings were also prescribed to help the womb 'return to its proper place' but in this instance the shavings were mixed with lees of ale and smeared on a cloth which the woman had to sit on.

Aromatic substances, including myrrh (currently being investigated for its antibiotic properties), were used as vaginal douches to stimulate menstruation. Another prescription containing myrrh, mixed with cumin, pine oil and stibium (another name for antimony, an extremely toxic metallic element used up to modern times as an emetic, an expectorant, and an antiparasitic agent), was recorded in the Edwin Smith Papyrus, c. 1600 BC, for the same purpose (Stevens, 1975 p. 950).

Another treatment mentioned in the Ebers Papyrus is 'milk of a woman who has given birth to a boy' (Eb.763) – this favorite recipe of the ancients was thought to be very powerful. Prescriptions to stimulate the flow of breast milk are detailed in Eb.836 and Eb.837.

The Ebers Papyrus also contains details of a medication for a crying infant (Eb.782): *Spn* seeds and fly dung were made into a paste, strained and fed to the baby on four successive days. The crying was meant to cease instantly. The *spn* seeds may have come from a species of poppy, possibly *Papaver rhoeas*. The active principle, opium, is present in much higher proportions in *Papaver somnifera* but this plant does not appear to have been used before the New Kingdom era.

A vaginal suppository of plant fiber dipped in a mixture of acacia, colocynth, dates and honey was prescribed as a contraceptive (Eb.783). It is now known that when this mixture ferments it produces lactic acid, a preparation currently used in vaginal contraception. Both acacia and colocynth have antifertility, and possibly abortifacient, effects.

The papyrus also contains instructions to 'loosen' a pregnancy, which Riddle (1992 p. 70) considers to be for abortion. The instructions are contained in Eb.797–799, Eb.801–807, and Eb.828–830, and were for topical or oral remedies. Among the agents mentioned are acacia, beans, beetle, date, and pine.

Riddle (p. 51) points out that estrogen-like substances are present in kidney beans. It is known that estrogens, progesterones and anti-fertility agents are also present in a large number of plants, e.g. acacia, apple seeds, castor oil plant, date palm seeds, pollen, pomegranate seeds, Scots pine, and willow flowers. The beetle may have contained cantharidin which causes intense urogenital irritation and which was later to become a well known aphrodisiac. It is possible, therefore, that some of the agents used to 'loosen' a pregnancy had a definite effect on the pregnant uterus and may indeed have caused abortion.

The Greater Berlin Papyrus

This papyrus was discovered by Heinrich Brugsch during excavations at Sakkara, and dates from c. 1300 BC. Walter Wreszinski translated the text which was published in 1909. Among the details relating to fertility is a prescription for human milk and watermelon. If the woman belched after drinking the mixture, she was thought infertile but vomiting was proof of fertility.

The papyrus contains an ancient pregnancy test (Bln.199) in which barley and emmer wheat were sprinkled with a woman's urine. If they germinated, the woman was deemed pregnant; if neither seed developed shoots, the woman was not pregnant. If only the barley germinated, a male child could be expected; growth of the emmer wheat predicted the birth of a female. It is quite remarkable how the Ancient Egyptians believed that pregnancy products were voided in the urine. Ascheim and Zondek did not describe their urinary pregnancy test until 1927 and prior to that the main 'pregnancy tests' available were visualization of the breasts and vulva or abdominal palpation and bimanual vaginal examination to detect increased uterine size (O'Dowd and Philipp, 1994 p. 21).

The authors of the Berlin Papyrus also advocated examination of the breasts, smeared with oil, to assess the blood vessels which would be affected by pregnancy. If dark green vessels were noted the woman was proclaimed pregnant and the prognosis was favorable. Sunken vessels indicated that a miscarriage was imminent. The woman with nice 'fresh' blood vessels was one who would give birth readily (page 1, lines 9 to 11). These ancient observations, which to a lesser

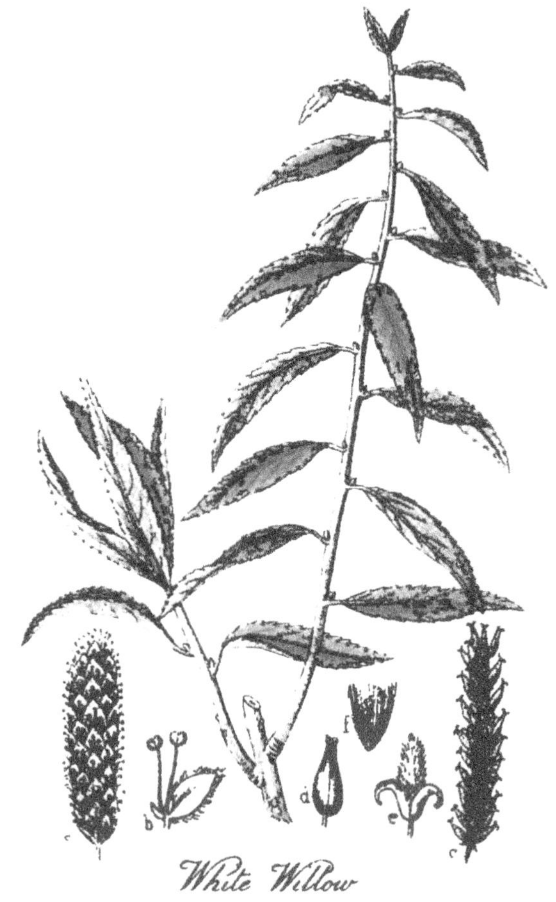

Figure 2 Willow (*Salix* sp.)

extent also appear in the Kahun Papyrus, could easily have formed part of the script for Montgomery in 1837, who wrote a definitive book describing breast changes in early pregnancy, illustrated with eight plates.

The Berlin Papyrus contains the first known reference to oral contraception. A mixture of beer, celery and oil was heated and prescribed as a potion to drink over four mornings; celery appears to have been the active principle. An alternative method of contraception was fumigation of the vagina with the smoke of burning emmer wheat seeds.

Other medical papyri

The Leiden Papyrus, which was written c. third century, AD, contains spells and recipes: powdered mouse was used as an aphrodisiac and plant products were prescribed which could be applied to the penis to arouse desire. The Hearst, Carlsberg and Brooklyn Museum papyri mention women's diseases and obstetric prognosis and prescriptions. Their contents are very similar and they may all be derived from the same source.

EXAMPLES OF WOMEN'S MATERIA MEDICA IN ANCIENT EGYPT

Uses

Abortifacients
Acacia, beans, beetle, bird dung, celery, date, juniper, pine, salt, turtle
Analgesics
Lettuce, linseed, mandrake
Antiseptics
Honey, malachite, mud
Aphrodisiacs
Banana, basil, bean (broad), garlic, lettuce, mandrake, milk, poppy, stallion's saliva and testicles
Birth prognosis
Barley, emmer wheat, watermelon
Breast conditions
Lotion for: vine;
For inflammation: willow
Childbirth
To induce: birthwort, bryony, castoreum, emmer wheat, fenugreek, juniper
To help: basil, beer, fir, honey, incense, madder, oil
Conception
Ale, dates, canal water, frankincense, *hprwr* plant, *hywy* liquid, mash (fermented), *mst*, oil
Contraception
Vaginal: acacia, celery, colocynth, crocodile dung, date, emmer wheat, honey, milk, natron
Oral: beer, celery, oil
Fertility
Ale (lees), carob, dates, juniper, lettuce, milk, oil, onion, pine, placenta, pomegranate, salt, testicles, watermelon
Galactagogues
Chickpeas, cucumber, fenugreek, garlic, sesame.
Libido
To reduce: lotus
To increase in women: milk, stallion's saliva
Menstruation
For excess: ale (lees), date juice
To induce: caper, cumin, dates, juniper, myrrh, oil, pine oil, rue, sesame, stibium (antimony)
To regulate: cedar, onion, parsley
To stop: flax tampon, onion, pea, tamarisk
Disorders of: cornflower
Miscarriage
Swallow's liver
Penile disorders
To soothe: cinnamon, honey, vine, spleen
Puerperium
Cumin, ergot (disputed), mother's milk
Pregnancy tests
Barley, emmer wheat, woman's urine, oil smeared on breasts
Prolapse
Ale, birthwort, cedar
Testicles
Sick: clover, willow
Uterus
For spasms: ass urine, frankincense, *h'wy* food, oil
To 'cool' contractions: celery, cumin, dill, hemp (marijuana)
Treatment for: acacia, liver
To contract: ergot (disputed)
Abnormal discharge: ale, almonds, ass liver, beans, frankincense, grass seeds, milk, mud, oil
Diseased (cancer): fumigation of roast meat.
Venereal disease
Apple
Vehicles
Drug vehicles were also diluents and solvents. Some had pharmacological effects: Ale, fat, honey, milk, oil, water, wax, wine
Vulva
Swollen after birth: malachite, milk, oil,
Warts (on private parts): leek

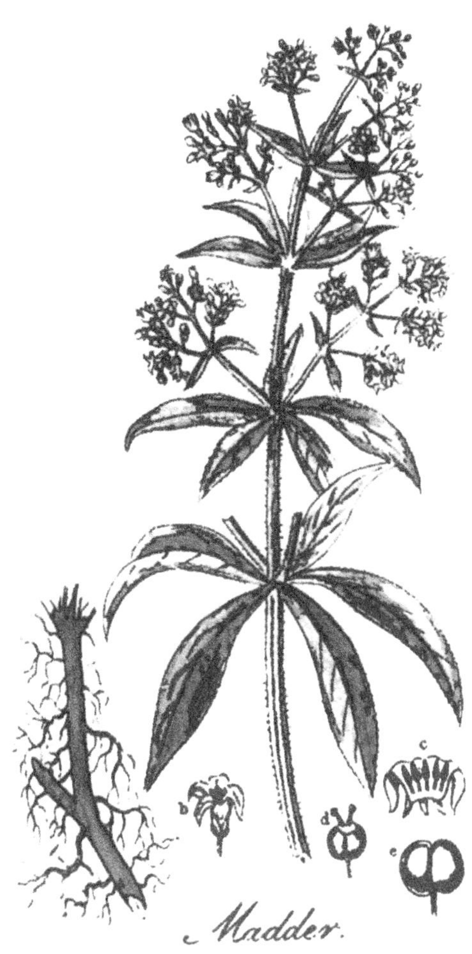

Figure 3 Madder

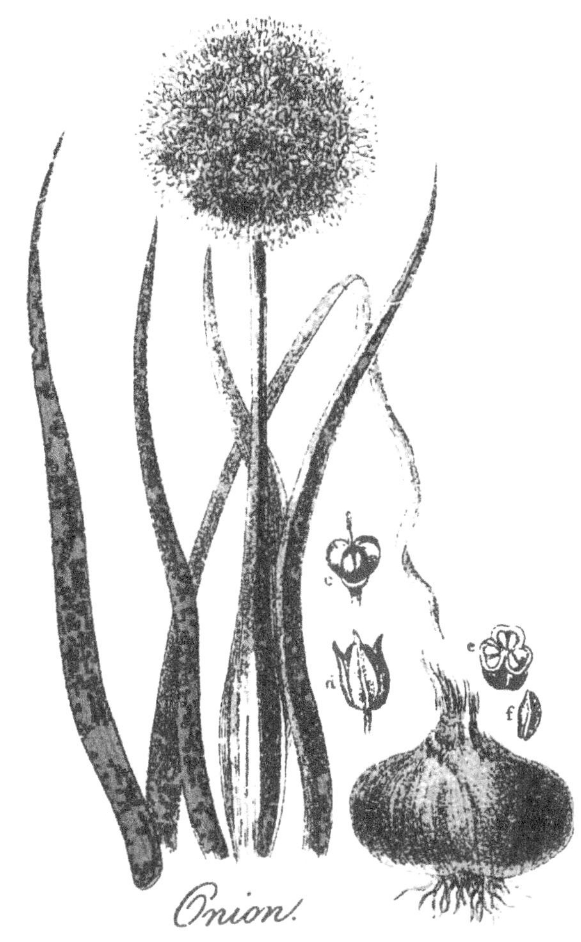

Figure 4 Onion (*Allium* sp.)

Birth injury: fresh meat applied daily
Hemorrhoids: fig
Herpes: coriander

Womens' disorders

The following were used for non-specified womens' ailments: castoreum, catfish, copper, lily, malabathron, malachite, oakum tar, paste-water, pine, pondweed, reed panicles, spelt wheat

Selected remedies

Absinthe, acacia, ale, almonds, apple, ass liver, ass urine

Banana, barley, basil, beans, beetle, ben, bird dung, birthwort, bryony

Caper, carob, castoreum, cedar, chickpea, cinnamon, colocynth, coriander, crocodile dung, cumin

Dates, dill, dough

Emmer, ergot (disputed)

Fat, fenugreek, fig, fir, flag (sweet), flax, fly dung, frankincense

Garlic, grain, grapes, grass seed

Hemp, honey, *hprwr* plant, *h'wy* fluid

Juniper

Leek, lees (of ale), lettuce, lily, linseed, liver, lotus

Madder, malachite, malabathron, mandrake, mash, meat, milk, mst, mud, myrrh

Natron (salt)

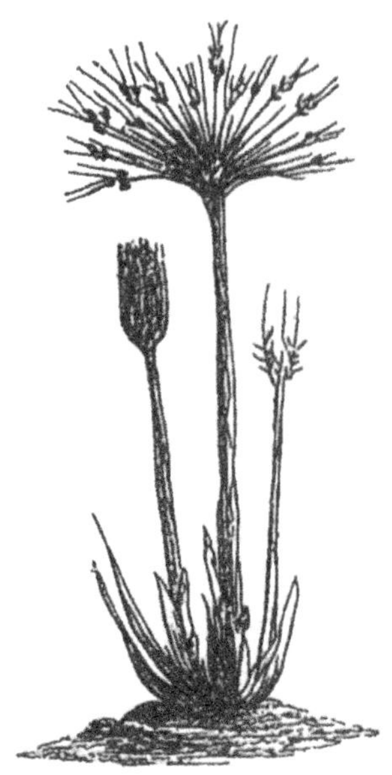

Figure 5 Papyrus reeds

Oakum tar, oil, onion

Papyrus, parsley, paste-water, pea, pine, placenta, pomegranate, pondweed, poppy, potsherd

Reed panicles, rue

Sesame, spelt wheat, spleen, stallion's saliva, stibium (antimony), sycamore fruit, swallow's liver

Tamarisk, terebinth, testicles (animal), *thwh* grain, turtle

Vine

Water, watermelon, wax, willow, wine

Acknowledgment

The lists of 'Uses and Remedies' are based on commentaries in English on the Ancient Egyptian Medical Papyri and in part on the texts of Estes, Leake, Manniche, Pinch, Reeves, Robins, Stetter and Tyldesley (see references).

GLOSSARY OF ANCIENT EGYPTIAN FERTILITY DEITIES

Amun A fertility god

Bes A god of luck, love and marriage, guardian of women in labor

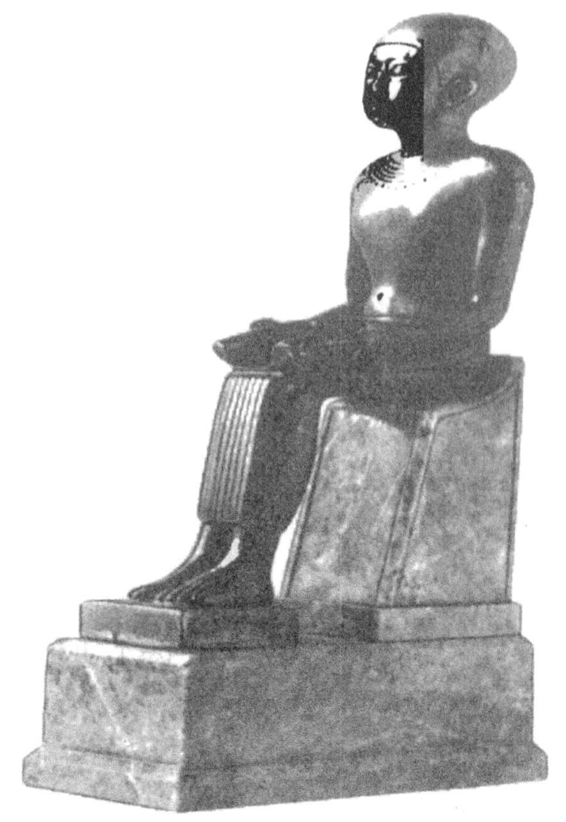

Figure 6 The Egyptian diety Imhotep (c. 2650 BC)

Hapy A god with sagging breasts and abdominal fat pad. He was the personification of the river Nile and was shown with a crown of water plants, papyrus or lotus

Hathor A goddess of love, identified with Horus

Horus Son of Isis and Osiris, born after his father's death

Imhotep The Egyptian god of healing. A deified human, he was the adviser and architect to the Pharaoh Djoser and was the builder responsible for the Step Pyramid at Sakkara

Isis Wife of Osiris and mother of Horus, the ideal mother figure

Khnum Granted health to the newborn

Meskhenet A birth goddess, later replaced by the god Shai.

Min The god of fertility, depicted with erect phallus, identified with Isia and Amun

Nephthys A midwife-goddess, sister of Isis
Osiris The husband of Isis and god of vegetation and corn
Renenutet Goddess of fertility and of children
Sakhmet A war goddess but also a guardian goddess against disease, and identified with Hathor
Serapis A god of land fertility and of healing
Shai A god of destiny and present at birth
Tauret The goddess of childbirth, depicted as a hippopotamus
Thoth The god of science, writing and wisdom.

References

Barnes, J. W. (1956). *Five Ramesseum Papyri*, pp. 28, 29. (Oxford: University Press)

Breasted, J. (1930). *The Edwin Smith Surgical Papyrus*, (Chicago: University of Chicago Press)

Ebell, B. (1937). *The Papyrus Ebers: The Greatest Egyptian medical document*. (Copenhagen: Levin and Munksgaard)

Estes, J. Worth (1989). *The Medical Skills of Ancient Egypt*, pp. 20, 59, 65, 69, 103, 114. (Canton, USA: Science History Publications)

Griffith, F. L. (1898). *Hieratic Papyri from Kahun, Gurob and Illahun*. (London)

Leake, C. L. (1975). *An Historical Account of Pharmacology to the 20th Century*, pp. 46, 75. (Springfield, IL: Charles C. Thomas)

Mahfouz Bey, N. (1957). Urinary Fistulae in Women. *J. Obstet. Gynaecol. Br. Emp.* 64(1), 23–33

Manniche, L. (1989). *An Ancient Egyptian Herbal*, pp. 61, 58. (London: British Museum Press)

Manniche, L. (1993). *An Ancient Egyptian Herbal* (Second Impression), p. 112. (London: British Museum Press)

Montgomery, W. F. (1837). *An Exposition of the Signs and Symptoms of Pregnancy*. (London: Sherwood, Gilbert and Piper)

O'Dowd, M. J. and Philipp, E. E. (1994). *The History of Obstetrics and Gynaecology*, p. 21. (London and New York: Parthenon Publishing)

Pinch, G. (1994). *Magic in Ancient Egypt*, p. 120. (London: British Museum Press)

Reeves, C. (1992). *Egyptian Medicine*, p. 19. (Buckingham, UK: Shire Publications Ltd.)

Riddle, J. M. (1992). *Contraception and Abortion from the Ancient World to the Renaissance*, pp. 51, 70. (Cambridge, MA: Harvard University Press)

Robins, G. (1993). *Women In Ancient Egypt*, pp. 77, 90. (London: British Museum Press)

Shaw, I. and Nicholson, P. (1995). *British Museum Dictionary of Ancient Egypt*, p. 91. (London: British Museum Press)

Stetter, C. (1993). *The Secret Medicine of the Pharaohs: Ancient Egyptian Healing*, pp. 89, 105. (Chicago, Berlin: Quintessence Publishing Co.)

Stevens, J. M. (1975). Gynaecology From Ancient Egypt: The Papyrus Kahun. A translation of the oldest treatise on gynaecology that has survived from the ancient world. *Med. J. Austr.*, 2, 949–52

Tyldesley, J. (1994). *Daughters of Isis, Women of Ancient Egypt*, p. 70. (London: Viking Press)

Biblical times 8

HISTORY OF THE BIBLE

The term 'Bible' comes from the Greek, *biblia* (books) meaning especially those of canonical nature which express ecclesiastical law. The Bible contains the sacred writings of the Jewish and Christian religions, and consists of the Old and New Testaments. Members of the Jewish religion accept the authority of the Old Testament which is sometimes referred to as the 'Hebrew Bible'. Christians accept both Old and New Testaments, and some of them also acknowledge a collection of writings called the Apocrypha (Greek, *apokryphos*, hidden) as part of the Bible. The 'secret' writings that constitute the Apocrypha consist of 15 books, or parts thereof. They date from 200 BC to AD 100, and are included in the Septuagint and Vulgate translations of the Old Testament. The Old Testament begins with an account of God's creation of the heavens and the earth, followed by the history and religious life of ancient Israel from about 1900 BC to the c. 330 BC. The New Testament deals with the time-span from the birth of Jesus Christ to the second half of the first century AD.

The 'holy books' officially accepted by a group of Jews or Christians as part of their respective bibles are called the 'canons'. The Old Testament Canon accepted by the Jewish faith comprises 24 books, the Protestant Canon consists of 39 books. The Roman Catholic Canon includes books of the Apocrypha in addition. The New Testament consists of 27 books which include the four gospel-writings ('gospel' derives from the Old English *godspell*, meaning good news).

With the dispersal of the Jews and the Persian domination of the Near East from the sixth century BC, the first translations of the scriptures from the original Hebrew were into Aramaic; these texts were known as the 'Targums'. During the third century BC, the Old Testament was translated into Greek and became known as the 'Septuagint'. The first Latin translations appeared in the second century AD. About AD 382 Saint Jerome revised the Latin Bible at the request of Pope St. Damascus I. Jerome used Hebrew, Greek and Latin translations to arrive at a new format. His version of the Bible was completed in AD 405 and became known as the 'Vulgate' (from the Latin word meaning 'popular'). For many centuries, the Vulgate was the only rendition of the Bible authorized by the Roman Catholic Church. In the mid-fifteenth century the Vulgate became the first version of the Bible to be printed using cold letter type. That text was produced by Johannes Gutenberg of Mainz, Germany, and was known as the 'Gutenberg Bible'.

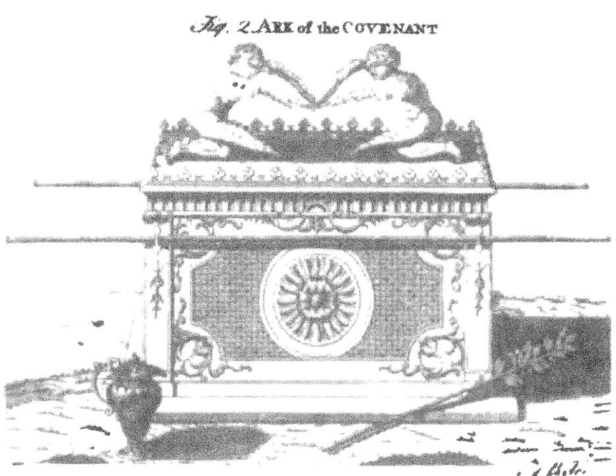

Figure 1 Depiction of the Ark of Covenant from the first edition of the *Encyclopedia Britannica* (1772)

The first complete English translation of the Bible was made by the English religious reformer, John Wycliffe, c. 1380. Almost two centuries later another Englishman William Tyndale rendered his translation of the Bible between 1525 and 1531, while living in Germany. Part of his text was based on a translation of the New Testament by Germany's Martin Luther (begun in 1521). Disagreement ensued as Luther was viewed as a controversial radical and Tyndale was accused of making 'untrue translations'. As a result of public hostility he was tried, sentenced to death, and executed in October 1536. Despite this dreadful outcome, other English translations of the Bible soon followed. The so-called Authorized Version of the

King James Bible was published in 1611, but no further translations of note appeared in English until the late nineteenth century. In 1973 an edition of the Revised Standard Version appeared as 'The Common Bible' and was approved by Greek Orthodox, Protestant and Roman Catholic religious leaders. The Biblical quotations in this Chapter that follows are taken from *The Revised Standard Edition of The Holy Bible* (1952), from *The New American Bible* (1970) and from the Revised Edition of *The Gideons International Holy Bible* (1982).

BIBLICAL MEDICINE

Douglas Miller of Glasgow wrote: 'In any approach to a study of medicine in the Bible three facts of fundamental importance should be borne in mind'. Miller's first point was that from the ancient days of Abraham, until the advent of Jesus of Nazareth, adversity and sickness were accepted as Divine visitations and the direct consequences of transgression. God was the one source of life and health and He was the only healer: 'At least until the end of Solomon's reign there were no physicians among the Hebrews. The priest was a divine agent and the health of the community was his exclusive province and responsibility'. The second fact was that the Mosaic laws were 'designed with the primary object of increasing the manpower and developing the health of the people'. The third point was that regulations were laid down in the form of divine edicts to ensure the health of the general population (Miller, 1953).

In the nineteenth century, Marinus de Waal, Dutch scholar and professor of comparative religion, wrote that due to the religious nature of the laws of Moses, the priests (Levites), in effect became health officials (de Waal, 1994). However, de Waal stated that physicians were also known at the time and in his book *Medicines from the Bible* he explored the role of the physician, the apothecary and the ancient methods of healing in Biblical Hebrew society. During New Testament times the physician was an integral part of society and we know that Luke, the gospel writer, practiced medicine.

Quotations from Ecclesiasticus support God's role as a healer but also acknowledge the presence of Biblical physicians, at least in the early third century BC. Ecclesiasticus is one of the books of the Apocrypha and is otherwise known as 'The Wisdom of Jesus ben-Sira', taking its name from its author. Written in Hebrew c. 180 BC, the text was translated into Greek c. 132 BC by the author's grandson. Chapter 38 deals with sickness and death:

Verse 1 Hold the physician in honor, for he is essential to you, and God it was who established his profession.
Verse 4 God makes the earth yield healing herbs which the prudent man should not neglect.
Verse 7 The doctor eases pain and the druggist prepares his medicines.
Verse 9 My son, when you are ill, delay not but pray to God, who will heal you.
Verse 12 Then give the doctor his place lest he leave; for you need him too.

In recent times, Margaret Lloyd Davies, BD, and Trevor Lloyd Davies, formerly professor of social medicine in the University of Malaya, have applied modern medical knowledge to study of the Bible in their book *The Bible. Medicine and Myth* (1991).

BOTANY OF THE BIBLE

The Bible opens with the book of Genesis:

> In the beginning God created the heavens and the earth. God said, 'Let there be light', and there was light … God said, 'Let there be a firmament between the waters to divide waters from waters … Let the waters under heaven be gathered into one place and let the dry land appear … Let the earth produce vegetation, various kinds of seed-bearing herbs and fruit-bearing trees with their respective seeds in the fruit upon the earth;' and so it was … And God saw that it was good … 'Let the waters teem with shoals of living creatures and let birds fly above the earth along heaven's firmament … Let the earth bring forth living creatures after their kind, livestock, reptiles and wild beasts after their kind' … Then God said 'Let Us make man in Our Image, after Our likeness, and let them bear rule over the fish of the sea, over the birds of the air, over the animals; over the whole earth' … God further said

'Behold, I have given you every seed-bearing plant over all the earth and every fruit tree, the fruit of which grows seeds; it will be your food'.

(Genesis 1: 1, 3, 6, 9, 11, 12, 20, 24, 26, 29)

Hippocrates of Kos, the renowned Greek physician of the fifth century BC, investigated food as medicine: to him is attributed the saying 'Let your food be your medicine'.

The Song of Solomon (Chapters 1–8) gives us valuable insight into the plant life and produce of King Solomon's gardens: apple trees, cedars, cypresses, fig trees, frankincense, henna, honey, lily-of-the-valley, milk, myrrh, ointment, pomegranates, rose of Sharon, spikenard, thistle, vine plants and wine. Solomon kept a special 'spice garden' where all the chief spices could be found: aloes, calamus, cinnamon, frankincense, henna, grapes, mandrake, myrrh, nuts, pomegranate, saffron, spikenard, and spiced wine.

Levinus Lemmens was the first author to attempt an analysis of the plants of the Bible in his book of 1566, which was translated from Latin into English by Thomas Newton in 1587. Over the following two centuries many other important works on the botany of the Bible were to appear. They all suffered from a scientific point of view, however, because their authors had never visited the Holy Land, basing their knowledge of Biblical botany on many differing (and often erroneous) translations of the Old and New Testaments, and on their belief that European plants were to be found in the Holy Land. In reality, Biblical plants differed from their European counterparts and many of them were quite unknown to these Biblical scholars.

The first scientific evaluation of Biblical plants was undertaken by Hasselquist who was a pupil of Carolus Linnaeus (1707–1778) the world-famous Swedish botanist. Hasselquist undertook a two-year exploration of the Holy Land and evaluated its plant life in relation to the Bible. His notes are contained in his *Iter Palaestinum* (1757) which was edited by Linnaeus and published after Hasselquist's untimely death. Soon afterwards, other naturalists visited the Holy Land and were to discover that many plants in the Bible were quite different from the indigenous plants of Europe.

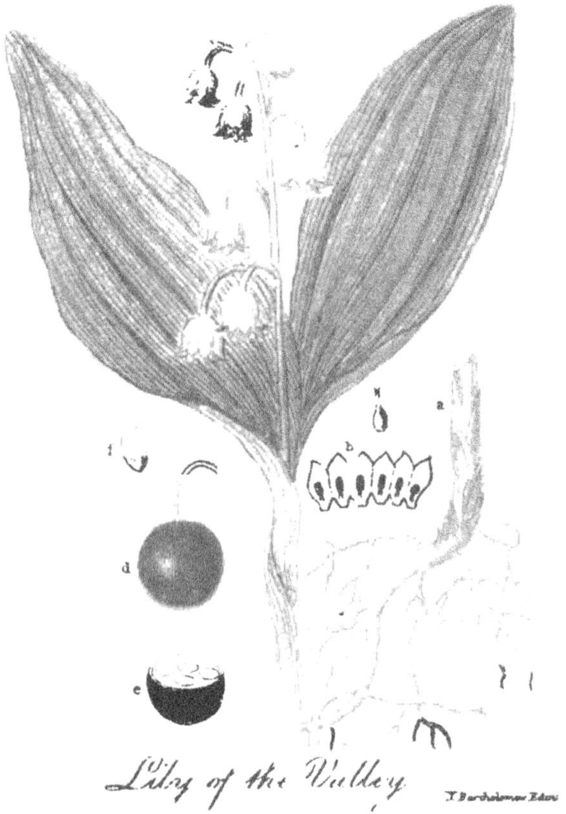

Figure 2 Lily-of-the-valley (*Convallaria majus*)

Harold Moldenke, curator and administrator of the Herbarium of New York's Botanical Gardens, and his wife, Alma Lance Moldenke (nee Ericsson), of the Biology Department, Evander Childs High School, New York City, wrote an authoritative history of the evolution of the many versions of the Bible and of accurate botany of the Holy Land in their *Plants of the Bible* (1952). More recently, Harrison has written an interesting book on *Healing Herbs of the Bible* (1966), and Duke followed with *Medicinal Plants of the Bible* (1983).

OBSTETRICS AND GYNECOLOGY IN THE BIBLE

The obstetrics and gynecology of the Bible begins with the story of Adam and Eve as related in Genesis: 'Then God said, "Let us make man in our image, after our likeness" ... so God created man in his image; in the image of God he created him; male and female he created them. God blessed them; God said to them, "Be fruitful; multiply; fill the earth and subdue it" (Chapter 1: 26–28). Levin, in his treatise on obstetrics in the bible (1960), wrote: 'This was the first commandment given by God to man. As a result thereof a goodly portion of the Bible concerns itself with reproduction, and by collecting and correlating these allusions to pregnancy and parturition, we can gain a fairly coherent view of the theory and practice of obstetrics in the Biblical area during the Biblical era'. Some tracts of that 'goodly portion' are quoted below and fall under recognizable (if somewhat contrived) headings.

Menstruation and sexual hygiene

The Biblical laws that dealt with menstruation and sexual hygiene are to be found in Leviticus 15: 1–33.

Verse 19 When a woman has a discharge, a flowing of blood of the body, then she shall be in separation for seven days. Whoever touches her shall be unclean till evening.
Verse 24 If a man lies beside her so that her menstruation comes on him, then for seven days he shall be unclean and so shall every couch on which he lies be unclean.
Verse 28 When she is cleansed of her issue then she shall count seven more days and after that she is clean.
Verse 16–18 When a man has an emission of sperm, he shall take a complete bodily water bath and be unclean until evening. Every garment and all leather on which sperm settle shall be washed in water and be unclean until evening. The woman and the man who has lain with her, if sperm is spilt, shall both take a water bath and be unclean until evening.

Fertility

When the waters subsided after the Great Flood, God's instruction to Noah was to 'be fruitful and multiply and replenish the earth' (Genesis 9: 1). Fertility was one of the many blessings promised by God to the ancient Hebrews (Deuteronomy 28: 2–4): 'All these blessings will overtake you and rest upon you if you obey the voice of the Lord your God.... Blessed shall be the fruit of your body'. Fertility was also promised in Exodus 23: 25–26: 'Serve the Lord your God and he will bless your food and your drink and I will remove sickness from among you. There will none be miscarrying or barren in your land...'.

When Rebekah left home to marry Isaac, a blessing was pronounced on her: 'you, our sister, may you become the mother of millions' (Genesis 24: 60). The good wishes were not fulfilled as Rebekah was relatively infertile and her only pregnancy resulted in the birth of the twins Esau and Jacob. Rebekah's husband, Isaac, blessed his son Jacob with the words: 'God Almighty bless you, make you prolific and multiply you so that you may become an association of peoples' (Genesis 28: 3). Psalm 113: 9 also contains blessings for fertility: 'He gives the barren wife a home to live in, now the joyous mother of children'. Psalm 127: 3, extols the virtues of fertility: 'Behold, children are a legacy from the Lord; the fruit of the womb is his reward'. So important was it to achieve pregnancy that Tamar, a widow and the daughter-in-law of Judah, disguised herself as a harlot so that she could conceive by him. She later gave birth to twins (Genesis 38: 14–19, 27).

Fertility aids in the form of aphrodisiacs and love potions were in use during Biblical times. The only occasion on which 'treatment' could be inferred was when Leah and Rachel sought the help of mandrake (*Mandragora officinalis*) to promote fertility, both sisters becoming pregnant (Genesis 30: 14–24). The mandrake plant was much sought after as an aphrodisiac in Biblical times and was mentioned in The Song of Solomon 7: 13, as the suitor offers his love to his bride, the Maid of Shulam: 'The mandrakes give forth their fragrance'. In a move mimicked by present-day *in vitro* fertilization experts, but then enacted by Divine intervention alone, God granted post-menopausal conception to Sarah (Genesis 18: 10–14) and Elizabeth (Luke 1: 36).

Infertility

Fertility was a primary aim of life during Biblical times and so sterility led to sorrow: 'There are three things that are never satisfied, four never say, "Enough". The nether world, and the barren womb; the earth that is never saturated with water, and fire' (Proverbs 30: 15–16). The greatest curse of the Old Testament was uttered by Jeremiah (22: 30): 'Write this man childless'. As childbearing was of paramount importance the fertile woman was honored while the barren woman was pitied. Rachel cried to her husband Jacob: 'give me children or else I die!' (Genesis 30: 1). God was judged responsible for 'closing the wombs' of Sarah (Genesis 16: 2) and Hannah (1 Samuel 1: 5) and 'Michal the daughter of Saul had no child to the day of her death' (2 Samuel 6: 23). Nevertheless, there are many instances in scripture of infertility followed by pregnancy in elderly primigravidae.

Conception

'The conception of Jesus Christ came about this way: When His mother Mary was engaged to Joseph, before they came together she was found to be with child from the Holy Spirit'. (Matthew 1: 18). Conception by divine intervention was not unusual in antiquity and Jesus, Buddha, and other important gods, Pharaohs and prophets of the era, were believed to have resulted from interaction of a mortal with the Almighty; in the more usual situation, human semen and egg were required. According to Levin (1960) the Biblical Hebrews probably concurred with the belief contained in the Talmud and the Koran that semen originated in the head and reached the genitals via the spinal column. Intercourse was not thought to be a prerequisite to achieve pregnancy as it was believed that the daughter of the prophet Jeremiah became pregnant having bathed in water containing seminal ejaculate. Once impregnated, by whatever means, the womb was viewed as a form of incubator for housing and nurturing the semen from which a child would develop.

Embryology

There are references to 'embryology' in Job 10: 8–9: 'Thy hands completely formed me and fashioned me ... remember that thou made'st me of clay'. Psalm 139: 13–16, exults:

> 'I praise thee because I am fearfully and wonderfully made; marvelous is thy workmanship, as my soul is well aware ... Thou did'st possess my inward parts and did'st weave me in my mother's womb ... My bones were not hidden from thee when I was made in secrecy and intricately fashioned in utter seclusion ... Thine eyes beheld my unformed substance, and in thy book always recorded and prepared day by day, when as yet none of them had being.'

In the Apocryphal work 'The Wisdom of Solomon' (7: 1–6) Solomon described his intrauterine existence and birth:

> 'in my mother's womb I was molded into flesh in a ten months period – body and blood, from the seed of man, and the pleasure that accompanies marriage. And I too, when born, inhaled the common air, and fell upon the kindred earth; wailing, I uttered that first sound common to all. In swaddling clothes and with constant care I was nurtured. For no King has any different origin of birth, but one is the entry into life; and in one same way they leave it'.

Pregnancy

The Bible considered that pregnancy was a precious gift bestowed by God (Ruth 4: 13–14) and Eve, when she gave birth to Cain, exclaimed: 'I have gotten the man with the Lord's help' (Genesis 4: 1). Fetal movements *in utero* were recorded by Rebekah: 'Then within her body the children jostled each other' (Genesis 25: 22). The encounter between Mary, the mother of Jesus Christ, and her cousin Elizabeth is related in Luke 1: 41–42: 'And as Elizabeth listened to Mary's greetings, the babe leaped within her. Then, filled with the Holy Spirit, Elizabeth spoke with a loud voice, "Blessed are you among women and blessed is the fruit of thy womb"'.

Antenatal care

Before the birth of Samson, his mother was given dietary advice by an angel: 'see that you do not partake of wine or strong drink or any unclean food for you shall conceive and bear a son ... [The woman] must carry out my instructions. She must not eat anything made from grapes, ... nor any unclean thing' (Judges 13: 4–5, 13–14).

Isaac prayed to the Lord that his wife would conceive and in due course Rebekah became pregnant. She experienced very strong fetal movements, 'so she went to the Lord' for advice and learned that she was carrying twins (Genesis 25: 21–23). The diagnosis was corroborated: 'when her days for delivery were completed there were indeed twins in her womb' (Genesis 25: 24).

Miscarriage and premature labor

Both of these complications of pregnancy are alluded to in a number of Bible passages. In Psalm 58: 8, we read of 'an untimely birth that never sees the sun'. Ecclesiastes 6: 3 tells the tale of the man who was given riches, wealth and honor, and he lacked nothing, 'yet God does not give him ability to enjoy it ... I say that an untimely birth is better than he'. Jeremiah cursed the day he was born 'because He did not kill me in the womb so that my mother should have been my grave and her womb for ever great' (Jeremiah 20: 17).

Injury to a pregnant woman could cause miscarriage: 'If in a quarrel between men a pregnant woman is hit, so that she miscarries ... the offender shall be fined' (Exodus 21: 22). Deliberate assault on pregnant women was mentioned when Elisha prophesied the downfall of Israel, and said to Hazael (who later became King of Syria): 'I know the calamity you will bring upon Israel ... their little children you will dash in pieces, and their pregnant women you will rip open' (2 Kings 8: 12).

Among the curses for disobedience was that of the prophet Hosea, 'Give them, Oh Lord: what wilt thou give? Give them wombs that miscarry, withered breasts' (Hosea 9: 14). Reference to pregnancy loss was made by the unfortunate Job when he cursed the day of his birth and called out, 'why was I not a miscarriage that is put away, as infants that never saw the light?' (Job 3: 16).

Normal labor

Labor usually had its onset after a full-term pregnancy: 'when her days to be delivered were completed' (Genesis 25: 24); 'Now Elizabeth's time to give birth had come and she bore a son' (Luke 1: 57); 'While they were there, her days were completed to give birth and she bore her first born son' (Luke 2: 6–7).

Childbirth was exclusively the prerogative of midwives who were available to help the laboring woman (Genesis 35: 17; 38: 28). Two midwives were named in Exodus 1: 15–16: 'The King of Egypt also gave his order to Shiphrah and Puah, the Hebrew midwives, "As you aid the Hebrew women in childbirth, watch them closely on the birthstool ..."' In the same chapter we read that Hebrew women 'are of quick delivery, they give birth before the midwife gets to them' (Exodus 1: 19) and that 'God treated the midwives well' (Exodus 1: 20). Not all women had fast labors. Maternal exhaustion or uterine inertia are referred to in 2 Kings 19: 3: 'for children who have come to birth but there is not strength to give birth' and also in Isaiah 37: 3: 'this day is a day of anguish, of rebuke and of disgrace; children have come to the birth, and there is no strength to bring forth'.

The placenta is referred to in Deuteronomy 28: 57 as 'the afterbirth from her womb', and also as the 'bundle of life' in 1 Samuel 25: 29. The care of the infant directly after birth with regard to cutting the cord, washing with water, rubbing the infant's skin with salt and swaddling with bands is mentioned in Ezekiel 16: 4. An angel announced the birth of Jesus: 'Today there was born for you in the city of David, a Savior, who is Christ the Lord' (Luke 2: 11).

The curse of Eve

The story of the fall from grace of Adam and Eve is related in Genesis, and from it we learn that because of their disobedience the Lord cursed them both: 'and to the woman he said "I will greatly increase your pregnancy troubles; in sorrow shall you bring forth children, you will suffer birth pangs, in pain shall you bring forth children" (Genesis 3: 16). For many centuries this Biblical passage was thought to indicate that pain in childbirth was fore-ordained.

The pain of labor implicit in the so-called 'Curse of Eve' is referred to on a number of occasions as a symbol of the extreme emotional and physical suffering women could experience in childbirth: 'panic seized them there, throes like those of childbirth' (Psalms 48: 6); 'As a woman with child writhes when the hour draws near for her delivery and cries out in her pangs' (Isaiah 26: 17); 'For I have heard the voice of a woman in labor, a cry as of one giving birth to her first child, the voice of the daughter of Zion, panting, begging for help' (Jeremiah 4: 31); 'then sudden destruction will come upon them like the birth-pangs of a pregnant woman, and there will be no escape' (1 Thessalonians 5: 3). Despite the forecast of doom, gloom and disaster, there was hope for the woman in childbirth: 'The mother in childbirth has anguish because her time has come, but when she has borne the child she no longer remembers her affliction, because a human being has been born into the world' (John 16: 21).

For many centuries the Curse of Eve was rigidly interpreted by clerics and medical-men alike, and women were denied access to analgesia in labor. Unnecessary pain and untold miseries were experienced by countless women in the name of religion. The exact wording of Genesis 3: 16, and its translation and interpretation gave rise to heated debate in the nineteenth century which was only concluded in the mid-twentieth century (Boss, 1962). (See Chapter 18).

The puerperium

Leviticus 12: 2–8 is devoted to the ritual purification of a woman following childbirth, related by God to Moses:

> 'Tell the Israelites when a woman has conceived and has given birth to a boy, she shall be unclean seven days, unclean as at the time of her menstruation. On the eighth day the flesh of his foreskin shall be circumcised. She shall then continue for thirty three days in the blood of purification. She shall contact nothing Holy and shall not attend the sanctuary till the days of her purification are completed. If she gives birth to a girl, then she shall be unclean [sexual relations were prohibited] for two weeks as in her monthly separation and for yet sixty six days, while bleeding, she shall stay at home, the purification period'.
>
> (verses 2–5).

After those days of purification the mother was to bring appropriate offerings to the sanctuary and thereby become ritualy clean.

Maternal mortality

Death of the mother in childbirth is recounted on two occasions. In Genesis 35: 16–20, the story of Rachel's giving birth to Benjamin tells us that she died after the delivery. In 1 Samuel 4: 19–21 it is written that the wife of Phinehas went into labor when she heard that her husband had died. She collapsed and gave birth to a son, but died soon afterwards.

Multiple pregnancy

The twin pregnancy and delivery of Tamar is described in Genesis 38: 27–30. During labor one baby presented by a hand. The midwife tied a crimson string around it but the child withdrew its hand into the womb. Soon afterwards, a boy named Perez was born, followed by his brother Zerah on whose hand was the crimson string.

Rebekah, wife of Isaac, gave birth to twin boys. At the time of delivery the second twin Jacob was seen to be holding his brother Esau's heel (Genesis 25: 24–26). This Biblical description of one twin holding the other's heel appears to have influenced artists in later generations: illustrations of twin pregnancy commonly depicted brothers *in utero*, one cephalic and one breech, the breech infant clasping the heel of his brother.

Perinatal mortality

Numbers 12: 12, refers to a macerated stillborn fetus as: 'one who is stillborn with half his flesh decomposed'. A case of early neonatal death, on day three, is described in 1 Kings 3: 18–21: 'The son of this woman died at night because she lay on it'. That was the beginning of the tragic story in which the wisdom of Solomon was required to decide which of two postnatal mothers should keep the surviving infant. Neonatal death was also recounted when the child born to David and Bathsheba, the wife of Uriah the Hittite, became ill: 'the Lord struck with sickness the boy whom Uriah's wife had borne to David … finally on the seventh day the boy died' (2 Samuel 12: 15–18).

Crimes against women

The relevance of 'spoiled' virginity, adulterous relationships, and the severe penalties involved are outlined in Deuteronomy 22: 13–30. The punishment for 'carnal union' with a married woman or with an engaged, but unmarried, woman (if the woman consented) was that both parties should be stoned to death. Criminal violation of a woman also carried the death penalty unless the assaulted woman was a virgin: in that instance the man who perpetrated the crime was compelled to pay her father fifty shekels of silver, after which he had to marry the woman. Incest was a major offense: 'And no child of an incestuous union could be admitted into the community of the Lord nor any descendent of his even to the tenth generation' (Deuteronomy 23: 2).

Rape

Several cases of rape are recorded in detail. The first one concerned Dinah the daughter of Jacob who was ravaged by Shechem, son of Hamor the Hivite, a local ruler. Both father and son paid for that deed with their lives (Genesis 34: 1–29). Another rape of a particularly brutal nature was described in detail in Judges 19: 22–30. The tragedy led to a civil war in which many thousands were slain. Another case of rape was the story of Tamar, the daughter of King David, who was ravaged by her half brother Amnon (2 Samuel 13: 1–4).

The 'fallen woman'

Proverbs 7: 10–27, deals with prostitution: 'And look, a woman comes to meet him, with the attire of a harlot, and a crafty mind … She has perfumed her bed with myrrh, aloes and cinnamon'. Another passage was meant to act as a deterrent to those who would seek the charms of the fallen woman: 'From the lips of a loose woman drop honeyed words and her palate is smoother that oil; but in the end she is bitter as wormwood, sharp as a devouring sword' (Proverbs 5: 3–4). Hosea attempted to persuade his unfaithful wife to 'clear her face of her marks of harlotry and remove her adulterous charms from her breasts' (Hosea 2: 2).

Venereal disease

The pleasures of indiscriminate couplings led to venereal disease, as recorded in Leviticus 15: 2: 'when a man has a burning issue out of his flesh, because of his issue his is unclean', possibly a reference to gonorrhea. Venereal disease is again mentioned in Deuteronomy 24: 1 when 'a man hath taken a wife and married her … when it come to pass that she finds no favor in his eyes, because he hath found some uncleanness in her; let him write her a bill of divorcement'.

A SELECTION OF BIBLICAL MATERIA MEDICA FOR WOMEN

Apothecaries in Biblical times were occupied with preparation of balms, fragrant oils, herbal mixtures, perfumes and spices as 'prepared as by a druggist' (Exodus 30: 25). In some translations the apothecary was known as *roqeah* now deciphered as 'perfumer'. Drugs were administered as decoctions of fresh or dried herbs, local applications, ointments, oral infusions and powders.

Balm of Gilead

A famous Biblical drug treatment known as balm of Gilead remained in the pharmaceutical literature right up to the twentieth century. Balm of Gilead is thought to have been the 'mastic' (resin) of *Pistacia lentiscus* or the resinous exudate from *Commiphora* sp., including *C. opobalsamum* and *C. meccanensis*, but is now commonly identified with a North American poplar tree, *Populus gileadenis*. A delicately odorous resinous substance of a dark-red color, it turns yellow as it solidifies. The balm has antiseptic and astringent properties. Gilead was a mountainous wooded country to the east of the River Jordan, which the Hebrews annexed from the Amorites.

Frankincense

Frankincense, a sweet-smelling gum-resin (Old French *franc encens*, pure incense) is also referred to as olibanum. Elfriede Abbe (1965 p. 177), the scientific editor in the Department of Botany of Cornell University, in *The Plants of Virgil's Georgics*, suggests that the Greek name for frankincense was *libanotis*, a word which the Romans transferred to rosemary (*Rosmarinus officinalis*). It is an exudate obtained from three *Boswellia* species, *B. carterii*, *B. papyrifera*, and *B. thurifera* (Moldenke and Moldenke, 1952 pp. 56–59). Frankincense is mentioned on at least 32 occasions in the Bible. The most notable reference to frankincense with regard to *Materia Medica Woman* was when the Wise Men from the East visited Mary after the birth of Jesus: 'Entering the house, they saw the little Child with His mother, Mary, and prostrating themselves they worshipped Him. And opening their treasure chests they offered Him presents; gold, frankincense and myrrh' (Matthew 2: 11). Frankincense was a constituent of the holy incense used in the temples. The holy incense also contained oil of myrrh, perfumes, Persian gum, powdered mollusk shells and salt (Exodus 30: 34).

Frankincense was a favorite remedy in obstetrics and gynecology. Burned in a pot, the fumes were conveyed to the 'privy parts' via a funnel to treat all manner of female complaints. In the second century AD, Soranus of Ephesus advocated its application for uterine hemorrhage and vaginal discharge (Temkin, 1956 p. 244). In his obstetric text *The Byrth of Mankynde*, Thomas Raynold (1545 pp. 71–81) wrote that frankincense was prescribed as a fumigation when the placenta was retained; it was applied to the newborn's navel; and was prescribed for excess lochia or menstruation. In his seventeenth-century obstetric book, *Speculum Matricis*, James Wolveridge (1671) wrote of medication with frankincense for premature labor, when the mother's 'throws' (contractions) came at an 'unseasonable' time: 'Let her sit over a suffumigation of frankincense; for that contributes no small strength both to the matrix, and to the infant also'. Wolveridge, author of the first book devoted to obstetrics in Ireland, prescribed frankincense in warmed date fruit to prevent abortion, and as a local fumigation to inhibit lactation, and to treat breast inflammation (pp. 113; 132; 139). Olibanum (frankincense) has been shown to have anti-inflammatory activity (Evans, 1996 p. 289).

Mandrake

The mandrake (*Mandragora officinalis*) takes its name from the Greek, *mandragoras*, which in turn is a corruption of the Assyrian, *nam tar ira*, or 'male drug of the plague god, Namtar'. The oval fruit of the mandrake is known by the synonyms, 'love-apple', 'devil's apple', or 'devil's testicles', alluding to its appearance and its supposed aphrodisiac properties. The plant is related to the other members of the Solanaceae family, including deadly-nightshade (*Atropa belladona*), potato and tomato. The mandrake has thick tap roots which resemble the lower portions of the human body. Legend relates that the plant should only be uprooted by a dog tied to the plant, after the surrounding ground had been sprinkled with menstrual blood, urine or semen. It was believed that the loud shrieking of the plant during its uprooting could kill a man. In the United States, the name mandrake has erroneously been applied to may apple (*Podophyllum pelatum*, American Mandrake) whose resin, podophyllin, is used to treat venereal and other warts.

In Song of Solomon 7: 13, the suitor declares that: 'the mandrakes give forth their fragrance ... these I have laid up for you'. Another mention of mandrake in the Bible is thought to refer to the amorous potential of the plant and is found in the story of the sisters Leah and Rachel, who both used the mandrake to achieve pregnancy with Jacob (Genesis 30: 14–24).

Mandragora was availed of in labor in ancient Assyria and it was known as an analgesic, emetic, poison and soporific in classical Greece and Rome. Dioscorides mentioned its application for menstrual disorders and both he and Pliny referred to its anesthetic properties. Shakespeare extolled the virtues of the plant in *Othello* (see Chapter 6) and also mentions mandragora in *Anthony and Cleopatra*, *Macbeth*, and *Romeo and Juliet*. Modern research has shown that the mandrake contains a mydriatic alkaloid, mandragorine, with similar analgesic and sedative effects to atropine and scopolamine (Evans, 1996 p. 358).

Myrrh

Myrrh is a bitter, aromatic, transparent gum resin, exuded from the bark of *Commiphora myrrha*, a tree native to North and East Africa. The name of this

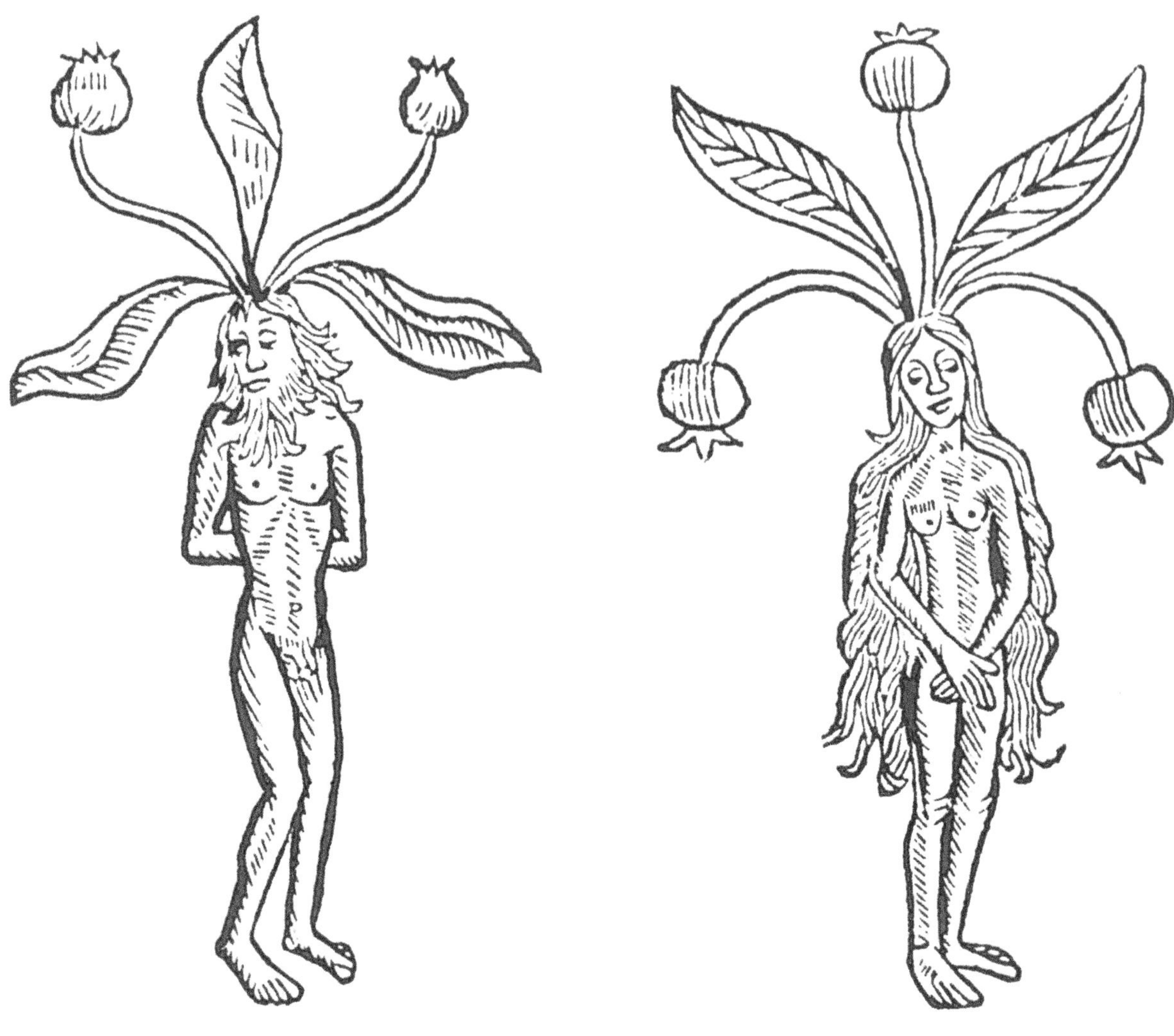

Figure 3 Fifteenth century depiction of the mandrake plant

well-known spice is practically the same in all languages (Arabic *murr*, Hebrew *mor*, Latin *myrrha* or *murra*, French *myrrhe* and Middle English *mirre*) so there is no doubt about its identity. In ancient legend it was related that the princess Myrrha was obsessed with love for her father Theias, King of Assyria. He returned her love and as a result of their incestuous relationship she bore a son, Adonis. Afterwards, in a state of grief and remorse Myrrha exiled herself to the barren deserts of Arabia and prayed for forgiveness. The gods transformed her into the myrrh tree, where she remains, weeping perfumed tears of repentance (Moldenke and Moldenke, 1952 pp. 82–84).

Myrrh was a component of the holy anointing oil prepared by Moses under instruction from the Lord (Exodus 30: 23–25). In The Song of Solomon 4: 14, the bridegroom boasts that his bride is like a garden of delightful fragrant plants that contained 'myrrh and aloes, with all the chief spices'. Myrrh was a favorite beauty aid for women and was employed in the 'purification' of the maidens who were led before King Ahasuerus (Xerxes), so that he could choose a Queen. The preparatory period involved 'six months with oil of myrrh and six months with balms and perfumes for beautifying the women' (Esther 2: 12–13). Myrrh was one of the three gifts of the Magi to Jesus after his birth (Matthew 2: 11) and was again offered to him on the cross (Mark 15: 23). Myrrh was used as an embalming agent and perfume for burial of the dead (John 19: 39–40).

Myrrh was employed as an abortifacient in Greco-Roman antiquity (Temkin, 1956 p. 231) and the classical scholar John Riddle has written an account of its application as an anti-fertility drug (1997 pp. 51–53). It was an important remedy for amenorrhea and leucorrhea, and as a labor oxytocic and treatment for uterine infection in the Middle Ages. Myrrh was employed as an aid to labor (possibly as an analgesic) by Thomas Raynold and was also applied to the stump of the newborn's cord (1545 p. 110). It is still prescribed in Ayurvedic medicine as an aphrodisiac and as a treatment for dysmenorrhea and irregular menstruation. It is not now advocated for female complaints in conventional Western medicine. Myrrh is an antiseptic (Evans, 1996 p. 289) and is available in conventional and herbal medical practice as an astringent and antiseptic (Reynolds, 1982 p. 315; *British Herbal Pharmacopoeia*, 1991).

Myrtle

The fragrant evergreen myrtle (*Myrtus communis*) takes its name from the Greek *myrtos* and Latin *myrtus*. Myrtle is frequently mentioned in the Old Testament. One such reference is found in Isaiah 41: 9: 'I will plant in the wilderness the cedar, the shittah tree, the myrtle and the oil tree'. Wood from the shittah tree was used in manufacture of Hebrew altars and the Ark of the Covenant. The plant symbolized purity and it's gum (gum arabic, highly esteemed in medicine) represented menstrual blood. The shittah is better known as the Acacia (*Acacia arabica*). A story is told that 'when Adam and Eve were expelled from Paradise they took with them wheat, chief of foods; the date chief of fruits and the myrtle, chief of scented flowers' (Moldenke and Moldenke, 1952 pp. 143–144). The plant was considered a symbol of love and immortality by the Greeks and Romans who crowned their heroes and poets with wreaths of myrtle and laurel, a ceremony known as the 'ovation'.

The myrtle was dedicated to Aphrodite and Venus, possibly because the aromatic leaves resembled the female pudenda. The myrtle berry, which contains a blood-red juice, was the common name for the clitoris in Greco-Roman antiquity. Plant extract was rendered into a perfume which was thought to be an aphrodisiac. Jewish brides carried myrtle twigs at their weddings and the custom spread to Europe. Queen Victoria's wedding bouquet contained myrtle when she married in 1840 and it is claimed by Roy Vickery (1995), curator of The Natural History Museum, London, that a sprig of myrtle grown from that bouquet was carried by Princess Anne at her wedding in 1973.

Myrtle found many uses in the obstetrics and gynecology of Soranus of Ephesus in the second century AD (Temkin, 1956 p. 231). It was prescribed in abortifacients, as a topical contraceptive, as an antihemorrhagic and as a local antiseptic for inflammation and venereal disease. Myrtle retained the same usage during the Middle Ages (Rowland, 1981). Twigs of myrtle were placed in babies' cots to keep them from crying. Myrtle is an antiseptic and astringent (Williamson and Evans, 1988) and its oil is used in soaps and skin care products. The fruit of the plant is still prescribed as a herbal medicine among the Asian community in England (Evans, 1996 p. 499).

Pomegranate

The pomegranate (*Punica granatum*) is an Oriental fruit much cultivated in warm countries. It takes its name from the Latin *pomum*, apple, and *granatum*, having many grains or seeds. 'Punic' refers to ancient Carthage (Latin *punicus* or *poeni*, the Carthaginians) and the 'Punic apple' was the pomegranate. The first reference to pomegranate in the Bible is found in Exodus 28: 33–34: 'A golden bell [a pomegranate flower] and a pomegranate, upon the hem of the robe round about'. The Lord here commanded Moses that the skirts of the priestly robes, or ephods, should be embroidered in blue, purple and scarlet in imitation of the flowers and fruit of the pomegranate. In The Song of Solomon there are a number of references to the pomegranate, one of which relates to the perceived aphrodisiac qualities of the plant: 'How beautiful you are my love ... let us [see] ... whether the pomegranates are come into flower; there will I give you my love' (7: 6–12).

The pomegranate came to be regarded as a sacred plant in Ancient Egypt and its characteristic flowers and fruits are easily recognized in Egyptian inscriptions and sculpture. Reverence for the plant spread to the surrounding civilizations. The Hebrew word for pomegranate is *rimmon*, derived from *rim*, to give birth. The flowers of red, scarlet, yellow or white hues served as patterns for the 'golden bells' of the Hebrews. The globular fruit contains numerous seeds and became a symbol of fertility in Biblical times. The calyx-like lobes of the fruit were the inspiration for Solomon's crown and all royal diadems since. Among the many myths about the plant is the story of a beautiful nymph who wished that she could wear a crown. One day she was transformed into a pomegranate tree by Bacchus, the god of wine, and a crown was placed at the top of the tree's fruit. A popular precious stone, the (red) garnet, is thought to take its name from *granatum*.

Although the pomegranate was a symbol of fertility, the fruit skin was applied as a contraceptive pessary 'with equal amounts of gum and an equal amount of oil of roses' by Soranus (Temkin, 1956 pp. 64–65). The theme of pomegranate's anti-fertility effects was explored by John Riddle. Based on scientific studies he concluded that extract of the plant resulted in fertility reduction in experimental animals of between 15 and 100% (1997 pp. 40–44). In *The Byrth of Mankynde* Thomas Raynold prescribed the 'flowre and rynde of pome granate [with eight other medicinal products] ... to Stynte and restrayne the outragyous flux of flowres [to reduce lochial or menstrual flow]'. He also prescribed the remedy for uterine prolapse which he described: 'Many tymes also it chanseth that the foundament gut cometh furth ... especially in women in this busynesse, by reason of they great labour and stryuyng with them self' (1545, *The Second Booke*, p. 83). In this instance, the prolapse was cleansed, replaced and held in place with linen soaked in herbs, including pomegranate.

Pomegranate rind, *pericarpium granati*, is still advocated for women's disorders in China. Known there as *shiliupi*, the drug is collected in autumn when the fruit is ripe, and dried in the sun. It is prescribed for abnormal uterine bleeding and leukorrhea in a dose of 3–9 gram. In addition traditional Chinese medicine physicians use the plant to treat intestinal worms (*Pharmacopoeia of the People's Republic of China*, 1992). This is in accord with Western medical practice – the pomegranate contains an alkaloid known as pelletierine which *Martindale, The Extra Pharmacopoeia* notes has a specific action against tapeworms (Reynolds, 1982 p. 102). It is rarely used nowadays because of its toxicity.

References

Abbe, E. (1965). *The Plants of Virgil's Georgics*, p. 177. (Ithaca, NY: Cornell University Press)

The Bible Societies (1952). *The Holy Bible containing the Old and New Testaments*, Revised Standard Edition. (Oxford: Oxford University Press)

Boss, J. (1962). The Character of Childbirth According to the Bible. *J. Obstet. Gynaecol. Br. Common.*, 69(3), 508–13

The British Herbal Medical Association (1991). *British Herbal Pharmacopoeia*, p. 73. (Bournemouth, UK)

The Confraternity of Christian Doctrine (1970). *The New American Bible*. Translated from the original languages with critical use of all the ancient sources by members of the catholic biblical association of America. (Washington DC)

de Waal, M. (1994). *Medicines from the Bible: Roots and Herbs and Woods and Oils*, English translation, 1984. (York Beach, ME: Samuel Weiser Inc.)

Duke, J. A. (1983). *Medicinal Plants of the Bible* (London: Tradco-Medic Books)

Evans, W. C. (1996). *Trease and Evans' Pharmacognosy*, pp. 289; 358; 499. (London: W. B. Saunders Company Ltd.)

The Gideons International (1982). *Holy Bible* (1982) Revised (ed.) (USA: National Bible Press)

Harrison, R. H. (1966). *Healing Herbs of the Bible*. (Leiden: Brill)

Hasselquist, F. (1757). *Iter Palaestinum; eller resa till Heliga Landet förrattad ifran ar 1749 til 1752*

Levin, S. (1960). Obstetrics in the Bible. *J. Obstet. Gynaecol. Br. Emp.*, 67(1), 490–8

Lloyd Davies, M. and Lloyd Davies, T. A. (1991). *The Bible. Medicine and Myth*. (Cambridge, UK: Allborough Publishing)

Miller, D. (1953). Res Obstetrica in the Bible. *J. Obstet. Gynaecol. Br. Emp.*, 60(1), 7–16

Moldenke, H. N. and Moldenke, A. L. (1952). *Plants of the Bible*, pp. 1–13, 56–9, 82–4, 143–4. (New York: The Ronald Press Co.)

Pharmacopoeia Commission of PRC (1992). *Pharmacopoeia of the People's Republic of China*, pp. 136–7. (Temple of Heaven, Bejing: Guangdong Science and Technology Press)

Raynold, T. (1545). *The Byrth of Mankynde, otherwyse named the Woman's Booke*, pp. 71, 81, 110. *The Second Booke*, pp. 81, 83. (London: Tho. Ray)

Reynolds, J. E. F. (ed.) (1982). *Martindale. The Extra Pharmacopoeia*, pp. 315, 102. (London: The Pharmaceutical Press)

Riddle, J. M. (1997). *Eve's Herbs. A History of Contraception and Abortion in the West*, pp. 51–3, 40–4. (Massachusetts and London: Harvard University Press)

Rowland, B. (1981). *Medieval Woman's Guide to Health. The First English Gynecological Handbook*, pp. 83, 85, 103, 105, 149. (London: Croom Helm)

Temkin, O. (1956). *Soranus' Gynecology*, pp. 244, 231, 64–5. (Baltimore: Johns Hopkins Press)

Vickery, R. (1995). *A Dictionary of Plant Lore*, pp. 251–2. (London: Oxford University Press)

Williamson, E. M. and Evans, F. J. (1988). *Potter's New Cyclopaedia of Botanical Drugs and Preparations*, pp. 198–99. (Saffron Walden, UK: C. W. Daniel Company Ltd.)

Wolveridge, J. (1671). *Speculum Matricis; or, the Expert Midwives Handmaid*, pp. 113, 132, 139. (London: E. Okes)

Greece and Rome 9

INTRODUCTION

The great age of ancient Greece and Rome is known as the 'Classical World' (c. 500 BC–c. AD 500). These two civilizations were responsible for shaping much of the developed world in which we live. Discoveries of the era form the basis of our knowledge of biology, literature, mathematics, medicine and therapeutics, obstetrics and gynecology, philosophy, politics and physics. In time, the all-conquering Greek general, Alexander the Great (356–323 BC) spread Hellenistic knowledge and culture throughout much of the known ancient world and the Romans later carried their civilization even further afield, past one of the 'Pillars of Hercules' (Gibraltar) to northern Europe.

By the first century BC the ancient world was divided into four great empires. The Roman empire was the most powerful and stretched from Europe to North Africa while the Han Dynasty controlled almost all of the Far East. The Middle East was ruled by the Sassand kings, while in India the Gupta family held power. Trade linked the empires and facilitated the spread of medical wisdom so that when the empires collapsed in the sixth century AD knowledge of botanical medicine and therapeutics was relatively similar throughout the ancient world. A healthy East–West trade in herbal medicines and spices continued through the centuries until the fall of the Byzantine empire in AD 1453.

MYTHOLOGY AND GRECO-ROMAN MEDICINE

Chiron the centaur

A mythical race of wild creatures inhabited the mountains of ancient Greece. Famous among them was Chiron the centaur, the fabulous creature who was half horse, half man. During his hunting escapades with Artemis (identified with the Roman goddess Diana) on Mount Pelion in Thessaly, the centaur discovered

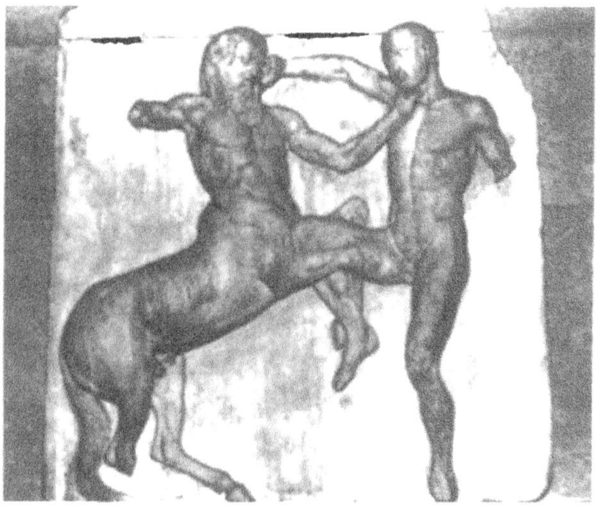

Figure 1 Grave steele showing a centaur applying carotid pressure

many medicinal plants and he became celebrated for his knowledge of 'simples', which were medicinal herbs of only one constituent. The centaury plant, or feverwort (*Erythraea centaurium*), is named after him. Centaury contains bitter glycosides, gentiopicrin and amarogentin and is useful as an antipyretic agent and for digestive disorders.

Apollo

The Greeks had several religions but a national Pantheon of gods and goddesses, many of whom were patrons to the healing arts. The principal deity of medicine was Apollo, a sun-god and also physician to the twelve gods who inhabited Mount Olympus. Apollo's favorite remedy was the peony, a plant of the genus Paeonia of the buttercup family, hence Apollo's epithet 'Paean', and 'Sons of Paean', was applied to physicians. Extract of *Paeonia officinalis* (common peony) and *Paeonia lactiflora* (Chinese peony) are known to stimulate the uterus. Apollo, who gained his knowledge of medicine from the centaur Chiron, could cause, or cure plagues and epidemics. Apollo, in turn, passed his knowledge to the hero Asclepius.

Asclepius

This legendary healer and his followers created a priestly order of healers known as the 'Asclepiadae. The temples of the cult were the famous Asclepieia, of which the most celebrated were at Cos, Epidaurus and Pergamum. Those who attended the sacred temples for healing were purified by bathing, anointing with soothing medications, massage, prayers and sacrificial offerings. They were then inducted into the special ritual of incubation or temple sleep.

Fielding H. Garrison remarked that 'Æsculapius was commonly represented as a handsome Jove-like figure (Jupiter), with a sacred snake entwined around a rod' (1929 p. 85). Among the legendary children of Asclepius and his wife Epione were his daughters Hygieia and Panacea. Hygieia represented health while Panacea presided over the administration of medicines. Two sons, Machaon and Podalirius were gifted healers skilled in drug treatments and were immortalized in Homer's *Iliad.*

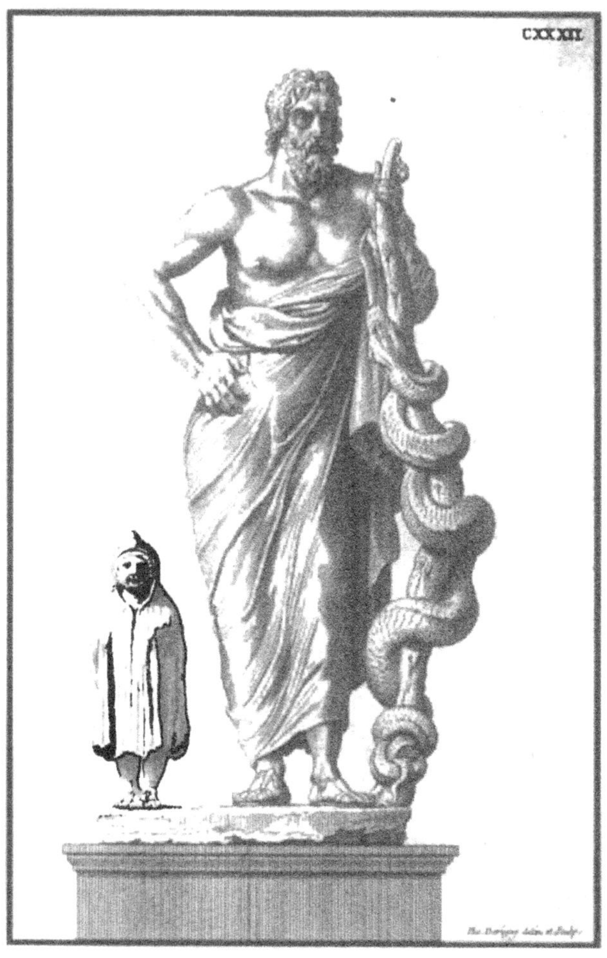

Figure 2 Asclepius, the Greek god of medicine (c. 1200 BC)

Prometheus

This Greek demi-god was a descendant of Uranus and Gaia and was thus one of the Titans. It is said that he created man from clay and stole fire from the heavens for the benefit of humankind. He also instructed mortals on how to prepare medicines for all ailments and is referred to as 'The First Pharmacist' (Wootton, 1910 vol. 1, p. 12).

Morpheus

Morpheus, son of the god of sleep (Hypnos), derived his name from ***morphe***, the Greek for form or shape, because of his ability to fashion the forms of dreams. Morpheus was usually represented with a poppy plant in his hand. It was from the poppy (***Papaver somniferum***) that the narcotic opium was derived. In 1806 Friedrich Wilhelm Sertürner (1783–1841) discovered the active principle of opium and in deference to his classical education he called the substance Morphium (morphine). An elixir which contained poppy juice as an essential ingredient became known in the Classical World as 'anodyna' or 'paregorica', giving rise to our terms 'anodyne' and 'paragoric' respectively. In the nineteenth century, paregoric elixir contained alcoholic solution of opium, benzoic acid, camphor and oil of anise, and was called 'Tincture Camphorae Co.'.

Nepenthe or Nepenthes (Greek ***ne***, not and ***penthos***, grief) was a legendary analgesic drug in Ancient Greece. The herb which contained the anodyne was imported from Egypt and although there is some doubt as to its identification it appears that the plant may have been *Papaver somniferum.* Nepenthe, in the guise of morphine, was a popular anesthetic premedication in the 1960s.

Pliny described incising the poppy plant to obtain opium: the copious poppy juice which exuded from the plant thickened sufficiently to be squeezed into lozenge shapes and left to dry in the sun. If the poppy heads were boiled down, the dark juice obtained was called 'meconium', a term later applied to the first dark-green intestinal discharge of newborn infants (Jones, 1989 book 20, p. 117). The scarlet ornamental poppy (*Papaver bracteatum*) contains thebaine, which can be converted to codeine and the important narcotic antagonist, naloxone, which is used to counter the effects of pethidine in the newborn and in infants born to heroin addicts.

Melampus and Agamede

Greek mythology also includes tales of humans who helped to shape medical evolution. Melampus, for instance, was a shepherd to whom we owe the medications hellebore (*Helleborus niger*) and iron. In one legend it is related that the women of Argos were stricken with disease and became insane. Melampus cured them by administering hellebore and goats' milk. In another story he cured the King of Phylacea of infertility by treating him with rust of iron in wine (*vinum ferri*). Women healers also offered medications and 'Agamede of the yellow hair who well understood as many drugs as the wide earth nourishes' was mentioned in Homer's *Iliad* (Garrison, 1929 p. 86).

MEDICINE IN THE EARLY CLASSICAL PERIOD

Hippocrates

European medicine began properly in the early classical period (460–136 BC). Its scientific spirit and ethical ideals owe much to Hippocrates (c. 460–370 BC) of Cos. Later dubbed the 'father of medicine', Hippocrates founded the art of bedside medicine with careful systematic clinical examination of the patient. His descriptions of disease processes are models of perfection and his views on many medical topics were accepted as authoritative until recent times. Hippocrates was the first physician to establish and set down a scientific system of diagnostic and prognostic medicine. Although influenced by Egyptian sources he dropped their elements of mystery and magic and dealt with disease as a natural phenomenon.

The four humors

Hippocrates believed in the doctrine of the four humors, later known as humoral medicine. The humors were the body fluids and he theorized that diseases were caused by imbalance of those fluids. In developing his theories of disease, Hippocrates was influenced by the basic principle of the Pythagorean universe which held that balance in all things should be the goal of correct behavior. Opposite pairs of substances and qualities could achieve that state of equilibrium. The number four was important because it also related to the four 'elements' of earth, air, fire and water. Corresponding to the four elements were the four 'qualities': dry, cold, hot and moist. Thus air was hot and moist; fire was hot and dry; earth was thought to be cold and dry and water was cold and moist.

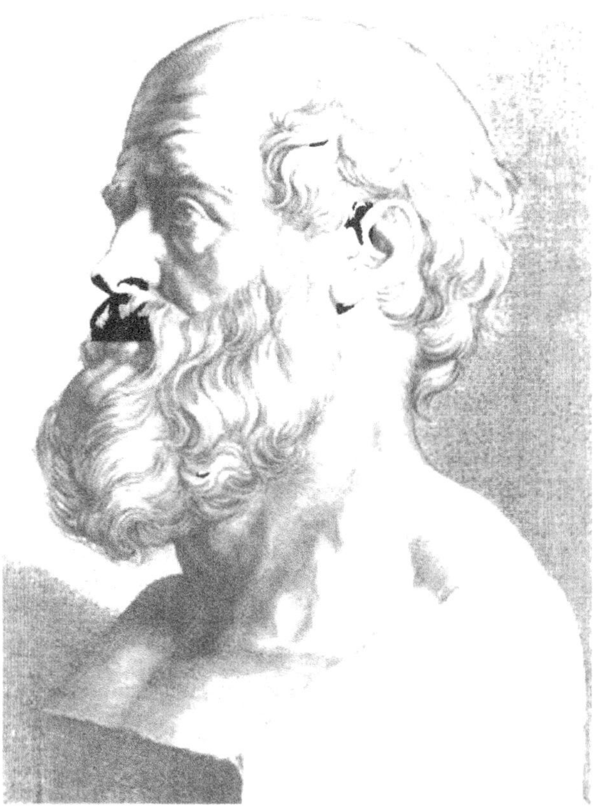

Figure 3 Hippocrates (c. 460–377 BC)

The four body secretions of blood, phlegm, yellow and black bile were the four humors. Blood was warm and moist while black bile was considered cold and dry. Yellow bile was warm and dry and phlegm was said to be cold and moist. Belief in the concept led to a hypothetical system of medicine which explained illness as resulting from alterations in the four basic humors of the body: if the humors were balanced the body was healthy but imbalance caused disease. The disease process had three stages, the first of which was a fever, followed by a 'crisis', after which the disease was resolved by discharge of excess humor or by death. The discharge of humors was manifested by the passage of blood, nasal phlegm, urine, sweat, vomit or fecal matter, and a cure was effected by restoring humoral balance.

The humoral concept of disease was perpetuated by the great Greek physician Galen (c. AD 131–201) who also classified personalities along humoral lines as phlegmatic, sanguine, choleric or melancholic. Other cultures, including the Chinese, were influenced by humoral doctrine although the Orientals developed a theory of disease based on *five* humors.

The Hippocratic Oath

The Oath was a code of ethics adopted by medical men throughout the ages and is regarded as a composite production rather than a genuine Hippocratic document. The only reference to drugs in the entire Oath reads: 'I will not give to a woman a pessary to cause abortion'. Greco-Roman physicians were aware of many herbs with supposed abortive properties and Dioscorides' great herbal mentions 50 remedies to use for abortion or miscarriage. The following rendering of the Hippocratic Oath is taken from Douglas Guthrie's *A History of Medicine* (Guthrie, 1945).

> 'I swear by Apollo the Physician, by Aesculapius, by Hygeia, by Panacea, and by all the Gods and Goddesses, making them my witnesses, that I will carry out according to my ability and judgment, this oath and this indenture. To hold my teacher in this art equal to my own parents; to make him partner in my livelihood; when he is in need of money to share mine with him; to consider his family as my own brothers, and to teach them this art, if they want to learn it, without fee or indenture; to impart precept, oral instruction, and all other instruction to my own sons, the sons of my teacher, and to pupils who have taken the physician's Oath, but to nobody else.
>
> I will use treatment to help the sick according to my ability and judgment, but never with a view to injury and wrongdoing. Neither will I administer a poison to anybody when asked to do so, nor will I suggest such a course. Similarly I will not give to a woman a pessary to cause abortion. But I will keep pure and holy both my life and my heart. I will not use the knife, not even, verily, on sufferers from stone, but I will give place to such as are craftsmen therein. Into whatsoever houses I enter, I will enter to help the sick, and I will abstain from all intentional wrongdoing and harm, especially from abusing the bodies of man or woman, bond or free.
>
> And whatsoever I shall see or hear in the course of my profession, as well as outside my profession in my intercourse with men, if it be what should not be published abroad, I will never divulge, holding such things to be holy secrets. Now if I carry out this Oath, and break it not, may I gain for ever reputation among all men for my life and for my art; but if I transgress it and forswear myself, may the opposite befall me.'

The Hippocratic Corpus and therapeutics

A group of medical texts written between 430 and 330 BC are collectively known as the *Hippocratic Corpus*. Although ascribed to Hippocrates the treatises appear to be the work of a number of medical writers. Among the writings are the *Aphorisms of Hippocrates* and the essays on *The Seed* and *The Nature of the Child*.

In the *Aphorisms*, the first medical truth, 'Life is short, science is long, opportunity is elusive, experiment is dangerous, judgment is difficult' introduces seven sections of medical principles. Sections four and five deal with the various afflictions which may beset the pregnant woman. The final aphorism of the seventh section reads: 'What drugs will not cure, the knife will; what the knife will not cure, the cautery will; what the cautery will not cure must be considered incurable' (Chadwick *et al.*, 1983).

The Hippocratic writings mention aromatic vapor baths as being useful for the treatment of 'female disorders' and advocate application of cupping glasses to the nipples to restrain heavy menstruation.

Hippocrates wrote about the act of procreation, and was of the opinion that intercourse improved a woman's health. Hippocrates included a fertility test in his aphorisms: the woman was wrapped in a cloak and incense was burned beneath her – if the odor passed through her body to her nose she was thought to be fertile. Hippocrates theorized on the male and female 'elements' which formed a pregnancy and offered an ancient Greek pregnancy test: a draught of hydromel (honey and water) was administered on a empty stomach and if the woman developed cramps she was judged to be pregnant.

Hippocrates also wrote about infertility, miscarriage, the 'attitude' of the child in the womb, and the initiation of labor. He believed that the fetus ruptured the amniotic membranes by spasmodic movements of its hands and feet, causing a flow of liquor and onset of labor. Drugs which cause sneezing were used to help expel the afterbirth. Hippocrates detailed cases of puerperal sepsis and referred to diseases of the newborn. He believed that medications could be taken by the mother from the fourth to the seventh month of gestation, but advised reduction in dosage from then until the end of the pregnancy.

Hippocrates knew that there was in most diseases a tendency to natural resolution, or *vis medicatrix naturae*, 'the healing power of nature', and made little use of drugs in treatment. Hippocrates believed that therapy should assist nature and he confined his treatments to fresh air, good diet, purgation with black hellebore (*Helleborus niger*), and vomiting induced with white hellebore (*Veratrum album*). Medical decoctions of barley gruel, barley water, hydromel (honey and water) and oxymel (honey and vinegar) were administered and complemented by massage and hydrotherapy. Hippocrates was aware of drug side-effects and warned that hellebore, used as an emetic or purgative, could cause convulsions if given in high dosage. He also thought that it was better *not* to treat those with internal cancers because they died sooner if treated.

With the death of Hippocrates, Greek medicine moved away from the open-minded and receptive spirit which characterized his teachings, towards a system of dogma noted more for its rigid adherence to dogma than for investigation and new ideas.

Aristotle

After Hippocrates came Aristotle (384–322 BC) of Stagira. Aristotle, son of a court physician and pupil of Plato the philosopher, was a great biologist and gave to medicine the beginnings of comparative anatomy, botany, embryology, psychology, physiology, and teratology. His writings were expanded by later authors and were popular until the early part of the twentieth century. The (pseudo) Aristotle works, the *Complete and Experienced Midwife* and the *Compleat Masterpiece* were commonplace texts with a wealth of detail on obstetrics and gynecology and the medications useful for female disorders. Although he was not a physician, Aristotle had a profound influence on medicine, particularly among later Arab authors. He left his library and his garden of medicinal herbs to his close friend and former pupil, Theophrastus of Eresus (see below).

Diocles Carystius

The earliest Greek herbal was written by Diocles Carystius who was born in the first half of the fourth century BC. He listed plants, noting their habitat and briefly described their medicinal properties. He classified plants according to their leaves, roots, seeds, stems, and growing season, and described varieties of medicinal plants which were found between the Atlantic coast and India. This was the beginning of a systematic analysis of plant remedies based on their individual characteristics (Leake, 1975). Only fragments of his writings remain available for study today.

Theophrastus

Theophrastus (c. 372–287 BC) of Eresus, on the island of Lesbos, studied philosophy at Athens, where he became a physician and follower of Aristotle. On Aristotle's death he took charge of the Lyceum (a gymnasium and grove close to the temple of Apollo at Athens, where Aristotle taught) and inherited Aristotle's library, manuscripts and medicinal herb garden. Theophrastus laid the foundations of modern scientific botany. He identified and classified plants in the *Historia Plantarum* and then described their characteristics in *Causis Plantarum*. The latter contains descriptions of some five hundred different plants and became the standard herbal textbook for many centuries. Theophrastus described not only the morphology and natural history of plants but also their use in therapeutics (Einarson and Link, 1976).

Theophrastus wrote that mandrake (*Mandragora officinalis*, an anodyne and soporific known to the Biblical writers of the Old Testament as the love apple) was suitable for use as an aphrodisiac. Several kinds of a plant known as all-heal (*Prunella vulgaris*, an astringent, and tonic; *Valeriana officinalis*, an analgesic and sedative; and *Stachys palustris*, an antispasmodic and antiseptic) were thought useful in a pessary for miscarriage. The roots of the plants were used during labor and for other 'diseases of women'. Root of cyclamen (sowbread, *Cyclamen hederaefolium* of the Primulaceae family, containing a saponin-like drug known as cyclamin) was used to induce rapid delivery and as a love-potion.

The root of the herb libanotis (its modern equivalent is unidentified) was used to promote lactation and also for 'diseases of women'. Birthwort (*Aristolochia clematitis*, a uterine stimulant, antibacterial and anti-inflammatory) was used as a lotion in cases of prolapsed uterus and for other 'disorders of the womb'. Flowers of the plant were seen to resemble a fetus and probably led to the herb's common name: according to the doctrine of signatures the shape or color of a plant indicated its purpose. The Cretan dittany plant (wild marjoram, *Origanum dictamnus*, an inducer of menstruation, rarely mentioned nowadays, and sacred to the goddess Dictyna of Mount Dicte, Crete) was used by women to ease the pains of childbirth. Cretan dittany apart, the other medications for women detailed by Theophrastus had proven efficacy and were still used in more modern times.

ALEXANDRIA

The great university and library of Alexandria were founded in 331 BC and Greek culture and science became firmly established in Egypt. A school of Empirics, who rejected all *a priori* knowledge, and relied solely on trial and experience, developed there in the second century BC. Its members experimented with medicinal drugs and toxicology. Mithridates VI (reigned from 120–63 BC), king of Pontus, in Asia Minor, was said to have developed the art of taking poisons without adverse outcome. He protected himself against the toxic effects of plants by developing a universal antidote, thereafter known as a 'mithridate' or 'theriac' (a mixture of medicines honey and other constituents later known as 'treacle').

Crateuas, a botanist and the earliest-known plant artist, lived during the reign of Mithridates. Crateuas wrote and illustrated a herbal known as the *Rhizotomikon*, and some of his artwork later found its way into the great herbal of Dioscorides (see below). The Alexandrian school attracted the foremost botanists, physicians and scientists from all over the Near East. The practices of these disparate groups were developed and extended through research and writing. A medical tradition evolved which was eventually transmitted to medieval Europe through the writers and scholars of the Arab world.

THE GRECO-ROMAN PERIOD

The Greco-Roman period lasted from 156 BC to AD 576. Corinth was destroyed in 146 BC and Greek medical men moved to Rome where they encountered a medical culture which was quite different from their own. The Romans relied mainly on votive offerings and superstitious practices. There was a household god for most diseases and each householder had a number of domestic herbal medicines for family use. A favorite at the time was cabbage (*Brassica oleracea*, which is now known to contain antibiotic substances). Initially slow to accept Greek medicine, the Romans were won over by the personality and abilities of the renowned physician, Asclepiades of Bithynia (born c. 124 BC), who introduced medicated enemas, internal medications, hydrotherapy and massage, and local applications. He also used occupational therapy and advised music and wine to promote sleep. As time went by the Romans enthusiastically adopted Hellenistic theories and treatment of disease.

Celsus

The new-style Roman medicine was recorded by Aulus Cornelius Celsus (fl. c. AD 30) who lived during the

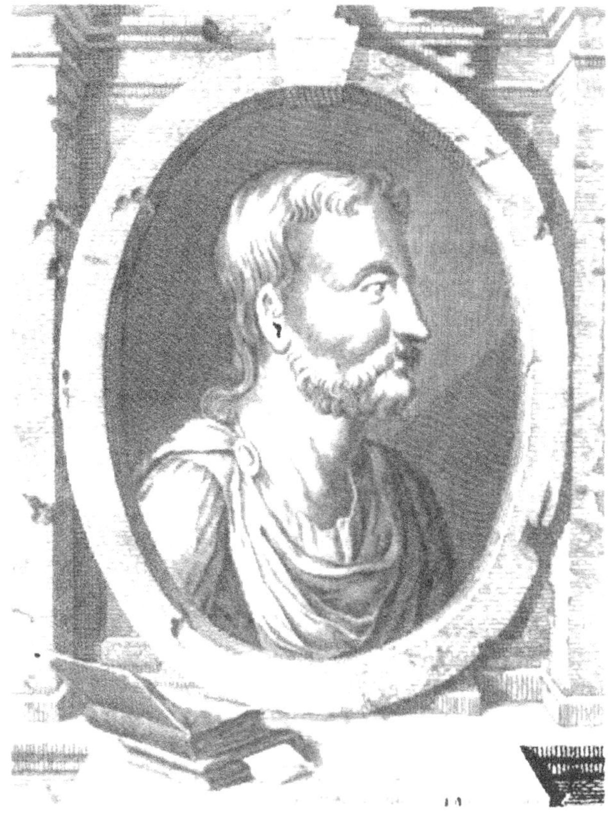

Figure 4 Cornelius Celsus (25 BC–AD 50)

reign of the Emperor Tiberius. Although he was not a physician, Celsus wrote an encyclopedia which included an eight-book treatise on medicine, *De re medicina*. The fifth book in the series is devoted to drug classification and description, pharmaceutical methods and weights and measures. *De re medicina* was written for lay readers and is based on information gained from Greek authorities on herbal medications and from Celsus' own experience of treating household members and slaves (Spencer, 1889). It became the first medical text to appear in print in 1478.

Soranus

Soranus of Ephesus was born in the second half of the first century AD. He studied medicine in Alexandria and later practiced medicine in Rome during the rule of the Emperors Trajan (AD 98–117) and Hadrian (AD 117–138). He is our leading authority on women's medications and the gynecology, obstetrics and pediatrics of Greco-Roman antiquity. His famous treatise *Gynecology* reflects the practice of his time, with some original observations.

The works of Soranus were perpetuated by later Greek compilers including Oribasius, Aetius of Amida and Paul of Aegina. The writings were translated into Arabic and the illustrated Latin edition by Muscio c. AD 500, was used in part by Eucharius Rösslin in 1513 for his famous obstetric textbook, *Der Schwangeren Frauen und Hebammen Rosengarten*, which was itself translated into many European languages. After Soranus there were no innovators in obstetrics and gynecology until the advent of Ambroise Paré some fourteen centuries later. Soranus' *Gynecology* was translated by Owsei Temkin of the Johns Hopkins University Institute of the History of Medicine and published in 1956.

Gynecology deals with gynecological conditions, pregnancy, labor and care of the newborn. Four sections relating to abscesses, ulcers, tumors and prolapse have been lost, but copies of the missing texts are to be found in the writings of Paul of Aegina, translated by Francis Adams (1864), and also in the works of Aetius (translated by Ricci in 1950). The contents list as laid out by Soranus was used as a template by other authors on obstetrics and gynecology for many centuries and is not dissimilar to the index lists in textbooks in the early part of the twentieth century. From an obstetric point of view, it is of interest that Soranus was aware of cephalic and podalic version and of breech extraction. The latter art was lost after his time until reintroduced to obstetric practice by Ambroise Paré (1510–1590).

What is not generally acknowledged is that *Gynecology* contains an extensive materia medica for women's diseases: over 250 medications are listed and used for a variety of gynecological and obstetric purposes. In some instances single drugs were used; in others multiple remedies (polypharmacy) were resorted to.

Dioscorides

Pedacius Dioscorides, of Anazarbus in Cilicia, was a Greek army surgeon in the service of the Emperor Nero (ruled from AD 54–68) and compiled the first materia medica. Dioscorides was first to write in detail on the therapeutics of medical botany and his text is the historic source of many herbal remedies. *De materia medica* was written between AD 50 and 70 and illustrated centuries later by a Byzantine artist in the year 512. The artwork was based on sketches by Crateuas. Dioscorides' materia medica was translated into English (but not published) by John Goodyer, a botanist of Petersfield, between 1652 and 1655. Robert Gunther edited that text and it was first printed in 1933 (Gunther, 1959).

The contents of *De materia medica* are set out in five books. The first relates to aromatics, oils, ointments and trees, while the second has sections devoted to living creatures, milk and dairy produce, cereals and 'sharp' herbs. Book three contains treatises on roots, juices and herbs, while the fourth deals with herbs and roots. The final book records the properties of vines, wines and metallic ores.

Dioscorides mentioned more than a thousand natural remedies, sourced mainly from the plant kingdom, although he also included drugs of animal or mineral origin. His work formed the database from which generations of physicians gained their knowledge of pharmacy. Dioscorides' text was widely and frequently translated into Latin, Arabic and Armenian. Dioscorides' descriptions and methodology were closely followed by all the best authors on medical botany and established the background for later pharmacopoeias (books of medicinal drugs). Many of the plants he described, such as aniseed (*Pimpinella anisum*), chamomile (*Anthemis nobilis*), cinnamon (*Cinnamomum camphorae*), dill (*Anethum graveolens*), ginger (*Zingiber officinale*), wild marjoram (*Origanum dictamnus*, Cretan dittany), pepper (*Capsicum annuum*), rhubarb (*Rheum palmatum*) and thyme (*Thymus vulgaris*), are still mentioned in modern sources. The study of materia medica eventually split into the specialties of botany, mineralogy, and pharmacy in the sixteenth century.

Dioscorides' text is very carefully organized and each plant is named, with a description of its botany, habitat, drug properties, indications and harmful side-effects. Quantities and dosages are given and special note is made of the harvesting, preparation and storage of the plants. Dioscorides also wrote about the veterinary uses, magical and non-medical uses, geographical locations, and possible adulterations of the plants. He classified medications according to their presumed physiological actions and his ideas were the origins of the sciences of pharmacology (the science of drugs) and pharmacognosy (a branch of pharmacology concerned with the study of crude drugs of plant and animal origin).

Dioscorides described single drugs or 'simples'; his contemporaries and successors prescribed a mixture of medications, or polypharmacy. This trend was challenged, with some success, in the sixteenth century when Paracelsus (1493–1541) observed that a single natural medication was itself a mixture of compounds (Riddle, 1985). Polypharmacy continued as the norm, however, despite Paracelsus' spirited opposition.

Pliny the Elder

Gaius Plinius Secundus, Pliny the Elder (AD 23–79), was a Roman of 'equestrian' rank (equivalent to a knight) who entered the army and later the navy. Born at Como in northern Italy, he was a compulsive reader, researcher and notetaker. His only surviving work is an encyclopedic series of 37 volumes, *Historia Naturalis*, a vast compilation of anthropology, botany, mineralogy, zoology and other subjects. These texts remained the great corpus of knowledge throughout the Middle Ages and were frequently copied over the centuries. *Historia Naturalis* contains over a thousand pages and original references to scurvy; the narcotic properties of mandragora juice, Mithridates' experiments with poisons, and many other original observations. His section on herbal medicine is partially derived from Theophrastus. His writings exerted a major influence on Anglo-Saxon medical plant-lore for many centuries. The manuscript of *Historia Naturalis* was purchased by London's Victoria and Albert Museum in 1896.

Pliny's curiosity about the ways of nature led to his death. In the early afternoon of 24 August 79, he entered the harbor at Misenum, on the Bay of Naples, as commander of the Roman fleet. Observing a cloud of unusual size and appearance, Pliny went ashore and was in time to experience the volcanic eruption of Vesuvius. He was overcome by noxious fumes and died on the beach before he had time to escape.

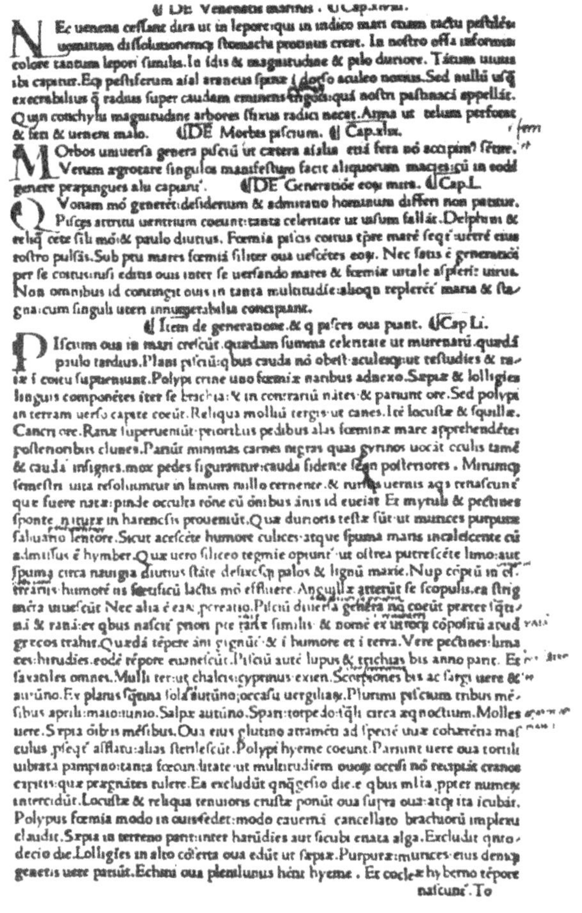

Figure 5 Page from a treatise by Pliny the Elder (AD 23–70)

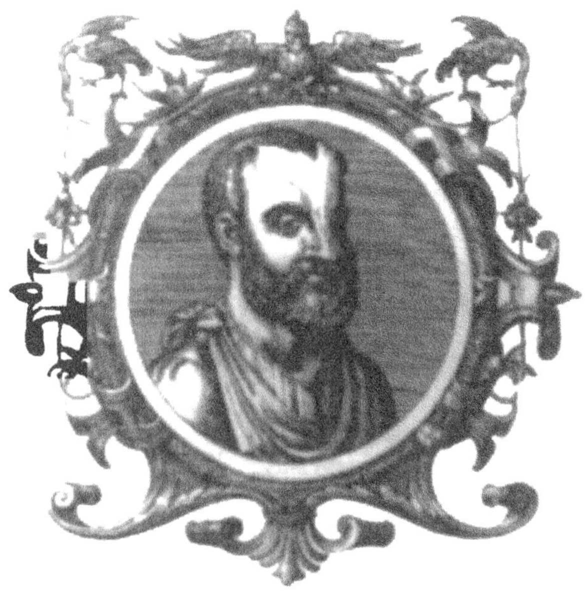

Figure 6 Galen (AD 129–200)

During Pliny's lifetime, medications were commonly prescribed by physicians, in sharp contrast to Hippocratic times when little use was made of drugs and *vis medicatrix naturae* was relied upon to effect a cure. The remedies mentioned by Pliny were chiefly herbal in origin, and designed for use by the layman as domestic medications (Jones, 1989). Unlike Dioscorides, Pliny attempted to explain drug actions on superstitious and magical grounds.

There is some similarity between certain passages in Pliny's *Historia Naturalis* and Dioscorides' *De materia medica* and it is likely that they had a common source, either Crateuas the first century BC herbalist, or the fourth century physician and herbalist, Diocles of Carystius (Jones, 1989). It was during Pliny's time that the doctrine of signatures originated, the theory that 'like could cure like'. The roots of the orchid plant, for example, which resembled testicles, were used to treat genital complaints and as an aphrodisiac. Although the various branches of medical men were well-versed in therapeutics the pharmacist's role had not yet evolved when the Roman Empire in the West came to an end (Cowen and Helfand, 1990).

Galen

Galen (c. AD 129–200) was born at Pergamum in Asia Minor. He studied medicine at Alexandria and then practiced as a physician in Rome. Galen followed Hippocratic methods and the humoral theory of disease. He employed diet, exercise and massage, but also used plant medications which became known as 'galenicals'. His herbal, *De Simplicibus* written in 180, was the only Greek herbal of importance compiled after Dioscorides' materia medica.

Galen wrote thirty books on pharmacy and among his prescriptions were barley-water, grape juice, honey with wine, colocynth (*Citrullus colocynthis*, a purgative), hellebore (*Veratrum album*, a sedative and emetic), henbane (*Hyoscyamus niger*, an analgesic and narcotic), opium (*Papaver somniferum*, an analgesic and sedative), and turpentine (*Terebintha canadensis*, a diuretic and counter-irritant). Galen visited the island of Lemnos and introduced its sacred earth as therapy for dysentery, gonorrhea, hemorrhages and infected wounds (Wootton, 1910) and as a binding agent for medicinal tablets. 'Lemnian earth' (*terra sigillata*) was a white or red greasy clay consisting of alumina, chalk and silica, and a little oxide of iron which gave it a red tint. *Terra sigillata* was also found on the islands of Melos and Samos.

Galen's writings were to make him more famous than Hippocrates and he was the foremost guide for the medieval physician. His teachings were not disputed until the sixteenth century. Galen popularized the remedy *hiera picra* which was a mixture of aloes (*Aloe socotrine*, a purgative), spices, herbs and honey, which Wootton claimed was the oldest known pharmaceutical compound (1910). Galen also used *theriac*, or treacle (a renowned version used during the late Middle Ages was known as Venice treacle) which contained anything up to 70 ingredients and was used as an antidote for poisons and a remedy for many illnesses. Theriacs, originally devised as an improvement on *mithridaticum*, were in common use until the mid-eighteenth century.

MEDICATIONS FOR WOMEN

The ancient Greeks and Romans were aware of many disorders which afflicted women and, through trial and error, developed a sophisticated knowledge of treatments based mainly on plant medications. For instance the myrtle (*Myrtus communis*), recommended by Soranus for cleansing the newborn, is now known to be an antiseptic and antiparasitic. The myrtle plant was sacred to the goddess Aphrodite, and the Greek word *myrtos* meant 'female genitals' (the myrtle berry was like the clitoris). Soranus identified at least 46 indications for drug use in women and the newborn under the main headings: abortion, breast, contraception, pregnancy problems, labor and the newborn, menstruation, tumors and venereal disease. There are 253 medications mentioned in the text of *Gynecology* of which 74% are of vegetable origin, 18.5% of animal origin and the remainder of mineral origin. Drug remedies were administered orally in oil or wine, medicated enemata and pessaries, or as ointments, emplasters and oily embrocations for massage.

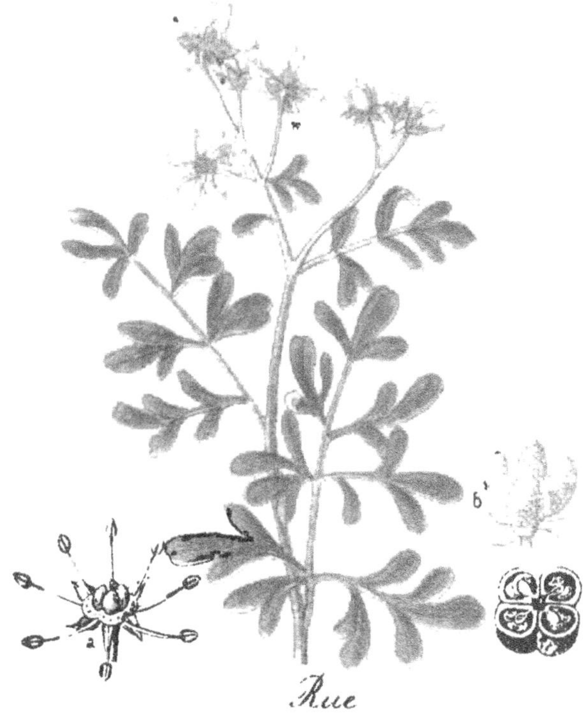

Figure 7 Rue (*Ruta graveolens*)

Soranus described many remedies which could be taken either alone or in combinations for each indication mentioned. For instance, he enumerated 19 forms of vaginal contraceptive (mainly of a gummy or obstructive type) and 13 contraceptive remedies which could be taken orally. Apart from the obstructive element of the vaginal preparations, at least two of these remedies, the pomegranate (*Punica granatum*) and rue (*Ruta graveolens*) have definite anti-fertility properties. For good reviews on contraception and abortion in the Greco-Roman world see Riddle (1992) and Riddle (1997).

Thirty remedies are offered in various combinations for 'hysterical suffocation' (convulsions) which Soranus defined as 'obstructed respiration with aphonia and a seizure of the senses caused by some condition of the uterus'. Many of the remedies are meant to relax the woman or to act by counter-irritation, or purgation to revive the comatose patient. White hellebore (*Veratrum album*), one of the remedies used to provoke vomiting in an effort to cure the hysterical suffocation, is known to have anticonvulsant effects.

The abbreviated materia medica which follows is a sample of the many medications listed by Celsus, Dioscorides, Pliny and Soranus. These remedies, chosen because of their frequent referrals, evolved during the classical Greek and Roman period and survived until modern times.

Artemisia

A number of the *Artemisia* species are mentioned in the ancient Greek sources. The name is derived from the most revered of Greek goddesses, Artemis. The mythological tale relates that the newborn Artemis helped to deliver her twin, Apollo the sun god, and from that time on she became known as the goddess of childbirth. Depicted as the many-breasted Artemis of Ephesus, she was the symbol of fertility and also the protector of children. She was also the goddess of the hunt, noted for her tall stature and strong physique. Forever chaste, it was Artemis who punished rapists and avenged the victims of infidelity. Athena (Minerva), another Greek goddess celebrated for her virginity, had a temple built in her honor, the Parthenon (meaning virgin-house, from *parthenos*, a virgin) at Athens. Several of the species were popular in Greco-Roman antiquity. Wormwood (*Artemisia absinthium*; wormwood, from the German *wermut*, preserver of the mind, and ***absinthium*** without sweetness) was used as an oxytocic by Soranus and Dioscorides to induce abortion, menstruation, miscarriage and placental delivery (Temkin, 1956; Gunther, 1959). Oil of wormwood was the source of absinthe, a toxic but addictive drink favored in nineteenth century France, which was introduced by Henri Pernod in 1797. Absinthe was still listed in major pharmacopoeias in this century as a cerebral stimulant. It contains flavanoids, thujone (responsible for its dramatic neurotoxicity) and other compounds. Absinthe (over 60% proof) stimulates the uterus and the brain, is anti-inflammatory, and aids digestion.

Southernwood (*Artemisia arborescens*) was noted by Dioscorides to stimulate menstruation (Gunther, 1959). Pliny agreed that it was beneficial to the uterus (Jones, 1989) but Soranus denied that it was an oxytocic (Temkin, 1956). Writing on 'the vertues' of southernwood in 1568, William Turner in *The Herbal*

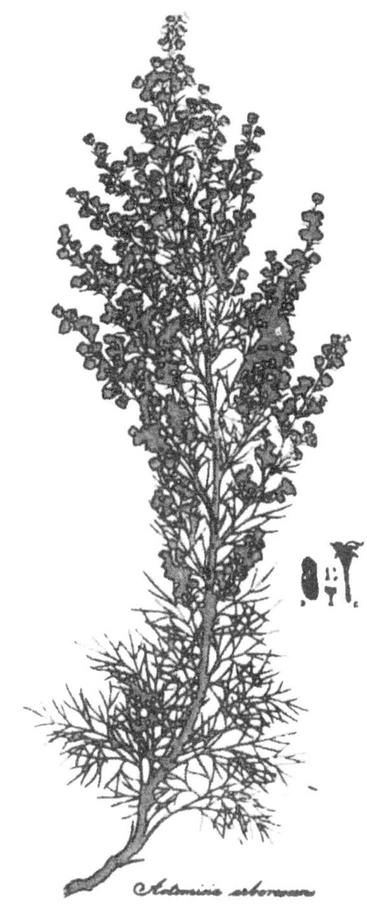

Figure 8 *Artemisia aborescens*

stated that 'some hold that this herbe layd but under a mannes bolster provoketh men to the multiplying of there kinde'. Not surprisingly, the plant later became known by the synonym 'maiden's ruin'. *The British Herbal Pharmacopoeia* (BHP) lists southernwood as an emmenagogue (1983).

Mugwort (*Artemisia vulgaris*), a related plant species, known by Pliny as 'parthenium', was an ingredient placed in a sitz-bath in which women sat to treat inflammation of the uterus (Jones, 1989 book 21, p. 285). The plant, also known as *mater herbarum* (Harris, 1916), was popular as an infusion for 'female complaints' during the sixteenth and seventeenth centuries. In traditional Chinese medicine the dried leaf, known as 'moxa', is burned on the skin over certain acupuncture sites. Mugwort is also advised for fungal infections. Another closely-related plant, tarragon (*Artemisia dracunculus*) is advocated in aromatherapy for menstrual disorders (Bown, 1996). The BHP lists mugwort as an emmenagogue (1983).

Field mugwort (*Artemisia campestris*) was identified by Dioscorides as ambrosia, the legendary food of the gods, referred to as either a drink or as a sweet smelling ointment 'for ye humors fallen down' (Gunther, 1959). Modern advocates of herbal medicine agree that wormwood, southernwood and tarragon are useful for menstrual disorders but should not be taken during pregnancy (Bown, 1996).

Cabbage

The sea cabbage (*Brassica oleracea*) is an ancestor of the garden cabbage and was domesticated from Mediterranean stock by the ancient Greeks and Romans, who viewed the wild cabbage as an apothecary's shop of medications and to a lesser extent as a food source (Grigson, 1996). Over-indulgent Romans ate raw cabbage to prevent drunkenness. The cabbage is closely related to the mustard and turnip plants.

Cabbage was advised as a remedy to induce menstruation and labor and to aid placental delivery. Pregnant women were advised to eat cabbage to increase their milk flow in the puerperium. Application of the plant was a remedy for breast congestion or abscess and Soranus mentions cabbage as an ingredient in a breast-binder for those mothers not intending to breastfeed. He also wrote of the Hippocratic treatment for hysterical suffocation (convulsions) with cabbage (Temkin, 1956). Pliny waxed poetically that '[It] would be a long task to make a list of all the praises of the cabbage' and enumerated its applications to women's materia medica while extolling its virtues 'for troubles of the testes and genitals' (Jones, 1989 book 20, pp. 47–55). Dioscorides wrote that 'the flower being applied in a pessum after child birth doth hinder conception' (Gunther, 1959 pp. 159–60).

Known as colewort in folk medicine (from Latin, *colis* or *caulis*, a stem, and Old English, *wyrt*, a root or herb), cabbage continued as a popular remedy through the years, and in the seventeenth century Nicholas Culpeper wrote that not only would cabbage juice 'help those that are bitten by an adder', but that a 'decoction of the [cabbage] flowers brings down women's courses' (1653).

Although not mentioned in the BHP of 1983, the cabbage, which has antibacterial and anti-inflammatory properties, is currently in vogue as a therapeutic agent – prepared leaves are applied to the breasts to relieve postnatal engorgement and mastitis (Ody, 1993).

The cabbage plant was important in the love-life of country folk and was used for love divination – owners of cabbage patches had to mind their gardens carefully for fear that their plants would go missing! The cabbage even featured on Valentine cards or in autograph books accompanied by a verse such as:

My love is like a cabbage,
Often cut in two,
The leaves I give to others,
The heart I give to you!

Castoreum

This animal product has a long association with women's materia medica and featured, with boar testicles, camel brain, crocodile dung and tortoise blood, in a list of medications by Serapion the Elder of Alexandria, c. 200 BC (Wootton, 1910 vol. 1, p. 217). Celsus of the first century AD mentions castoreum in his list of medicaments in his *De re medicina* (Spencer, 1989). Soranus related that castoreum was applied to the nose and ears of hysterical (convulsing) women as a pungent ill-smelling unguent: the displaced uterus, which was thought responsible for the fits, was believed to flee from the evil smell and find its way back to the pelvis. Castoreum was also smeared on the prolapsed uterus to encourage replacement. Soranus disagreed with the use of castoreum.

Castoreum, or castor, was the secretion and the dried preputial follicles (Latin, *praeputium*, prepuce or foreskin) of the beaver (*Castor fiber*). The musk secretion was reddish-brown, with a strong unpleasant smell and a bitter and nauseous taste. The product was popularly prescribed as an oxytocic to induce labor, particularly in cases of intrauterine death and was mentioned in obstetric texts through the years until the nineteenth century.

According to J.A. Paris, physician to the Westminster Hospital, London, the substance was antispasmodic and 'seems to act more particularly on the uterine system. It certainly proves beneficial as an adjunct to anti-hysteric combinations' (Paris, 1822). The remedy was prescribed so frequently that it ran into short supply and was sometimes counterfeited with a mixture of dried blood, gum ammoniacum, and a little real castor stuffed into the scrotum of a goat. The fraud could only be detected by comparing the taste and smell with those of real castor.

Ernest Mann (1915) detailed the chemical analysis of castoreum and stated that it contained castorin, volatile oil, bitter resin, fat, and traces of benzoic acid, salicin and phenol. Castoreum was an 'official' product in the pharmacopoeias of most European countries in this century and still featured in Dorland's medical dictionary in 1932. It was to be administered in a dose of 300–600 mg, as a stimulant and antispasmodic. More recently, castoreum was reduced to the status of a fixative in perfumery (Reynolds, 1982).

Leeches

Leeches are aquatic segmented worms of the class Hirudinea, which have a sucker at each end of their bodies and feed on the blood or tissues of other animals. Soranus of Ephesus advised the application of leeches, with cupping and scarification, to remove blood from congested parts, as treatment for painful menstruation and inflammation of the uterus, and for molar pregnancy (Temkin, 1956).

The process of bloodletting was a recognized form of therapy from Hippocratic times until the early twentieth century. Blood was thought to contain all the body humors and bleeding to help restore humoral balance. The most common method of bloodletting was to open an engorged vein with a knife and drain blood into a bowl, a form of treatment much used in eclampsia. Another less dramatic method was known as 'cupping': a heated cup with a greased rim was placed over a scarified portion of skin, and blood or pus was drawn through the skin opening by the suction which developed. Leeching was an easier method, as the blood loss was more controlled and quantifiable.

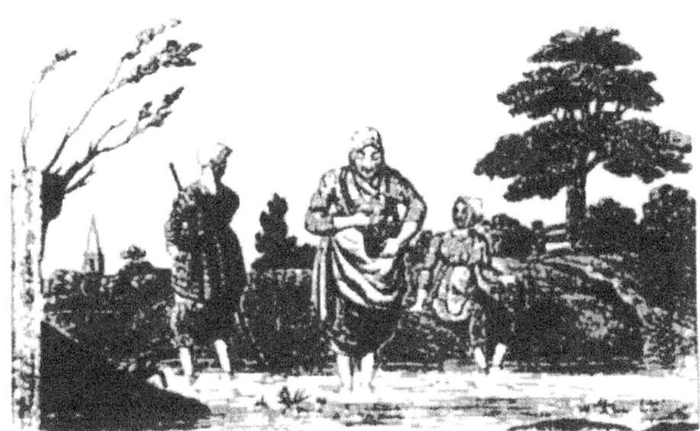

Figure 9 Leeches being collected from a pond

According to Wootton, in his *Chronicles of Pharmacy* (1910 vol. 2, p. 139), the physician who introduced leeches to medicine was Themison of Laodicea who practiced in Rome around 50 BC. The application of leeches to treat disease was to become so popular that physicians themselves became known as 'leeches', while the art of medicine became known as 'leechcraft' and a remedy or prescription as a 'leechdom'. Various forms of leeches were used, including the speckled Leech (*Sanguisuga medicinalis*); the green Leech (*Sanguisuga officinalis*) and later on the five-striped or Australian Leech (*Hirudo quinquestriata*).

The leech was applied to a clean, hairless, non-greasy part of the body and if it was slow to latch on, an application of cream, milk or sugar could be used to encourage suction. A good specimen could extract up to 2 drachms, which is quarter of a fluid ounce or approximately 8 ml (see Table 1). A large number of leeches were applied to areas of inflammation, pain or suspected illness. In women the vagina was a favorite target for leech treatment but insertion and later removal of all of the leeches proved difficult. In more modern times a tubular 'leech glass' was employed for internal use so that only one leech head could feed at a given time. When sated and heavy with blood a leech would simply fall off; if it failed to do so the application of a strong salt solution made it disengage. After feeding, the leech was placed in salt (camphor water was used in later times) so that it vomited the ingested blood, and after 10 days' rest in clean water it was ready for action again (Squire, 1908). Leeches remained in popular use until the nineteenth century in the treatment of vaginal discharge, cervical cancer and uterine prolapse. In the nineteenth century, leeches were also applied to treat a condition referred to as 'exquisite sensibility' of the clitoris, a less drastic procedure than removal of the organ which had become a popular operation for all manner of female complaints at that time (Dally, 1991).

In general medicine, the physician Francois Broussais (1772–1838) so swayed medical opinion that in 1833 almost 42 million leeches were imported to France (Garrison, 1929). The archivist of St Thomas' Hospital, London wrote that '[The] use of leeches was in high favor with physicians and surgeons alike ... accounting for 8% of the hospital's total expenditure in 1823 ... the last leech vanished from surgery about 1956' (McInnes, 1963).

The lowly leech (which secretes the anti-clotting agent, hirudin) was, however, reintroduced into medicine in the 1980s to help remove venous congestion of tissues following delicate microsurgery (Reynolds, 1996).

Mallow

The mallow used by the Greeks, *Malva sylvestris*, was the common or blue mallow. The name derives from *malakos*, Greek for 'soft', a reference to the plant's emollient effects as a medicine (Le Strange, 1977). Soranus mentions its application as a decoction, and as a pessary or poultice for: abortion; mastalgia; convulsions; the induction of labor; cleansing of the newborn; relief of dysmenorrhea; and prolapse (Temkin, 1956 pp. 229–39). Pliny's script is similar but also states that mallow is an aphrodisiac (Jones, 1989 book 20, pp. 129–35).

Marsh mallow (*Althaea officinalis*, derived from the Greek *altho*, to cure) is of the same family, but somewhat different, and is often confused with mallow. Together with the common mallow and other plants of the Malvaceae family, it was a favorite medicinal remedy for centuries. Dioscorides indicated that Marsh mallow was useful in inflammation of the breasts and uterus, stating that 'it is good for enflamed duggs ... for ye inflammations and preclusions of ye matrix ... and expelling also ye so-called after-purgaments' (Gunther, 1959 p. 388). His sentiments were shared by

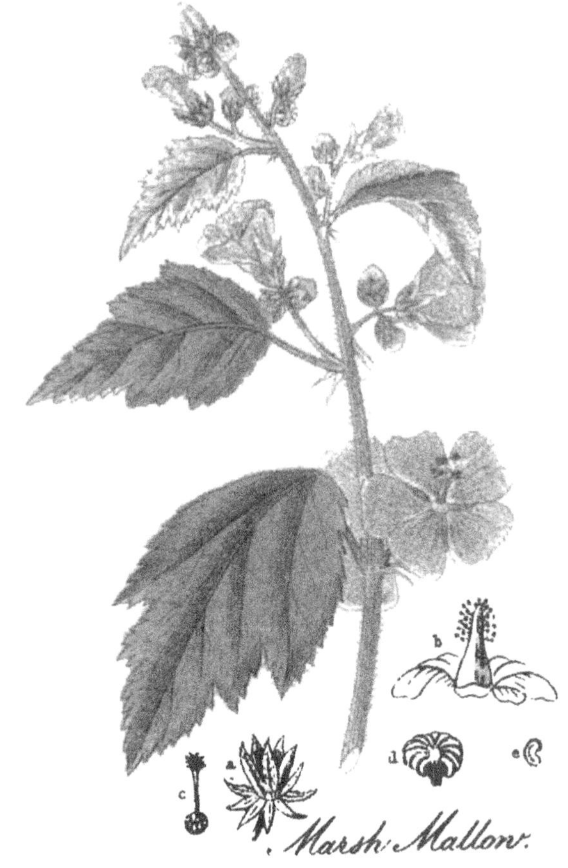

Figure 10 Marshmallow (*Malva* sp.)

Nicholas Culpeper (1653 p. 156) some 15 centuries later, and mallow still featured in the materia medica of the *Pharmacopoeia of the Royal College of Physicians of London* in the nineteenth century (Powell, 1815).

Marsh mallow contains mucilage, flavanoids, salicylin and other chemicals. It is noted for its anti-inflammatory, expectorant and demulcent actions and is still available as a herbal medicine (Wren, 1989).

Olive oil

Olive oil, obtained from the fruits of the evergreen tree (*Olea europaea*), was one of the most precious products of the ancient Eastern nations. In addition to its use as food, oil was applied as a body cleansing agent and was burnt in the sacred temples lamps. A crown of olive leaves was bestowed on victors in the Olympic Games.

Anointing with holy oil was an important religious ceremony and the word 'Messiah' means 'anointed'. The name 'Christ' in turn is the Greek equivalent of the Hebrew word for 'anointed' (Wootton, 1910).

Dioscorides documented that '[The] juice doth stay ... ye fluxum muliebrem ... move the urine and menses ... and doth expel the partus' (Gunther, 1959 pp. 74–7). Pliny noted the use of a woollen pessary impregnated with oil for excess menstruation and that lees (sediment) of oil was applied to genital ulcers (Jones, 1989 book 23, pp. 461–77). Soranus advised the application of olive oil to anoint midwives' fingers and to lubricate the genital tract while extolling its virtues as a medication for abortion, breast abscess, vaginal contraception, induction of labor, painful menstruation, cleansing of the newborn, uterine hemorrhage and other conditions (Temkin, 1956 pp. 233–4). The three authors agreed on its use as a vehicle for other medications.

Olive oil contains glycerides of oleic acid, and of linolenic, palmitic and stearic acids. It is a nutritive demulcent with a mild laxative action (Evans, 1996).

Rue

Rue (*Ruta graveolens*) is an evergreen plant native to southern Europe. The name of the genus Ruta comes from the Greek *rute* to set free (from illness), and was given because of its reputation for treatment of various diseases. Rue remained popular as a medicinal and magical drug through the ages. Sprigs of the plant were used to sprinkle holy water during religious ceremonies, and the plant became known by its synonym 'herb of grace'.

Rue was the most popular of the many medications utilized as an abortifacient and emmenagogue from Greek times onwards. Gunther's 1959 translation of Dioscorides reads: 'It [Rue] moves also ye menstrua ... but kills ye embrya' (pp. 286–8). Pliny agreed, noting that rue 'brings away the afterbirth and the fetus that has died before delivery'. He also stated that 'its use as food hinders the generative powers' (Jones, 1989 book 20, pp. 77–85). Soranus debated the differences between abortives and contraceptives and agreed that Rue was used for both purposes (Temkin, 1956 pp. 62–8).

Rue contains rutin and a large number of other active constituents. Not advised for use in pregnancy, it is still advocated as treatment for 'atonic amenorrhea' in the BHP (1983).

Wine

Wine, the fermented juice of the grape *Vitis vinifera* (and others) has an alcoholic content of up to 15%. Known to the Greeks as *oinos* and *vinum* to the Romans, wine was important commercially. Apart from its recreational use, it was used as a solvent and as a vehicle for numerous medications. The grape vine itself was a remedy for the heartburn and vomiting of pregnancy and the grape-skin and the lees were used for breast inflammation (Jones, 1989 book 23, pp. 435–61). The fruit was advised as a suitable food for pregnancy although wine was to be avoided in the early stages (Temkin, 1956 pp. 243–4). Grape seeds were thought suitable for the treatment of excess menstruation. Dioscorides' text contains a learned dissertation on the various sorts of wines and claims that Lesbian wine 'is good for ye ... lustful women'. He wrote of honey-wine or mead, oxymel (a vinegar and honey mixture) and medicated wines. Among the latter he mentions *oinos phthorios embruon*, abortion wine, which contains veratrum, wild cucumber and/or scammonie, and which is 'a wine destructive of embrya' (Gunther, 1959 pp. 607–23).

Medicated wines were an important part of the therapeutic armamentarium until 1930. In that year an 'International Agreement for the Unification of Pharmacopoeial Formulae for Potent Drugs' became operative (*British Pharmacopoeia*, 1932). The agreement contained the following statement: 'no potent drug shall be prepared in the form of a medicinal wine' – thus ending almost two millennia of medical history.

EXAMPLES FROM SORANUS' MATERIA MEDICA

Uses

Abortion

Absinthium, cardamom, cucumber, fenugreek, hellebore, iris, mallow, myrtle, rue, wormwood.

Application to cord
Heated pipe, warp, wool.

Breast abscess and inflammation
Bread, cabbage, celery, cumin, fenugreek, fig, linseed, saffron, sea sponges.

Painful breast
Fenugreek, linseed, mallow, olive oil, sea sponges, water.

To suppress milk
Alum, coriander, fleawort, heat, purslane, pyrite.

Candida, or oral thrush
Anthera remedy, black mulberry, cyperus, frankincense, honey, iris, lentils, myrrh, oak gall, plantain, pomegranate peel, poppyheads, rose, saffron, tamarisk.

Oral contraception
Cow parsnip, cyrenaic balm, myrtle, panax, pepper, rocket seed, rue, vinegar and honey, wallflower, wax.

Vaginal contraception
Balsam, cimolian earth, fig, gum, honey, natron, olive oil, panax, pomegranate peel, wool.

Convulsions
Castoreum, cedar, fenugreek, henna oil, mallow, mustard plasters, radish, sitz baths, spikenard, storax.

Diarrhea
Millet, plantain.

Labor, analgesia
Apples, bread, ground grain, gruel, liquid barley, melon, olive oil.

Labor, difficult
Fenugreek, linseed, mallow, olive oil.

Labor, oxytocic
Anise/aniseed, cedar resin, cucumber, dates, dittany, southernwood, sweet bay, olive oil.

Labor, induction
Cerate, fomentations, goose fat, hydromel, linseed, mallow, marrow, oily sitz bath, olive oil, sea sponges, sitz bath, water.

Menstruation, disorders of
Intense heat, mustard, natural water, radish, sitz bath.

Menstruation, for excess
Apples, grape seed, hare, lotus, myrtle, pine, pomegranate peel, quinces, samian earth, tart wine.

Menstruation, painful
Absinthium, bayberry, cumin, dill, leeches, linseed, marjoram, pitch plaster, sitz baths, tragos, warm fomentations.

Menstruation, to induce
Cucumber, cyrenaic balm, hellebore, panax.

Milk supply and quality
Bat, brine, caper, eggs, fish, garlic, leek, onion, owl, pig, pine, radish, sweet bay, vinegar.

Miscarriage
Absinthium.

Placenta delivery
Absinthium, cantharides, cassia, dittany, galbanum, myrrh, lilies, salvia, soapwort, spikenard.

Prolapse
Dates, dry cupping, fenugreek, mastich, moistened ashes, mustard, natron, pomegranate peel, salt, sea sponges, willow plasters.

Uterine hemorrhage
Acacia, cumin, frankincense, henbane, mastich, myrtle, nightshade, opium, sea sponges, sitz bath, willow.

Uterine inflammation
Bitumen, bread, butter, castoreum, leeches, nightshade, olive oil, rue, vinegar, warm fomentations.

Uterine tumor
Centaury, dittany, fig, goose fat, hyssop, iris, leeches, lily, natron, pennyroyal, radish.

Venereal disease
Acacia, bramble, cerate, chaste tree, dates, hemp, mastich, quince, rose, rue.

Selected remedies

Absinthium (wormwood), acacia, aloe, anise, antelope, aphronitre, apple, asparagus, asses' milk, assian stone.

Balsam, barley, bayberry, bitumen, black cumin, black mulberry, blackbird, bramble, bread, brimstone, brine, butter.

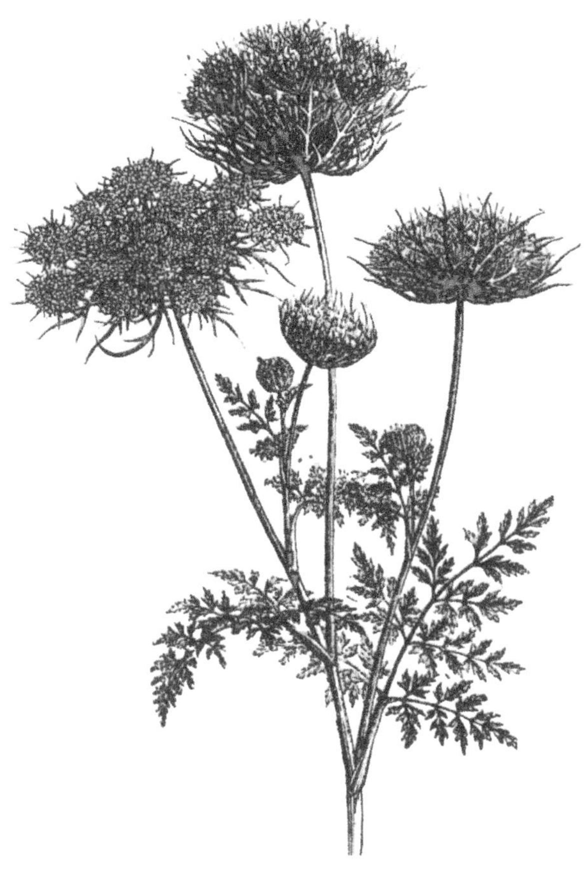

Figure 11 Carrot (*Daucus* sp.)

Cabbage, cantharis, carrot, cassia, castoreum, centaury, chaste tree, cimolian earth, coriander, cumin, cyclamen (sowbread), cyperus.

Dates, date salve deer, dill, diospolis remedy, dittany, duck.

Egg, endive.

Far wheat, fat, fenugreek, fig, fireweed, fish, fleabane, fleawort, flock, fowl, francolin, frankincense.

Galbanum, garlic, germander, ginger, goat's marjoram, goose fat, grapes, grape seed, ground grain, gum laudanum.

Halikakabon, hartshorn, hellebore, hemp, henbane, henna oil, honey, horehound, houseleek, hyssop.

Iris, ivy.

Kid, knotgrass.

Table 1 Greek and Roman weights and measures. Each of the weights and measures had symbols which indicated the quantity to be used

Dry measures	
Name	*Weight (g)*
Libra/Pondus	336.00
Uncia	28.00
Denarius/drachma	4.00
Scripulum	1.16
Obolus	0.66
Liquid measures	
Name	*Volume (l)*
Amphora	30.000
Sextarius	0.500
Heminae	0.250
Acetabulum	0.063
Cyathus	0.042

Lamb, lead, leek, lemon, lentils, licorice, lily, linseed, litharge, lotus, lupins.

Mallow, marjoram, mastich, medlars, melilot, melon, millet, mustard, myrrh, myrtle.

Narcissus, nard oil (spikenard), natron, natural water, navelwort, nettle, nightshade, nosemart.

Oak gall, olive oil, omphakion, onion, opium, owl, ox bile, ox fat, ox meat, oxymel.

Parsley, partridge, pellitory, pennyroyal, pepper, pine, plantain, pomegranate, poppy, pulses, purslane.

Quince.

Radish, raisin, red mullet, rennet, resin, ring-dove, roasted fowl, rocket, rose, rue.

Saffron, samian earth, sea sponges, sesame, soapwort, southernwood, spikenard, storax, sweet bay (laurel bay), Syrian unguent.

Tamarisk, tanning sumach, tart wine, Theban dates, thrush, tragacanth, tragos, tribulus, trumpet shell, turpentine.

Urine.

Vaginal suppositories, vegetables, vine, vinegar.

Wallflower, warm fomentations, waters natural, wax, wheat, white lead, willow, wine, wool, wormwood.

GLOSSARY OF GRECO-ROMAN MEDICAL TERMS

The earlier Greek and Roman physicians prepared the medicines they prescribed for their patients. As time went by many other workers became involved in the collection and preparation of medications. There were often several names for those connected with medicine and pharmacy.

Apotheke Greek for 'storehouse', giving rise to the term 'apothecary'. The original apothecaries were pounders and mixers of herbs. Apothecaries' weights and liquid measures based on the 'troy ounce' (Troyes, France) were in use until 1965 and converted the pound into 5760 grains, divisible into 12 ounces of 20 pennyweight (one pennyweight corresponds to 24 grains of Troy weight).
Botanologoi herbalists.
Medicae, female healers.
Medicamentarii Latin, the group of Greek physicians whose history corresponds closely with that of the English apothecaries. In Alexandria and in Rome they gradually assumed the position of general practitioners.
Medici, Roman physicians.
Migmatopolos seller of mixtures.
Myropoeos maker of ointments.
Obstetricie midwives.
Pharmacopaei professional poisoners and those who sold philters and abortifacients.
Pharmacopeus Greek, a handler of drugs, who occasionally sold philters or poisons.
Pharmacopolae drug peddlers.
Pharmacopoli druggists.
Pharmacotribae drug grinders.
Pharmakeia Greek, the preparation of medicines or poisons, giving rise to the term 'pharmacy'.
Pharmakon Greek, and **medicamentus**, Latin, could mean either 'medicine' or 'poison'.
Pharmakopoeos maker of remedies.
Pharmakopolos itinerant drug seller.
Pigmentarii maker of cosmetics.
Rhizotomi root gatherers who collected vegetable simples.
Sagaer wise-women.
Seplasia or **Medicina** Roman name for a druggist's shop.
Seplasiarii and **Ungentarii** ointment makers.

References

Adams, F. (1864). *The Seven Books of Paul of Aegineta*. (London: The Sydenham Society)

Bown, D. (1996). *The Royal Horticultural Society Encyclopedia of Herbs*, pp. 243–4. (London: Dorling Kindersley)

British Herbal Medicine Association (1983). *British Herbal Pharmacopoeia*, pp. 183–4. (Bournemouth, UK)

The General Medical Council (1932). *British Pharmacopoeia*, pp. xxi–xxv. (London: Constable and Co.)

Chadwick, J., Mann, W. N., Withington, E. T. and Lonie, I. M. (1983). *Hippocratic Writings*, pp. 206–36. (London: Penguin Books)

Cowen, D. L. and Helfand, W. H. (1990). *Pharmacy. An Illustrated History*, p. 36. (New York: Harry N. Abrams Inc.)

Culpeper, N. (1653). *The English Physician, Enlarged*, Wordworth Edition (1955), pp. 52, 156. (UK: Wordsworth)

Dally, A. (1991). *Women Under the Knife*, p. 161. (London: Hutchinson Radius)

Dorland, W. A. N. (1932). *The American Illustrated Medical Dictionary*, p. 249. (Philadelphia and London: W. B. Saunders Co.)

Einarson, B. and Link, G. K. K. (1976). *Theophrastus. De Causis Plantarum*. (London: Heinemann Ltd. & Cambridge MA: Harvard University Press)

Evans, W. C. (1996). *Trease and Evan's Pharmacognosy*, pp. 185–6. (London: W. B. Saunders Co.)

Garrison, F. H. (1929). *An Introduction to the History of Medicine*, pp. 79–120, 409. (Philadelphia and London: W. B. Saunders Co.)

Grigson, G. (1996). *The Englishman's Flora*, pp. 53–4. (Oxford: Helicon Publishing Ltd.)

Gunther, R. T. (1959). *The Greek Herbal of Dioscorides*, pp. 74–7, 159–60, 286–8, 388, 607–23. (New York: Hafner Publishing Co.)

Guthrie, D. (1947). *A History of Medicine*, p. 54. (London: Thomas Nelson & Sons Ltd.)

Harris, J. R. (1916). *The Origin of the Cult of Artemis*, p. 20. (Manchester: The University Press)

Hort, A. (Sir) (1980). *Theophrastus. Inquiry into Plants and Minor Works on Odours and Weather Signs*. (Cambridge, MA: Harvard University Press & London: Heinemann Ltd.)

Jones, W. H. S. (1989). *Pliny. Natural History*, Vol. 6, book 20, pp. 20, 47–55, 77–85, 117, 129–35; book, 21, p. 285, Vol. 6, book, 23, pp. 461–77, 435–61. (Cambridge, MA and London: Harvard University Press)

Le Strange, R. (1977). *A History of Herbal Plants*, pp. 171–2. (London: Angus and Robertson)

Leake, C. D. (1975). *An Historical Account of Pharmacology to the 20th Century*, p. 60. (Springfield, IL: Charles C. Thomas)

Mann, E. W. (1915). *Southall's Organic Materia Medica*, p. 333. (London: J. and A. Churchill)

McInnes, E. M. (1963). *St. Thomas' Hospital*, p. 90. (London: George Allen and Unwin Ltd.)

Ody, P. (1993). *The Herb Society's Complete Medicinal Herbal*, p. 42. (London: Dorling Kindersley)

Paris, J. A. (1822). *Pharmacologia*, Vol. 2, pp. 129–30. (London: W. Phillips)

Powell, R. (1815). *The Pharmacopoeia of the Royal College of Physicians of London*, Third edition, p. 35. (London: Longman, Hurst, Rees, Orme and Brown)

Reynolds, J. E. F. (ed.) (1982). *Martindale. The Extra Pharmacopoeia*, p. 1692. (London: The Pharmaceutical Press)

Reynolds, J. E. F. (ed.) (1996). *Martindale. The Extra Pharmacopoeia*, p. 898. (London: Royal Pharmaceutical Society)

Ricci, J. V. (1950). *Aetius of Ameda. The Gynecology and Obstetrics of the 6th Century AD*, Translated from the Latin edition of Cornarius, 1542 and fully annotated. (Philadelphia: The Blakiston Co.)

Riddle, J. M. (1985). *Dioscorides on Pharmacy and Medicine*. (Austin, Texas: University of Texas Press)

Riddle, J. M. (1992). *Contraception and Abortion from the Ancient World to the Renaissance*. (Cambridge, MA: Harvard University Press)

Riddle, J. M. (1997). *Eve's Herbs. A History of Contraception and Abortion in the West*. (Cambridge, MA: Harvard University Press)

Spencer, W. G. (1989). *Celsus. De Medicina*, Vol. 2, p. xxv. (Cambridge, MA: Harvard University Press & London: Heinemann Ltd.)

Squire, P. W. (1908). *Squire's Companion to the latest edition of the British Pharmacopoeia*, pp. 597–8. (London: J. and A. Churchill)

Temkin, O. (1956). *Soranus' Gynecology*. Translation. pp. 62–8, 138, 147, 160, 229–39, 233–234, 243–44. (Baltimore, MD & London: The Johns Hopkins University Press)

Turner, W. (1568). *The Herbal*, p. 16. (Imprinted at Collen by Arnold Birchman)

Whalley, J. I. (1982). *Pliny the Elder. Historia Naturalis*. (London: Victoria & Albert Museum)

Wootton, A. C. (1910). *Chronicles of Pharmacy*, Vol. 1, pp. 12, 58–60, 217, Vol. 2, p. 139. (London: Macmillan & Co.)

Wren, R. C. (1989). *Potter's New Cyclopaedia of Botanical Drugs and Preparations*, pp. 184–5. (Essex, UK: C. W. Daniel Company Ltd.)

Byzantium 10

INTRODUCTION

The ancient Greek city of Byzantium was founded on the Bosphorus c. 660 BC. Constantine I restored the city to its former glory in AD 330 and thereafter the metropolis became known as Constantinople, present-day Istanbul. In the fourth century AD the Emperor Diocletian divided the Roman Empire into two portions for administrative purposes. The western region had its capital at Rome, while Byzantium was chosen as the chief city in the east. When the last Roman emperor was deposed in AD 476, the Byzantine Empire came into being and it flourished until the fall of Constantinople in 1453.

The Byzantine period of medicine flowered from AD 476 to 732. According to the eminent American medical historian Fielding H. Garrison (1929), the medical history of Byzantium was chiefly concerned with the four prominent physicians who practiced medicine during the first three centuries of the Byzantine era: Paul of Aegina, Oribasius of Pergamum, Aetius of Amida, and Alexander of Tralles. The four physicians were also known as encyclopedists because they compiled anthologies of the medical works of their illustrious predecessors. Centuries later when medicine went through its dark ages in Europe the Byzantine medical writings were translated into Arabic and Western medical tradition was kept alive.

ORIBASIUS OF PERGAMUM (AD 325–403)

The first of the eminent Byzantine medical compilers, Oribasius, was born in the city of Pergamum, the birth place of Galen, the most renowned of all Greco-Roman physicians. Oribasius studied medicine in Alexandria and moved to Constantinople, where he became physician to Julian the Apostate, a grand-nephew of Constantine the Great. When Julian became emperor he entrusted Oribasius with the task of compiling the medical works of authors dating from ancient Greece until his own time. As a result, Oribasius produced an encyclopedia of medicine which consisted of 72 books. Much of his remarkable anthology was eventually lost but Oribasius epitomized his work in a small book, *Synopsis*, which he wrote for his physician son, and a *Euporista*, a treatise on diet, hygiene and household medical lore for laymen.

The *Euporista* contained a chapter entitled 'De Partu' which gave a detailed description of postnatal care. Oribasius discussed the three terms used by the ancients to describe the uterus: the delphos, the hysteros and the matrix. The term 'delphos' came about because the womb engendered males or brothers. The uterus was called 'hysteros' because it functioned later (after the menarche). It was called 'matrix' for two reasons: first, it was the 'mother' because it engendered offspring, and second, it 'measured the menstrual cycle'. Oribasius was aware of a relationship between the breasts and the uterus, noting that during regular menstrual cycles lactation did not occur, and that during breastfeeding the menses ceased. Oribasius followed Galenical tradition and wrote of food or medications (of which he offered 14) which increased lactation or induced the menstrual flow.

In his book *The Genealogy of Gynecology*, James V. Ricci, professor of obstetrics and gynecology, New York Medical College, gave a résumé of the gynecological references in the *Collectio Medicinalia* of Oribasius, extracted from French and Greek translations. The following materia medica is compiled from Ricci's text (1943 pp. 171–80).

Amenorrhea

If amenorrhea continued despite bandaging of the lower limbs, bloodletting, diet, massage of the pubes and legs, and purgation, specific medications were resorted to:

Decoctions (boiled extracts) of cabbage roots, castoreum, leek, myrrh, pepper and rue in honey or sweet wine

Pessaries (aperient tampons) containing aromatic oils, ashes of dried grape-pulp, ass and goose-fat, blossoms of wild glasswort, cyperus plant, mandragora juice, mouse-dung, oil of narcissus, ox-gall, powdered quince, salt, storax, wormwood
Vaginal douches with lily water followed by tampons or plasters of mustard to the pubic area.

Contraception

Application anointing the male parts with a juice of hedyosme
Potion extract of leaves of cabbage, male fern roots or leaves of the willow tree in sweet wine
Tampon powdered cabbage flowers introduced into the vagina after intercourse to 'prevent the semen from coagulating'.

Medicated tampons

Aperient tampons (laxatives) were used to provoke menstruation, to remedy cervical occlusion or to relax a contracted uterus
Astringent tampons (to contract tissues and stop bleeding and discharge) were used for contraception, to 'contract' the uterus and for utero-vaginal discharge or prolapse
Emollient tampons (to soften and relax tissues and protect sensitive areas) were used when the uterus was 'cold', displaced, inflamed, or swollen with gas. These tampons were prepared with oil or a fatty base such as chicken fat, goose grease, oil of henna or lily, reindeer marrow, sweet butter, or wax.

Menorrhagia

Diet of acacia, juice of pomegranate flowers and dried green raisins
Vaginal sponge with acacia cinders soaked in tar
Woolen tampons with oil of myrtle leaves, rose oil and wine.

Uterus

Carcinoma
Tampons of saffron and opium in woman's milk to alleviate pain.
Inflammation
A cataplasm made with flowers of fenugreek.
Prolapse
A fumigation with malodorous substances such as (burnt) feathers, hair, leeches, sponges and wool (to force the uterus to flee back into the pelvis).
Suffocation
Castoreum diluted with vinegar.
Suppuration
Applications of fenugreek, linseed or barley seeds and pigeon dung.

Vulva

Fissures
Powdered lilies, honey and turpentine applications
Inflammation
Enemas of linseed meal or milk.

AETIUS OF AMIDA (SIXTH CENTURY AD)

According to James Ricci, 'Aetius of Amida [in Mesopotamia] was the first eminent Christian physician of antiquity. He studied medicine at Alexandria and practiced at Byzantium where he became the royal physician to Emperor Justinian the First' (1943 pp. 180–95). Aetius wrote an extensive compilation, *Tetrabiblion*, which contained a mixture of Greek medical tradition and Christian mysticism. The sixteenth book of the series dealt with women's disorders and was a summary of the accumulated gynecological knowledge of the Greco-Roman world rather than an original work. Aetius' epitome was used by Paul of Aegina in the following century, and was the authoritative text on gynecology until well after the twelfth century.

Aetius' tract on gynecology consisted of 123 short chapters. He described the pelvic anatomy and methods for examining the uterus and its appendages. Sections on diseases of the external genitalia, the vagina and the cervix were included. Regarding the uterus, he wrote on abscess, cancer, hydrops, inflammation, malposition, prolapse, ulceration and other disorders including leukorrhea. Aetius wrote about normal menstruation and the problems of amenorrhoea and menorrhagia. According to Ricci, Aetius of Amida was the first author among the ancients to mention cloves and camphor as drugs.

Amenorrhea

Aetius believed that amenorrhea resulted from a 'hot temperament' and advised 'cooling' foods such as cucumber, fish, fowl, grapes, lamb, lettuce, milk, ptisan (decoction of barley), and weak white wine. Suitable medications included calamint, cassia, savin, spikenard or thyme, drunk in old white wine, as well as vaginal suppositories and purgatives. If these various preparations failed, venesection was resorted to, provided that the patient was plethoric.

Contraception

Aetius quoted 18 contraceptive prescriptions, including wool tampons soaked in wine containing pine bark and tanning fluid, applied two hours before coitus; pomegranate rind in water or mixed with acorns in wine; wine with myrrh, dried and used as a suppository; and pulp of dried figs soaked in wine. If taken on a regular basis coriander seeds were thought to produce permanent sterility.

Menorrhagia

In the treatment of menorrhagia, Aetius advised anointing the limbs with myrtle oil, quince oil, rose oil or wine, and then the application of constrictive bandages to the limbs in an effort to reduce blood flow to the uterus. Cupping of the breasts was also deemed useful.

ALEXANDER OF TRALLES (AD 525–605)

This much-traveled medical practitioner settled in Rome and according to Garrison (1929), although mainly an encyclopedist, he was 'the only one of the Byzantine compilers who displayed any special originality. While Alexander was a follower of Galen, his *Practica* [first printed at Lyons in 1504] contained descriptions of disease and some prescriptions which seemed to be his own ... [he was] said to have been the first to mention rhubarb'. Alexander of Tralles is frequently mentioned by later writers. He was the first to fully describe worms and their treatment with vermifuges, for which he was accorded the appellation 'The first parasitologist'. Among the medications he used for women were fenugreek, linseed, pomegranate oil, poppy heads, rose oil and turpentine. In his major treatise, *The History of Ancient Gynaecology*, W.J. Stewart McKay of Sydney (1901) wrote that Alexander had copied from Aetius of Amida.

Alexander was the first to mention the sponge-tent, for dilating the cervix, a technique that was still practiced for dysmenorrhea in the early twentieth century. Other forms of treatment mentioned by him were: bleeding, cataplasms, counter-irritation, cautery, cupping, fomentations, fumigations, and massage. He also recorded use of rectal irrigation, rectal pessaries, sitz-baths, sponge-tents, vaginal irrigation, vaginal pessaries, vaginal plugs.

PAUL OF AEGINA (AD 625–690)

Paul of Aegina, or Paulus AEgineta as he was known until the twentieth century, was the last of the great Byzantine medical compilers and was born on the island of Aegina, close to Athens. Paul became a physician and surgeon of high repute but had a special interest in gynecology and obstetrics. Paul's treatise *Epitome medicae libri septum* was a link between Soranus of the second century (who wrote the finest treatise on diseases of women during the Greco-Roman period), Aetius, and the Arabian authors. In their own works the Arabian authors quoted Paul repeatedly. After the death of Paul of Aegina, the influence of Byzantine medicine continued, but was sterile and imitative. Later, as related by James Ricci, 'The revival of learning in Christian Europe, instigated in a great measure by the wholesome translations of the Arabic manuals into Latin, kept Paul's gynecology in the fore. And when, following the capture of Constantinople in 1453, the Greek originals reached Italy, Paul of Aegina again rose to merited heights' (Ricci, 1943 pp. 195–207).

Paul was of the opinion that the ancient authors had written all that was required about the art of medicine. His own desire was to produce a compendium useful to himself and to those of his contemporaries who did not wish to read the elaborate treatises of the ancient authors. Oribasius' encyclopedia of 70 books was much too bulky and expensive, while his *Synopsis* and his *Euporista* were too brief. Paul wrote a medium-sized seven-volume treatise to fill the void and his text included the existing knowledge of medicine, surgery, obstetrics, gynecology and pediatrics. *The Seven Books of Paulus Aegineta* were translated by Francis Adams for the Sydenham Society in the nineteenth century. Francis Adams' own treatise ran to three volumes, with 1847 pages, and commented on the opinions of the Greek, Roman, Byzantine and Arab writers on all the subjects discussed by Paul of Aegina. Francis Adams' first volume was published in 1843 and re-issued in 1844. The remaining volumes were published in 1846 and 1847.

There are a hundred chapters in Paul's first book with titles such as:- 'On the complaints of Pregnant Women, and their Diet'; 'On the Nurse'; 'On the Milk of the Nurse'; 'How to correct the bad qualities of Milk'; 'On Venery'; 'On Impotence'; 'On Inordinate Venery'; 'On Redundance of Semen'; 'On Emmenagogues' and 'Diagnosis of the Temperaments of the Testicles'. Paul's third book dealt with various medical complaints, including the chapters: 'On Affections of the Breasts'; 'On Inflammation of the Testicles and Scrotum, and on the other diseases of these parts'; 'On Gonorrhea and Libidinous Dreams'; 'On Satyriasis'; 'On Priapism' and 'On Impotence of the Parts'. There were a further 17 chapters regarding uterine disorders and a final one entitled 'On Difficult Labor'.

Paul's seventh book, which is contained in Francis Adams' third volume, dealt with materia medica and the 'Powers of Simples Individually'. There is a valuable appendix of 56 pages entitled 'On the Substances introduced into the Materia Medica by the Arabians'. In the section 'On Pessaries' Adams quoted from the work of Antyllus (one of the most daring and accomplished surgeons of the era. Most of his works are lost but are known through the compilations of Oribasius) and pointed out that pessaries of Greco-Roman times were medicated tampons as distinct from the more modern pessaries, which were designed to prevent prolapse.

Medicated vaginal pessaries

A number of vaginal pessaries and their constituents and uses were detailed by Paul of Aegina, They included the Egyptian pessary 'for when the parts were foul' but without inflammation; the golden pessary as an emollient; the Libian pessary, an emmenagogue; the pessary called 'genitura', for conception; the pessary enneapharmacus, a cure-all; the saffron pessary for inflammations; and the titian emollient pessary' (Adams, 1847 pp. 601–2).

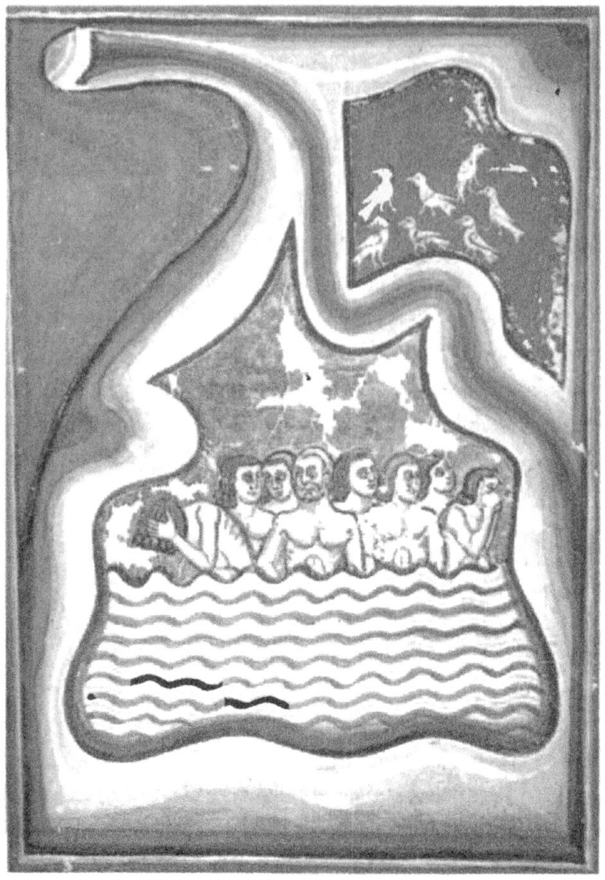

Figure 1 Bathing as a form of medical treatment

The saffron tampon contained calf marrow, fowl grease, goose grease, honey, mastich, oesypium, rose oil, saffron, stag marrow, and white wax.

The Libian tampon contained bulls tallow, fowl grease, fresh hog lard, goose grease, nard ointment, oesypium, ointment of amaracus, ointment of lilies, stag marrow, Tuscan wax, and turpentine.

The genitura tampon contained aloes, butter, cassia, fowl grease, goose grease, honey, myrrh, oesypium, oil of rose, spikenard, stag marrow, Tuscan wax, turpentine.

Emollient pessaries or tampons, for use in 'inflammations of the womb', were prepared from burnt rosin, fat from geese and fowl, fenugreek, oil of privet and of lilies, stag marrow, Tuscan wax and unsalted butter.

Anastomotic pessaries (to 'open the mouths' of vessels) were used to induce menstruation. They were prepared from dittany, honey, juice of cabbage, juice of horehound, liquorice, mugwort, rue, and scammony.

Astringent pessaries were applied to 'restrain' female discharge and contained acacia, alum, juice of plantain, juice of roses or omphacium.

The **emmenagogue pessary** contained birthwort, castoreum, cumin, ginger, honey, musk, pulp of colocynth and rue mixed with suet or wax.

Adams noted that the most prolific writer on the subject of pessaries was Myrepsus who had described the preparation of 45 pessaries.

A SELECTION OF BYZANTINE MATERIA MEDICA FOR WOMEN

Alum

Alum takes it's name from the Latin, *alumen*. In its basic form, alum exists as crystals of a double sulfate of aluminum and potassium. Alum is obtained from a shale consisting of alum, clay, coaly aterial and iron pyrites. (Alum should not be confused with alum root, which is an American plant of the Saxifrage family, with astringent properties.) Francis Adams described three forms of alum: stone alum, round alum and liquid alum (Adams, 1847 vol. 3, pp. 360–1). The substance was used as a medication from earliest times and Hippocrates prescribed application of alum for ulceration of the uterus. Dioscorides wrote of its astringent qualities and apart from alum being 'smeared on for ye Oedemata and for ye rank smells of ye armpits and ye groins', he advised that the medication 'co-operates to inconception, being laid before conjunction on ye mouth of ye matrix, and it expels ye Embrya'. Dioscorides also found that it was a useful preparation for 'excrescencies' of the privities' (Gunther, 1959 pp. 642–3).

During the Byzantine era Paul of Aegina advised powdered round alum with herbs as an application for hemorrhoids and described its use: as a vaginal contraceptive; for soothing genital lesions; for uterine hemorrhage; and for fissures or condylomata in the genital area (Adams, 1844 vol. 1, p. 603). Alum retained its popularity as a medication in obstetrics and gynecology through the centuries. James Wolveridge advised a *tutia* of burnt alum, red lead, pompholyx, and sugar candy for application to the breast to suppress milk formation and to prevent inflammation (1671 p. 139). In France, the most famous obstetrician of the seventeenth century, François Mauriceau, the Parisian accoucheur, wrote in 1683 of painful nipples during breastfeeding 'to these sore nipples desiccative Medicines may be applied, as Allum ... but especially care must be taken, that nothing be applied to disgust the Childe, wherefore many content themselves to use only Honey of Roses'. Mauriceau prescribed alum for application to bleeding hemorrhoids in pregnancy, and also to the newborn's cord.

At the beginning of the twentieth century, William Wyatt Squire in his *Companion to the British Pharmacopoeia* described alumen or alum as salts of potash alum and of ammonia alum. He wrote that alum was an astringent that could be prescribed 'as an injection for leucorrhoea and gonorrhoea, 60 grains in a pint of water ... also for menorrhagia' (1908 pp. 125–7). Alum was also advised for leukorrhea in *Dorland's Medical Dictionary* (1932 p. 60). Alum products are still used as astringents to check exudative secretions and minor hemorrhage. Reynolds, editor of *Martindale, The Extra Pharmacopoeia* (1982), noted that alum may be used as an antiperspirant, as a foot powder, and as a pediatric 'alum and zinc dusting-powder' to be applied to the umbilical cord (p. 283).

Cantharides

Cantharis is Latin for the Spanish fly or blister beetle of the order Coleoptera (Evans, 1996). The medicinal *cantharis* of the ancients, found in corn or wheat, was the *Mylabris Cichorii* or *Mylabris Fusselini*. The ancient Greeks prepared the beetles for medicinal use by killing them with heated vinegar fumes. The bodies were allowed to dry out and were powdered (forming 'cantharides') before being added to a prescription.

The Greek tradition of preparing cantharides continued until the middle of the twentieth century.

In Greco-Roman times, Dioscorides detailed the preparation of cantharides and wrote of the 'Buprestes': 'a kinde of the Cantharides ... They provoke the Menses, being mixed with mollifying Pessums' (Gunther, 1959 p. 106). Galen (AD 130–200) copied Dioscorides, and eight centuries later, the Arab writers borrowed from both. The dried bodies of the beetles were also availed of to induce blistering, in an effort to relieve pain by counter-irritation. Alexander of Tralles was the first to use cantharides, as a blistering agent in the treatment of gout (Wootton, 1910).

Cantharides was included in love potions and cooked in biscuits, cakes and pastries or inserted into candies and chocolates and ingested by budding Casanovas or their unwitting consorts. The French have long favored Spanish fly and Madame Pompadour is said to have used tincture of cantharides to regain the love of Louis XV (Warburton, 1995). Cantharides exerted irritant and stimulatory effects on the urogenital system and because of ... 'the sympathy existing between the genitary and urinary tracts ... [cantharides] often produced erection of the penis [useful in the impotence of] old age, and in that resulting from self-abuse or sexual excess'. The intense congestion and irritation of the urethral mucosa far outlived the ejaculatory act and the cantharides abuser suffered wretchedly for many hours. Perhaps that was why cantharides was prescribed for unauthorized 'Seminal Emissions' (Ringer, 1888). The ultimate in trivia knowledge on cantharides was related by Walter Dixon in 1913 in his *Manual of Pharmacology* where he wrote that the hedgehog was immune to the effects of Spanish fly!

At the dawn of the twentieth century, Hobart Amory Hare of Philadelphia opined that 'When given by mouth the tincture [cantharides] is used as a uterine stimulant [to relieve amenorrhoea and] is of value in incontinence of urine of a minor degree' (1901). Peter Wyeth Squire (1908) referred to cantharides as *Cantharis vesicatoria* (related to *Mylabris phalerata*) and of its medicinal properties he noted that an ***emplastrum*** or ***liquor epispasticus*** was used to relieve inflammation, pain and swelling 'in deep parts.... Internally in small doses it is diuretic and aphrodisiac. It is given in gleet [mucus discharge], in impotence, and incontinence of urine due to paralysis'. Squire listed seven official preparations (1908 p. 317). W.A. Newman Dorland wrote that 'Cantharides are applied externally as powerful rubefacient and blistering agents; in moderate internal doses they are diuretic and stimulant to the urinary and reproductive organs; they are highly poisonous in large doses. Dose of the tincture, 1–20 minims (1.3 cc)' (1932 p. 237).

Powdered cantharides was gray-brown in color with shiny green particles and had a strong disagreeable odor. The active principle, cantharidin, was found to be a lactone. When taken internally it acted as a very powerful irritant. Cantharidin plasters contained 0.2% of the lactone and were employed to cause blistering and redness in restricted areas of the skin. Application of cantharidin to the mucus membranes caused intense irritation, pain and blistering. Cantharides owed its reputation as an aphrodisiac to profound irritation of the urethra caused by the passage of urine containing dissolved cantharidin (Lewis, 1964). Cantharidin was found to be highly toxic and the fatal dose was less than 60 mg. It was nephrotoxic and had multiple constitutional effects. Cantharides was prescribed to remove skin lesions such as warts and was in common medicinal use until the mid-twentieth century.

Fig

The fig is the dried fleshy receptacle of *Ficus carica* and takes its name from the French, *figue*. The fig was cultivated from earliest times in ancient Greece. Fig was an old name for a hemorrhoidal tumor or for the venereal wart, condyloma acuminata. The fig leaf was used to veil the naked 'private parts' of humans or human images as statues or in pictures: 'Then the eyes of both were opened and they realized that they were naked. So they sewed fig leaves together and made themselves skirts' (Genesis 3: 7). Dioscorides was aware that figs 'loosen the belly' and that figs applied locally in a plaster reduced inflammation. They were 'mixed also in Cataplasmes of barley-meal for women's fomentations with Foenigreec' (Gunther, 1959 p. 90). Soranus of Ephesus mentioned fig as a locally-active contraceptive; as an inhibitor of milk secretion; and as a medicinal suppository in uterine infection (Temkin, 1956 pp. 223–4).

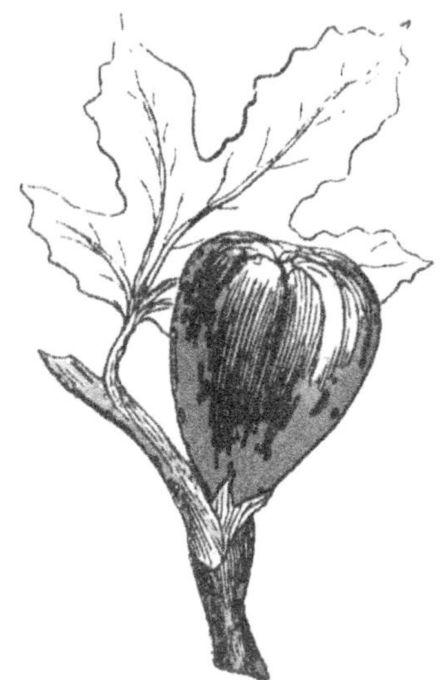

Figure 2 Fig (*Ficus* sp.)

Paul of Aegina applied a cataplasm of dried figs with rue, frankincense and other medications for cancer of the uterus (Adams, 1844 vol. 1, p. 257) and also mentioned the use of fig for constipation, uterine inflammation and penile swelling. In the Middle Ages, figs were thought to 'increase the seed' and were an important component of medications for disease of the uterus (Rowland, 1981 pp. 95; 117). The fig was one of a number of medications present in an ointment for 'hard and difficult births' prescribed by James Wolveridge 'in a posset to facilitate the birth, drive out the secundine, false conception or dead child'. He also prescribed figs in a suppository for convulsions (1671 pp. 126; 130; 160).

Squire confirmed that the fig was demulcent, laxative and nutritious: 'cheaply used medicinally in constipation. Cut open and heated, it forms a convenient cataplasm' (1908 p. 538). Officially it was contained in *confectio sennae* and also compound syrup of figs, a mixture of figs and senna. Figs were prescribed for pregnant women at term to relieve constipation and to induce labor. The fig is still in use today as a demulcent and laxative.

Gall

A gall (Latin, *galla*) is an abnormal growth on a plant caused by parasitic infestation. The oak galls of commerce and medicine are excrescences on the *Quercus infectoria*, a small oak indigenous to Asia Minor and Persia. The galls result from the puncture of the bark of the young twigs by the female gall wasp, *Cynipis gallae-tinctoriae*, which lays its eggs inside. The larvae of the hatched eggs feed on the plant tissues and secrete a fluid which stimulates rapid growth of the tissue and formation of a gall, or gall nut. The galls are hard, heavy and globular and measure 12 to 18 mm in diameter. The Aleppo or Turkey galls were the most esteemed and were found in blue, green and white varieties. Other galls in commercial use were the English, Chinese and Mecca galls (also known as Dead Sea apples). The galls contain gallo-tannic and gallic acids and were used as powerful astringents (Mann, 1915).

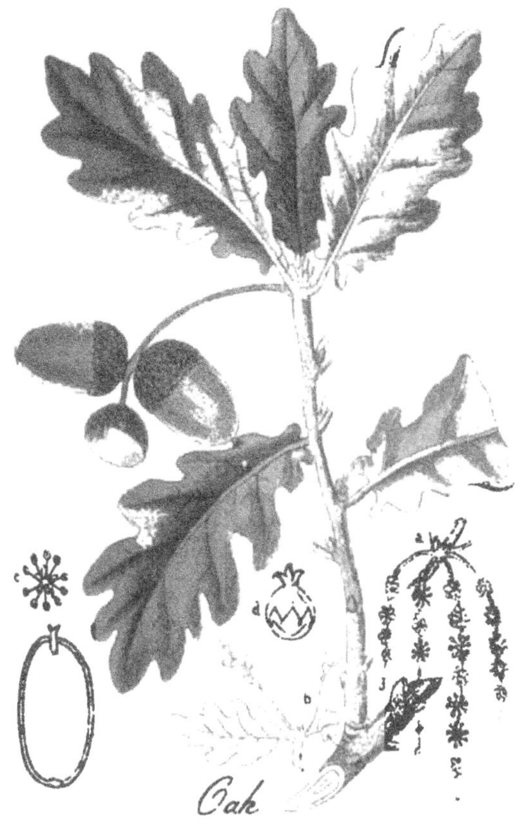

Figure 3 Oak (*Quercus* sp.)

Dioscorides described the gall as 'the fruit of the Oake, somme of it is called Omphacitis ... the decoction of them is good by insession, for ye procidentes vulvas and ye fluxes' (Gunther, 1959 pp. 77–8).

Soranus of Ephesus used *omphakitis* (oak gall) in the treatment of uterine hemorrhage (Temkin, 1956 p. 234). The oak galls should not be mistaken for gall or bile obtained from gallbladders of various beasts. The bile was dried, powdered, and used in an ointment for maternal convulsions (Wolveridge, 1671).

Medicinally, galls are the most powerful of all vegetable astringents and were much used to treat gleet (excess mucous discharge) gonorrhea and leukorrhea. *Ungentum gallae* (gall mixed with benzoated lard) was a popular medication for painful hemorrhoids (Squire, 1908). Gall extract was available as a decoction or tincture, and in suppositories and unguents. Commercially, galls are employed in tanning and dyeing and gallic acid, obtained in crystalline form from gall nuts, was once used for making ink.

Linseed

Linseed, also known as lintseed or flax seed, is the dried ripe seed of *Linum usitatissimum*, a medicinal herb that was cultivated from earliest times. Linseed contains mucilage, and an oil which can be obtained by expressing the seed. Extract of linseed was found to be emollient and demulcent and was much used to treat superficial or deep seated inflammation in the form of a poultice to relieve irritation and pain and to promote suppuration (Grieve, 1931).

Dioscorides, the ancient Greek authority on materia medica, thought that linseed was aphrodisiac and commended it as an enema for 'erosions of the bowells and the wombe … [and] being taken by way of incession for the inflammations which are in the wombe' (Gunther, 1959 p. 136). Paul of Aegina used cataplasms laced with linseed, barley, fenugreek, and other herbal medications to promote suppuration of uterine abscess, for uterine cancer (Adams, 1847 vol. 3, p. 230), for sore testicles and as an aid in difficult labor. During the Middle Ages, linseed was prescribed for similar indications but also for the excessive and painful menstruation that was 'concerned with inflammation of the uterus, that is very sore' (Rowland, 1981 p. 115).

Linseed oil mixed with an equal quantity of limewater was known as 'carron oil' and was applied to burns and scalds. When exposed to oxygen, linseed oil formed a hard transparent varnish and was used in fine arts for its properties as a drying oil. Flax was used for cord and sail cloth and a finer version became known as linen, the cloth from which Biblical garments were fashioned. Until cotton came into ready supply in the eighteenth century, flax and hemp were the most important vegetable fibers. The term 'flax' is derived from old English *flaex* and the German *flachs*.

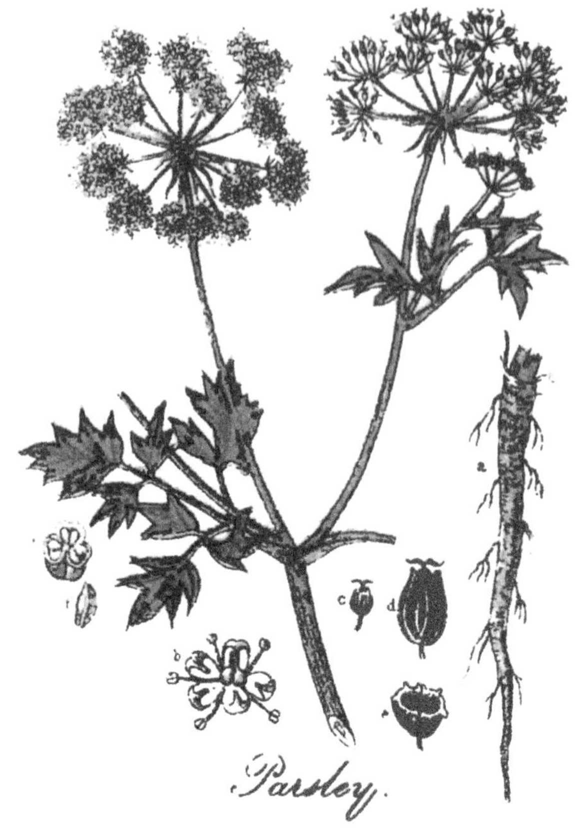

Figure 4 Parsley (*Petroselinum* sp.)

Modern observers agree with ancient belief in the curative properties of linseed: an entry in *Martindale* reports that linseed is demulcent and can be used as a bulk laxative (Reynolds, 1982 p. 957) and in the *British Herbal Pharmacopoeia* (1991 p. 132) the actions of *Linum* or flax seed are recorded as anodyne, demulcent, and emollient.

Parsley

Parsley is named from the French, *persil*. Its botanical name, *Petroselinum*, is derived from the Greek, *petroselinon: petros*, a rock, *selinon*, parsley. The Greeks held parsley in high esteem and during the Isthmian games (held on the isthmus of Corinth) the victorious athletes were awarded crowns of parsley. In Roman times, parsley was associated with the goddess Persephone, queen of the underworld.

During the Hippocratic era, parsley was prized for its medicinal properties being advocated as an aphrodisiac and as a treatment for menstrual disorders. It had a reputation as a remedy for leukorrhea and as a fertility aid. Nursing mothers were advised to take fennel, lettuce and parsley when their milk was deficient (Adams, 1844 vol. 1, p. 8). Many centuries later the Arabs followed suit.

In his Greek herbal, Dioscorides indicated that parsley grew 'in rockie and mountainous places. [and] Both ye seed and ye root have a ureticall faculty, being drank in wine it also expels ye menstrua' (Gunther, 1959 p. 310). Soranus of Ephesus mentioned parsley oil infusion as a remedy for uterine inflammation but rejected the nostrum as it was too irritant (Temkin, 1956 p. 148). In her studies of gynecology in the Middle Ages, Beryl Rowland found that parsley was an important medication for women. She recorded that the herb was prescribed: to induce purgation of the uterus and menstruation; to stimulate labor; and to assist with placental delivery; and as an application for a prolapsed uterus (Rowland, 1981 p. 67).

Although popular in Mediterranean areas, parsley was not introduced into Britain until 1548, where it soon gained a reputation in the treatment of women's disorders (Chevallier, 1996). However James Wolveridge (1671) cautioned against its inclusion in the diet or medications of wet-nurses. According to him there was no doubt that parsley provoked lust in wet-nurses and that it had 'a peculiar malice to the increase of milk [but was] an enemy to the growth of infants'. A late edition of Nicholas Culpeper's classic text *The English Physician, Enlarged* (1792) advised medication with parsley to provoke women's 'courses' and added that, 'applied to women's breasts that are hard through the curdling of their milk, it [parsley] abates the hardness quickly'.

John Lindley in his *Flora Medica* (1838) wrote that parsley leaves acted as a diuretic (by inference also as an emmenagogue, as both properties were thought similar) and that 'the fruit is a deadly poison to parrots'. Parsley root was still advised as a treatment for functional amenorrhea in the *British Herbal Pharmacopoeia* of 1991 (p. 155). Parsley contains apiole and myristicin which have diuretic properties. The volatile oil of parsley is a strong uterine stimulant.

MEDICATIONS FOR WOMEN PRESCRIBED BY AETIUS OF AMIDA

Abrotonum (southernwood); acetum (vinegar); adiantum (maidenhair fern), *Allium* (garlic); *Althaea* (marshmallow); amaracus (marjoram); ambra (amber); amygdala (almond); *Anethum* (dill), anisum (anise); apium (parsley); *Aristolochia* (birthwort); *Asarum* (wild spikenard).

Baca (berry); balaustium (flower of wild pomegranate); *Basilicum* (garden basil); basilicus (a kind of wine); bdellium (an Asiatic plant); betis (beet); bitumen; *Bryonia* (a wild vine); bupthalmos (oxeye plant); butyrum (butter).

Cannabis, cannabum (hemp); *Cardamomum* (cardamom); caryophyllum (true clove tree); castorium (castor); centaurium (centaury plant); chamaemelum (chamomile); *Cicuta* (hemlock); colocynthis (colocynth); coriandrus (coriander); crocinum (oil of saffron); cyclaminon (sowbread plant).

Daucus (carrot family); diachylon plaster, diacodion (a medication from poppy juice); *Dictamnus* (dittany plant); diospoliticum; diphryges; dropax (pitch ointment); dyonysia (ivy).

Elaterium; enneapharmacus; epithymon (thyme flower); eruca (colewort); ergi grana (kernels of bitter vetch); ervum (bitter vetch); *Euphorbia* (gummy thistle).

Faba (a bean); faex vini (lees of wine); farina (ground corn); farina ordei (ground barley); fel (gall); *Ferula* (fennel-giant); *Ficus* (fig tree); flos iuncus (bulrush flower); *Foeniculum* (fennel); foenum graecum (fenugreek).

Galbanum (a resinous sap); galla (gall nut); gallarum omphacitidum (juice of unripe grapes with sugar);

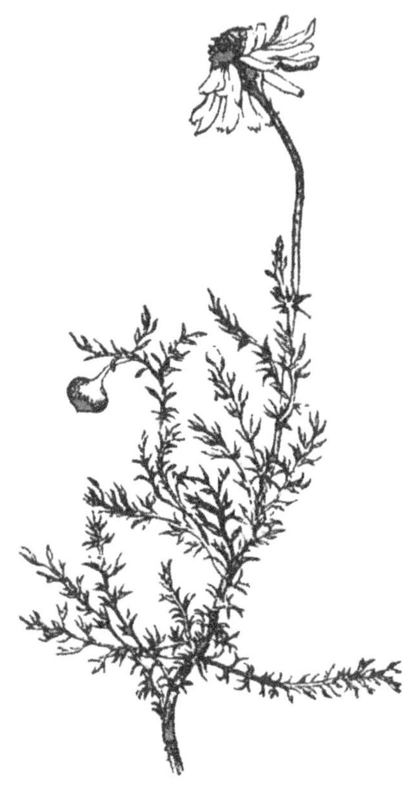

Figure 5 Chamomile (*Athemis nobilis*)

Gentiana (gentian); gingidium (toothpick chevril); glaucion (celentine plant); glaesum (amber); gleucinum (oil of must); gramen (field grass); granum cnidium (seed of mezereon).

Haematites (bloodstone); *Hedera* (ivy); *Helleborus* (hellebore); *Helenium* (elecampane plant); hiera (purgative); *Hordeum* (barley); horminum (wild clary); hydromelum (apple, honey and water); hydrorosatus (rose water); *Hyoscyamus* (henbane).

Icesii emplastrum, intubus (endive); iridis calamus (iris reed); iridis illyricae (illyrian iris); irinum (iris ointment); irio (bank cress); *Iris* (sword lily).

Juncus (rush); *Juglans*, juglans nux (walnut).

Lac (milk); ledanum (resin from the lada shrub); *Laurus* (bay tree); laver (a water plant); lemnium sigillum (aluminum silicate); lenticula (lentil); lentiscinum (mastic-tree resin or oil); *Lilium* (lily); lini semen (linseed); *Lolium* (darnel, rye grass, cockle, or tare); *Lotus* (Egyptian water lily).

Malabathron (betel or base cinnamon); mala (apple); mala punica (pomegranate); *Malva* (mallows); *Mandragora* (mandrake); melilotum (kind of clover); *Mercurialis* (dog's mercury); *Mespilus* (fruit of the medlar tree); *Morum* (mulberry); murrha (myrrh tree).

Narcissus (daffodil); nardus celtica (spikenard); *Nigella* (gith); nitrum (niter); *Nux indicum* (Indian nut); *Nymphaea* (water lily).

Oenanthe (grape of wild vine); oesypum (unscoured wool); olea (olive); oleum omphacinum (oil or juice of unripe grapes or olives); opium (poppy juice); opobalsamum (juice of the balsam tree); *Opopanax* (juice of herb panax); hordeum (barley); *Origanum* (wild marjoram); ossa (bones).

Paeonia (peony); *Panax* (all-heal, from *Heraclium* sp.); parathenis (also called *Artemisia*); parthenium (a group of unknown plants); pepo (pumpkin); perdicium (pellitory); *Petroselinum* (rock parsley); *Piper* (pepper); *Plantago* (plantain); *Polygonus* (knotgrass); pompholyx; *Portulaca, purslane Punicum malum* (pomegranate tree); *Pyrethrum* (Spanish chamomile).

Resina (resin); *Rhamnos* (buckthorn); rhaphanus (radish); rheum (*rha*, rhubarb); *Ricinus* (castor oil tree); rosae (roses); *Rubia* (madder); *Rubus* (blackberry bush); *Rumex* (sorrel); *Ruta* (rue).

Sabina (savina); *Salvia* (sage); *Sambucus* (elder tree); sarcocolla (Persian gum); satyrios (ragwort); scammonia (scammony, or purging weed); scordion (water germander, *Scordium*); *Sesame* (an oily seed); sideritis (vervain); *Solanum* (nightshade).

Tamarix (tamarisk); tarus (aloes); terebinthus (terebinth); terra (earth); thymelaea (spurge); thymum (thyme); tragacantha (goats thorn); *Triticum* (wheat); troglodyta (sparrow); thuris (incense).

Veratrum (hellebore); *Verbenacea* (irio); vinum (wine); vinum hadrianum; *Viola* (violet); virgultum (brushwood); viridium (green plants herbs or trees); vitex (chaste tree); vitis (vine).

References

Adams, F. (1844). *The Seven Books of Paulus Aegineta*, Translated from the Greek, Vol. 1, pp. 8, 257, 603. (London: The Sydenham Society)

Adams, F. (1846). *The Seven Books of Paulus Aegineta*, Translated from the Greek, Vol. 2. (London: The Sydenham Society)

Adams, F. (1847). *The Seven Books of Paulus Aegineta*, Translated from the Greek, Vol. 3, pp. 153–5, 230, 360–1, 601–2. (London: The Sydenham Society)

The British Herbal Medicine Association (1991). *British Herbal Pharmacopoeia*, pp. 132, 155. (Bournemouth, UK)

Chevallier, A. (1996). *The Encyclopaedia of Medicinal Plants*, p. 244. (London: New York: Dorling Kindersley)

Culpeper, N. (1792). *The English Physician, Enlarged*, pp. 214–5. (London: A. Law & W. Millar & R. Kater)

Dixon, W. E. (1913). *A Manual of Pharmacology*, p. 12. (London: Edward Arnold)

Dorland, W. A. Newman (1932). *The American Illustrated Medical Dictionary*, pp. 60, 237. (Philadelphia & London: W. B. Saunders Co.)

Evans, W. C. (1996). *Trease and Evan's Pharmacognosy*, p. 54. (London and Philadelphia: W. B. Saunders Co.)

Garrison, F. H. (1929). *An Introduction to the History of Medicine*, pp. 85, 86, 121–5. (Philadelphia and London: W. B. Saunders Co.)

The Gideon's International (1982). *The Holy Bible*, The Revised Berkeley version in modern English, p. 2. (USA: National Bible Press)

Grieve, M. (1931). *A Modern Herbal*, Vol. 1, pp. 317–9. (London: Jonathan Cape)

Gunther, R. T. (1959). *The Greek Herbal of Dioscorides*, pp. 77–8, 90, 106, 136, 310, 642–3. (New York: Hafner Publishing Co.)

Hare, H. A. (1901). *A Text-Book of Practical Therapeutics*, pp. 127–9. (London: Henry Kimpton)

Lewis, J. J. (1964). *An Introduction to Pharmacology*, p. 585. (Edinburgh & London: E. & S. Livingstone Ltd.)

Lindley, J. (1838). *Flora Medica; A Botanical Account of all the More Important Plants used in Medicine, in different parts of the World*, p. 36. (London: Orme, Brown, Green & Longmans)

Mann, E. W. (1915). *Southalls Organic Materia Medica*, Eighth edition, pp. 209–10. (London: J. & A. Churchill)

Mauriceau, F. (1683). *The Diseases of Women with Child, And in Childbed*, Translated by Hugh Chamberlen MD, p. 350. (London, John Darby)

Reynolds, J. E. F. (ed.) (1982). *Martindale, the Extra Pharmacopoeia*, pp. 283, 957. (London: The Pharmaceutical Press)

Ricci, J. V. (1943). *The Genealogy of Gynecology*, pp. 171–207. (Philadelphia: Blakiston Co.)

Ringer, S. (1888). *A Handbook of Therapeutics*, pp. 381–3. (London: H. K. Lewis)

Rowland, B. (1981). *Medieval Woman's Guide to Health, The First English Gynecological Handbook*, pp. 67, 95, 115, 117. (London: Croom Helm)

Squire, P. W. (1908). *Squire's Companion to the British Pharmacopoeia*, 18th ed., pp. 125–7, 317, 538, 550. (London: J. and A. Churchill)

Stewart McKay, W. J. (1901). *The History of Ancient Gynaecology*, pp. 179–222. (London: Balliere, Tindall and Cox)

Temkin, O. (1956). *Soranus' Gynecology*, pp. 148, 223–4, 234. (Baltimore: The Johns Hopkins Press)

Warburton, D. (1995). *A–Z of Aphrodisia*, p. 90. (London: Thorsens)

Wolveridge, J. (1671). *Speculum Matricis; or The Expert Midwives Handmaid*, pp. 114, 126, 130, 139, 160, 145. (London: E. Okes)

Wootton, A. C. (1910). *Chronicles of Pharmacy*, Vol. 1, p. 216. (London: MacMillan & Co.)

The Arab influence 11

INTRODUCTION

The mighty Arabian empire was founded by the prophet Mohammed (AD c. 570–632) and his emirs (the name given to independent chieftains and descendants of his daughter Fatima). The successors of the great prophet were known as 'caliphs'. After the death of Mohammed the empire was divided into kingdoms or caliphates, and in those provinces the arts and sciences flourished. According to Fielding Garrison, the principal service of Islam to medicine was 'the preservation of Greek culture'. The Saracens also added algebra, chemistry, geology and many other improvements or refinements to civilization. The medical authors of the Mohammedan era were called 'Arabic' because this was the language they used for their writings, but most were born in Persia or Spain and many were Jewish (Garrison, 1929).

Mohammedan physicians gained their medical knowledge from a persecuted Christian sect known as the Nestorians. Nestorius became the patriarch of Constantinople in AD 428 but taught that the Virgin Mary should not be styled the 'Mother of God', as was the custom, but should be revered as the 'Mother of Jesus Christ'. The new teaching was deemed to be heretical and Nestorius and his followers were banished to the desert. In time they took up the study of medicine and established a renowned medical school at Edessa in Mesopotamia. The Nestorian practitioners were, however, driven out of the empire by the orthodox Bishop Cyrus in AD 489. They fled to Persia and formed the medical school of Gondisapor (Jundishapur). It was at Gondisapor that Arab medicine began.

The Arab physicians 'translated the Greek authors, commented upon them, popularized them and, to their lasting glory, transmitted Greek Medicine – augmented with their own clinical experience – to the Europeans' (Garrison, 1929). One of the principal Arab translators was Johannes Mesue the Elder (AD 777–837). While the Arabs derived their knowledge of Greek medicine from the Nestorian monks they also assimilated many practical details from the Jews, and astrological lore from Egypt and the Far East.

Edward G. Browne, Professor of Arabic at the University of Cambridge, related the story of Arabian medicine in a series of 'Fitzpatrick Lectures' delivered at the College of Physicians between November 1919 and November 1920 and published in 1921. In his view, the main Arabian medical era was 'the first century or two of the 'Abbasid Caliphate of Baghdad (from AD 750 onwards)' and Browne wrote: 'The Caliphate was overthrown and its metropolis sacked and laid waste in AD 1258, and though the surviving scholars of the younger generation carried on the sound tradition of scholarship for a while longer, there is, broadly speaking a difference not only of degree but of kind between the literature and scientific work done before and after the thirteenth century throughout the lands of Islam' (Browne, 1921).

Excellent source material for the lives of the great Arabian physicians may be found in the *Bibliography of Medieval Arabic and Jewish Medicine and Allied Sciences* written by Rifaat Y. Evied, R.Y. and that of Donald Campbell in his two-volume work *Arabian Medicine, and its Influence on the Middle Ages* (1926).

ARABIAN OBSTETRICS AND GYNECOLOGY

Although there were many recipes for women in the Arabian materia medica, it appears that female disorders were primarily taken care of by midwives. The references to obstetrics and gynecology contained in the Arabic medical literature reflect the views of the Greco-Romans transmitted through the texts of Hippocrates and Galen and the later works of the great medical compilers, Oribasius, Aetius, and Paul of Aegina (Ricci, 1943).

ARABIAN MATERIA MEDICA

The pharmacy and chemistry of the Arabs, combined with the simples (medicines of one constituent) known by them from the works of Dioscorides, Pliny and the other great medical and botanical authors of Greece and Rome, formed the basis of later European pharmacopoeias. Arabian descriptions of materia medica and their methods of drug preparation became the standard authority throughout the Middle Ages. The most important Persian works on pharmacology were the materia medica of Abu Mansur (c. 970), which contains descriptions of 585 drugs; the *Grabadin* or Apothecaries Manual (*Antidotarium*), a mysterious Latin compilation of the tenth or eleventh century by a pseudonymous Mesue (now known as 'Pseudo-Mesue'); and the *Jami* of Ibn Baitar of the thirteenth century which describes some 1400 drugs, of which about 300 were said to be new at the time.

In the Arabian schools of medicine, the principal courses held were clinical medicine, pharmacology and therapeutics. Arabian medicine gave birth to alchemy and these early chemists explored the notion of an 'elixir of life' that would cure all diseases and confer immortality. That elixir came to be known as the *Aurum potabile* (drinkable gold). According to Garrison, the Arabian pharmacists (sandalani) introduced a number of new drugs to Western medicine (see below), and described alcohol, aldehydes, juleps and syrups, all of which are named from the Arabic. They also introduced flavoring extracts made of lemon peel, orange, rosewater, tragacanth and other ingredients.

Medications introduced to Western medicine by Arabian physicians

Aconite, ambergris, camphor, cassia, cloves, colocynth, cubebs, ?ergot, hashish, Indian hemp, mercury, musk, myrrh, nutmeg, rhubarb, sandalwood, senna, strychnine, tamarind.

SERAPEON THE ELDER (AD 802–849)

Serapeon the Elder, also known as Jakie Ben Serabi, was a Christian physician of the medical school of Gondisapor. His main treatise was the *Kounnach*, the Latin version named the *Brevarium*. The *Kounnach* included details on the care of pregnant women and the management of difficult labor. Gynecological chapters included sections on abortion, menstrual disorders, prolapse, sterility and the uterine problems of abscesses, growths and hemorrhage. In uterine inflammation, for example, he advised laxatives and venesection accompanied by application of fomentations or plasters containing barley flour, chamomile, dill, endive, fenugreek, figs, fleawort, pigeon dung and pomegranate rind. Serapeon also prescribed sedatives if pain was severe (Ricci, 1943).

RHAZES (AD 860–932)

Abu Bakr Muhammad ibn Zakariyua, known as Rhazes wrote an encyclopedia of medicine, the *Al Hawi or Liber Continens*, a 25-volume compilation from many sources. The twelfth book of the *Al Hawi* contained a resumé of gynecology. The ninth book,

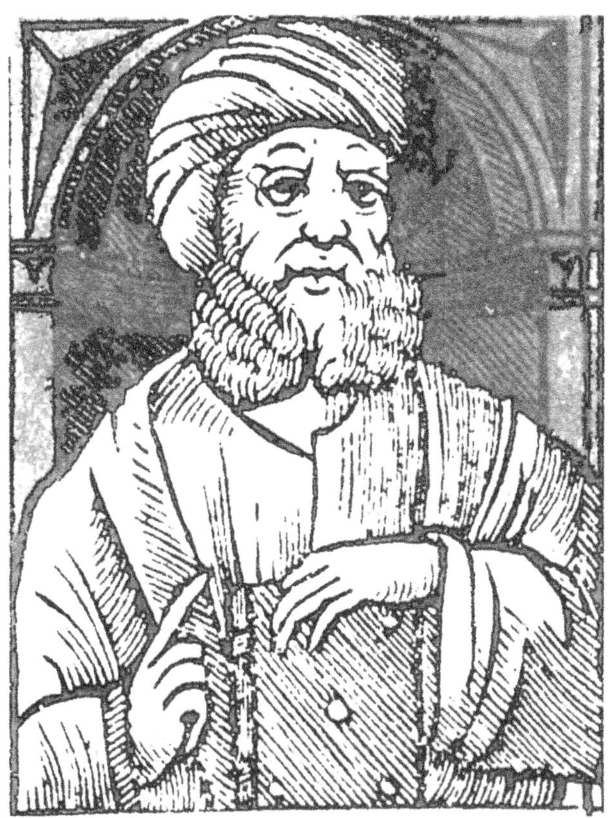

Figure 1 Rhazes (860–932)

revised by Vesalius, was the main source of therapeutic knowledge until long after the Renaissance (Garrison, 1929). Rhazes was the first to introduce chemical preparations into the practice of medicine (Campbell, 1926 vol. 1). His materia medica included over 760 items (Adams, 1847 vol. 3).

A selection of Rhazes' materia medica for women

Retention of the menses Massage, hot baths, purgation, venesection, and medication with suppositories of black hellebore, hiera and savin
Menorrhagia Venesection and astringent vaginal pessaries of acacia, alum, antimony, frankincense, gall and wild pomegranate flowers.
Sterility Tampons of honey, myrrh and oil.

HALY BEN ABBAS (DIED AD 994)

Ali ibn al Abbas al-Majusi, or Haly Ben Abbas, was Persian by birth. The *Al Maliki* (royal book) written by Haly Ben Abbas was generally regarded as one of the best works of the Arabian period (Campbell, 1926). The *Al Maliki* contained an account of the anatomy of the female genitalia, and of impregnation and fetal development. In the treatment of amenorrhea he advised bull's gall, chamomile, colocynth, fennel, hellebore, myrrh, parsley, rue, savin and wormwood (Ricci, 1943).

AVICENNA OR IBN SINA (AD 980–1037)

Abu Ali al-Husayn ibn 'Abdullah ibn Sina, or Avicenna, the 'prince of physicians' was born at Afshena near Bokhara. His five-volume *Canon of Medicine* (*al-Qanun-fi't-Tibb*) was the main authority on medicine throughout the Middle Ages. The *Canon* was translated into Latin by Gerard of Cremona in the twelfth century. Maimonides translated Avicenna's *Canon* to Hebrew. Approximately half of Avicenna's medical works are versified treatises (Browne, 1921)

O. Cameron Gruner translated the first volume of Avicenna's *Canon* in 1930 and a close connection between Arabian and Chinese medicine began to appear obvious. He wrote that Avicenna had quoted from various sources, notably Dioscorides. About 760 drugs were named in the materia medica but there was some duplication as a number of medications were included under several names. Mazar H. Shah, in his book *The General Principles of Avicenna's Canon of Medicine* (1966) related that 'It appears that for well over 600 years no medical book ever written had been studied so thoroughly over such a long period ... [the *Canon*] is still being used as the vade-mecum [or pocket-companion book] of Unani-Tibb [Greco-Arabic] Medicine'.

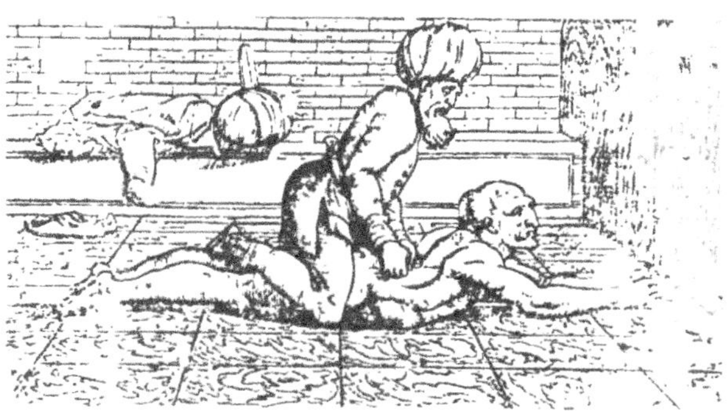

Figure 2 Avicenna (980–1037) applying physical therapy

Avicenna's famous *Canon* dealt with anatomy, physiology, medicine, surgery, gynecology, obstetrics and materia medica. There were almost 70 chapters related to gynecology, the largest volume written on the subject by any Arabian author. In cases of sterility, for example, Avicenna wrote that the semen would float in water if it was defective, and that the urine of an infertile woman, poured at the roots of lettuce, would cause the plant to shrivel up. Alternatively, the urine of an infertile woman voided onto grains of wheat barley or beans planted in earthen pots would fail to induce sprouting at the end of seven days. Avicenna related the ancient version of a tubal patency test: the vagina was fumigated, and if the aromatic odor was exhaled from the mouth or nose the woman was deemed fertile.

It is claimed that Avicenna wrote the definitive gynecological treatise of his day and that he enumerated the signs, symptoms and treatment of many gynecological disorders. Apparently, he was also the first physician to use a mirror to reflect ambient light between the blades of a vaginal speculum. Avicenna substituted the use of cautery for the knife and it appears that he was aware of the antiseptic effects of alcohol for he recommended that wounds should be washed with wine. Unfortunately, a full English version of the entire *Canon* is not available but Shah's book contains an index of the 179 'simple drugs' mentioned by Avicenna in the first volume of the work.

Book One of Avicenna's *Canon* contained instructions for: the management of infancy; infant feeding; qualifications of a good wet-nurse; and lactation and weaning. When the infant was delivered the umbilical cord was cut 'at four-finger distance from the umbilicus and then tied ... and dressed with a piece of clean linen soaked in olive-oil'. The wound was also dusted with anzaroot (similar to tragacanth, an astringent), cumin seeds, Indian kino, lichen and turmeric. Dietary measures were outlined to ensure good lactation. If the milk was deficient, the breasts were massaged and the following medicinal herbs were administered: black cumin, blue meliotus, carrot, clover, dill, fennel, fenugreek and leek. They were powdered and mixed with fennel water, fresh honey and clarified butter, to be taken when required. Excessive lactation was treated by application of a plaster consisting of clay, cumin, lentils and vinegar (Shah, 1966). Book One also contained interesting tracts on leeches and the techniques of cupping and venesection. Francis Adams should be consulted for an excellent overview of these procedures (1846 vol. 2).

Soheil M. Afnan of Pembroke College, Cambridge, in his treatise *Avicenna, His Life and Works*, noted that Book Two of the *Canon* dealt with materia medica, while Book Five was devoted to pharmacology: '[this was] a subject of some importance when it is remembered that Islamic pharmacology comprised a good deal of original work, and survived in Europe down to the beginning of the nineteenth century' (1958). Afnan's work contains a valuable bibliography on the life and times of Avicenna, and his successors and commentators, and outlines Avicenna's beliefs on logic, medicine, metaphysics, natural sciences, psychology and religion.

ALBUCASIS (AD 936–1013)

Abu'l-Qasim Khalef ibn Abbas al-Zahrawi, or Albucasis, was born in Zahra, near Cordoba, in Andalucia, Spain. He was the author of the *Tasrif* ('Collection'), based on the work of Paul of Aegina, which became a leading textbook on medicine and surgery in the Middle Ages. Albucasis' treatise contained descriptions of a number of surgical procedures for gynecological disorders and he indicated that, where possible, gynecological operations 'are to be performed by midwives or female attendants possessing a medical knowledge'. If, however, female attendants were not available, the help of a physician was permissible provided he was well mannered, and had a working knowledge of gynecology.

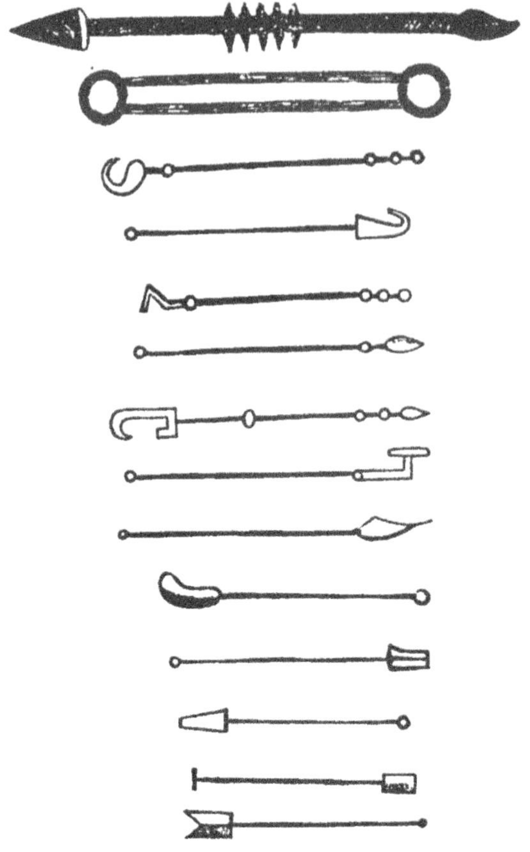

Figure 3 Surgical instruments used by Albucasis (936–1013)

Albucasis wrote on the surgical treatment of imperforate hymen with acacia and dragon's blood and incense mixed with egg white to hand for hemostasis. He offered surgical extirpation of the male organs in hermaphroditism and a similar procedure for clitoral enlargement. Albucasis reported an interesting case of secondary abdominal pregnancy: a pregnant woman suffered a stillbirth but the fetus was not expelled. Some time later the patient developed an umbilical abscess which ruptured and expelled a large number of fetal bones. He described the vaginal speculum and an early version of the Walcher position for childbirth, and he invented a piston syringe. It is doubtful, however, whether or not he ever practiced midwifery himself (Ricci, 1943).

AVENZOAR (AD 1113–1162)

Abu Merwan Abdal-Malik ibn Abu'l-Ala Zuhr, or Avenzoar, was a Spanish–Arab physician and surgeon, born (possibly of Jewish parents) near Seville. Obstetrics was entirely omitted from Avenzoar's chief work, the *El Teisir* ('Assistance'). The *El Teisir* contained a summary of the diseases of the female genitalia, including sterility, uterine displacements and disturbances of menstrual flow. According to Ricci (1943), his book contains the earliest reference to perineal repair: the wound was drawn together with silk thread and sprinkled with 'healing powder'.

AVERRÖES (AD 1126–1198)

Abu-al-Walid Muhammad ibn Ahmed ibn Muhammad ibn Rushd, or Averröes, was Avenzoar's most distinguished pupil and author of the *Colliget*, a commentary on the *Canon* of Avicenna. The *Colliget* contains only three short paragraphs relating to gynecology: one on the anatomy of the breasts; one on the female genitalia, and one on the diseases of the vulva. Averröes related the case of a woman who became pregnant while taking a bath 'in the same warm water in which bad men had previously had orgasms'.

SAFAVID MEDICAL PRACTICE (1500–1750)

Cyril Elgood's book *Safavid Medical Practice* (1970), described the practice of medicine, surgery and gynecology in Persia during the Safavid dynasty (1501–1750). He devoted seven chapters to the obstetrics and gynecology of the era under the headings: Women in Safavid Days, Anatomy of the Female Pelvis, Diseases of the Pelvis, Birth Control and Abortion, Sterility, Pregnancy, and Lactation and Infant Welfare.

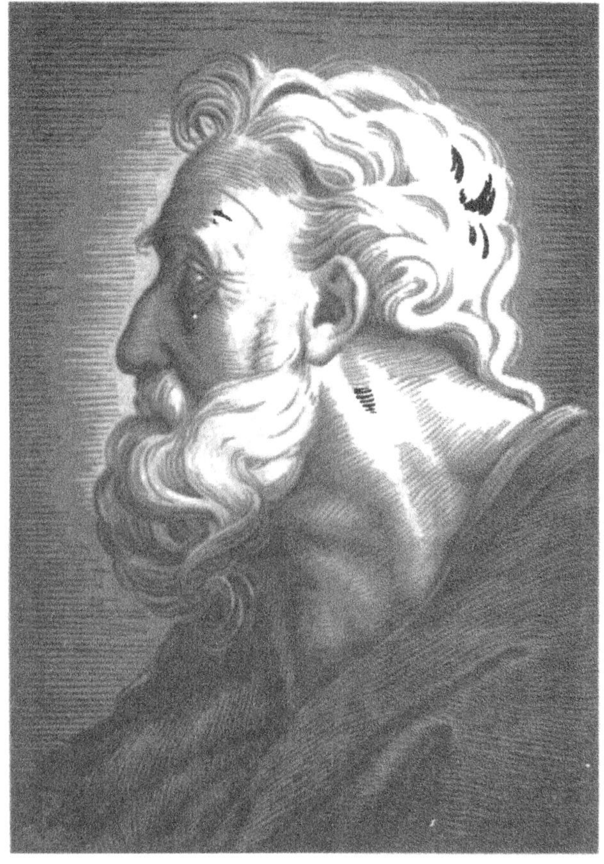

Figure 4 Avenzoar (1113–1162)

ARAB MEDICINE IN THE EARLY TWENTIETH CENTURY

M.W. Hilton-Simpson of Oxford, in his book *Arab Medicine and Surgery* (1913) wrote how he was admitted to some of the secrets of the reticent Berber and Arab doctors of Algeria. He made notes on medications for gonorrhea and swollen testicles; remedies for use in obstetric medicine; nostrums for excessive menstruation; and aphrodisiac herbs.

Family planning Conception could be prevented (or abortion procured) by insertion of madder root into the vagina. Alternatively the vagina was fumigated with sulfur or castor oil seeds and 'foam from the mouth of a male camel in the rutting season' were swallowed.

Heavy periods Excess menstruation was treated by infusion of blackberry or fenugreek seeds with burnt oil, sugar and wheat.

Labor oxytocics Hilton-Simpson wrote that when the child was 'badly placed and delivery accordingly impeded' a mixture of powdered carrot seeds, the body of the beetle *Mylabris oleae* and a plant of *Euphorbia* was administered in water, as an expulsive.
Love potions Aphrodisiacs were available in the form of ajuga eva, butter, garlic, honey, nuts, olive oil, *Pyrethrum* and sheep testicles.
Pregnancy test To test whether a woman was pregnant, she drank liquid madder (*Rubia tinctorum*). If her urine turned red she was deemed not to be pregnant; if her urine was clear she was considered *enceinte*.

A SELECTION OF ARABIAN MATERIA MEDICA FOR WOMEN

Ambergris

The *Encyclopaedia Britannica* (1771) defines ambergrease or ambergris as 'a solid, ash-colored, fat, inflammable substance ... greatly used by perfumers on account of its sweet smell ... In medicine it is used for nervous complaints ... [and] is found in great quantities in the Indian Ocean, near the Molucca isles, also near Africa, and sometimes near the northern parts of England, Scotland, and Norway'. Ambergris takes its name from the Arabic, *anbar* and the Latin, *ambare*, and *grisa*, gray. Ambergris is a strongly scented substance produced by the spermaceti whale and was variously believed to be the semen, indurated feces, or vomitus of the whale. Its odor is derived from the squid (*Saepia moschata*) on which the whale feeds.

Ambergris was apparently unknown to the Greeks and Romans but there is a theory that the ancients confused ambergris with amber (their name was *electrum*), the fossilized tears of the pine tree. Ambergris was used by the Arabs as an antispasmodic and went on to hold a special place in the materia medica of women for many centuries. During the Middle Ages ambergris was prescribed for 'suffocation' of the uterus (Rowland, 1981 pp. 93, 95, 97). In his 1651 *Directory for Midwives*, Nicholas Culpeper, the English 'physician, divine and gent', advised ambergris for 'The After-Pains ... Boyl an Eg soft, and powr out the Yolk of it, with which mix a spoonful of Cinnamon Water and let her drink it; and if you mix two grains of Amber greece with it, it will be the better'.

James Wolveridge the author of the *Speculum Matricis*, Ireland's first textbook on obstetrics and one of the rarest books on midwifery, distinguished between amber and ambergris. He prescribed oil of amber as an oxytocic to facilitate childbirth and placental delivery and to help deliver a stillborn infant (1671 pp. 130–1). Wolveridge also advised ambergris for the nausea of early pregnancy and as a general cordial or broth, to prevent miscarriage (1671 pp. 129, 131). In the nineteenth century ambergris was used as a cure for sterility (Pseudo-Aristotle c. 1830) and to relieve after-pains and uterine prolapse. It was also prescribed during pregnancy.

Richard Hoblyn, in his *Dictionary of Terms used in Medicine* (1878), had little of a positive nature to write about ambergris but noted (in italics) that the Japanese called it 'whales dung'. Ambergris was still in use as a medication in the early twentieth century and Dorland wrote of it as 'A grey substance from the sperm whales intestines: used as a perfume and as a stimulant in low fevers, chronic catarrh, hysteria, and other nervous infections. Dose 1–3 grains' (1932 p. 70).

Camphor

Camphor is a solid essential oil of the camphor laurel (*Cinnamomum camphora*) and is also available as a white crystalline substance. The name is derived from the Arabic *kafur*, the Latin *camphora* and French *camphre*. Camphor was obtained from China, Formosa and Japan until a synthetic substitute became available.

According to Francis Adams, Serapeon is the ancient authority who gave the fullest account of camphor and other Arabian authorities agreed with his analysis (1847 vol. 3, pp. 427–9). Regarding its medicinal virtues, camphor was availed of to relieve inflammation and was prescribed as a sedative, as an antihemorrhagic, and as an anti-aphrodisiac. The medication was commonly used in fumigations and ointments. Arab physicians prescribed camphor to cause impotence and to 'coagulate' (stop) nocturnal seminal emissions. Over the years, many expressions were used for the involuntary loss of reproductive fluid, including *oneirogmus, pollutio nocturni somni, somnia veneris* (Adams, 1844 vol. 1, p. 595). In

Oriental medicine nocturnal emissions are still judged to be detrimental to health, a belief that was shared in the West until the mid-twentieth century.

Camphor was prescribed during the Middle Ages in Europe for menorrhagia (Rowland, 1981 p. 79) and to relieve uterine pain, inflammation and ulceration. It was also availed of to treat venereal disease, and to 'restrain' sexual intercourse. In the seventeenth century James Wolveridge (1671 pp. 139, 148) advised the use of camphor to suppress lactation and to prevent breast inflammation. Camphor was still used to control excessive menstruation in the nineteenth century (Pseudo-Aristotle, 1830). Hobart Amory Hare, professor of therapeutics and materia medica at the Jefferson Medical College of Philadelphia advised camphor for dysmenorrhea, and menopausal symptoms, to promote sleep in 'hysterical females', for spermatorrhea, and as a nervous sedative. He also reported that it acted as a sexual stimulant if taken in large doses (1901 pp. 121–5).

Camphor was found to have definite sedative properties and for a time was advocated to suppress eclamptic convulsions. Unfortunately the medication itself could cause fits if administered in large doses. It was available as an aqueous solution, a spirit, a tincture, and a liniment (Mann, 1915). In *Martindale. The Extra-Pharmacopoeia* it is related that camphor is a mild analgesic and rubefacient, long used as a counter-irritant. Formerly administered as a respiratory and circulatory stimulant, there is little evidence of its value for this purpose nowadays (Reynolds, 1982 p. 351). *Cinnamomum camphora* is used as an internal preparation in Ayurvedic medicine to treat painful menstruation (Bown, 1995 p. 262). In pharmacognosy camphor is regarded as a mild antiseptic and carminative (Evans, 1996 p. 278) and is known to be an antiparasitic.

Cubebs

Cubebs (*cubebae fructus*) are the dried, unripe, nearly full-grown fruits of *Piper cubeba*, a climbing pepper shrub, found in Java and Sumatra. The name 'cubeb' came from the Arabic *kababah* and French *cubebe*. It is thought that the plant was introduced into Europe by the Arabs who used the fruit as a pepper. Cubebs are extensively grown in coffee plantations where they are well shaded and supported by the coffee trees.

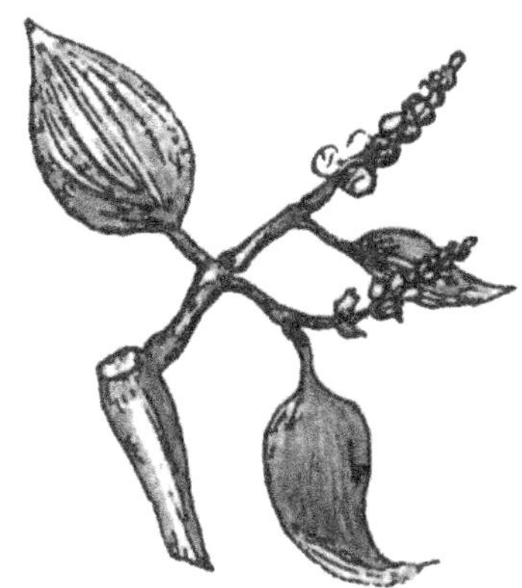

Figure 5 Pepper (*Piper* sp.)

Dioscorides did not include cubeb pepper in his second-century herbal but mentioned *Piper nigrum* which he noted was used to 'drive out the embryum' and as a contraceptive pessary (Gunther, 1959 p. 199). The Arab authors wrote that cubebs rendered 'the breath fragrant and cured affections of the bladder' and that eating cubebs 'enhances the delight of coitus' (Adams, 1847 vol. 3, p. 456). Rhazes included cubebs in a long list of substances with supposed aphrodisiac properties (Adams, 1844 vol. 1, p. 47). Serapeon recommended aromatic spices such as cardamom and cubebs for the disordered appetite (pica) of early pregnancy. The term 'pica' was derived either from the name of a bird of the magpie or jay family which gathers unsuitable objects as food items, or from the name for ivy (*Hedera helix*): 'as Ivy entwines itself about various plants, so does this appetite in pregnant women fasten upon a variety of improper articles of food' (Adams, 1844 vol. 1, p. 2).

Nicholas Culpeper wrote in the *London Dispensatorie* that cubebs were 'hot and dry in the third degree ... they cleanse the head of flegm and strengthen the brain, they heat the stomach and provoke lust' (1654 p. 58). A later edition (1826) informed the reader that 'the Arabs call them Quabebe, and Quabebe Chine: they grow plentifully in Java, they stir up venery ... and are very profitable for cold griefs of the womb'.

William Wyatt Squire was of the opinion that cubebs 'act specifically on genito-urinary mucous membrane. [They are] given in all stages of gonorrhea'

(1908 p. 462). There were various preparations of cubebs including *oleum cubebae* (oil of cubebs), tinctures, fluid extracts, oleo-resin compounds, lozenges and vapors (used for throat complaints). Information printed in *The National Botanic Pharmacopoeia* (1921) indicated that cubebs were 'an excellent remedy for flour albus or whites' (Scurrah, 1921 p. 34). W.A. Newman Dorland was in agreement and wrote in his *The American Illustrated Medical Dictionary* that cubebs were a 'stimulant diuretic ... used in gonorrhea, leucorrhea, urethritis, etc.' (1932 p. 336). In more recent times Reynolds wrote that cubeb oil was 'formerly employed as an emulsion or in capsules, and as a urinary antiseptic. It is used as a flavoring agent' (1982 p. 675). Demi Bown noted that the cubeb (*Piper cubeba* or tailed pepper) is a bitter, antiseptic, stimulant herb used in throat and genito-urinary infections (1995 p. 330). The cubeb plant is not listed in the 1991 *British Herbal Pharmacopoeia.*

Mercury

Mercury, or Quicksilver, is a silvery metallic element which is liquid at room temperature. It takes its name from the Latin *mercurius*, probably from *merx, mercis*, meaning merchandise. In Ancient Egypt the metal was identified with Thoth, the ibis-headed god of art, medicine and science. The metal is named after Mercury, the Roman god of merchandise, theft and eloquence, who was also messenger to the gods and identified in Greek mythology as Hermes. The word 'mercury' is of modern origin and dates from the seventh AD century. It is also used for the planet nearest to the sun, whose name and sign, date from the same period (Wootton, 1910 vol. 2, pp. 304–11).

Quicksilver was known to the Ancient Egyptians, and to the Chinese and Oriental Indians of antiquity. The metal was mentioned in Greek writings in the fourth century BC. In his great herbal of the second AD century Dioscorides described the metal as being derived from the sulfide, kinnabari or cinnabar, a substance that was often mistaken for red lead. His name for mercury was hydrargyrum, or 'fluid silver'. Dioscorides was of the opinion that mercury had the same virtue as hematite (iron ore) and that it was good for 'blood-stanching ... and ye breaking out of [skin] pustules'. He was aware that mercury had a 'pernicious faculty' when drunk, relieved by drinking milk or wine infused with herbs (Gunther, 1959 p. 637). Dioscorides' description of the method of preparation of mercury from cinnabar is probably the first account of the process of distillation that we possess. The Greek physicians made little use of mercury in the practice of medicine (Adams, 1847 vol. 3, p. 385). Both Pliny and Galen called the substance ***argentum vivum*** and considered it to be a dangerous poison.

The Arabs, through their knowledge of Greek, Chinese and Indian medicine, were interested in the potential therapeutic benefits of mercury. Geber, the Arabian physician, considered by many to be 'The First Chemist', investigated the mercurial compounds, red precipitate and corrosive sublimate. Mesue Senior recommended mercurial ointments for skin diseases, and Avicenna, Haly Abbas, Rhazes and Serapeon recommended the metal for local treatment of scabies and 'malignant' skin ulcers. They were aware of the toxic effects of mercury if taken orally although Avicenna cast doubt on the poisonous nature of the metal.

When the European knights returned from the Crusades they brought with them a mercury salve for skin disorders, popularly referred to as ***unguentum Saracenium***, but it was in 1496 that the Veronese physician, Georgio Sommariva, first applied the ointment to the skin sores of syphilis. The word 'syphilis' was derived from a poem by the physician Girolamo Fracastoro (1478–1553) entitled *Syphilis sive morbus Gallicus.* The word syphilis first appeared in an English medical book in 1717 when Daniel Turner published his *Syphilis; a Practical Dissertation on the Venereal Disease* (Oriel, 1994). Prior to that, the devastating venereal disease was known as 'the great pox' (***lues venerea***), the French pox (***morbus gallicus***) and many other appellations.

Theophrastus Bombastus von Hohenheim, better known as Paracelsus (1493–1541), popularized the general use of mercury as a medication. ***Emplastrum vigonium*** was a compound of mercury in olive oil, spread on calico, and the plaster was applied for syphilitic skin eruptions from the mid-fifteenth century onwards. Peter Andrew Methiolis (1500–1577), physician to Archduke Ferdinand of Austria, gained the credit for first prescribing mercury by oral administration. As time went by the medication was applied in large quantities as an ointment or oral preparation, and in vapor baths.

Mercury treatment was sometimes referred to as the 'salivations' or 'the salivary cure' (Quetel, 1990): the aim of the treatment was to induce a heavy flow of saliva in order to eliminate poisonous phlegm. Unfortunately, the excessive salivation was also a symptom of mercury poisoning and so the treatment was as damaging as the disease itself. The first formula for mercurial pills was sent by Barbarossa, the second king of Algiers (and a famous pirate), to Francis, the first king of France, in the second quarter of the sixteenth century. The pills contained agarick, aloes, amber, canella, mastic, musk, myrrh, quicksilver, rhubarb, rose juice and Venice turpentine. The original mercurial pills were superseded by those compounded by Belloste, a French army surgeon, who devised a new formula c. 1700.

Calomel, a milder formulation of mercury, was introduced into medical practice in about 1608. The name (from the Greek *kalos* beautiful and *melas* black) related to its physical appearance and was coined by Theodore Turquet de Mayerne. Another form of mercury known as 'corrosive sublimate' was introduced in the middle of the eighteenth century, and was also used as a remedy for syphilis: the original formula was 24 grains of corrosive sublimate dissolved in two quarts of whisky, a tablespoonful to be taken night and morning. A compound called 'catholicon', thought to be a universal panacea, was a preparation of gold and corrosive sublimate and known as *aurum vitae*, the gold of life. Precipitated mercury (red precipitate) was at one time used as a purgative (Wootton, 1910 vol. 1, pp. 408–22).

Bismuth was introduced by Felix Balzer in 1889. The medication killed the syphilitic spirochetes and was less dangerous than mercury. However, mercury remained the main treatment for syphilis until the early twentieth century. In his *Companion to the British Pharmacopoeia* Squire included 33 pages of mercurial preparations for use in the treatment of syphilis and skin disease (1908 pp. 601–34). In 1904 Paul Ehrlich of Frankfurt developed the arsenic-based compound named '606' or 'salvarsan' and this new remedy gradually replaced the mercury treatments. Almost 40 years later, John F. Mahoney and associates of New York (1943) introduced effective and relatively non-toxic treatment of syphilis with penicillin.

Nutmeg

Nutmeg is the aromatic kernel of an East Indian tree (*Myristica fragrans*) much used as a seasoning in cookery. Its name comes from the Middle English *notemuge*, nut, and Old French *mugue*, musk. The native habitat of the nutmeg was the Spice Islands (the Moluccas), an area that was annexed by the Portuguese soon after their invasion of 1512, but later colonized in turn by both the Dutch and the English. It was the search for the Spice Islands which led to the discovery of the Americas.

Nutmeg (and mace, an extract of the husk of nutmeg) was included in the pharmacopoeia of Chinese medicine from ancient times for the treatment of nausea and vomiting. It also had a reputation as an aphrodisiac. In the Ayurvedic medical tradition nutmeg was used specifically to control premature ejaculation. Nutmeg and mace were first introduced into Europe by Arabian physicians in the middle of the twelfth century (Evans, 1996). They described the use of nutmeg in an analgesic pessary (Adams, 1847 vol. 3, p. 437).

In the Middle Ages nutmeg was used for 'ache' of the uterus: 'sometimes due a stillborn child being born before his time … the distress caused the ache of the uterus'. Nutmeg was mixed with other herbs in a small linen bag and placed as a pessary in the vagina to correct uterine prolapse. Mace was a remedy for excess menstruation, and was useful in the treatment of uterine mole, uterine suffocation (convulsions) and the vomiting of early pregnancy (Rowland, 1981 pp. 81, 101, 119).

The English naturalist William Turner wrote an outstanding three-volume herbal in 1568 in which he compiled the knowledge of Western botanical medicine from Greco-Roman times to the sixteenth century. In the third part of his expertly researched treatise, Turner indicated that nutmeg was an aphrodisiac: 'it is also profitable for cold housbandes that would fayne haue children, but not for lecherous bores and bulles'. He also wrote that it would be a useful remedy for uterine disease (Turner, 1568, part 3 pp. 40–1).

Demi Bown recorded the fascinating instance of the first recorded case of nutmeg poisoning, in 1576, when a 'pregnant English lady' became deliriously inebriated after she ate ten to twelve fruits (Bown, 1995).

James Wolveridge (1671) advised nutmeg with meat in the diet of 'breeding women'. Nutmeg was also a component of his remedies for the prevention of miscarriage and for the treatment of convulsions. He included mace in nostrums designed to aid placental delivery and to increase milk supply. Wolveridge favored mace ale as a purge and as a remedy for uterine prolapse (1671 pp. 93, 111, 132, 148). Nutmeg continued in popularity right through the nineteenth century when it was thought of as a primary treatment for 'the whites', the term used at the time for excess vaginal discharge. The Pseudo-Aristotle (c. 1830) contains a full chapter devoted to 'the False Courses, or Whites' and nutmeg was one of 134 different medications (some of which were compound) for treatment of the condition.

At the dawn of the twentieth century, Hare concluded that nutmeg was a soporofic and nerve sedative (1901 p. 305). Soon afterwards Squire opined that nutmeg, in large doses, caused similar symptoms to those of *Cannabis indica*, and that nutmeg was aromatic, carminative and stimulant. The distinctive flavor was availed of to disguise the tart taste of rhubarb and other medicines. Nutmeg was available in a range of official preparations in many national pharmacopoeias in this century (Squire, 1908) and was included in nourishing drinks for convalescents (Grieve, 1931 p. 592).

Nutmeg appears to inhibit prostaglandin synthesis (Reynolds, 1982 p. 679) but is currently used as a carminitive, gastric secretory stimulant and spasmolytic (*British Herbal Pharmacopoeia*, 1991). The nutmeg seed and seed covering (mace) are rich in volatile oils and contain safrole, as found in *Sassafras albidum*, and also myristicin, a hallucinogenic compound. Nutmeg and mace have an antibacterial action and may be prescribed in infantile diarrhea (Evans, 1996 pp. 273–4).

Rhubarb

Rhubarb takes its name from the Greek *rha*, and Latin *barbarum*, foreign. *Rha* was the ancient name of the Volga along whose banks the plants grew; an alternative explanation is that the name derives from the Greek *rheo*, to flow, referring to the purgative properties of the root. Rhubarb is a member of the genus *Rheum*, of the dock family, and a number of rhubarb varieties were used as medications.

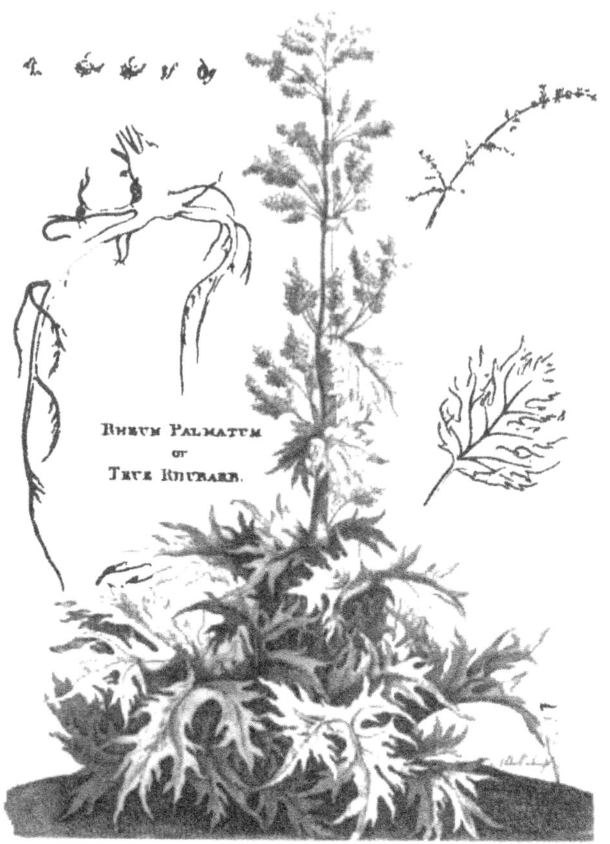

Figure 6 Rhubarb (*Rheum sativum*)

The use of rhubarb as a therapeutic agent in China can be traced back to 2700 BC (Evans, 1996 pp. 242–5) and it was a popular remedy during the Han Dynasty (206 BC–AD 23). Chinese rhubarb was known as *Da Huang*. The plant was an important article of commerce and it was carried from China along the trade routes via Turkey and Russia to Europe. Rhubarb was known to the Arabian physicians and was included as a therapeutic agent in Avicenna's *Canon* in the eleventh century AD (Shah, 1966). At some later date the rhubarb plant was introduced into Europe by the Arabs and it has been grown in the West since the early eighteenth century (Chevallier, 1996). According to the *Encyclopaedia Britannica* (1771), rhubarb was introduced into England in 1762 by a Dr Mounsey who brought the seeds from Russia. He

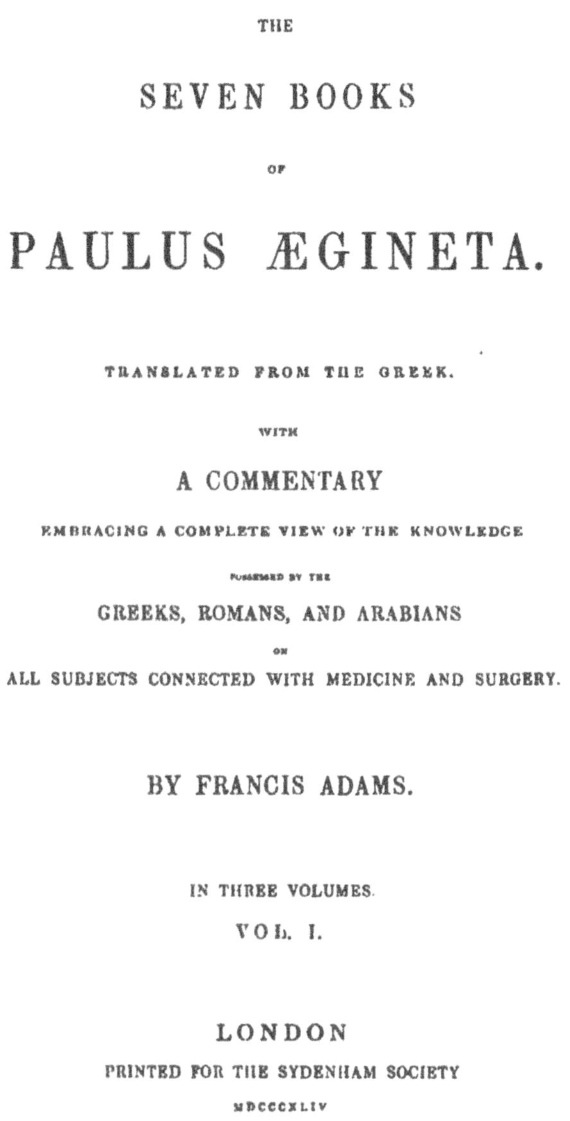

THE

SEVEN BOOKS

OF

PAULUS ÆGINETA.

TRANSLATED FROM THE GREEK.

WITH

A COMMENTARY

EMBRACING A COMPLETE VIEW OF THE KNOWLEDGE

POSSESSED BY THE

GREEKS, ROMANS, AND ARABIANS

ON

ALL SUBJECTS CONNECTED WITH MEDICINE AND SURGERY.

BY FRANCIS ADAMS.

IN THREE VOLUMES.

VOL. I.

LONDON

PRINTED FOR THE SYDENHAM SOCIETY

MDCCCXLIV

Figure 7 Frontispiece from Adam's *The seven Books of Paulus Aeginata*

passed the seeds to Dr Hope, professor of medicine and botany at Edinburgh who sowed them in his physic garden. Maps of the garden from 1777 show large areas devoted to rhubarb cultivation.

Although not yet grown in the West, rhubarb was used as a medication during the Middle Ages to provoke menstruation. It was one of many remedies taken in pills for 'the mola of the womb … the cure for this malady is very difficult and takes a long time before it is effective' and for 'excessive flowing of blood at the wrong time; and this sickness weakens a great number of women' (Rowland, 1981 pp. 75, 141, 153). It is of interest to note that rhubarb was not mentioned in *The Byrth of Mankynde* (Raynold, 1545), the most important book on obstetrics to appear in almost 1500 years, nor in the seventeenth century midwifery texts at my disposal. Monks rhubarb (*Rumex alpinus*, a dock) did find a place in the *London Dispensatoria* (Culpeper, 1654) for the treatment of liver disorders, and it was known to have a purging action.

Rhubarb was very popular in gynecological practice in the nineteenth century when rhubarb pills were prescribed for vaginal 'whites', for fertility and menstrual disorders, and for uterine inflammation. In nineteenth century medicine, rhubarb was classified as an 'alternative', a medication that changed the character of the blood through its action upon the organs of nutrition. Rhubarb (*Rheum palmatum*, Turkish rhubarb) was thought to be anti-syphilitic (Scurrah, 1921 p. 115). Maud Grieve, the best twentieth-century writer on herbal medications, related that rhubarb was used extensively in the treatment of both gout and syphilis (1931 p. 675). The various forms of rhubarb contain anthraquinones (laxatives) and tannins (astringents) which act on the alvine (from the Latin *alvus*, belly) secretion. Extract of Chinese rhubarb (Chinghai rhubarb, *Da Huang*) is thought to stimulate the uterus and is currently used in traditional Chinese medicine for amenorrhea and menstrual problems (*Pharmacopoeia of the Peoples Republic of China*, 1992). Only the rhubarb roots are used as the leaves may be poisonous. Rhubarb remained as an medication in the British pharmacopoeia until late in the twentieth century.

ARABIAN DRUGS AND THEIR USES RECORDED IN FRANCIS ADAMS' *PAUL OF AEGINA*

Abortion
Artamita

Aphrodisiac
Berberis, buzeiden, camphor, cubebs, galanga, granum kelkel (alkelkel), horon (bombax), musk, nux henden (banden), secacul, vertz

To soften the breast
Cassia fistula (senna)

Unspecified
Horon (bombax)
Cramp
Ambra grisea
Emmenagogue
Lapis lazuli, usnen, zerumbeth (cassumunar root)
Hemorrhage (unspecified)
Camphor, gum vernix (sandraracha), margaritae
Hemorrhoids
Coconut oil, fel, gum vernix, myrobalans, raspberry
To cause impotence
Camphor
To cause an erection
Berberis, galanga
For excess menstruation
Gum vernix, raspberry
Pregnancy (for fetal growth)
Musa
For sperm
Berberis, buzeiden, coconut oil, galanga
To stop semen
Camphor
Disease of the uterus
Berberis, horon (bombax), mace
Uterine purge
Dende, manna, myrobalans, turpeth
Uterine swelling (dropsy, inflation)
Zerumbeth (cassumunar root)

References

Adams, F. (1844). *The Seven Books of Paulus Aegineta*, translated from the Greek. Vol. 1, pp. 2, 47, 595. (London: The Sydenham Society)

Adams, F. (1846). *The Seven Books of Paulus Aegineta*, translated from the Greek. Vol. 2, pp. 316–28. (London: The Sydenham Society)

Adams, F. (1847). *The Seven Books of Paulus Aegineta*, translated from the Greek. Vol. 3, pp. 5, 385, 425, 427–9, 437, 456. (London: The Sydenham Society)

Afnan, S. M. (1958). *Avicenna. His Life and Work*. (London: Allen & Unwin Ltd.)

Bown, D. (1995). *The Royal Horticultural Society Encyclopaedia of Herbs and their Uses*, pp. 262, 330. (London: Dorling Kindersley)

British Herbal Medicine Association (1991). *British Herbal Pharmacopoeia*, pp. 147–8. (Bournemouth, UK)

Browne, E. G. (1921). *Arabian Medicine. Being the Fitzpatrick Lectures delivered to the College of Physicians in November 1919 and November 1920*. (Cambridge: University Press)

Campbell, D. (1926). *Arabian Medicine, and its Influence on the Middle Ages*, Vol. 1, pp. 65–75. (London: Kegan Paul, Trench, Trubner & Co.)

Campbell, D. (1926). *Arabian Medicine, and its Influence on the Middle Ages*, Vol. 2, pp. 1–12. (London: Kegan Paul, Trench, Trubner & Co.)

Chevallier, A. (1996). *The Encyclopedia of Medicinal Plants*, p. 124. (London: Dorling Kindersley)

Culpeper, N. (1651). *A Directory for Midwives: or, A Guide for Women, in their Conception, Bearing, And Suckling their Children*, p. 198. (London: Peter Cole)

Culpeper, N. (1654). *Pharmacopoeia Londoninsis: or The London Dispensatorie, Further Adorned by the Studies and Collections of the Fellows now living of the said Colledge*, pp. 58, 75. (London: Peter Cole)

Culpeper, N. (1826). *Culpeper's Complete Herbal and English Physician*, p. 47. (Manchester: J. Gleave & Son)

Dorland, W. A. N. (1932). *The American Illustrated Medical Dictionary*, pp. 70, 336. (Philadelphia & London: W. B. Saunders Co.)

Elgood, C. (1970). *Safavid Medical Practice*. (London: Luzac & Co.)

Encyclopaedia Britannica (1771). *Encyclopaedia Britannica or a Dictionary of Arts and Sciences, compiled upon a new plan*, Vol. 1, pp. 132, 642. (Edinburgh: A. Bell & C. MacFarquhar)

Evans, W. C. (1996). *Trease & Evans Pharmacognosy*, pp. 278, 273–4, 242–5. (London: W. B. Saunders Co.)

Evied, R. Y. (1971). *Bibliography of Medieval Arabic and Jewish Medicine and Allied Sciences*. (London: Wellcome Institute of the History of Medicine)

Garrison, F. H. (1929). *An Introduction to the History of Medicine*, pp. 126–39. (Philadelphia & London: W. B. Saunders Co.)

Grieve, M. (1931). *A Modern Herbal*, pp. 592, 675. (London: Jonathan Cape Ltd.)

Gruner, O. C. (1930). *The Canon of Medicine of Avicenna*, Translation of the First Book. p. 592. (London: Luzac & Co.)

Gunther, R. T. (1959). *The Greek Herbal of Dioscorides*, pp. 637, 199. (New York: Haffner Publishing Co.)

Hare, H. A. (1901). *A Textbook of Practical Therapeutics*, pp. 121–5, 305. (London: Henry Kimpton)

Hilton-Simpson, M. W. (1913). *Arab Medicine and Surgery*. (London: Oxford University Press)

Hoblyn, R. D. (1878). *A Dictionary of Terms used in Medicine and the Collateral Sciences*, p. 25. (London: Whittaker & Co.)

Mahoney, J. F., Arnold, R. C. and Harris, A. (1943). Penicillin Treatment of Early Syphilis – a preliminary report. *Am. J. Public Health* 33, 1387–91

Mann, E. W. (1915). *Southalls Organic Materia Medica*, pp. 287–8. (London: J. and A. Churchill)

Oriel, J. D. (1994). *The Scars of Venus. A History of Venereology*, p. 14. (London: Springer-Verlag)

Pharmacopoeia of the People's Republic of China (1992). English edition of The Pharmacopoeia of the People's Republic of China, 1990 ed., p. 161. (Beijing. China: Guang Dong Science and Technology Press)

Pseudo-Aristotle (c. 1830). *The Works of Aristotle, the Famous Physician*, p. 66. (London: Miller, Law & Cater)

Quetel, C. (1990). *History of Syphilis*, pp. 29–30. (Cambridge: Polity Press)

Raynold, T. (1545). *The Byrth of Mankynde*, English Translation. (London: T. Ray)

Reynolds, J. E. F. (ed.) (1982). *Martindale the Extra Pharmacopoeia*, 28th ed., pp. 351, 675, 679. (London: The Pharmaceutical Press)

Ricci, J. (1943). *The Genealogy of Gynaecology*, pp. 211–37. (Philadelphia: Blakiston Co.)

Rowland, B. (1981). *Medieval Woman's Guide to Health*, pp. 75, 79, 81, 93, 95, 97, 101, 119, 141, 153. (London: Croom & Helm)

Scurrah, J. W. (1921). *The National Botanic Pharmacopoeia*, 2nd ed., pp. 34, 115. (Bradford: Woodhouse, Cornthwaite & Co.)

Shah, M. H. (1966). *The General Principles of Avicenna's Canon of Medicine*, p. 435. (Pakistan: Naveed Clinic)

Squire, P. W. (1908). *Squire's Companion to the latest edition of the British Pharmacopoeia*, 18th ed., pp. 462, 601–34, 797–800. (London: J. and A. Churchill)

Turner, W. (1568). *The Herbal*. Part 3, pp. 40–1. (Collen: Arnold Birckman)

Wolveridge, J. (1671). *Speculum Matricis; or the Expert Midwives Handmaid*, pp. 93, 111, 129, 130, 131, 132, 139, 148, 148. (London: E. Okes)

Wootton, A. C. (1910). *Chronicles of Pharmacy*, Vol. 1, pp. 408–22; Vol. 2, pp. 304–11, 304–11. (London: MacMillan & Co.)

The late Middle Ages 12

INTRODUCTION

The long-established medical school at Salerno in southern Italy came to prominence in the eleventh century. It was at Salerno that the Arabic medical manuals were translated and brought to the attention of educated Europeans, so reviving the ancient Greek and Latin medical teachings. Prominent among the translators was Gerardo of Cremona (1114–1187), an Italian who went to Toledo to learn Arabic and who became the principal translator of the Toledan Arabic medical and scientific texts.

The Arabic texts described in detail the concepts of Greco-Roman medicine of 1000 years previously. They included some new drugs, and also brought astrological medicine to the fore. Belief in the influence of the planets and stars was prevalent in Babylonian culture but was less so among the Greeks and Romans. Through the Arabian influence, however, astrology reached the dignity of a science and during the Middle Ages became an integral part of medicine, holding a place in Europe until the eighteenth century.

During the Salernitan era of medicine there were a number of important practitioners whose works were copied and translated into the European languages. These texts, based on Greco-Roman medicine (derived from Arabic sources) and complemented by the influences of Chinese and Indian medicine, were the beginnings of a new era in medicine. The medical centers of the Levant went into decline and European medicine began to flourish.

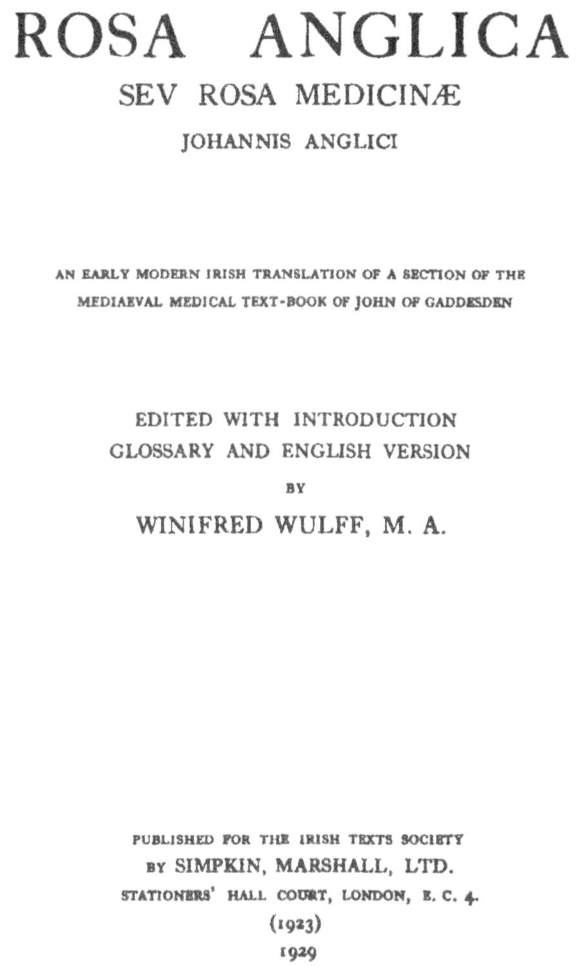

Trotula of Salerno

Although there is some dispute as to her identity, it is claimed that Trotula of Salerno wrote *Curandarum Aegritudinem Muliebrium, Ante, In et Post Partum*, better known by its short title, *De Passionibus Mulierum*, which dates from about 1050. The first printed version of the book was produced by Schottus of Strasburg in 1544 (Ricci, 1943). Elizabeth

ROSA ANGLICA

SEV ROSA MEDICINÆ

JOHANNIS ANGLICI

AN EARLY MODERN IRISH TRANSLATION OF A SECTION OF THE MEDIAEVAL MEDICAL TEXT-BOOK OF JOHN OF GADDESDEN

EDITED WITH INTRODUCTION GLOSSARY AND ENGLISH VERSION BY

WINIFRED WULFF, M. A.

PUBLISHED FOR THE IRISH TEXTS SOCIETY BY SIMPKIN, MARSHALL, LTD. STATIONERS' HALL COURT, LONDON, E. C. 4. (1923) 1929

Figure 1 Frontispiece from Wulff's *Rosa Anglica*

Mason-Hohl translated the text into English in 1940. The booklet was devoted to gynecology, obstetrics and care of the newborn. Most of the text is devoted to medications for female disorders. Trotula prescribed fumigation with ginger, laurel and savin for oligomenorrhea. For 'uterine suffocation' she advised asafetida. Her text includes a discourse on the repair of perineal lacerations with silk thread. The technique was closely followed by Mauriceau in the seventeenth century.

The term 'flowers' was used to describe the menstrual period for the first time: 'In women there is not enough bodily heat for proper consumption and elimination of humors as in men; the excess accumulation is eliminated by the menstrual flow, which by the rabble is called the flowers. Just as the tree does not bear fruit without blossoms, so a woman without menses will not bring forth an issue' (Ricci, 1943). It was through the name Trotula that the term 'Dame Trot' evolved for a woman involved in maternity care.

Nicolas Salernitanus

In the early part of the twelfth century Nicolas Salernitanus (also known as Nicolas Praepositus), dean of the medical school at Salerno, wrote a manuscript entitled *Antidotarium*. It was the first drug formulary of the era and centuries later, in 1471, it became one of the first medical books in print. The *Antidotarium* contained 139 prescriptions, laid out in alphabetical order, and listed many of the new Arabic drugs. It was famous for its original formula for the *spongia somnifera*, the medieval anesthetic sponge. A small number of prescriptions were included for gynecological problems.

Hildegard of Bingen

In the twelfth century St Hildegard (1098–1179), the abbess of Rupertsberg, was the first female natural scientist and physician in Germany. Between 1151 and 1158 she completed two books, *Physica* and *Causae et Curae*. *Physica* dealt with plants, animals and medicine and over half of the book was related to botany. *Causae et Curae* was a book of general medicine and therapeutics that included tracts on gynecological disorders. For failure to menstruate she advised the use of aniseed, cloves, diptam, feverfew, heidelberries, honey, lilies, rue, white pepper and yarrow. The herbs were either mulled in wine and taken after breakfast, or placed in a bath in which the woman immersed herself. Excessive menstruation was treated with an oral preparation of betony or by placing cold celeriac in wine on the thigh and navel. For painful birth Hildegard advised fennel and hazelroot applied to the back and thighs.

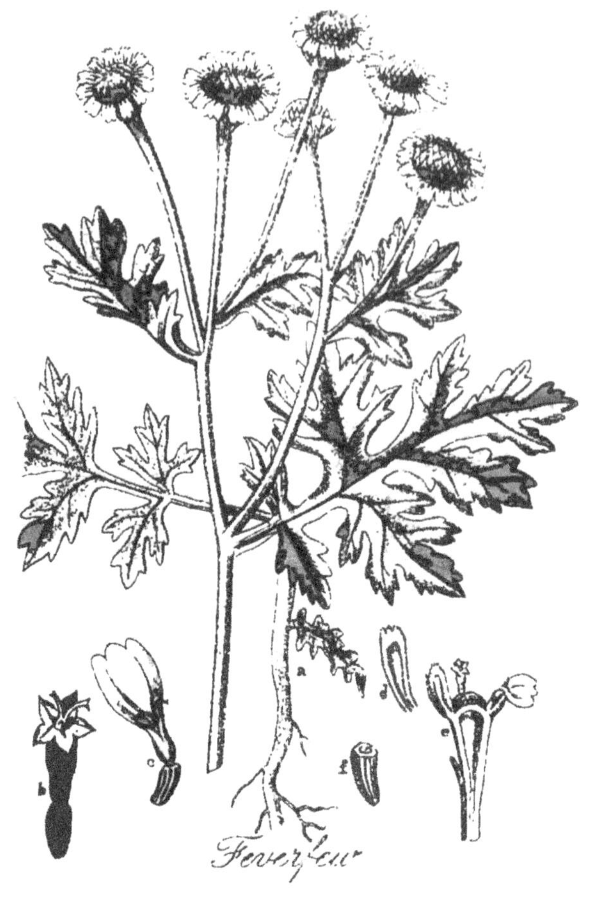

Figure 2 Feverfew

Albertus Magnus

Albertus Magnus (1193–1280), was a Dominican monk and eminent naturalist of the thirteenth century, who taught at Paris but settled in Cologne. His *De vegetalibus et plantis* was based on his personal botanical observations and a further work, *De animalibus*, was a commentary on the works of Aristotle. Of more importance to obstetrics and gynecology was the work reputed to have been written by Albertus Magnus, *De secretis mulierum*. Although mainly a work on cosmetics the manuscript contained a large amount of astrological medical lore, and included a piece regarding the planetary influence on the formation of the fetus. Magnus detailed a test for chastity in his text: the woman to be tested was fed powder of yellow lilies – if she was not a virgin she would pass urine immediately, those who were virginal would not. In another test, if non-virginal urine was poured over mallow herb, the plant dried up and died. Virgin's urine was thought to be clear and bright, but that of sexually experienced women was turbid due to adulteration with seminal sediment.

Three important manuscripts

In the latter part of the Middle Ages the three manuscripts of most prominence were John of Arderne's *De Arte Phisicali et de Cirurgia* of 1412, *A Leech Book or Collection of Medical Recipes* of c. 1443 and the undated but early fifteenth century *Medieval Woman's Guide to Health*. This last text was translated by Beryl Rowland in 1981 and was in reality a book of therapeutics for women. The *Medieval Woman's Guide to Health* is the most important book of the era from the *Materia Medica Woman* point of view.

JOHN OF ARDERNE'S *DE ARTE PHISICALI ET DE CIRURGIA*

Master John Arderne (1307–1360) Chirurgion of Newark in the county of Nottingham, is the best-known of the early English surgeons (Garrison, 1929). He practiced in Newark from 1349 until 1370 and then traveled extensively in Europe before settling in London (Power, 1922). Arderne was well-versed in astrology, religion and wort-cunning and he prescribed medicinal herbs, and animal and mineral treatments, while invoking the aid of the Almighty and His heavenly retinue. His text contains 28 treatments for reproductive health.

John of Arderne was well-read in medicine and surgery and in his own writings he quoted from the works of Avicenna, Almansor, Serapeon and Alexander of Tralles. The existing manuscripts contain different combinations of his treatises. One of his works, *Treatises on Fistula* (in Ano) was printed by John Read of Gloucester in 1588 but the bulk of his work remains unpublished. Nicholas Culpeper, in his translation of *The Pharmacopoeia Londinensis*, mentioned the compound medications tapsimel, tapsivalentia and valentia scabiosae: 'these three last was stolen out of the manuscripts of Mr. John Arderne for a Chyrurgian at Newark upon Trent, though now the College have the honesty to conceal his name' (1654 pp. 304–5). Culpeper's translation into English of the second *London Pharmacopoeia* was not authorized by the College of Physicians, and led to considerable annoyance among its members. Sir D'Arcy Power wrote: [John Arderne] 'somewhat of a pharmacist and his name lived longer in this connection than as a surgeon. Three of the preparations he invented appear in the second issue of the first *London Pharmacopoeia* of 1618 and some of them were certainly in use as late as 1733'.

John of Arderne's manuscript, *De Arte Phisicali et de Cirurgia*, is an abbreviated version of his works, made some years after his death, and dates from c. 1412. The original copy is in the Royal Library at Stockholm. Eric Millar made a replica of the Stockholm manuscript for the Wellcome Historical Medical Museum and Sir D'Arcy Power's translation of the document was published in 1922. In reality John of Arderne's *De Arte Phisicali et de Cirurgia* was a compilation of drug treatments for various 'surgical' disorders, although a small number of surgical procedures were outlined. Included with the manuscript was a tract entitled 'Of Those who are Pregnant and of Labour' which contained instructions for midwives was illustrated by birth figures in the style of Muscio (fifth century).

John of Arderne's obstetrics and gynecology

Arderne advised the midwife that she should carry out her manipulations gently and without roughness: 'She should, therefore, frequently pour over the parts themselves warm oil or juice of fenugreek, or boiled linseed and mallows'. He instructed that at all times the baby should be born safely 'for we have known very many children born after a difficult labour and we have seen them live'. Arderne briefly described 'natural' and 'unnatural' forms of the birth process. Seventeen birth figures (one was duplicated) showed the fetus inside an inverted flask-like uterus and illustrated various fetal malpresentations.

John of Arderne's medications and their uses

Uses

'Against Bleeding Piles or to Restrain the Menses'
Arderne noted that 'all authors say that remedies which restrain the piles also restrain the menses'.

Accordingly he offered the following prescription: 'Moisten the finest wheaten flour (Ador or Pyrus) with juice of Millefoil and make into pills and give three or four of them daily in the morning moistened with wine of the decoction of Millefoil or of Plantain or of Shepherd's purse, or of Nettle or of Periwinkle'. Alternatively, phlebotomy could be performed on the basilic vein of the arm, or from the saphenous vein of the outer ankle.

'For the disease which is called *Chaude pisse*'
Chaude pisse (hot piss) was the French term for gonorrhea. The patient was advised to 'Take Parsley and boil it in water until it is turned into a mucilage. Let it be well shaken with oil of roses or violets and then add to it the milk of a nursing woman in which camphor is dissolved, and inject with a syringe'. An alternative remedy ... 'Against Gonorrhoeal inflammations' included: 'Psidium, Purslane seed, Water-lentil, and Water-lily'. 'Make a syrup'.

'When the penis or vulva is inflamed'
Medications for inflammation included bran, egg yolk, henbane, mallows, oil of roses, violets, warm milk and warm water.

'Affections of the testicles and their Purses'
Barley meal, bean meal, egg, honey, oil of roses, powdered tannin, rotten oak wood, vinegar and violets; were used by local application or enema.

Selected remedies

Barley meal, bean meal, bran,
Camphor,
Egg,
Fenugreek,
Henbane, honey,
Linseed,
Mallows, millefoil, milk, mother's milk,
Nettle,
Oil of roses,
Parsley, periwinkle, plantain, powdered tannin, psidium, purslane seed,
Rotten oak wood,
Shepherd's purse,
Vinegar, violets,
Water, water lentil, water lily, wheaten flour, wine.

A LEECH BOOK OR COLLECTION OF RECIPES

> 'Here beginneth good medicines for all manner of evils that every man hath, that good Leeches have drawn out of the books of those who men called Archippus (Æsculapius) and Hippocrates, for these were the best leeches of the world in their time: and therefore who so will do as this book will teach him, he may be secure to have help for all evils and wounds and other diseases and sickness both within and also without'.

Thus began the *Leech Book or Collection of Medical Recipes* of the fifteenth century transcribed by Warren R. Dawson (1934), Fellow of the Royal Society of Medicine and librarian at Lloyd's. The *Leech Book* dates from 1443 or the following year.

The content of the manuscript was a large collection of recipes for ailments, affections, and injuries of all kinds. The recipes include 86 products for reproductive health. Unlike most manuscripts of its era, the usual charms and incantations were lacking but some magical elements were present. The drugs were mainly herbal in origin although animal and mineral preparations were also used. Bloodletting and cupping were mentioned and there were passages devoted to the preparation of confections, potions, salves and other forms of medication, and to the gathering of herbs.

Dawson wrote that the recipes in the *Leech Book* were drawn up in a manner similar to those contained in the Ancient Egyptian hieratic medical papyri. First came the titles; then the drugs with their quantities and directions for preparation; and the directions for administration, either separately or in a vehicle. Some remedies had alternatives, offered as 'another remedy' or 'another' or 'another for the same'. Many of the recipes end with the words 'until he be whole' or remarks such as 'a good remedy' or by the colophon 'It is proved; *Probatum est*'. Some remedies are specifically stated to be 'for a man or a woman'.

Another indication of Egyptian influence was the medicinal use of the milk of a woman who had borne a male child. This remedy was mentioned a number of times in the *Leech Book* and was characteristic of Egyptian medicine. Medication which included mother's milk was cited twelve times in the Ebers

Papyrus, thrice in the London medical papyrus, twice in the Berlin medical papyrus and once each in the Hearst, Berlin 3027 and Cairo Coptic medical papyri.

Medications and their uses in the *Leech Book*

The *Leech Book* consists of 1074 passages, in paragraph form, of which 55 relate to women's materia medica. Many of the prescriptions below are quoted directly from the book to give a flavor of the text. The remedies are cataloged here into groups but retain their original paragraph numbers for those interested in further research. The paragraph reference numbers for the mother's milk prescriptions are included.

Uses

Breast disorders

Cancer

'For canker in the paps ... [Take] pigeon's dung, honey, virgin wax, flour of barley and of beans and linseed; and seethe them in vinegar or wine, and put there two ram's tallow; and make in the manner of a plaster, and lay thereon (#213).
'For the canker in the teats' use 'celandine juice and goose-dung, stamped on and laid on the breast (#903).
'Another': beans, barley flour, duck's dung, honey, linseed and ram's tallow mixed and 'laid on the breast as a plaster' (#904).

Congestion

'For milk that has hardened in a woman's teats ... Seeth [boil] Mint in wine and oil, and lay them upon the teats in a plaster' (#620).
'For women's teats that be swollen': white of egg, Juice of smallage and linseed 'and lay thereto. And if she loses her milk, give her to drink the juice of vervain, and she shall have enough' (#898).
'For rankling teats that come of too much milk': powder of hempseed was added to the mother's food (#900).
'To make teats small': the breast was anointed with seed of hemlock and vinegar (#901).
Another; incense and vinegar (#902).

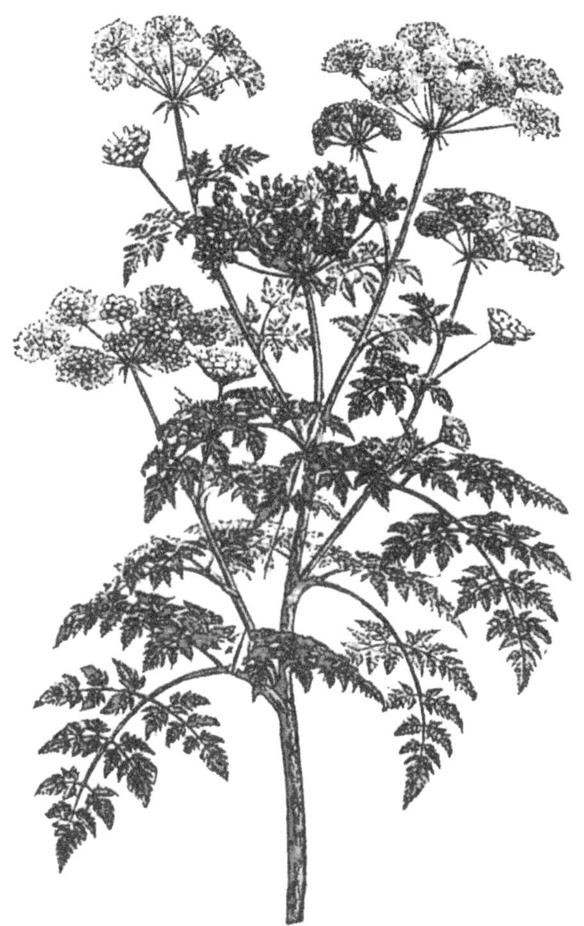

Figure 3 Hemlock (*Conium maculatum*)

'Another for aching of teats that cometh of too much milk. Make powder of hempseed and give it her in all her meat and drink' (#49).

Galactagogue

For 'woman's milk that faileth ... [take] crystal and pound it, and give it her to drink, with the milk of another woman; but let her not know what milk it is' (#621).
'Another for the same': vervain in lukewarm white wine ... and she shall have milk enough, on warranty' (#622).

Inflammation

For 'Ache of women's breasts or teats that are rankled [inflamed]. Take groundsel and daisies, and wash

them and stamp them; and drink them first and last [morning and evening] (#47).
'Another': 'Take senvey [mustard seed] and stamp well in a mortar, and take thereto the third part of crumbs of white bread; and baste thereto dry figs, honey and vinegar, according as the ache waxeth and the quantity of the sore sufficeth' (#48).
'To make a healing entrete for broken and open teats ... [take] a herb that men call alla [wood sorrel] and wrap it in red cabbage leaves; and lay it under hot ashes half a mile-way [the time taken to walk half mile], and then [take] these herbs out of the fire and stamp it as well as thou may'st with good honey and vinegar, and mingle it well together, and put them in a box; and lay first to the pap a plaster made of ga [*sic*] and of flour of wheat sodden with vinegar; and lay this plaster twice on the sore and afterwards lay the entrete [thereto]' (#297).
'For an imposthume [abscess] in a woman's teats ... [take] the juice of morell [nightshade], and take the white of eggs, and flour of beans; and mingle them together and lay it cold to the teats' (#717).
'For teats that ache'. Mint in wine and olive oil bound to the breasts (#899).
'For boils on women's teats': egg oil, bean meal and juice of nightshade, in a plaster (#916).
'Another for aching teats ... [take] mint and stamp it, and lay thereto in the manner of a plaster, all hot' (#917).

Convulsions

'For the suffocation of the mother ... [Let her] receive the smoke of turpentine laid on the coals through her mouth' (#589).

Lechery

'Kynd [lechery] of man to stop it. Take heavy blue cloth and burn it in a red pot or upon a red tile-stone; and make powder thereof, and take good ale; and beat it in the pot, and cast therein the powder and give him to drink three days; and that is medicinable [curable]' (#542).
To avoid lechery: 'Take nettle-seed and bray it in a mortar with pepper, and temper it with honey or with wine, and it shall destroy it. And if thou wilt prove it, give it to a dog that goeth on the scent, and he will forsake the bitch, and she will go mad' (#577).

Man's privy member

'For the palsy in a man's privy member. Seethe castoreum and wine, and wash him therewith about the pubic region, and wet the cloth therein and [lay it] upon the organ in the manner of a plaster. *Probatum est*' (#741).
'For a privy member that is chafed [excoriated] ... [Take] the juice of morell bruised linseed and barrow's grease; and boil together, and lay thereon hot' (#892).

Menstruation

To induce

'For women's flowers ... [take] the roots of gladyne [iris], and seethe them in wine or vinegar; and when it is well sodden, set in on the ground, and let her stride or stand thereover that the fumes may steam up to her, so that there may be no air but even up. Unless she be with child, this medicine failed never' (#313). A further three compound prescriptions are offered as plasters or potions to provoke menstruation. The remedies contained ale, alexanders, bay, bran, chamomile, fennel, fern roots, frankincense, goat dung, horehound, hyssop, lily oil, mace, mugwort, sheep grease, southernwood, sow thistle, withy leaves, and wormwood (#314–316).
'For to make a woman have her flowers red when they have ceased to flow ... [this] medicine faileth never, but beware that she is not with child'. Iris, vinegar and wine in a 'fume' or a honey and madder suppository (#321–322).
'Another for to bring them ... [take] the juice of mercury, honey, flour and cockle, of each equal quantities; and make little balls thereof, and give her one or two or three; and that night she shall have them [the terms] and be disposed to conceive' (#325).
[A cockle may be one of several plants, in particular, the corncockle, which grow as a weed in cornfields. Tony Hunt in his *Plant Names of Medieval England* (1989) identifies corncockle as *Agrostemma githago* but Dawson indicated that the cockle was ergot, thus relating it to *Ustilago maydis* (corn smut or

corn ergot) which is a uterine stimulant. A tract in the *Medieval Woman's Guide to Health* shows that the cockle was availed of to 'purge' the uterus, and that 'the uterus smarts inside because of the sharpness of the Cockle' (Rowland, 1981 p. 111). It is generally held that the first reference to ergot was in a German book, the 1582 edition of Adam Lonicer's *Kreuter Buch*. The history of ergot is dealt with in Chapter 3.]

For excess flow

'For too many flowers': four compound medications were offered which contained ale, antidotum emmenagogum, comfrey, gelt's grease, hare's foot, honey, horse dung, milk, sheep droppings, vinegar, wheat flour and wine (#317–320).

'To dissolve flowing flowers': two compound medications of madder in sweet wine or juice of waybread 'in the privity, or drink it', were offered to check menstrual flooding (#323–324).

'An ointment to dissolve women's flowers, if she be anointed therewith from the navel downwards; and it is good for sore teats, and it is called ungentum lilium. Take oil of olive and stop it full of lily flowers, and let it stand open in the sun nine days; and then strain it through a cloth, and let it stand again to clear another nine days, and then put it in a glass or join-pot [a jar with a lid] and let [it] stand long in the sun, and keep it' (#660).

For dysmenorrhea

'For the mother, of the evil cake [clotting dysmenorrhea]'. Onion, anise and cumin were cooked and eaten (#588).

Disorders of the uterus

To cleanse

'A suppository made of cotton and anointed with turpentine cleanseth the mother' (#590).

To purge

'The matrix, to purge it of wicked humours and to help make more easy mala matricis': conduct fumes of celandine, gladden, mugwort, and vervain boiled in white wine to 'the place and let the breath [steam] go well in; and then lay thereto all hot a plaster thereof' (#591).

For leukorrhea

'For to dry the superfluities of the mother [leukorrhea]. Seethe calamint in water, and therewith wash her from beneath' (#592).

For inflammation

'The virtues of Nept [catmint]. Take Nept and seethe it in red wine and lay it to a woman's navel when she is lying in; and that shall bring out all manner of corruption, and make her small, and do away [reduce] the mother [womb]' (#643).

'Oil of hillwort ... anoint about the liver, about the navel, and about the womb-piece of a woman that is sick in the mother' (#671).

Oxytocics

'For deliverance of a dead child ... [take] leek blades and scale them, and bind to the womb about the navel; and it shall cast out the dead child; and when she is delivered, take away the blades or she shall cast out all that is in her' (#256).

Other oxytocic potions contained dittany, hyssop, roses in wine, or madder roots and honey in a suppository and savory in wine (#357–359).

Woman's privy member

'A drink of wine oft tempered with the juice of southernwood for it doth good against the cough and whooping-cough and against all the grievance of a woman's privy member' (#269).

Fertility test

For '[knowing] the default of conception, whether it belong to the man or the woman', the woman and her partner urinated into two separate earthen pots. Into each, a small quantity of wheat bran was placed and left to stand for ten days after which the results were read: 'Thou shall see in the water that is in default small live worms; and if there appear no worms in either water, then they be likely to have children in process of time when God will' (#523). This antique fertility test had been developed in Ancient Egypt.

Mother's milk prescriptions

In the *Leech Book*, mother's milk was prescribed for 'broken bones in the Head': a soft linen cloth was laid over the wound '[and] afterwards let woman that feedith a male child, if it be a man that is wounded, milk her pap softly on the flour that is strewn on the cloth'. In another recipe for the same condition the mother's milk was mixed with betony and vervain, and the head was covered until the following day (#93). Mother's milk was also prescribed: with leeks to treat cough (#201); with yarrow 'for the white that over groweth the apple of the eye' (#509); as a sleeping potion, applied to the temples with leek seed and the white of an egg (#851); and as a treatment 'To cease weeping ... [make] a little plaster of small powder of henbane seed, and of the white of eggs, of vinegar, and of woman's milk, and of a little incense, and lay it to the head and to the stomach' (#960).

Selected remedies

Ale, alexanders, anise, *antidotum emmenagogum*
Barley, barrow grease, bay, beans, betony, blue cloth, bran
Calamint, chamomile, castoreum, catmint, celandine, cockle, comfrey, cotton, crystal, cumin
Daisies, dittany, duck dung
Eggs
Fennel, fern roots, figs, frankincense
Ga (*sic*), gelt grease, gladden, goat dung, goose dung, groundsel
Hare's-foot, hemlock, hempseed, henbane, hillwort, honey, horehound, horse dung, hyssop
Incense, iris
Leek, lily, linseed
Mace, madder, mercury, milk, mint, mother's milk, mugwort, mustard
Nettle, nightshade
Olive oil, onion
Pepper, pigeon dung
Ram's tallow, red cabbage leaves, roses
Savory, sheep droppings, sheep grease, smallage, southernwood, sow thistle
Turpentine
Vervain, vinegar
Water, wax, waybread, wheat, white bread, wine, withy leaves, woman's milk, wood sorrel, wormwood
Yarrow

Quantities used in prescriptions

Quantities were measured in units of a pound, half a pound, half a quartron, an ounce, half an ounce, a drachm, half a drachm, a scruple (20 wheatcorns making a scruple): 'A scruple weigheth a penny; three scruples maketh a drachm; eight drachms maketh an ounce and sixteen ounces make a pound'. Another unit of measurement was the handful (written as 'm'.).

MEDIEVAL WOMAN'S GUIDE TO HEALTH

The *Medieval Woman's Guide to Health* is the name used for the Sloane Manuscript No. 2463 which dates from the early fifteenth century and was concerned with obstetrics and gynecology. The Middle English text was translated into modern English by Beryl Rowland, professor of English at York University, Toronto. According to Rowland, the manuscript was the first English gynecological handbook, although it was not available in printed format until recently (Rowland, 1981).

The recipes of the *Medieval Woman's Guide to Health* include 267 of herbal origin, and 17 medicaments which contain more than one ingredient. Recipes including metals, minerals and precious stones number 37; animal parts are 78; and 12 forms of alcohol are mentioned. Twelve related items such as ointments are added. I have endeavored to summarize, over the next few paragraphs, the author's advice, chapter by chapter, beginning with an extract from the introductory remarks:

'Because there are many women who have numerous diverse illnesses – some of them almost fatal ... [women] are ashamed for fear of reproof in times to come and of exposure by discourteous men who love women only for physical pleasure and for evil gratification ... and so, to assist women, I intend to write of how to help their secret maladies so that one woman may aid another in her illness and not divulge her secrets to such discourteous men'.

'The first chapter is concerned with the stopping of the blood that women should have in purgations and be purged of'

The author dealt with the 'signs and general indications of this sickness ... retention of this blood so that they cannot have their purgations at the proper times'. During their 'courses' some women 'have a desire to consort with men' and produce children that are 'lepers or have some other such evil sickness'. The author concluded that corrupt humors, which she or he identified as phlegm, bile and black bile, were the cause of menstrual disorders. Treatment involved bloodletting, cupping under the nipples, and hot baths with herbal medications or medicated wine. A medicated suppository (a type of medieval tampon) was availed of and was 'fastened with a thread bound round one of her thighs, in case the suppositories should be drawn completely into the uterus'. Various forms of cordials, electuaries and pills were prescribed, or medicated plasters were laid on the woman's genitalia. There was a special medicated pillow that women would sit on when bathing '[to reduce painful] retentions and soften the processes of the womb'. When all else failed, the lancet was employed to let 'a considerable quantity of blood'.

'The second chapter is concerned with excessive flowing of blood at the wrong time; and this sickness weakens a great number of women'

Explanations were offered for excessive utero-vaginal blood loss and cures of cupping, scarification, powders, suppositories and all the usual methods were offered. The author was careful to point out that based on results previously obtained, the various remedies were efficacious. The first two chapters contain in excess of 150 medications that were used to inhibit or induce the menses.

'The third chapter is concerned with the suffocation of the uterus'

The author defined 'suffocation of the uterus' in the following manner: '[suffocation] is when a woman's heart and lungs are thrust together by the uterus so that the woman seems dead except for her breathing ... this sickness is due to various reasons ... such as the retaining of blood or of corrupt and venomous uterine humours'. Treatment for the ailment involved purging the uterus and, dependent on the type of suffocation, 'it is helpful to have relations with a man'. The patient was fumigated 'underneath' with sweet smelling things and was allowed to smell stinking things. These measures forced the malign humors back to the uterus from whence they could be purged. The third chapter combined almost 90 remedies for uterine suffocation.

'The fourth chapter is of the precipitation of the uterus'

This ailment was thought to result from paralysis of the uterus which fell, either sideways or downwards, from its natural position. 'Let the midwife put it in again with her hand. Let her anoint her hand first with oil and afterwards make a fumigation underneath of stinking camomile or of dry ox-dirt thrown on the coals and let her smell fragrant things'. For precipitation of the uterus, the patient was offered cupping, fumigation, bathing in herbs, an ointment to apply to the vulva, suppositories or a special plaster applied to the vulva. In excess of 100 remedies were availed of to treat uterine prolapse.

'The fifth chapter is concerned with wind in the uterus'

Uterine pain was experienced due to swelling of the uterus, thought to be due to retained wind, for which 33 nostrums were available. An electuary, a bath, and medicines for 'stitches' and 'winds' were used. The patient was also asked to abstain from windy foods.

The remainder of the chapter was concerned with excessive bloody discharge, distress following childbirth, and 'dropsy [edema] of the uterus'. There was no sixth chapter.

'The seventh chapter is concerned with a rawness that occurs when the uterus seems to be excoriated'

'[To] cure women of this complaint have them purge themselves with the electuary of rose juice, and afterwards have the patient make a bath of cold herbs, and then bleed her on the vein under the ankle inside the foot.' Fumigation, pessaries and powders of cloves, frankincense, myrrh and rose leaves were employed: '[Let] a discreet woman put it where the rawness is and this powder will heal it'. There were 23 remedies offered for ulceration of the uterus.

'The eighth chapter is concerned with inflammations of the uterus that is very sore'

'Inflammation of the uterus occurs in various parts of it; sometimes it is in the innermost parts of the uterus and sometimes at the mouth of it.' The author continued with a detailed explanation of the causation and symptoms of the disorder. The illness resulted in an abscess, which, when 'broken down', voided purulent discharge. Thirty herbal remedies were used to treat this condition.

'The ninth chapter is concerned with aching of the uterus'

'The ache of the uterus is sometimes due to a stillborn child being born before its time. Because the mother has great contentment and happiness from the child inside her, when she loses it she naturally mourns and grieves just as a cow does when she has lost her calf, and that distress causes the ache of the uterus.' Sometimes, however, the uterus was thought to ache due to cold or heat. Details of 28 paregorics (analgesics) were given.

The remainder of chapter nine was concerned with establishing whether or not a woman was pregnant, without examining the urine: the woman was advised to drink mead and retire to bed. If she developed great discomfort 'in her belly' it was considered a definite sign of pregnancy. The author then went on to list a number of compound medications which were prescribed in order to expel a dead child from the womb.

'The tenth chapter is concerned with the sicknesses that women have in childbearing'

The author wrote that 'when it is natural [cephalic presentation] the child comes out in twenty pangs or within those twenty ... and [when] the child comes out unnaturally ... that may be in sixteen ways'. The medications for labor are shown below. Of particular interest was the use of cockle flour as an oxytocic.

'The eleventh chapter is concerned with the secundine that is retained in women after childbirth'

The secundine (placenta) was sometimes retained *in utero* 'because of the great weakness of her womb'. The midwife was advised to anoint her hands with oil and to attempt a manual removal. If that intervention failed she was instructed to use herbal fumigations, medicated baths and herbal potions 'that will draw out the secundine ... [and] do the same for stoppage of the menstruation'. There were 33 medications used to expel the placenta.

'The twelfth chapter is on how to make woman conceive a child if God wills'

The woman was first purged of any retained menstrual blood. Herbs were boiled in wine to make a fertility potion for consumption. Alternatively, a plaster was prepared from four raw egg yolks, half an ounce of powdered cloves and one drachm of saffron. The woman was anointed with hot oil of roses before lying on the fertility plaster. Altogether there were 34 drugs to aid fertility.

'The thirteenth chapter is concerned with excessive bleeding after childbirth'

Excess blood loss after delivery was considered to be due to decaying matter present in the uterus, causing a bloody discharge, or was due to blood that required to be 'purged'. Hot powdered thyme was placed in a bag of sufficient breadth and length to cover the 'privy parts' and fastened securely to the vulva. An alternative remedy was a mixture containing ceptfoil, cinqfoil, watercress and water parsnip and wine placed on hot coals for fumigation of the privities.

The thirteenth chapter also contained information on uterine cancers, ulcers and sores; on remedies for 'swelling of women's legs when they were pregnant; on remedies 'to restrain sexual intercourse'; 'concerning hardness of the womb and its roughness'; on 'painful discharge of urine and hindrance from urination'; 'concerning the swelling of the testicles'; and 'concerning tumor of the breast due to copious milk'. There was also a list of medications 'for women only' and finally there were tracts concerning menstruation and medicines for 'palsy' and 'the stone'.

Medications used to aid labor in the *Medieval Woman's Guide to Health*

Acorns, agrimony, artemisia, asafetida, athanasian creed (a latin charm)
Balm, beaver gland, bishop's weed, black hellebore, black olive oil, bull gall
Calamint, caraway, cassia fistula bark, castory powder, cinnamon bark, cockle flour, colocynth, cyclamen (sowbread)
Dill, dittany, dried beaver gland
Electuary
Furze
Galbanum, gall, girdle, gladiola, goat's milk, gum ammoniac
Hazelwort (asarabacca), hemagoge, honey, hyssop
Iris, ivy
Jasper, juice of balsam tree, juice of beech tree, juice of hyssop, juice of iris, juice of vervain, juniper
Laurel, leeks, lettuce, linseed, little pellitory, loadstone, lupin
Mallow, malmsey, marjoram, may butter, mercury, milkwort, mountain willow, mugwort, myrrh
Nasturtiums
Oil, oil of laurel, of lilies, of musk, of roses, of violets, ointment of aragon, orchis, ox gall
Parsley, pellitory of Spain, pennyroyal, pepper, precious balm
Quicksilver
Red chick peas, red coral, root of smallage and of iris, rosemary, round birthwort, rue
Salt, savin, savory, scammony, snake skin, southernwood, spikenard, spurge, stavescare, sweet smelling things
Terebinth resin, thyme
Unsalted butter
Vine roots, vinegar
Water (from man's skin in which he has washed), white wine, wild celery, wild mint, wild thyme, wine, woman's milk, woodruff, wormwood
Yellow iris roots

A SELECTION OF MEDIEVAL MATERIA MEDICA FOR WOMEN

Ætites the eagle stone

The ætites or eagle stone was an important amulet for women during Greco-Roman times and until the eighteenth century. In the Middle Ages the ætites was recommended by the female physician Trotula of Salerno as a precious stone that would shorten the pangs of childbirth. Indeed, its powers of traction were such that if overused it was thought likely to cause uterine prolapse at delivery (Rowland, 1981 p. 33).

The eagle stone is a small, round, encrusted nodule of iron oxide mixed with argil (from the Greek ***argillos***, white clay or alumina as used by potters). It was formerly supposed that eagles carried the stones to their nests to help them lay eggs. The golden eagle lays white eggs spotted with reddish-brown or gray, similar in appearance to the ætites. Dioscorides of Anazarbus in Cicilia wrote a section devoted to the properties 'of all metallic stones' in his first century AD Greek herbal. Of the 99 stones and earth forms that he enumerated, 21 were useful for the materia medica of women. In his discussion on the eagle stone (***ætites lapis or ætites lithos***) Dioscorides wrote that 'on being shaken [the stone] sends out a sound as if it were great [pregnant] with another stone. It is an holder in of ye Embrya when ye wombs are slippery, being tied about ye left arm; but in the time of deliverance, taking it from ye arm tie it about ye thigh, and she shall bring forth without pain' (Gunther, 1959 p. 656).

The intriguingly 'pregnant' eagle stone was further described by Nicholas Culpeper 1500 hundred years later in his translation of the *Pharmacopoeia Londinensis* (1654 pp. 70–1): 'Etites or the stone with child' wrote Culpeper, 'because being hollow in the middle, it contains another little stone within it, it is found in eagles nests, and in many other places, this stone being bound to the left arm of women with child, stays their miscarriage or abortion, but when the time of their labour comes remove it from their arm, and bind it to the inside of their thigh, and it brings forth the child, and that (almost) without any pain at all'. Culpeper quoted Dioscorides and Pliny (AD 23–79), the great Roman encyclopedist, as his sources. The *Encyclopaedia Britannica* (1771) confirmed that eagle stones have a 'loose nucleus rattling in them'.

Frances Adams wrote that ætites or eagle stone is a type of iron oxide (1847 pp. 227–8). It was used frequently by the ancients and the great Arabian physicians 'who confirmed in the strongest terms, the imaginary efficacy of the Eagle-stone, when used as an amulet ... it accelerated the delivery of women in tedious labour ... we have often regretted that such innocent modes of working upon the imagination of women in labour has given place to more dangerous methods of practice in such cases'. The Eagle-stone was retained in the English Dispensatory with all its ancient characters as late as Quincy' – John Quincy's dispensatory was published in 1721 (Matthews, 1962).

Hematite, the blood stone

Hematite is a valuable iron ore, often blood-red in color. It is also called 'blood stone', which is a green silica with blood-like spots of red jasper (from the Greek *Iaspis*, of Eastern origin), an opaque quartz containing clay or iron compounds. The name 'blood stone' may have been given because of its appearance or because hematite was used in Galenical medicine as a styptic agent used to stop bleeding. Hematite (*aimatites lithos* or *haematites lapis*) was described by Dioscorides who wrote that 'it is drank with wine for ye Dysurie, and for women's fluxes; and for spitting of blood with Pomegranate juice ... with women's milk it is good for ... bloodshotten eyes'. A second form of hematite, referred to as 'schistos', was found in Spain, and 'it hath the same force that Haematites hath'. Mixed with woman's milk it was used to treat various eye ailments (Gunther, 1959 p. 652).

The Arabians physicians of the tenth and eleventh centuries AD recommended hematite for the treatment of menorrhagia (Adams, 1847). In Europe hematite was prescribed during the medieval era in a potion, or in a pessary 'cast into her privy member' for 'excessive flowing of blood at the wrong time; and this sickness weakens a great number of women ... it staunches if the condition is curable' (Rowland, 1981 p. 85). John of Arderne advised hematite in a compound syrup for 'a flux of blood' (Power, 1922). In an accompanying note describing the efficacy of hematite and other 'medicinal' stones, Power (1922) wrote: 'The loadstone (magnetite) was thought to be preferable to steel (chalybs) for medicinal purposes as an astringent and to increase the momentum of blood. It was a powerful deobstruant and greatly promoted the menstrual discharges'. Thomas Raynold in the *Byrth of Mankynde* (1545), advised hematite for women who suffered an 'outragyous flux of flowres' during the puerperium.

Hematite consists principally of iron oxide (60 to 80%). It was mainly used in the obstetrics and gynecology of olden days as an astringent or styptic. Various oral iron preparations were prescribed for women as treatment for anemia and iron salts were prescribed for the anemia of chlorosis (Ringer, 1888). Chlorosis was defined as a 'Distemper in young women which is called the Green-sickness, because they are generally of a wan, sallow complexion' (Quincy, 1775). The treatment for the 'green sickness' was chalybeate medicine (containing iron) but 'if these will not suffice ... matrimony is a certain cure' (Encyclopaedia Britannica, 1771).

Dr G. Lovell Gulland wrote an article on chlorosis for *Green's Encyclopedia and Dictionary of Medicine and Surgery* (1906). He indicated that tight corsets, inadequate diet and menorrhagia were 'exciting causes' of the ailment. Chlorosis only occurred in women, and the first attack came on between 14 and 20 years of age. The condition was accompanied by secondary amenorrhea, and a host of anemia-related symptoms. The hemoglobin level was commonly reduced to 40%.

Treatment was with Blaud's pills (containing ferrous sulfate). When all else failed, the 'special' treatments of bloodletting of four ounces, or a fifth of a pint (to stimulate the marrow!), or arsenic in water, were advised. Perhaps matrimony was a better option! In modern times, red ferric oxide is used to tint medications and saccharated iron oxide is used in the treatment of iron-deficiency anemia (Reynolds, 1982).

Dragon's blood

Dragon's blood is the resin obtained from the *Calamus draco* or *Dracaena draco* tree. Entirely different from dragon's blood is dracunculus (dragon herb or *Draconitum*), an astringent herb which was thought to be an aphrodisiac and a promoter of the menses (Adams, 1847 p. 97). There are several varieties of the tree, including the Canary, East Indian, Socotrine and South American (*Pterocarpus draco*) varieties. According to Wootton, 'Dragon's blood was first obtained from Socotra and taken with other merchandise by the Arabs to China ... the shrewd Arabs invented the name Dragon's blood to please their Chinese customers' (1910). In olden pharmacy dragon's blood was used as a mild astringent to arrest bleeding, and it was also used as a varnish for violins. In some parts of Europe dragon's blood had a reputation as a charm to restore love: 'Maidens whose swains are unfaithful or neglected procure a piece, wrap it in paper, and throw it on the fire saying: "May he no pleasure or profit see, till he come back again to me"' (Wootton, 1910).

Dragon's blood was used by Master John Arderne in the treatment of 'dropsy from hot and cold cause' and was applied in a plaster with bole-ammoniac, egg white and incense (Power, 1922). An alcoholic solution of dragon's blood was advocated by James Wolveridge (1671) to treat 'immoderate flux of the courses' and also 'convulsion-fits in infants newly born'. Use of dragon's blood continued until the nineteenth century when it was advised, with other medications, 'to strengthen the fruit of the womb' (Pseudo-Aristotle, c. 1830).

John Lindley, professor of botany at University College, London, wrote in his *Flora Medica* of a Mexican variety of dragon's blood, '*sangre del drago*'

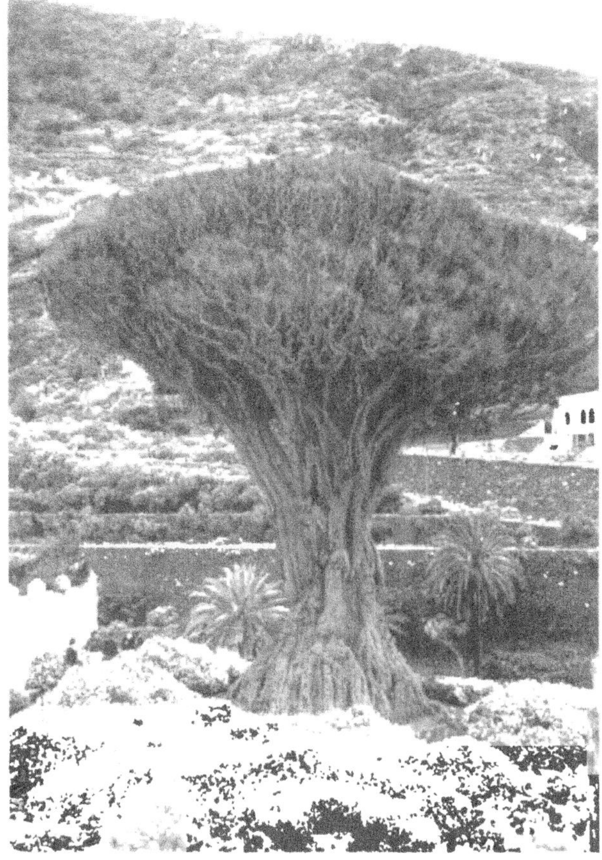

Figure 4 Dragon's blood (*Dracaena* sp.)

and noted that it was used as an astringent and vulnerary (a treatment for wounds) (1838 pp. 582–3). William Rhind, a member of the Royal College of Surgeons, Edinburgh, related that 'At certain times the trunk [of the *Dracaena draco*] cracks in various parts, and emits a gum which concretes into tears, and is the red substance commonly known as dragon's blood'. One ancient specimen of the *Dracaena draco* tree, found in the Canary Islands, had a circumference of 45 feet. 'Dragon's blood was at one time highly esteemed in medicine ... for its astringent properties ... but is now little used' (Rhind, 1870).

A very full account of the dragon's blood tree may be found in Maud Grieves' *A Modern Herbal*. She wrote that its resin was valued for its astringent action and that it was prescribed in the treatment of diarrhea (1931 pp. 262–3). The resin was also used in a compound medication as a treatment for 'severe syphilis'.

Recent research has confirmed the wound-healing properties of *sangre del draco* (Evans, 1996).

Iris

The iris is one of the oldest cultivated plants. Its name came from the Greek, *Iris*, the Rainbow goddess, messenger to the gods, because it appeared in many different colors. The iris was also dedicated to Juno and the flower, with its stem, gave rise to the scepter. In her *Flowers and their Histories*, Alice Coates (1956) wrote that an iris (possibly *Iris florentina*) was among the plants brought from Syria to Egypt by Thutmose III (1501–1447 BC) and is recognizably represented in bas-relief on the wall of the 'Botanical Chamber' in his temple at Karnak. The yellow water flag, *Iris pseudacorus*, is the origin of the fleur-de-lis. First adopted as an emblem in the sixth century by Clovis, the first king of the Francs, the iris flower was chosen by Louis VII as his blazon during the Crusades in the twelfth century. The iris flower thus became the Fleur de Louis, but in time became known as the 'fleur de luce' or 'fleur de lis'.

In classical Greece and Rome the iris was prized for its medicinal uses. Dioscorides began his famous herbal with a tract on the iris which he identified as *Iris florentina* or *Iris germanica*. He noted that '[irises] dranck with wine, they bring out the menses, yea, and the decoction of them is fitting for women's fomentations which do mollify and open the places ... being applied as a Collyrium [an eye ointment] with honey, they draw out the Embryons' (Gunther, 1959 pp. 5–6). Soranus of Ephesus advised iris in oil as an abortifacient; with honey, or on its own, for vaginal discharge; in oil or as suppositories, for inflammation of the womb, and also as a preparation for induction of miscarriage in mole pregnancies (Temkin, 1956 pp. 227–8).

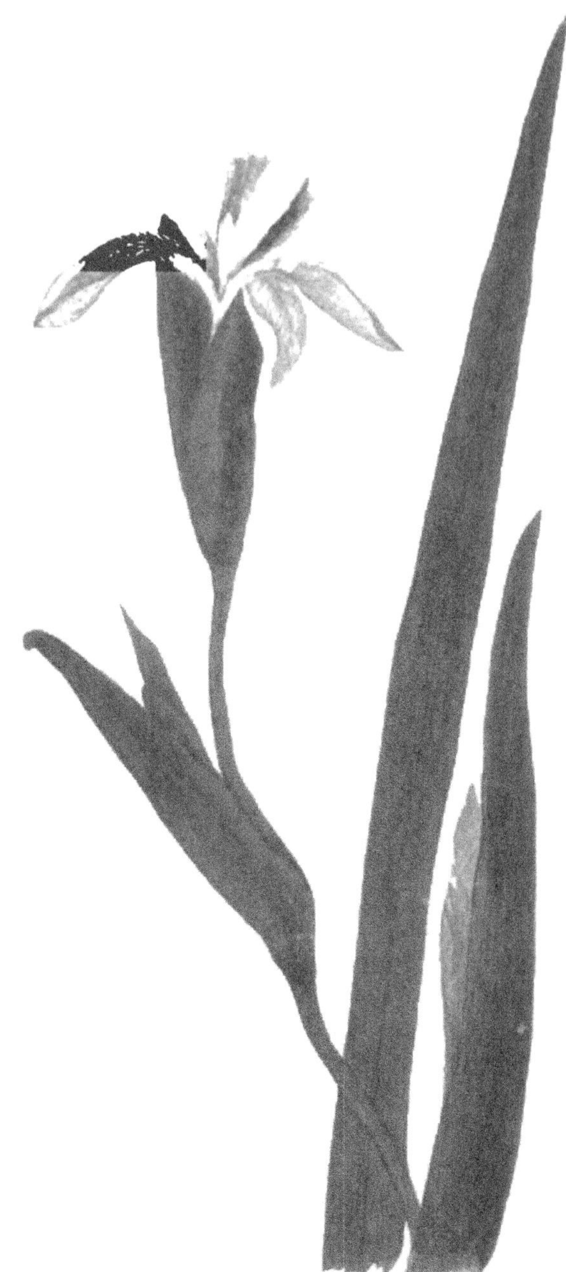

Figure 5 Iris

Iris was offered as a treatment for menstrual disorders in the *Leech Book* (see above). It was prescribed to induce menstruation and miscarriage for molar pregnancy. The iris was availed of as a labor oxytocic in the *Medieval Woman's Guide to Health*: 'for even if there was a dead child in her womb, it would bring it out. And the root of yellow iris has the same virtue' (Rowland, 1981 p. 69). Lindley included *Iris versicolor, Iris florentina* and *Iris pseudoacorus* in his *Flora Medica* (1838) and wrote that they possessed emetic, diuretic and purgative properties. According to Frances Adams, in his translation of *The Seven Books of Paulus Aegineta*, the iris was used by Avicenna to treat gonorrhea and the 'pollutio nocturnia somni' (Adams, 1847 pp. 111, 145–6). At the time Adams was writing, the iris was still availed of in the practice of medicine 'and is still kept in apothecaries shops'.

Iris versicolor (blue flag iris) was a commonly-used medicinal plant of the North American native Indians, and was listed in the *Pharmacopoeia of the United States* until 1895. The iris still held a place in *Southall's Organic Materia Medica* of 1915 (Mann, 1915). Maud Grieve classified iris as a powerful cathartic; its sap had been employed in dropsy (edema) and 'It is reputed of value in dysmenorrhoea and leucorrhoea and also found use in the treatment of syphilis' (Grieve, 1931 pp. 434–40).

Iris florentina was identified in the *British Herbal Pharmacopoeia* (1991) as being a demulcent and antidiarrheal agent, while *Iris versicolor* was noted to be a laxative, diuretic, and dermatological agent, and had anti-inflammatory effects. The rhizome of the *Iris versicolor* may be used for pelvic inflammatory disease but should not be prescribed to pregnant women (Bown, 1995). The dried root of iris, known as 'orris', contains a volatile oil which remains important in perfumery.

Savin

Savin (*Juniperus sabina*), a species of juniper, takes its name from Old French *sabine*, which in turn came from the Latin *sabina*. Savin yields an irritant volatile oil which is abortifacient and antihelminthic, characteristics which are shared by the related Virginian juniper (red cedar). Juniper berries were added to gin, giving it the distinct flavor much favored by some midwives in days of yore. They used the liquid as an internal 'lubricant' and mixed it with castor oil to stimulate labor.

Dioscorides recorded that savin was used to treat skin disease; as an oxytocic in labor; to induce menstruation; and 'being anointed around the Genitall before Conjunction, it doth cause sterilitie' (Gunther, 1959 p. 57). During the Middle Ages, extract of savin was used as an emmenagogue; to cause miscarriage of uterine mole and as an oxytocic in labor (Rowland, 1981 p. 667). Many similar citations of savin for these indications followed through the centuries. James Wolveridge found savin useful for 'hard and difficult births ... [as] an ointment or in a potion'. He also prescribed it for 'retention of the lochia' and for 'after-pains' (1671 pp. 117, 127, 133). In the same century, Nicholas Culpeper wrote that savin was 'hot and dry in the third degree, potently provokes the Terms, expels both birth and after-birth'. In his *English Physician Enlarged* (1792 edition) it was also related that 'being applied to the place, [savin] may happily cure venereal fores [sores]'.

John Lindley wrote that 'it [savin] acts as a powerful emmenagogue, and in pregnancy has a strong tendency to produce abortion' (1838 p. 575). Frances Adams recorded that savin was the most certain and powerful emmenagogue of the whole materia medica (1847 p. 77). William R. Wilde, surgeon to St Mark's Hospital, Dublin and father of Oscar Wilde, penned *A Short Account of the Superstitions and Popular Practices relating to Midwifery, and some of the Diseases of Women and Children in Ireland.* He found that the actions of savin and rue (*Ruta graveolens*) were well known to Irish women (Wilde, 1849). Savin was still in general use in obstetrics in the late nineteenth century.

Maud Grieve related in her *Modern Herbal* that savin, mixed with verdigris, was used as an efficacious application for the removal of venereal warts (1931 p. 718). Verdigris, from the Old French *vert de Grece*, green of Greece, is cupric acetate, which forms the green coating on brass, bronze or copper. *Martindale, The Extra Pharmacopoeia* noted that savin oil (*oleum sabinae*) 'was formerly used as an emmenagogue ... it may cause haematuria and violent gastro-intestinal irritation. Serious and fatal cases of poisoning have resulted from its use as a supposed abortifacient' (Reynolds, 1982 p. 683).

Savin (*Juniperus sabina*) is now considered too poisonous for internal use because it contains podophyllotoxin as found in *Podophyllum pelatum* (known as American mandrake, May apple, wild lemon). Podophyllotoxin has antimitotic and antiviral effects, and is a drastic purgative. Podophyllum is used as a medicinal 'paint' in the topical treatment of soft venereal and other warts. Savin is subject to legal restrictions in most countries and cannot be prescribed to pregnant women (Bown, 1995).

Shepherd's purse

Shepherd's purse (*Capsella bursa-pastoris*, also known as *Thlaspi bursa-pastoris*, witches pouches or, pick-pocket.) is so-called because its seed-bearing pouches

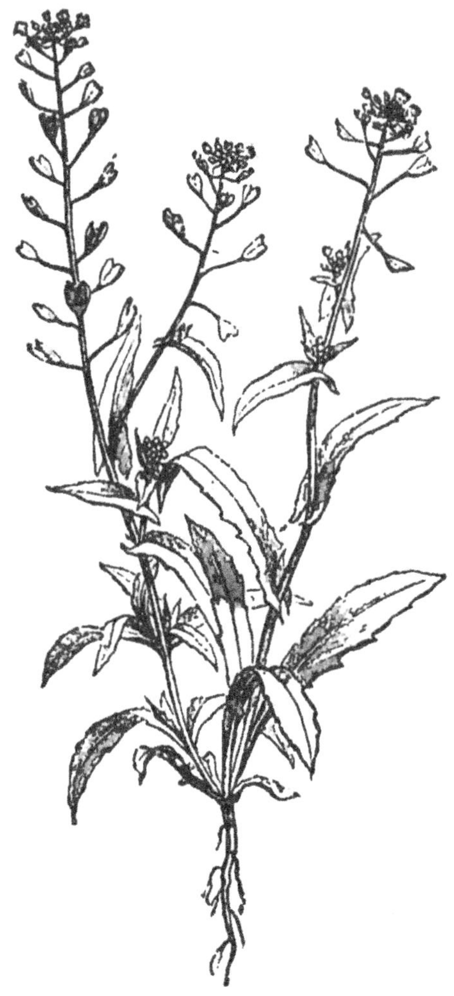

Figure 6 Shepherd's purse (*Capsella bursa pastoralis*)

resemble a leather purse. The heart-shaped seed pods give rise to the alternative common name, 'mother's hearts' (Ody, 1993). Shepherd's purse is a persistent and common weed of fields, gardens and waste-ground, and has been used as a food product for thousands of years. Found all over the world, except in tropical areas, the plant was carried to America by the Pilgrim Fathers.

Shepherd's purse was traditionally used as a domestic remedy to staunch both internal and external bleeding and to check hemorrhage in childbirth. The plant was mentioned by John of Arderne, for the treatment of excess menstruation 'all Authors say that remedies which restrain the piles also restrain the menses and visa versa'. He advised a decoction of 'millefoil, or of plantain, or of shepherd's purse'.

According to William Turner's *Herbal* (1568), 'the Bursa Pastoris is cold and drye\and bindinge ... it is also good to stoppe weomens floures with all\if they runne to muche out'. In his *Byrth of Mankynde* Thomas Raynold (1545) advised: 'of Bursa Pastoris, of each ii. handfules: beat all these to powder ... fethe them together in rayne water ... let the woman bathe herselfe in this water up to the nauyll ... when the flowres issue more aboundantly then neadeth'. In his herbal of 1636, John Gerard wrote that shepherd's purse was '[the] Poore man's Parmacetie [pharmacy]' (Woodward, 1927).

The hemostatic properties of shepherd's purse are said to equal those of ergot (*Claviceps purpurea*) and golden seal (*Hydrastis canadensis*). During the First World War a liquid extract of shepherd's purse was used both to control bleeding from wounds and as a substitute for ergot (Grieve, 1931 pp. 338–9, 738–9). According to George MacDonald Hocking, professor of pharmacognosy, Alabama Polytechnic Institute, shepherd's purse contains an ergot substitute (Hocking, 1955). The specific indication for shepherd's purse in the *British Herbal Pharmacopoeia* (1991) is for uterine hemorrhage. It may be combined with birth root (*Trillium erectum*) and hydrastis for menorrhagia. Shepherd's purse is astringent, diuretic, a urinary antiseptic and antihemorrhagic. The herb contains acetylcholine, choline, and other agents acting as vasoconstrictors and hemostatics (Chevallier, 1996) and is oxytocic and uterotonic (Kenner and Requena, 1996).

Wax

According to Dorland's medical dictionary (1932), wax is any one of a series of plastic substances deposited by insects or obtained from plants. They are esters of various fatty acids with higher (usually monohydric) alcohols. The wax used in pharmacy is principally beeswax, the material which honeycomb is made from. It consists chiefly of ceran and myricin. Chinese wax is a hard white wax of insect origin procured from *Fraxinus chinensis*, a Chinese ash tree while Japanese wax comes from the fruit of bayberry (*Myrica cerifera*) and other species of the same genus. Beeswax is obtained by melting the walls of the honeycomb of the bee (*Apis mellifera*) with hot water and removing the foreign matter. Cerason or mineral wax is obtained by purifying ozokerite, a naturally-occurring solid paraffin. It is used as a substitute for beeswax or hard paraffin. *Cera alba* or white beeswax is a somewhat translucent solid obtained by air-bleaching wax and 'being of moderate temperament, forms the basis of many other medicines' (Adams, 1847 p. 169). Wax was contained in ointments, pills, plasters and suppositories.

In classical Greece and Rome, Etruscan wax, with olive oil, was used to anoint the newborn, or for coating pills (Temkin, 1956 p. 243). Cerates with myrtle oil, wax and white lead were used as topical contraceptives (Temkin, 1956 p. 220). Wax salves were applied for amenorrhea, breast inflammation, dysmenorrhea, gonorrhea, hemorrhage, physometra, and skin sores. Galen's wax is described as white beeswax, mixed with almond oil, borax and distilled rosewater (Reynolds, 1982 p. 1065).

In the Middle Ages, wax mixed with common oil and purslane was applied for swellings of the penis; to ulcers and inflammation; to reduce uterine pain; and was applied with other herbs in a plaster to the patient's abdomen and low back for 'distress after childbirth'. A wax salve with asafetida and six other herbal remedies was applied to the prolapsed uterus (Rowland, 1981). James Wolveridge advised white wax in an 'emplaister' for sore nipples and to prevent breast engorgement (1671 pp. 137–8).

An alternative name for wax is 'cere' or 'cerate' which means a paste or stiff ointment containing wax (Latin *cera*, wax). A 'cerecloth' was a cloth dipped in melted wax that was impregnated with medicinal herbs and was applied to various parts of the body. There were many forms of 'cerecloths' including *ceratum de galbano* which contained asafetida, bdellium, galbanum, myrrh and other herbs and was used to treat maternal convulsions and retained placental products after childbirth (Culpeper, 1654 pp. 314–6). Other 'cerecloths' were *ceratum oesypatum*, *ceratum santalinum* and Galen's *unguentum refrigerans* all of which were used to treat women's disorders.

Cerates were softer than a traditional plaster and could be spread on the skin without melting. In more recent times there were various forms including a 'blistering cerate' which contained cantharides, and a 'spermacetic cerate' containing olive oil, spermaceti and white wax. Spermaceti (from the Latin *sperma*, sperm and *cetus*, or the *Greek ketos*, a whale, originally but incorrectly thought to be whale's sperm) is white crystalline fat which derives from the head of the sperm whale, *Physeter macrocephalus*. Dorland (1932) indicated that it was a demulcent and was an ingredient of various cerates and ointments.

Lanolin

Lanolin (from the Latin *lana*, wool and *oleum*, oil) was also used extensively as a base for ointments. John of Arderne mentioned lanolin in his *De Arte Phisicali et de Cirurgia*. Sir D'Arcy Power quoted a crude method of obtaining lanolin from Arderne's 'Treatises on Fistula': 'Lana succida [is] wolle that groweth atwixt the legges of an ewe, about the udder, full of sweat, not washed' (1922 p. 9). Lanolin was known as 'oesypum' in Hippocratic medicine and was defined as the sordes (dirty sweat) of unwashed wool. Dioscorides described how it was prepared by collecting the scum from the surface of water. He advised the use of lanolin (wool fat or oil) for treatment of vulval ulcers and as an emmenagogue and oxytocic (Gunther, 1959 pp. 112–3). Lanolin is still obtained from sheep wool and contains a mixture of oleate, palmitate and stearate of cholesterol.

References

Adams, F. (1847). *The Seven Books of Paulus Aeginata*, Vol. 3, pp. 77, 97, 111, 145–6, 169, 227–8, 222. (London: The Sydenham Society)

Pseudo-Aristotle (c. 1830). *The Works of Aristotle the Famous Philosopher*, p. 66. (London: Miller, Law & Cater)

Bown, D. (1995). *The Royal Horticultural Society Encyclopaedia of Herbs and their Uses*, pp. 297, 299. (London: Dorling Kindersley)

The British Herbal Medicine Association (1991). *British Herbal Pharmacopoeia*, pp. 46–7, 119–20. (Bournemouth, UK)

Chevallier, A. (1996). *The Encyclopaedia of Medicinal Plants*, p. 181. (London: Dorling Kindersley)

Coats, A. (1956). *Flowers and Their Histories*, pp. 126–34. (London: Adam and Charles Black)

Culpeper, N. (1654). *Pharmacopoeia Londonensis: or The London Dispensatory. Further adorned by the studies and collections of the Fellows, now living of the same Colledge* ...', pp. 50, 70–1, 304–5, 314–6. (London: Peter Cole)

Culpeper, N. (1792). *The English Physician Enlarged with 369 Medicines, Made of English Herbs*, pp. 272–3. (London: Printed for A. Law, W. Millar and R. Cater)

Dawson, W. R. (1934). *A Leech Book or Collection of Medical Recipes of the 15th Century*. (London: Macmillan & Co.)

Dorland, W. A. N. (1932). *The American Illustrated Dictionary*, p. 1433. (Philadelphia and London: W. B. Saunders Co.)

Encyclopaedia Britannica (1771). *A Dictionary of Arts and Sciences, Compiled Upon a New Plan*, Vol. 1, p. 35. (Edinburgh: A. Bell and C. Macfarquhar)

Evans, W. C. (1996). *Trease and Evans' Pharmacognosy*, p. 230. (London: W. B. Saunders Co.)

Garrison, F. H. (1929). *An Introduction to the History of Medicine*, pp. 158–9. (Philadelphia & London: W. B. Saunders Co.)

Grieve, M. (1931). *A Modern Herbal. The Medicinal, Culinary, Cosmetic and Economic Properties, Cultivation and Folk-Lore of Herbs, Grasses, Fungi, Shrubs and Trees with all their modern scientific uses*, pp. 262–3, 338–9, 434–40, 718, 738–9. (London: Jonathan Cape)

Gunther, R. T. (1959). *The Greek Herbal of Dioscorides*, pp. 5–6, 57, 656, 652, 112–3. (New York: Hafner Publishing Co.)

Hocking, G. M. (1955). *A Dictionary of Terms in Pharmacognosy, and, Other Divisions of Economic Botany*, p. 40. (Springfield, IL: Charles C. Thomas)

Hunt, T. (1989). *Plant Names of Medieval England*, p. 262. (Cambridge: DS Brewer)

Kenner, D. and Requena, Y. (1996). *Botanical Medicine. A European Professional Perspective*, p. 178. (Brookline, MA: Paradigm Publications)

Lindley, J. (1838). *Flora Medica; A Botanical Account of all the more important Plants used in Medicine in different parts of the World*, pp. 182, 582–3, 575. (London: Orme, Brown Green & Longmans)

Lovell, G. (1906). *Green's Encyclopadia and Dictionary of Medicine and Surgery*, Vol. 2, pp. 109–14. (Edinburgh and London: William Green and Sons)

Mann, E. (1915). *Southall's Organic Materia Medica*, 8th (ed.) pp. 77–8. (London: J. and A. Churchill)

Mason-Hohl, E. (1940). *The Diseases of Women by Trotula of Salerno*, Translation. (Los Angeles: Ward Ritchie Press)

Matthews, L. G. (1962). *History of Pharmacy in Britain*, pp. 86–7. (Edinburgh: E. & S. Livingstone)

Ody, P. (1993). *The Herb Society's Complete Medicinal Herbal*, p. 45. (London: Dorling Kindersley)

Power, Sir D'Arcy (1922). *John Arderne's 'De Arte Phisicali et de Cirurgia' of 1412*, a translation. pp. 9, 22, 25, 28, 30, 32, 33, 36, 37. (London: John Bale, Sons and Danielsson Ltd.)

Quincy, J. (1775). *Lexicon Physico-Medicum: or, A New Medicinal Directory*, 9th (ed.) p. 80. (London: T. Longman)

Raynold, T. (1545). *The Byrth of Mankynde*, English Translation, Folios 80, 81. (London: Tho. Ray)

Reynolds, E. F. (1982). *Martindale. The Extra Pharmacopoeia*, pp. 683, 875–81, 1065, 1366–7. (London: The Pharmaceutical Press)

Rhind, W. (1870). *A History of The Vegetable Kingdom; Embracing the Physiology Classification, and Culture of Plants: with their various uses to man and the lower animals; and their application in the Arts Manufactures, and Domestic Economy*, p. 479. (Glasgow: Blackie & Son)

Ricci, J. V. (1943). *The Genealogy of Gynaecology*, pp. 248–52. (Philadelphia: Blakiston & Co.)

Ringer, S. (1888). *A Handbook of Therapeutics*, p. 213. (London: H. K. Lewis)

Rowland, B. (1981). *Medieval Woman's Guide to Health. The First English Gynecological Handbook*, a modern English translation, pp. 33, 67, 85, 69, 105, 106, 111, 161. (London: Croom Helm)

Temkin, O. (1956). *Soranus' Gynaecology*, pp. 220, 227–28, 243. (Baltimore & London: The Johns Hopkins University Press)

Turner, W. (1568). *The Herball*, Part 3, p. 17. (London: Arnold Birkman)

Wilde, W. R. (1849). A short account of the superstitions and popular practices relating to midwivery, and some of the diseases of women and children in Ireland. *Mon. J. Med. Sci.* 150, New Series 35, 711–26

Wolveridge, J. (1671). *Speculum Matricis*; or *The Expert Midwives Handmaid*, pp. 129–35, 117, 127, 133, 137–8. (London: E. Okes)

Woodward, M. (1927). *Gerard's Herball. The Essence thereof Distilled by Marcus Woodward from the Edition of Th. Johnson 1636*, p. 61. (London: Spring Books)

Wootton, A. C. (1910). *Chronicles in Pharmacy*, pp. 31–3. (London: Macmillan and Co.)

The sixteenth century 13

INTRODUCTION

A 'renaissance of midwifery' occurred in the sixteenth century, and this new era in maternity care was signaled by the appearance of a series of books designed for the instruction of midwives. In previous centuries the knowledge of midwifery was handed down as an oral tradition from one generation of midwives to the next with little, if any, supervision. With the introduction of printing, books on medical matters had become more commonplace, and for the first time the texts were printed in the mother-tongue rather than in Latin. The general populace could now gain knowledge that was previously only available in Latin or Greek manuscripts owned by physicians, clerics and the well educated upper classes.

Although some aspects of obstetrics had been covered by surgical books, there appeared in print in 1476 a brief text written by Albertus Magnus entitled *De secreta mulierum* which was devoted entirely to obstetrics. Soon afterwards the *Buechlein der Schwangeren Frauen* by Ortolff von Bayerland was published. Both short texts were obstetric monographs. Then followed the first book to appear on obstetrics in over thirteen centuries, *Der Schwangern Frauen und Hebammen Rosengarten*, of 1513. Soon afterwards, in 1554, came another German text better known by its Latin title *De Conceptu et Generatione Hominis*. These printed obstetric and medical books were complemented by texts on medicinal herbs which brought the knowledge of the apothecary and herbalist to public attention.

As enlightenment spread, concern was voiced about the poor state of midwifery of the time, and laws were introduced to raise standards in obstetric practice. The first guidelines issued to midwives in Germany came from Emperor Charles V's 'Carolina' issued by the Reichstag of Regensburg, in 1532 (Ingerslev, 1909). Another public document in German, containing legislation governing midwives, appeared in 1555 and Adam Lonitzer published a treatise on the subject in Frankfurt in 1573. The status of medical men also came under scrutiny and in England, for instance, the physicians established their College in 1518, during the Tudor period. A generation later the surgeons and barbers came together to form the United Company of Barber–Surgeons. Lectures and examinations were introduced in an effort to modernize the old system of apprenticeship and gradually medical standards were raised.

The attendance of a physician at childbirth became popular during the Greco-Roman era but lapsed in the fourth century AD. From then onwards a medical (almost always male) presence on such occasions was frowned upon by society, except in extreme cases where a midwife requested a physician or surgeon to conduct a delivery because all usual maneuvers to effect the birth had failed. In 1522 a Dr Wertt of Hamburg disguised himself as a woman in order to witness a childbirth but was discovered and burned to death. It was not until Ambroise Paré's time in the seventeenth century that the physician–obstetrician regained the right to be present in the birth chamber. François Bouchet officiated at the delivery of La Valliere, the mistress of Louis XIV, and in 1682 Jules Clement was present at the birth of the dauphin and received the title 'accoucheur'. However, the position of men in midwifery remained controversial and gave rise to much debate concerning the role of the 'man-midwife' (this term, common in the seventeenth century, persisted until the nineteenth century [Gordon, 1931]).

During the sixteenth century the foundations of obstetric science became established with the study of human anatomy and 'physiology' of reproduction. The art of midwifery slowly developed and the processes of pregnancy and childbirth, so long steeped in superstition and ignorance, were questioned. It is a chastening thought to realize that no innovations were made in the entire area of maternity care in the 1300 years from the era of Soranus of the second century AD to the sixteenth century. In fact much of the Greco-Roman knowledge of obstetrics and gynecology was forgotten and only regained later from translations of Arabic medical tracts which contained most of the writings of the Classical authors.

The maternal and neonatal mortality and morbidity figures for the period were unacceptably high. Little help was available for the pregnant mother and her unborn child and for the complications of pregnancy, labor and the puerperium. Obstetric forceps still awaited invention, there was scant knowledge of analgesia, no anesthesia and of course no antisepsis or antibiotics. Onto a scene such as this came von Bayerland's monograph, *Buchlein der Schwangern Frauen*, soon followed by Rösslin's epoch-marking midwives' handbook, of 1513. What has never been acknowledged is that the obstetric texts of the time are a valuable source for women's materia medica, over half of the books' contents dealing with drug treatments for the ailments which befall both pregnant and non-pregnant women. The remainder deal with basic anatomy and the conduct of childbirth but these portions tend to be the most often quoted.

THE LITTLE BOOK FOR WOMEN

The *Buechlein der Schwangeren Frauen* (c. 1495–1500), often known by its English title, *Little Book for Women*, was written by Ortolff von Bayerland, a physician of Würzburg. Although only 13 pages long, the book was the first obstetric text printed in the German language. Von Bayerland also wrote the first German pharmacopoeia, *Artzneibuch* (1477), which was an important German text of popular medications.

On the title page of the *Little Book for Women* the author wrote: 'I, Ortolff, Doctor of Medicine, was asked by honorable women to write a short instruction how the pregnant woman has to behave during her pregnancy and after the delivery, and also of the duties of the midwife'. The book contained clear instructions for the mother and the midwife. These concerned regulation of the bowels, diet (the avoidance of bitter foods), exercise and baths. The expectant mother was advised against vigorous exercise and was to beware falls or injuries.

Oil of chamomile (from *Chamomilla recutita*, or German chamomile, an analgesic and antispasmodic) was applied to the pregnant woman's thighs in late pregnancy, to facilitate labor. In the management of delayed labor the midwife was advised to blow sneezing powder into the woman's nose and to anoint the genitalia with oil or fat containing saffron (from *Crocus sativus*, which has oxytocic properties) and barleycorn (*Hordeum vulgare*, a demulcent for irritated tissues). Sneezing powders were also used to facilitate delivery of the placenta. Extract of the rue plant (*Ruta graveolans*, an oxytocic) was administered to enable evacuation of any retained placental products from the uterus, thus avoiding 'rotten vapors to the heart, liver and stomach which make the woman perish'. The author advised the pregnant woman of the benefits of sunlight and warned against bloodletting, a common practice of the times.

DER SCHWANGERN FRAUEN UND HEBAMMEN ROSENGARTEN

On 24 September 1513, Maximilian, the Holy Roman Emperor, granted a copyright to a little book, *Der Schwangern Frauen und Hebammen Rosengarten*, later known by its short title, the *Rosengarten*. The book was written by Eucharius Rösslin, Stadtartz or city physician of Worms (Power, 1927). Rösslin became an apothecary at Freiburg in 1493 and was elected physician to the city of Frankfurt-am-Main in 1506. Two years later he entered the service of the court of Catherine, Duchess of Brunswick and Lüneburg, Saxony. It appears that Rösslin was an able obstetrician and his book was published on the encouragement of 'E.F.G.' (*Euer Fürstlicher Gnade*, Your Grace) and also the support of his patroness, Catherine. The identity of 'E.F.G.' is uncertain but may have referred to Emperor Maximilian, or to Princess Catherine's deceased husband, Sigmund of Austria. It is much more likely, however, that 'E.F.G.' was Erik 1, Duke of Brunswick and Lüneburg, who was Catherine's second husband. The *Rosengarten* was dedicated to Catherine and written in an easy style. It proved an immediate success, and went through over a hundred editions, including translations.

Rösslin's introduction

In the Introduction to his *Rosengarten* Rösslin wrote an open letter to Princess Catherine.

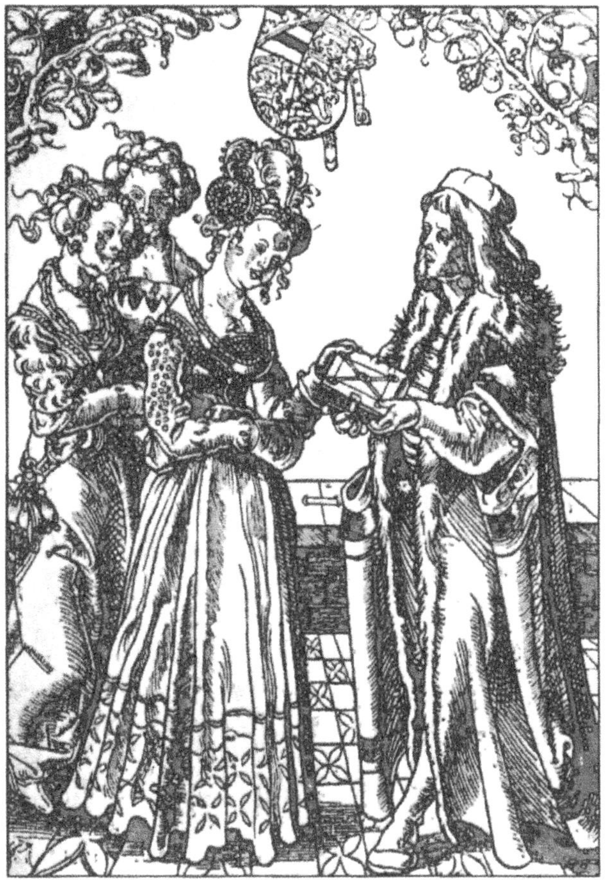

Figure 1 Rösslin presenting his book to the Duchess of Brunswick and Lüneberg

> 'Dear Serene Highness Princess Katharina of Saxony, Duchess of Brunswick and Lüneburg, I, Eucharius Rösslin, Doctor of Medicine, would like to send my respects and kind regards to you and your ladies....[the] omnipotent God had cursed our first mother, because of a disregard of a commandment, to give birth to her children in great pain, and all women have inherited this from her. Although this pain can not be completely healed by any sense, wisdom, or art, it could be eased if the pregnant woman would remember some rules'.

Rösslin explained to the duchess that 'E.F.G.' had asked him a few years previously to write a book for pregnant women, midwives and doctors. He hoped that 'E.F.G.' would distribute the book in his and other German counties as Rösslin was sure that those who read it would find good cheer and good advice within. He mentioned that some details were not to be found in his book, as they were not suitable to be written down, but that he would be pleased to pass them on by word of mouth to 'E.F.G'.

Rösslin wrote his book: 'for the honor of women' so that they would be 'better prepared' for labor'. Rösslin extolled the virtues of herbal remedies contained in his book in rhyme:

> Darinn yr kreutter/brechen graben
> Die leyb/seel/und leben haben
> [In it you find herbs to use
> Which have body, soul, and life]
>
> Sollich rosen die yr hand genommen
> Fur Gottes angesicht werden kommen
> [Such roses which you took in your hand
> Will come to God's face]
>
> Darumb yr sollet haben acht
> [That's why you should pay attention]

(Forward slash marks were used at this time as punctuation marks, where we would use commas.)

Origin of the title

The origin of the curious title *Der Schwangern Frauen und Hebammen Rosengarten* (The Garden of Roses for Pregnant Women and Midwives) was thought by Palmer Findley (1939) to have been a play on the name of the author – Roesslin or Rösslin, meaning 'rose' – or it may have been a reference to the Rose Gardens at Worms, the home of the author. In his treatise on the *Rosengarten*, Ingerslev of Copenhagen wrote that textbooks with exotic titles relating to botanical, medical, and pharmacological subjects were popular in Germany at that time. He believed that Rösslin's title was chosen to appeal not only to midwives, physicians and pregnant women but also to apothecaries, herb collectors, quacks and distillers, and to the general public, so achieving popularity and a widely-based audience for his book (Ingerslev, 1909).

Rösslin's sources

The *Rosengarten* appears to be a compilation of material from ancient Greco-Roman sources and Rösslin refers to the writings of Hippocrates, Galen, Aetius, Avicenna, Albertus Magnus and others. It is also believed that Rösslin may have used a translation by Muscio (c. AD 500) of the works of Soranus of Ephesus (of the early second century AD) as the main source for his book, although neither are mentioned by Rösslin. It is known that a copy of the Soranus manuscript, complete with illustrations, was contained in the library of the castle at Heidelberg during Rösslin's professional lifetime, and it is probable that Rösslin saw it there while on a visit. Copies of the Muscio manuscript from Heidelberg were taken to Rome in 1622 and later became known as the *Codex Palatinus*. There were at least three editions of the *Rosengarten* produced in 1513 and on the front page of one version there is an illustration of two women in Old German dress with a child in swaddling clothes. One of the women (possibly a midwife) holds a rose tree in her right hand. In a different edition the rose is replaced by branches of an acanthus plant. A dedicatory illustration shows Rösslin presenting his book to Princess Catherine, who was attended by two ladies-in-waiting.

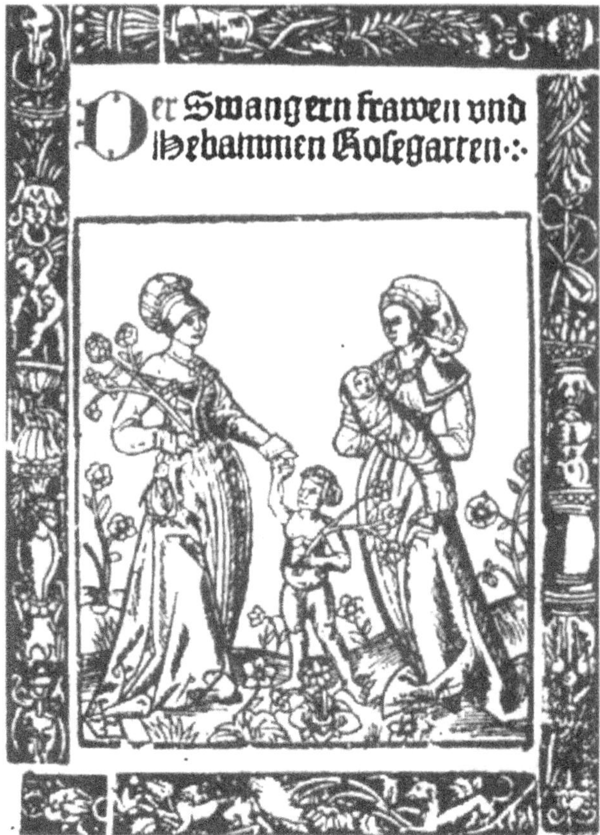

Figure 2 *Der Schwangern Frauen und Hebammen Rosengarten*

Contents and significance

The *Rosengarten* was the earliest printed book devoted exclusively to obstetrics and contained the earliest obstetric figures printed from woodblocks. According to Alfred M. Hellman the significance of the *Rosengarten* was that it resumed a tradition of treatises related to obstetrics which had been broken for almost 1500 years. In his essay on early obstetric books Hellman (1952), wrote that Rösslin established the necessity for thorough instruction of midwives. His book had an enormous influence on the obstetric practice of both the midwives and surgeons of the time because it was written in the vernacular, German; Latin, the universal language of scholars and books of the period, was unknown to Rösslin's public. The *Rosengarten* was introduced at the time when the practice of midwifery was based solely on tradition and 'clinical' observation and was beset with superstition and religious bigotry.

In the *Rosengarten* Rösslin brought to public attention those obstetric secrets which had never before been open to general knowledge or debate and the importance of his treatise can, therefore, never be surpassed. *Der Schwangern Frauen und Hebammen Rosengarten* is the most important obstetric book of all time. Imagine, for the first time in history, an interested woman could read about the normal position of the fetus *in utero* with its placenta and membranes; about various pregnancy-related problems; about the signs of labor and difficult delivery; recommendations for a half-sitting position for the woman in labor, preferably on a special birth stool; instructions for midwives about the conduct of labor; and about the care of the newborn. The book also contains a large number of prescriptions for women's ailments, and nostrums in the book's materia medica account for over half of the text. Medicinal herbs were identified mainly by their Latin names but occasionally also appeared in German. Rösslin included an eight-page drug index in his book which listed most, but not all, of the remedies mentioned. The 206 medicinal herbs and other treatments are identified by their Latin name and (often multiple) German synonyms, in tabular form. Not all are easily identifiable with their modern equivalent.

In his *Rosengarten*, Rösslin reintroduced, but did not particularly emphasize, the knowledge of podalic version which had been almost forgotten since the time of Soranus. This obstetric maneuver was popularized by Ambroise Paré and his pupil Jacques Guilleameau later in the sixteenth century, and by François Mauriceau in the seventeenth century. Podalic version was a major advance on the much more difficult cephalic version which was employed from the time of Aetius in the sixth century until the rediscovery of the works of Soranus, and their revival by Eucharius Rösslin in the sixteenth century.

The great number of editions and reprints of *Der Schwangern Frauen und Hebammen Rosengarten* testified to the popularity of Rösslin's text. This is also shown by the large number of translations of the text into other European languages which were undertaken soon after the original publication. In addition, other obstetric textbooks were to be published soon afterwards which reproduced the text and illustrations from the *Rosengarten* in more or less modified form.

Eucharius Rösslin Junior, translations and later editions

The *Rosengarten* was translated into Dutch in 1516 and Czech in 1519, but further developments in the history of the *Rosengarten* were to depend on Rösslin's own son, also called Eucharius Rösslin, who became a physician like his father. Rösslin Junior studied medicine in Cologne, Freiburg and Leipzig and succeeded his father as town physician in Frankfurt. Their identical names and similar professional identity created confusion so the younger Rösslin took the Greek form of his name, *Rhodion*, or 'little rose'. After his father's death in 1526, Rösslin Junior re-issued the *Rosengarten* in German, with some additional material from ancient sources, but under the title *Ehestands Artzneibuch*. He also published a Latin translation of the *Rosengarten* with the title *De Partu Hominis* which was printed by Christian Egenolph at Frankfurt in 1532. The Latin edition went through numerous reprints and was used mainly for translations into other European languages (in preference to the German edition).

Rösslin's illustrations

Rösslin's diagrams of the positions of the fetus *in utero* closely resemble those from manuscripts of antiquity and from Muscio's sixth century AD catechism for women's diseases and midwifery, which was, in turn, largely based on the *Gynecology* of Soranus of Ephesus. Illustrations common to the early editions of Rösslin's book are twenty small woodcuts which include images of a birth stool (the birth stool was employed from ancient times until the seventeenth century when its use was largely replaced by childbirth in bed) and diagrams of twins connected at the chest. Of the remaining eighteen which show the various positions of the fetus *in utero* two are duplicated so that there are sixteen altogether, the same number found in the illustrated Muscio manuscripts. The uterus was represented as an inverted flask or cupping-glass containing an unnaturally, mature-looking fetus. The famous woodcut artist Erhard Schön of Nuremberg (a pupil of Albert Dürer) made the woodcuts for Rösslin's book of 1513 although Ingerslev (1909) wrote that Conrad Merckel, a painter from Ulm, and a friend of Dürer's could have been responsible. Later editions of the book in the 1560s contained illustrations copied from Vesalius', *De Humani Corporis Fabrica* of 1543.

THE BYRTH OF MANKYNDE

The first English translation of the *Rosengarten* appeared in 1540 with the title *The Byrth of Mankynde newly translated out of Laten into Englysshe*. This was a literal translation '[By] a certayne studious and dilygent clarke at the request, and desyre of dyuers honest and sadde matrones beynge of his acquayntaunce' of the *De Partu Hominis*, the Latin version of *Der Schwangern Frauen und Hebammen Rosengarten*. The diligent clerk in question was one Richard Jonas, of whom nothing is now known (Ballantyne, 1906). *The Byrth of Mankynde* was dedicated to Queen Catherine of England 'most gracious and in all goodnesse most excellent vertuous Lady Quene Katheryne [Howard], wyfe and most derely belovyd spouse unto the moste myghty sapient

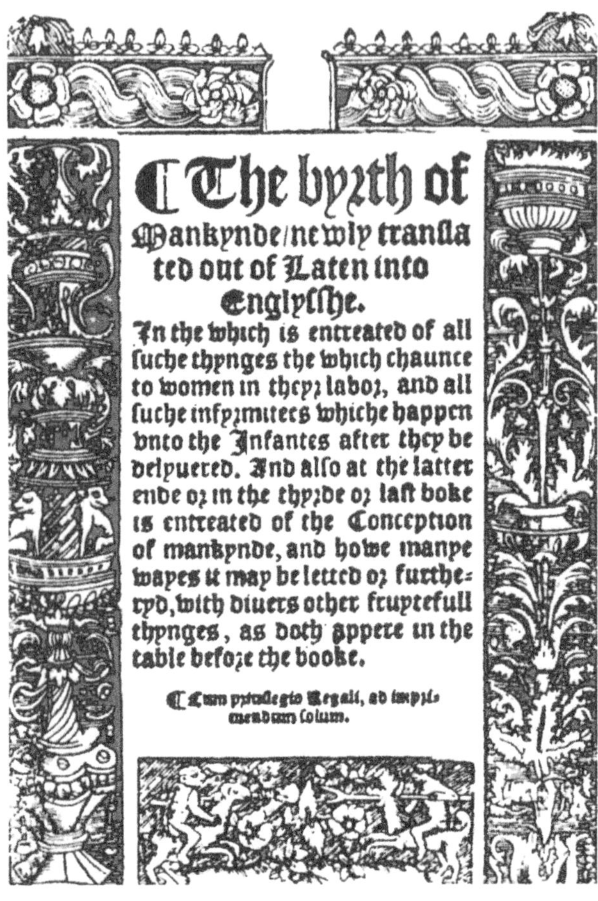
The byrth of
Mankynde/newly transla
ted out of Laten into
Englysshe.
In the which is entreated of all
suche thynges the which chaunce
to women in theyr labor, and all
suche infyrmitees whiche happen
vnto the Infantes after they be
delyuered. And also at the latter
ende or in the thyrde or last boke
is entreated of the Conception
of mankynde, and howe manye
wayes it may be letted or furthe-
ryd, with diuers other fruytefull
thynges, as doth appere in the
table before the booke.

Cum priuilegio Regali, ad impri-
mendum solum.

Figure 3 Title page from *The Byrth of Mankynde*

Christen Prynce, Kynge Henry the VIII'. The 1540 edition is very rare and J.W. Ballantyne of Edinburgh (1906) and Charles Gordon (1931) of New York have written interesting reviews of the text.

The next English edition of *The Byrth of Mankynde* was published in 1545 and was 'newly set furth, corrected and augmented' by Thomas Raynold, 'Phisition', and referred to by him as *The Woman's Booke*. Raynold's was a freer translation which, while including some original observations, adhered to the original format and paid respect to the works of Aristotle, Avicenna, Galen, Hippocrates, Rhazes and 'divers others' – but not to Rösslin, whom Raynold failed to mention.

The Byrth of Mankynde was a larger work with a long prologue added. This edition was illustrated with birth figures copied from *Der Schwangern Frauen und Hebammen Rosengarten* and two 'new' copper plates illustrating the muscles of the anterior abdominal wall and the abdominal contents covered by omentum. Apart from the fact that the illustrations (from copies made by the anatomist Thomas Geminus in 1545 of illustrations from Andreas Vesalius' 1543 *De Humani Corporis Fabrica*) are of a male torso, the special interest of the figures is that they were the earliest copper plates to be printed in England by a roller press. Raynold described a further nine figures which were supposed to illustrate his text but they did not appear in most of the 1545 editions (Crummer, 1926).

The Byrth of Mankynde was copied and reprinted many times over the next two hundred years. English midwives and physicians were entirely dependent on the book for guidance in the practice of obstetrics until the scientific treatises of William Smellie (1697–1763), 'The Master of British Midwifery', and of his contemporary, William Hunter (1718–1783), appeared in the eighteenth century (Findley, 1939). *The Byrth of Mankynde* comprises 322 pages with an additional prologue of 35 pages and a contents list of six pages. The main body of the text is subdivided into four 'Bookes'.

A Prologue to the women readers

In the introduction to the 1545 edition Raynold's aim was 'set furth and evidently declarid, all the inward partes of woman ... and that not onely in wurdes, but also in lyuely and expresse figures ... when a person is syck or diseased in any part, it is halfe a comfort, ye halfe his helthe, to understande in what part the disease is, and howe that part lyeth in the body'.

Raynold invoked the gods and goddesses of medicine and the Muses of Mount Helicon to help him in his task: Apollo, Aesculapius, witty Mercury and the sweet Suada (the three Sudice goddesses of Eastern Europe were said to attend at childbirth, to cast the fate of the newborn) were all called upon as was Christ. Raynold was proud to present his 'lytell booke' in the mother tongue but feared that his motives might be misconstrued. He stressed that writing about 'wemens priuitiees' was not a mortal sin although he was aware that 'euery boy and knaue had of these bookes, readyng them as openly as the tales of Roben hood'.

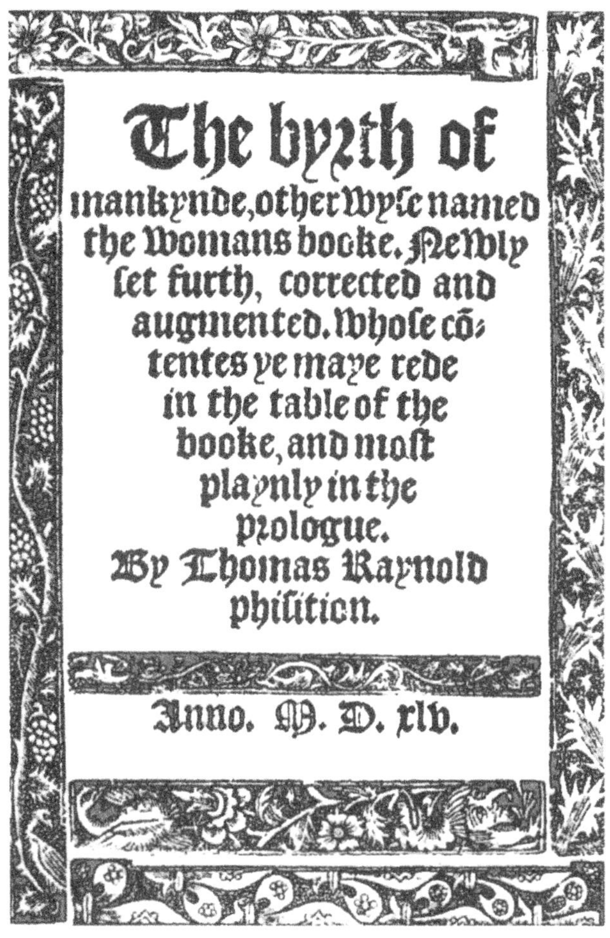

The byrth of
mankynde, otherwyse named
the womans booke. Newly
set furth, corrected and
augmented. Whose cō-
tentes ye maye rede
in the table of the
booke, and most
playnly in the
prologue.
By Thomas Raynold
phisition.

Anno. M. D. xlv.

Figure 4 Prologue page from *The Byrth of Mankynde*

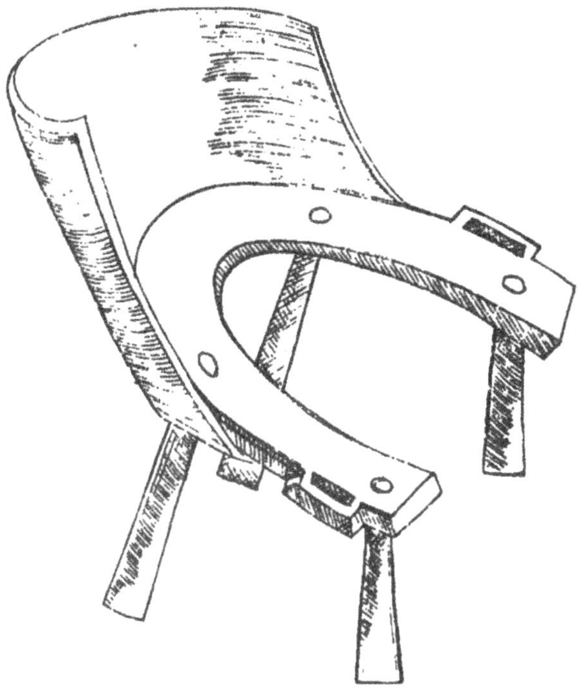

Figure 5 Birthing chair from *The Byrth of Mankynde*

The Fyrst Booke

This portion of the text is devoted to the female anatomy. 'The matrix, the mother, and the wombe, do signifie but one thing; that is to saye, the place, wherein the seede of man is conceauyd, fetifyid, conseruyd, nourishyd, and augmentyd, unto the time of deliuerance'; and he disposed of the old idea that the uterus contained seven separate chambers – 'the matrix hathe but one holoness'. He referred to the ovaries as 'the vesselles of seede called the woman's stones … wherein is engendryd the seede and sparme that cumeth from the woman'. Raynold referred to the Fallopian tube as the 'wormye bodye' but he was unaware of its function. He wrote that the purpose of the seed in women was to moisten the genital passage 'as it were with a dewe'.

The 'termes', 'flowres' or *menstrua* 'happen alwayes to womankinde, after xiiii or xv. years of age passed' and recurred 'at certaine seasons, times and terms' when menstrual blood was 'poured into the uterus'. It was also thought that the menstrual blood which was not shed during pregnancy was used to nourish the fetus. However Raynold did not subscribe to the ancient theories of Pliny that menstrual blood was a fatal poison and he denounced such notions as 'but dreams and plane dotage'. He wrote that the menstrual flow was diverted to the breasts to create milk after childbirth.

The Second Booke

'Of the tyme of byrth, and which is called naturall or unnaturall'

Raynold wrote that 'naturall byrthe is when the child is borne both in due season and also in due fashion … about XL wekes after the conception'. Raynold dealt with natural, unnatural, and difficult births. There are remedies for hard labor, placental delivery, and repair of a torn perineum. Instructions were included for the mother post-delivery and 'expert medicines' to induce menstruation, abortion and delivery of dead infants.

'Of easy and uneasy, difficull, or dolorous delyueraunce...' Regarding difficult labor Raynold enumerated various causes including a 'child ... of a fuller and greater growth' and advised about 'narrow passage', abnormal presentations or tumor masses obstructing the birth canal. He regarded constipation as a deterrent to labor.

'How a woman with chylde shall use her self, and what remedies be for them that haue harde labor'
Raynold wrote that the pregnant woman must keep two diets, one for the month before labor and the other during her laboring. She was advised to avoid foods which would hinder the birth. It was important to avoid constipation and a list of foodstuffs was advised which would 'loose the belly without parell'. Certain foodstuffs such as meat, rice, hard eggs, beef and chestnuts (*Castanea sativa*, an astringent) were thought to constipate and were to be avoided. If necessary a clyster (enema) was allowed but should be very gentle. Any infirmity, disease or swelling of the privy parts was to be 'loked unto and cured before the tyme of labor commyth, by the aduise of some experte surgion'. As labor approached, constipation could be eased by a clyster of egg yolk, hollyhock (*Althea rosea*, soothing and diuretic), honey, lard, mallows (*Malva sylvestris*, a mucilaginous laxative), dog's mercury (*Mercurialis annua*, a mucilaginous laxative), salt, soap and sugar, in a pint of water. If the woman 'waxe faynt or sickly' then she must be comforted with good meat and wholesome drinks accompanied by 'noble electuaries...such thinges the whiche maye laxe, open, and mollify the nature and passage, so that byrth may more frely procede'.

Older women were thought to be drier and more rigid and therefore required hot and moist medications, applied by anointing, in baths, by fomentation, or as suppositories. Grease from ducks, geese and hens or the oils of fenugreek (*Trigonella foenum-graecum*, a uterine stimulant), hollyhock and linseed (*Linum usitatissimum*, a mucilaginous laxative) were applied to the genital area. Alternatively the woman was advised to bathe in water to which was added chamomile (probably German chamomile, *Chamomilla recutita*, an analgesic and anti-inflammatory), fenugreek, hollyhock, linseed, maidenhair (*Adiantum capillus-veneris*, a soothing herb), dog's mercury and mallows 'to mollifie and suple'. If the woman was unable to bathe, the herbal water was applied with a sponge to the 'privie parts', followed by anointing with oils or grease. It was also thought profitable to 'suffume [fumigate] the nether places with muske, ambre [*Liquidambar orientalis*, oriental sweet gum, an anti-inflammatory and antiseptic] and *Gallia muscata* [probably galls of muscatel sage or clary, *Salvia sclarea*, a uterine stimulant]' which were placed on hot embers.

In early labor 'when the stormes and thronges begyn to come on ... and the humors ... flowe furth' the woman was advised to have her special labor diet ready and to prepare herself for the trial to come. She was advised at first to sit still for an hour but then to begin crying or wretching out loud. She was to hold her breath for periods of time in order to thrust the abdominal contents downwards. She was then ready to receive some medicine to induce the birth. Raynold wrote of the special midwives' stools which were used 'for the nonce' in France and Germany, which had a hole in the seat.

At this stage the midwife was to anoint the genitals with oil of almonds (*Amygdalus communis* var. *dulcis*, a demulcent) or white lilies (*Lilium candidum*, astringent and soothing). Offering good meat and drink and 'with swete wurdes' of encouragement the midwife extolled the value of patience and tolerance and gently stroked the belly above the navel to depress the birth downward. As the labor progressed the privy parts were again anointed with oil of white lilies and the midwife was advised to stretch, relax and loosen the 'straytes and not to be afrayde ne asshamed to handle the parts'. Raynold gave advice on rupturing the membranes with the fingernails or with a knife and advised that the woman should not be encouraged to push before she was ready. If the woman was very dry, the white of an egg, together with the yolk, were poured into the birth canal to supply natural emollient 'humidity'.

If the amniotic fluid had escaped too early and a dry labor resulted, the midwife was to apply oil of white lilies or grease obtained from hens, ducks or geese. The white of an egg was also used as a lubricant. To facilitate delivery of the 'secondyne' or second birth (placenta) the midwife could provoke maternal

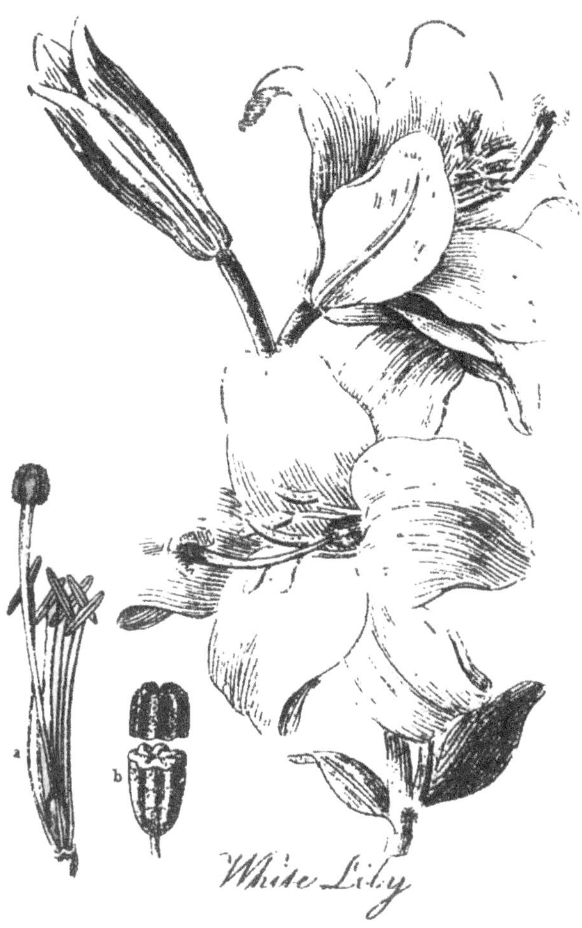

Figure 6 White lily

sneezing by the administration of powder of eleborus (*Helleborus niger*, a powerful sneezing agent and purgative) or pepper (*Piper nigrum*, a sneezing agent) and if this failed, he advised that the placenta should be manually removed.

'*Remedies and Medicines by the which the Labor may be made more tollerable, easy, and without great payne*'
Raynold offered a number of remedies which would ease the woman in labor. These could be applied by anointing and massage, by fumigation, in pessaries, pills, and plasters or by encouraging sneezing. The following are some examples:

Fumigation '[Taking] yelowe brymstone, myrrhe [*Commiphora myrrha*, an anti-inflammatory], madder [*Rubia tinctorum*, an antiseptic], galbanum [*Ferula galbaniflua*, an anti-inflammatory and antiseptic], opponacum [*Opopanax chironium*, an antispasmodic], of eche lyke muche, and temper all these together, makynge of them pylles: and with those also ye may make fume to be receaued underneth.'

Drink 'canell [*Cinnamomum cassia*] dronke with wine is very good.'

Sneezing This was provoked with 'powder of Eleborus, or els of pepper'.

Annoyntynge '[The] Priuities with oil [of almonds or white lilies] or other such grese': to these could be added musk, saffron (*Crocus sativus*, a uterine stimulant) and other remedies.

Pylles Containing 'myrrhe, galbanu, castoreum [secretion of, or the dried, preputial glands of the beaver, *Castor fiber*, antispasmodic and stimulant]'.

'Certayne pylles the which make the labor easye and without payne'
One analgesic mixture contained *Aristolochia rotunda* (a form of birthwort, a uterine stimulant), canell, cassia lignea, myrrh, opium (*Papaver somniferum*, analgesic, and sedative), savin (*Juniperus sabina*, a uterine stimulant, and also contains podophyllotoxin), and storax (*Liquidambar orientalis*). These were to be administered with good old wine.

'Meanes to helpe and provoke the byrth' Safrane (saffron) or silver montanum (*Seli massiliense*) were said to provoke 'the byrth of any liuyng thyng'. Other remedies in this section include, ammoniacum (*Dorema ammoniacum* gum, an antispasmodic), asafetida (*Ferula asafoetida* gum, known in German as teuffelkot, or as devil's dung, an antispasmodic, laxative and stimulant), juniper berries (*Juniperus communis*, a uterine stimulant), pennyroyal (*Mentha pulegium*, a uterine stimulant), rue (herb of grace, *Ruta graveolens*, a uterine stimulant) and savin. A 'playster to prouoke the byrth' was laid on the woman's 'belly betwene the nauel and the nether part'. The plasters contained barley meal (*Hordeum vulgare*, a demulcent), colocynth (bitter apple, bitter cucumber, *Citrullus colocynthis*, an aperient, hydragogue and cathartic), myrrh and rue.

'How the secodyne or second byrth shall be forsed to yssue furth, if it come not frely of his owne kynde'
Raynold wrote about the woman who was weakened with 'trauell, dolour and payne' and who did not have the strength to expel the placenta. The placenta could

be 'entangled' within the matrix or the walls of the uterus were thought to have closed down and encased it. If the placenta was not expelled, Raynold wrote that it was likely that it would putrify and the 'yll noysom and pestiferous vapours' would ascend to the heart and brain and 'many tymes [a woman] is playnly suffocated, stragled, and dead of it'. A nutritious broth of bird flesh, egg yolk, fat and wine was fed to the woman to build up her strength. Ointment or oil of white and blue lilies (astringent) and oil of marjoram (*Origanum dictamnus*, a carminative and stimulant) were applied to the matrix in an effort to provoke placental delivery.

Remedies thought to have expulsive properties were drunk as a decoction with lukewarm wine. These included galbanum, juniper berries, pennyroyal and southernwood (*Artemisia abrotanum*, a uterine stimulant). Fumigation to 'suffume the secreates with perfumes' was also thought good for the purpose, but if the 'odoriferous and swete smellynge thynges: as ambre' (amber, the resin of various coniferous trees, antispasmodic and stimulant), 'muske' (dried secretions from the preputial glands of the deer, *Moschus moschiferus*, antispasmodic and stimulant), frankincense (olibanum from *Boswellia* species, an antiseptic and used to relieve menstrual pain in traditional Chinese medicine), or *Gallia muscata* were unsuccessful then fumes of 'such thynges, the whiche stynck or haue abbominable smel: as asafetida, castorum, mans here or woman's here burnt, pecockes fethers burnt' were conducted to the birth canal. Sneezing was provoked with powder of hellebore or pepper. Once the placenta appeared, the midwife was to receive it tenderly and softly 'leste it breake'.

'Howe that many thynges chaunse to the women after theyr labor, and howe to auoyde, defende, or to remedy the same'

'Lacke of due purgation of the flowres' Raynold offered remedies which could be taken by mouth; by application of lotion or washing of the feet; by decoction of herbs; by emplasters; by fumigation of odors; by ointments; by purgations or by sneezing powders. He wrote that methods which provoke urination also cause 'the flowres to departe' and that then were to be used only under the supervision of an expert physician. When all remedies failed bleeding was resorted to and the 'saphena vayne' at the ankle was the chief target.

'Yf the woman haue the ague after her labor' The ague or puerperal fever was thought to be due to retention of the lochia. In addition to remedies which provoked the lochia the woman was advised to drink a decoction of beaten barley and cicers (chick pea, *Cicer arietinum*, an astringent), cullis (strong broth) of a cock, milk whey, pomegranates (*Punica granatum*, an antiparasitic and astringent) and tamarind (*Tamarindus indica*, an antiseptic, laxative and stimulant) in water 'where these thynges do prouoke the flowres, and mitigateth the immoderat heate'.

'If the body after labor do swel and inflate' 'If the body after labor do swel and inflate' or there was 'fretting and knawyng of the guttes and payne of the matrice, and other secret partes thereabout' medication was required: a number of anointings, clysters, drinks infused with herbs, electuaries, fumes, pessaries and plasters were used. A linen bag containing sodden herbs, conveyed to the 'secret parts' was also thought helpful.

'After the labor the flowres yssue more vehemently' A number of explanations were advanced for excessive post-delivery loss which led to a state of 'langour and painfullness in the woman'. The midwife was advised to seek the counsel of an 'expert phisitias' who, by his learning and experience, would 'consyder the true cause of it, and the very remedy to amend it'. One such remedy involved binding the woman's arms, thereby reducing general blood flow back to the body, followed by the use of a 'ventose, boxe, or cuppynge glasse, with fyre which is called boxyng under [the] brestes without any scarification'.

A large number of remedies were offered for: anointing; to add to baths; to apply in linen bags; as medicinal potions; and as electuaries, ointments, plasters, powders or trochiskes (lozenges). 'Farthermore there be at the apothecaries trochiskes which help greatly in this case, as the trochiskes of kerabe [*Ceratonia siliqua*, carob contains mucilage, and is a demulcent and laxative] or ambar and the trochiskes of bole armoniake [Armenian earth containing alumina, chalk, silica and iron oxide, used to treat hemorrhages] which must be ministred a dram or more of either of them, with four or five sponefulles of plantayne water [*Plantago asiatica* or *Plantago major*, anti-inflammatory, and styptic]'.

'Yf it be that there be engendred any apostume...' Apostumes (abscesses) or other swellings which developed in the privy places after labor were cleansed, purged and healed, and the pain mitigated with juice of berries or leaves of nightshade (*Atropa belladona*, an analgesic, and antispasmodic), of plantain (*Plantago major*), and oil of roses (astringent) and 'the places annoynted therewith'. Abscesses were to be opened only by a surgeon or expert physician. Prolapse of the uterus or vagina was likely to occur after delivery and a large number of remedies were offered for application as ointments or in sitz baths. Once treated the prolapse was reduced and replaced.

'How that sumtyme the privy parte and fundament become one' Rupture of the perineum sometimes occurred as a result of the birth: 'many tymes it chanseth that thorowe the greate difficultie and thronges of labor the preuye parte and the foundament become one, by reason of rupture and breakynge of the same parte in the delyueraunce of the chylde'. Raynold described in great detail how to cleanse the area and repair it with silken thread. A linen bandage soaked with a little liquid pitch (the resin of fir, pine, spruce, also called turpentine, an adhesive, and anti-inflammatory) was applied to the wound to help healing.

'Of deade byrthes...' Raynold enumerated the various clinical symptoms and signs present in a case of intrauterine fetal death and wrote that 'yf her handes put into very warme water, and then layde on the woman's belly, and the chyld steare not, is a signe that it is deade'. He advised that there were two ways to expel 'deade byrthes': the use of medicines or of instruments. Numerous herbal medications were used in the hope that the patient would labor. These included rue and other herbs thought to have expulsive properties and also plant remedies known to exert a purgative effect. However, when 'medicines profette not, then must be used more seuere and harde remedyes, with instrumentes, as hokes, tonges, and suche other thynges made for the nonce'. Raynold detailed such deliveries and then wrote about the release of hydrocephalus with a sharp penknife and the birth of the abnormal infant. If a woman died in labor he advised that 'the chylde hauynge life in it; then shall it be mete to kepe open the woman's mouth, and also the nether places, so that the chylde maye by that meanes boche receaue and also expelle ayre and brethe, whiche otherwyse might be stopped to the destruction of the childe: And then to turne her on her lefte side, and there to cutte her open, and so to take out the childe: They that be borne after this fashion are called Cesares, for because they be cutte out of theyr mothers bellye: whereuppon also the noble Romayn Cesar the first, toke his name'. People born by cesarean section in these circumstances were also known as 'caesones' – *a caeso matris utero.*

'Certayne experte medicines which be most requisite...' In the final chapter of the second book Raynold wrote about 'certayne experte medicines ... compendiously set furth ... whereby the woman's labore maybe made the more easye'. There followed seven pages devoted to the medications available to hasten labor. Certain lozenges and emplasters described by Raynold could be found 'at the signe of the Dooues in Boucklar's bery in London: the name of the good man of this house is Wyllyam Normeuyll, in whose shoppe I have caused the sayde thinges faithfully to be made, for because that I am certayne that he is one of the moost fydell and faithfullest Apothecaries in London and suche as will not spare for any cost to acquire and obtayne of the best and moost syngular symples and droges in there kynde, that may be gotten for monye'.

The Thyrde Booke

According to Raynold, the third book 'entreatyd what is to be done to the infant borne, and how to choose a nource, and of her office, with manifolde medycynes and remedies agaynst sundry infyrmytees which eftsones happen to infantes in theyr infancie'. He advised that the navel should be cut three-fingers breadth from the belly and tied. The 'powder of bole armeniacke, and *sanguis draconis* [dragons' blood; gum from the *Dracaena draco* tree, an adhesive] with sarcocolla [*Buxus* species, an antipyretic], myrrhe and cumyne [cumin, *Cuminum cyminum*, an antibacterial and astringent]' was then applied on a piece of cotton wool dipped in olive oil (oil from *Olea europaea*, a demulcent). He went on to write how the various wrinkles, or lack of them, on the cord could portend the mother's obstetric future. Thereafter followed general advice for cleansing and swaddling the baby.

A long treatise on the 'nourse, and her mylke: and howe longe the chyld shulde sucke' with various remedies for increasing milk flow are offered. The advice appears quite similar to the guidance given by Soranus. The final section of the third book three deals with 33 ailments of the newborn and contains 40 pages of remedies, the last of which being for 'google eyes or that it loke squynt'.

The Fourthe Booke

The fourth book deals with conception, with fertility tests, and with remedies to assist conception or determine the sex of the offspring. Finally, there are remedies for enhancing a woman's beauty, including the treatment of dandruff; the removal of unwanted hair, freckles or spots; the treatment of warts; skin clarification; softening of hard skin; treatment for pimples; dental hygiene; treatment for halitosis; and finally, treatment of 'the ranke sauour of the armeholes'.

DE CONCEPTU ET GENERATIONE HOMINIS OR *THE EXPERT MIDWIFE*

Jacob Rueff's *Trostbuechle* or 'midwives' book was published in 1554, four years before his death. The text was revised in 1559 and further editions of the book were published. Rueff (1500–1558) was the town surgeon and teacher of obstetrics in Zurich from 1532, responsible for the instruction and examination of midwives in the area. He was also a poet and playwright who wrote on astronomy and history and advocated the notion of religious freedom. His obstetric book was published in both German and Latin editions in the same year (Le Fanu, 1976), a marvelous achievement when one remembers the complexity of the writing and printing processes of the era. The German edition was known by the short title *Trostbuechle* and the more popular Latin edition was entitled *De Conceptu et Generatione Hominis*. The Latin edition of 1554 contains a dedicatory passage from Conrad Gesner (Gesner, 1516–1565, is often referred to as the German Pliny) in which he praises Jacob Rueff, the celebrated surgeon.

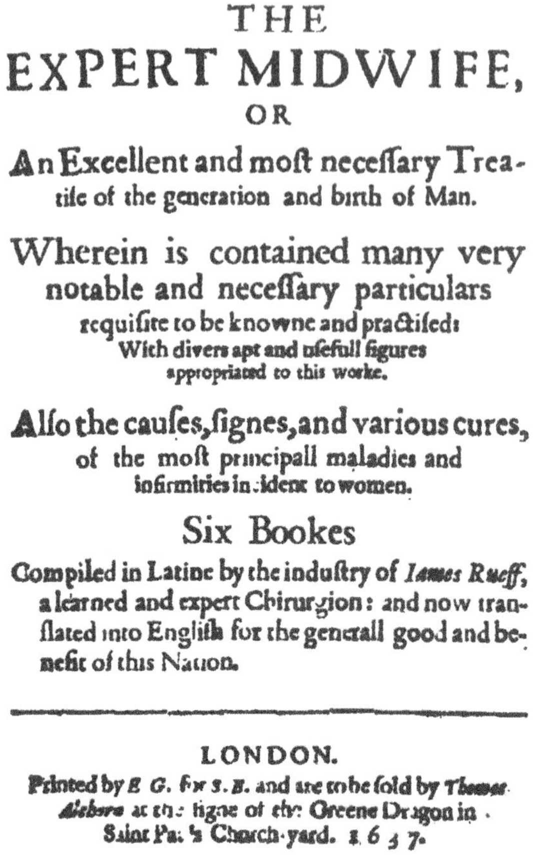

THE
EXPERT MIDWIFE,
OR
An Excellent and moſt neceſſary Treatiſe of the generation and birth of Man.
Wherein is contained many very notable and neceſſary particulars requiſite to be knowne and practiſed: With divers apt and uſefull figures appropriated to this worke.
Alſo the cauſes, ſignes, and various cures, of the moſt principall maladies and infirmities incident to women.
Six Bookes
Compiled in Latine by the induſtry of *James Rueff*, a learned and expert Chirurgion: and now tranſlated into Engliſh for the generall good and benefit of this Nation.

LONDON.
Printed by E. G. for S. B. and are to be ſold by *Thomas Alchorn* at the ſigne of the Greene Dragon in Saint Pauls Church-yard. 1637.

Figure 7 Frontispiece from *The Expert Midwife*

Rueff's text was subdivided into six 'Bookes' with further divisions into chapters. The work was highly illustrated, with 69 diagrams throughout the text. An English translation entitled *The Expert Midwife* was published in 1637: no translator's name is acknowledged in the text but it is essentially similar to the German and Latin editions of the previous century. Jacob Rueff identified his sources as being chiefly ancient Greco-Roman and Arabic: Ariston, Aristomymus, Aristotle, Augustinius, Averröes, Avicenna, Cassianus, Fulvius, Galen, Hippocrates, Paul of Aegina, Pliny, Plutarch, Rabi Moses, and Vincentius.

Rueff also referred to the work of Albertus Magnus and that of his contemporary, Andreas Vesalius, some of whose anatomical figures were used in the text. Vesalius (1514–1564), although better known for his

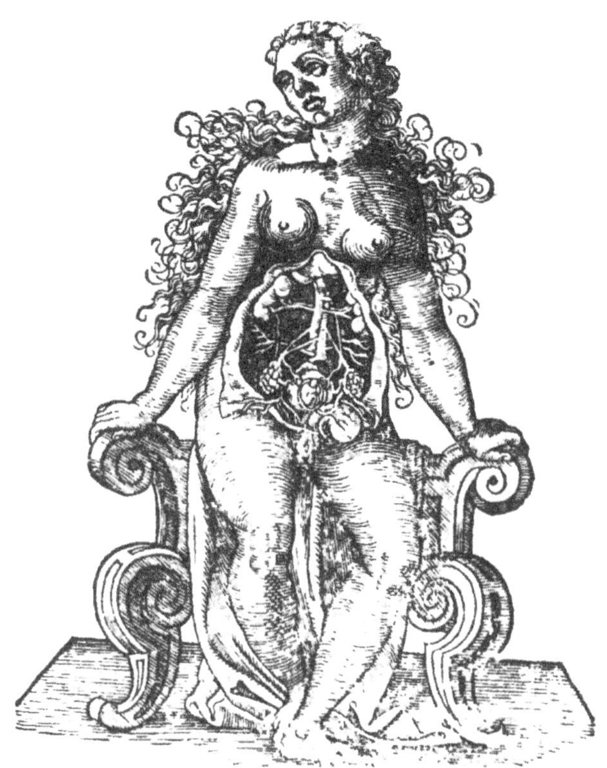

Figure 8 Female anatomy from *The Expert Midwife*

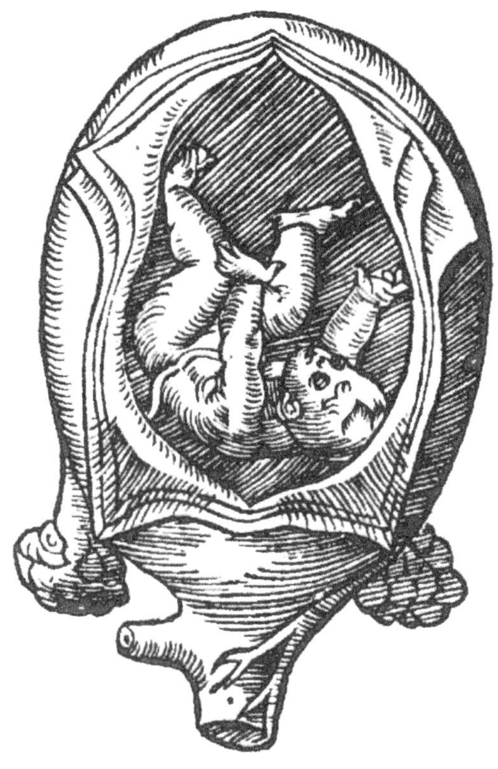

Figure 9 Fetus *in utero* from *The Expert Midwife*

anatomical works, described the therapeutic use of china root (*Smilax china*) in the treatment of syphilis. Jacob Rueff also refers, in passing, to Emperor Maximilian. It was inevitable that Rueff would have read Eucharius Rösslin's *Der Schwangeren Frauen und Hebammen Rosengarten* of 1513 (see above) but he made no mention of his illustrious predecessor.

Illustrations in *The Expert Midwife*

Rueff was convinced of the importance to midwives of anatomical knowledge of the internal female organs. He was the first to use true anatomical pictures in an obstetric book: the *barmutter* (uterus) is displayed as part of a female figure in one of the 69 illustrated plates with a full description. Other illustrations depict scenes from the birth chamber, formation of the fetus, obstetrical instruments and fetal malformations. The Frankfurt publisher, Sigmund Feyerabendt, published an edition of *De Conceptu...* in 1580 which contained much more lifelike figures (woodcuts) by the celebrated artist Jost Amman (Hagelin, 1989).

Materia medica of *The Expert Midwife*

In common with Eucharius Rösslin's book on midwifery, less than half of Jacob Rueff's text is devoted to the anatomical aspects of conception and childbirth. The remainder, and the larger portion of the book, is a compendium of drug treatments for use in pregnancy, childbirth, the puerperium, and for fertility and menstrual disorders. Rueff's book contains larger numbers of both indications and medications that are found in Rösslin's *Rosengarten*. In the German edition of Rueff's book almost all the medications are named in Latin but a few are called by their German name. The medications are prefixed by the *Rx* (recipe sign) and consist of a mixture of drugs, compounded for administration by divers methods. Most of the compounds contain six to ten items but there is one recipe which contains over 35 individual components. Most of the recipes containing large numbers of individual ingredients were used for the cure of sterility or to stimulate or inhibit menstruation. In the English edition of Rueff's work the drug names have been

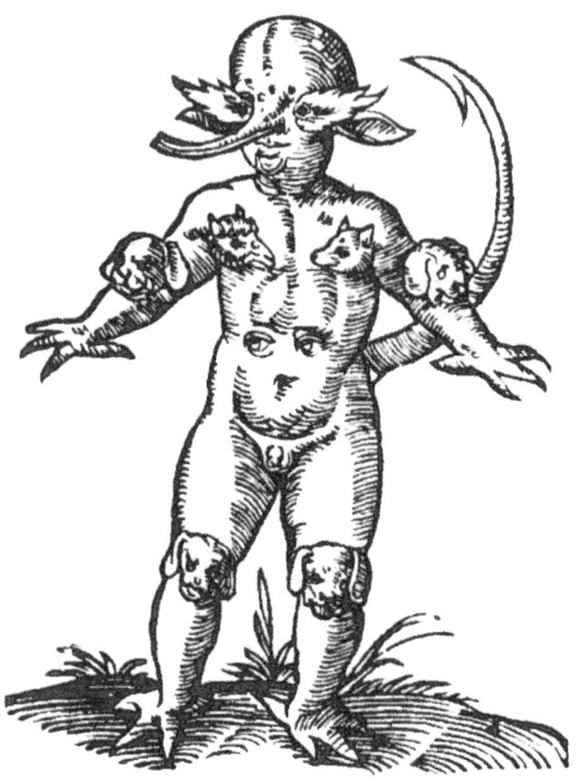

Figure 10 Fetal malformations from *The Expert Midwife*

translated into their English equivalent although some Latin terms remain. The English and German texts are easier to read because or their superior layout.

The drugs were prescribed with instructions such as *fiat decoctio* (let a decoction be made), or *fiat haustus* (let a draught be made). Medications were administered in water, in a *balneum* (bath) or by decoction, *electuarium* (syrup), *emplastrum* (medicated plaster), *epithema* (medication in alcohol), *fomentu* (fomentation), or *infusio* (infusion); *as pessariu* (pessaries), *piluae* (pills), *potioa* (potions), or *pulvius* (powder); as a purgation; by *sufficus* (fumigation), *syrupus*, or *tabulis* (tablets); or as an *unguentum* (ointment). One oxytocic prescription from *The Expert Midwife reads*

Rx *Castorei*
Sulphuris
Galbani
Opopanacis
Stercoris Columbini
Assae foetidae

Misce cum succo Rutae et fiant trochisci ad formam nucis auellanae. His fumigia facere proderit.

Liber Primus – *De Generatione Hominis*, the 'Generation of Man and Women'

Rueff declared that menstrual blood was the matter of woman's seed and went on to write that the 'termes' are called *menstruum* in Latin and the 'monthly purgation', *mensis lunaris* (or 'flowers' in German). The appearance of menstruation on a regular basis meant that women were fertile. If the 'flowers' did not appear, then women were unfruitful, like trees that did not develop flowers in their due season'. When the woman was pregnant, the 'termes' were not shed and Rueff quoted Hippocrates, 'prince of physicians', who (like Galen) wrote that the menstrual blood was altered to milk for the newborn: '[the] Dugges or Paps ... alter and change the blood into milke; further, two veines doe descend from the Paps into the Matrix, which draws blood from thence to be digested and turned into milk'.

Liber Secundus – *De Matrice et Eius Partibus*

Rueff cautioned that women should not be bled or cupped, and that they should abstain from taking pills or purges in early pregnancy without the counsel of an expert physician. He advised a special diet for the pregnant woman which included white and red meats, cinnamon, nutmeg (*Myristica fragrans* or *Nigella sativa*) and sugar, and cautioned that certain meats, fruits and vegetables were best avoided. 'If they be bound [constipated] and cannot goe orderly to stoole', lettuce (*Lactuca sativa*) with butter, salt, spinach (*Spinacia oleracea*), vinegar or wine were advised. If these remedies failed, mild purgation was allowed using suppositories of egg with Venice soap (olive oil soap) or, if necessary, a potion containing a decoction of cassia leaves with senna (another form of cassia) could be taken.

If the woman was subject to 'fainting and swooning' in early pregnancy she was advised to drink sorrel water (from *Rumex* species) and rosewater mixed with cinnamon and other herbs such as wild cloves (*Pimenta acris*) and saffron. Further medications were offered to alleviate vomiting; to 'strengthen the stomach'; to avoid preterm birth; and for bleeding in pregnancy. Rueff also advised a special diet to hasten the onset of childbirth in women who had a tendency to prolonged pregnancy.

Liber Tertius – *De Partu, et Parturientium Infantium et Cura Omnifaria.*

The conduct and requirements for midwives was discussed in detail. Always important to have at hand were oil of lilies or sweet almonds, hen's grease and white of egg for application to the birth canal. A powder compound of bole armeniac, *sanguis draconis* and myrrh was required for application to the newborn infant's navel. A large number of remedies were available to the midwife for application in cases of difficult or prolonged birth and could be administered as baths, electuaries, emplasters, pessaries, pills, potions or unguents. If the placenta was retained after the delivery, remedies were offered to stimulate its expulsion.

Suffocation of the matrix (eclampsia) was described and one recommended treatment was hellebore powder, used to induce sneezing (American hellebore contains antihypertensives). Medications were offered to induce childbirth when the infant was dead, but if the woman failed to labor she was placed in bed in a head down position (an early form of the Walcher position) and instruments were applied. These included the three-bladed *speculum matricis* ('the mirror or looking-glass of the matrix') and the *apertorium* ('an opener'), a double bladed instrument used to stretch the cervix. Once visualized, the *rostrum anatis* ('the duck- or drakes-bill'), a toothed forceps, was used to 'take hold of the dead childe' to effect delivery. Then the forceps called the *longa et tersa* ('long and smooth') were used so that 'she may easily pull out that which is to be drawne forth'. Rueff went on to describe a vulval hematoma and how it should be incised with a clean knife and anointed with oil of roses.

Liber Quartus – *De Differentiis non Naturalis Partus, et Earundem Curis.*

This book is mainly devoted to the mechanical aspects of various forms of fetal presentation and birth and is also noted for a reference to combined external and internal manipulation to achieve version (Findley, 1939). If the uterus should prolapse after the birth, warm oil of chamomile (*Chamaemelum nobile* or *Matricaria recutita*), roses or violets (*Viola odorata*) were to be gently applied. Should the woman's 'flowers cease oversoone, as it often chanceth then powder of Elleborus or Peper, shall be blown into her nostrills ... to provoke the flux'. Other confections with a similar purpose were mentioned.

Liber Quintiis – *De Mola.*

What we now term hydatidiform mole was known to Rueff as the 'false conception' or *mola* and he wrote that the word was probably derived from *molon*, a Greek term for a round object or possibly from the Persian word *moli*, a 'misshapen thing or disordered lump'. The Greeks also used the term *mylon* and the Latin word was *mola*. Having considered the difference between a *mola* and a normal pregnancy, Rueff enumerates many remedies, mostly of plant origin, to help purge the tumor from the matrix.

Rueff also wrote of 'unperfect children, also of monsterous Births'. These he attributed to judgments of God (for venery, immoderate desire or lust) or to corruption of the seed. In the section devoted to congenital fetal malformations he describes cleft-lip and a number of other well-known congenital abnormalities, including conjoined twins.

Liber Quintiis continued with the causes and signs of abortion and the treatments which were available to avoid miscarriage, followed by a section which described coitus of men and women with devils and the conception of devil-children (although Rueff himself was skeptical of such stories). The evil female spirit was named a *succubus* and the male an *incubus*: 'wherefor, that the Divell, named in Latine, Succubus, may be able to conceive with men, and being changed into the Divell, termed Incubus, may cast forth the same seede conceived into women, and begat a man, is not only a fabulous thing to be spoken, but also impius, wicked, and odious to be believed'.

Liber Sextus – *De Sterilitatis causis diuersis.*

Having frightened the reader into a state of celibacy, Rueff concerned himself with sterility, its causes and investigations. With echoes from ancient times, Rueff informed the reader that if barley sprouted within ten days after urine had been poured onto it, the donor could be assured of their fertility or 'fruitfullness'. Rueff also mentioned Hippocrates' 'fumigation test' and others which were used to determine whether or not the matrix was 'open' for pregnancy.

The cure of sterility depended on the cause, which could be related to a number of factors including 'Phlegme or Cholericke humidities and moistures of the Matrix'; 'superfluous bloody humors of the Matrix'; 'melancholy humor'; 'over-much heate and drinesse'; or 'moistere and coldnesse'. Different medications were required for sterility resulting from different causes. Among the remedies to increase 'fruitfulness' were stones (testicles) of a fox or of a bull, stones of a lecherous goat, whether or boar, 'of each three ounces'. These were dried, powdered and mixed with various herbs and dried priapus or 'pissle of a bull ... or goat' to be taken daily by the couple in an electuary (a mixture of medicine with honey).

The next portion of Jacob Rueff's book continued with treatises on 'suffocation and choking of the matrix [eclampsia] ... precipitation or falling downe of the matrix' (uterine prolapse) and menstrual disorders, including 'superfluities of the termes' (here meaning heavy lochial loss). A large number of medicinal products were mentioned, with *mumia* (mummy medicine) being suggested for the first time in the book.

The final section of *The Expert Midwife* also dealt with 'the termes' and how they may be cured or stopped. Rueff mentioned here, among other remedies, immersion in The Baths. He wrote of the famous Baths of Badina in Germany, which contained brimstone (sulfur) and were thought most efficacious in curing overabundance of the termes. When all other methods failed, the ancient remedy of bleeding was resorted to: 'veines, named Saphenae, shall be opened in both feete, the Moone going downe'.

WALTER CARY'S *A BOKE OF THE PROPERTIES OF HERBES*

Around 1560, Walter Cary wrote: 'A boke of the properties of herbes called an herball, where unto is added the time of herbes, floures, and sedes shold be gathered to be kept the whole yere, with the virtue of y herbes when they are stilled. Also a general rule of all manner of herbes drawen out of an ancient boke of physeck by W.C'. Cary quoted Constantine, Dioscorides, Galen and Hippocrates and, while he detailed 210 medicinal herbs and their value for general ailments, only 28 were used for women's diseases. Men's reproductive organs were mentioned, with betony (*Stachys officinalis*, an astringent and sedative) being offered for when 'Mannes Yarde be swolen'. To avoid such a disaster Carey advised the use of hemlock (*Conium maculatum*, an analgesic and narcotic), writing that the 'ioyce of this herbe kepeth maydes testes smal and destryth the great aptyte of lecherye'.

The English terminology of Cary's text was initially somewhat confusing for this contemporary reader. Plant remedies were offered for 'wormes in the wombe', and references to the breast appeared out of context. After initial confusion it became obvious that the 'wombe' in question was in fact the intestines, and that 'breast' meant the chest, and not the mammary glands. The word 'womb' is derived from Old English *wamb* and Middle English, *wambe*, meaning belly, stomach or bowels, and could refer to the anatomy of either sex but eventually came to signify the uterus. The term 'breast' comes from Old English *breost*, which referred to the forepart of the human body between the neck and the belly but now almost exclusively refers to the mammae. On the final page of his *Boke of the Properties of Herbes*, Walter Cary offered this 'general rule of all maner of herbes':

It is a general Rule,
that from the eyght: ka
lendes of the moneth of
April: unto the moneth
of Julye, all maner of
leaves of herbes be best, and from
the. VIII. Kalendes of July unto
the. VIII. Kalendes of October: the
stalkes have mooste vertue. And
from the. VIII. Kalendes of Octo
ber: unto the VIII eyght kalendes
of April: all maner
of Roots of Her
bes be in their
full strength.

FINIS.

Cary's materia medica for women

Anti-aphrodisiac
eruca, dragancia, hemlock

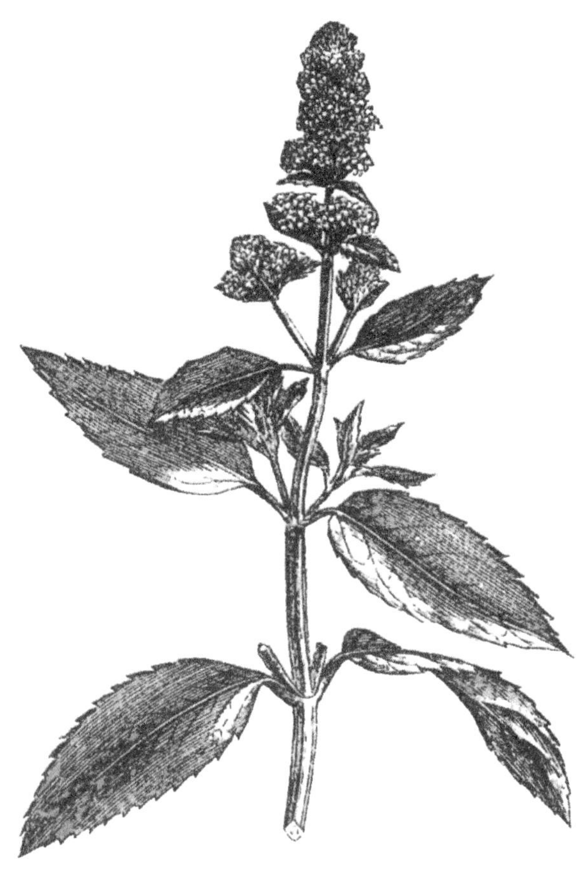

Figure 11 Mint (*Mentha* sp.)

Breast disorders
Anti-lactation agnus castus, marjoram
Caked (mastitis) celandine
Galactagogue fennel

Childbirth
Oxytocic geniacus, horsehelm, polegium, savin
Oxytocic for dead child basil, mint, dittany, lolium, peony

Convulsions
peony

Fertility
To increase motherwort, olibanum
Contraceptive agnus castus

Menstruation
Emmenagogue motherwort, mustard
Menorrhagia plantago, shepherd's purse

Postnatal purge
mint, motherwort, onion, sage

Sedative
poppy

'Swollen yard'
betony

Uterine pain or disease
agrimony, baume, olibanum, wormwood.

WILLIAM TURNER'S *HERBAL*

William Turner (1510–1568) was a botanist, cleric and physician. A native of Northumberland, he was born during the reign of King Henry VIII and attended Pembroke Hall, Cambridge (under the patronage of Thomas Lord Wentworth) where he remained until 1540 when he became a peripatetic preacher traveling the highways and byways of the English countryside. Later on, he traveled extensively throughout Italy, Germany and Holland. He studied botany under the guidance of Luca Ghine at Bologna and proceeded to an MD degree. Turner subsequently developed a close and lifelong friendship with Conrad Gesner, the famous Swiss naturalist. During his time in Germany Turner advanced his interest in plants and conducted extensive botanical experimentation. He returned to England as the dean of Wells but continued with his plant research.

In her book, *The Old English Herbals* (1922), Eleanour Sinclair Rohde recounted that Turner was the first Englishman 'who studied plants scientifically, ... his herbal marks the beginning of the science of botany in England'. Turner's *Herbal* was indeed the first original work on botany written in English and such was his academic stature that Turner became known as the 'father of English botany' to generations of plant enthusiasts. The *Herbal* was published in three parts, the first printed in 1551, the second in 1561 and the 1568 edition containing all three sections. Turner's *Herbal* contained a large number of woodcut illustrations, at least 400 of which were 'borrowed' from the 1542 *Herbal* of the renowned Bavarian physician, Leonhard Fuchs (1501–1566), to whom we owe the plant genus name, *Fuchsia*.

In the introduction to his text Turner castigated the English physicians who relied on apothecaries' medicines to treat their patients, while the apothecaries in turn trusted 'old wives' to gather their medicinal herbs. Turner argued that many physicians were not present when their remedies were compounded and 'many a good man by ignorance is put in jeopardy of his life, or good medicine is marred to the great dishonesty both of the phisician and of Goddes worthy creatures'. Now that he had presented them with a herbal in English, Turner hoped that physicians and apothecaries alike would mend their ways and become involved in the lengthy business of collecting and preparing the medications they prescribed.

Turner's *Herbal* names herbs in apothecaries' Latin (which often differed from 'true' Latin), French, German, Greek, Latin, and sometimes in Italian. Turner quoted extensively from the works of Aetius, Avicenna, Dioscorides, Galen, Paul of Aegina and Theophrastus, and refers to more than 36 authoritative sources in his books. Not blind to the risks involved in preparing and ingesting the plant medicines, Turner cautioned against the excessive use of any herb, and in some instances offered an antidote for overdosage. Each medicinal herbal entry in his books described in great detail the particular plant in question and indicated where it could obtained, whether in England, Europe or the Levant. Many of the plants were illustrated. Following the plant's description came an exposition of the 'vertues' or medicinal (or other) properties of the particular herb as they related to the various bodily systems and their diseases, as understood at that time.

William Turner's materia medica

The *Herbal* had 667 pages, with references to 365 plant remedies, of which 195 related to reproductive ailments. The medicinal herb with the most applications in women's disorders was the chaste tree (*Vitex agnus castus*) which could be used to increase milk flow, reduce fertility, reduce menstrual loss, treat uterine disease or induce a state of chastity. Unlike the obstetric texts of the era which merely mentioned a remedy by name, Turner dealt with each medicinal herb in great detail and he did not describe compound medications.

Turner wrote of aphrodisiacs and anti-aphrodisiacs. Nutmeg (*Myristica* species, used in Ayurvedic medicine for premature ejaculation) was 'profitable for cold husbandes that would fayne haue children, but not for lecherous bores and bulles' while hemlock (*Conium maculatum*, a highly poisonous narcotic analgesic and sedative) was said to 'febleth the member of generetion'. Gender-specific contraceptives were also described. Some herbs were said to promote or to stop menstruation. Plants which were claimed to act as diuretics were also used as emmenagogues (Turner mentions 17 inducers of menstruation), a feature shared with other texts of the time. Twenty-one oxytocic herbs are recommended to stimulate childbirth or to expel a dead fetus, while 17 other plants with expulsive powers were advised for delivery of the placenta. Nine herbal medications were offered for 'strangulation' of the womb (eclampsia) some of which were used 'to stereth up weomen' after the convulsion. Other remedies were used for 'whyte flowres' (vaginal discharge), for inflammations, and for other diseases of the uterus. Sex selection was considered possible, and Turner advocated the application of arsemart (or smartweed, *Polygonum hydropiper*, sometimes used as a remedy for venereal disease) if a 'man-child' was desired.

Turner's herbal includes four indications for breast treatment and the remedies for each are specific to the category: seven remedies 'Bringeth milke to the toppes'; 'Fore pappes ... after a woemen's byrthe puffed up and do swell' six herbs were recommended; there were seven medications for 'Burning impostume of the pappes'; and for 'Breasts ... loose and hanging down' lady's mantle (*Alchemilla mollis*) was to be used.

Of the books reviewed for this chapter only Turner mentions St Anthony's fire and the 'French Poxe' both of which were important medical problems of the era. St Anthony's fire, with burning and pain in the extremities, was caused by the ingestion of rye bread contaminated with ergot. The same contaminant caused uterine spasms and although in use as a labor stimulant by European midwives of the time, ergot is not referred to in the sixteenth century obstetric books or herbals. Turner offered nine different herbal remedies to alleviate the symptoms of 'the fire'.

The 'French Poxe' (syphilis) which had erupted in the fifteenth century continued to wreak havoc among

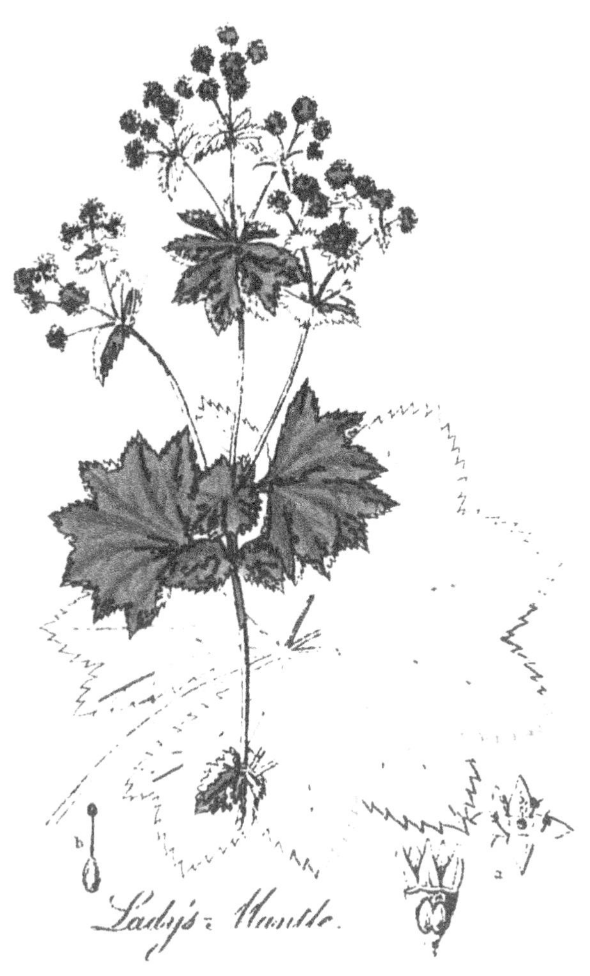

Figure 12 Lady's mantle (*Alchemilla mollis*)

those who indulged in 'lechery' and congenital *Lues Venereum* devastated the health of the offspring of their couplings. Turner suggested the European herbal remedies of dog's-tongue (*Cynoglossum officinale*, an analgesic and anti-inflammatory) and tamarind (*Tamarind indica*, or Indian date, which contains methyl salicylate, an analgesic and anti-inflammatory also used for 'womene that are vexed with theyr unmeasurable isshue' and for uterovaginal prolapse). Turner wrote of the American imports, *lignum-sanctum* (*Guajacum officinale*, anti-inflammatory and diaphoretic) and sarsaparilla (*Smilax* species, with antibiotic and anti-inflammatory properties), which became the main treatments of the 'Great Poxe' until the advent of mercury (see Chapter 26). Other venereal diseases were featured and Turner opined that

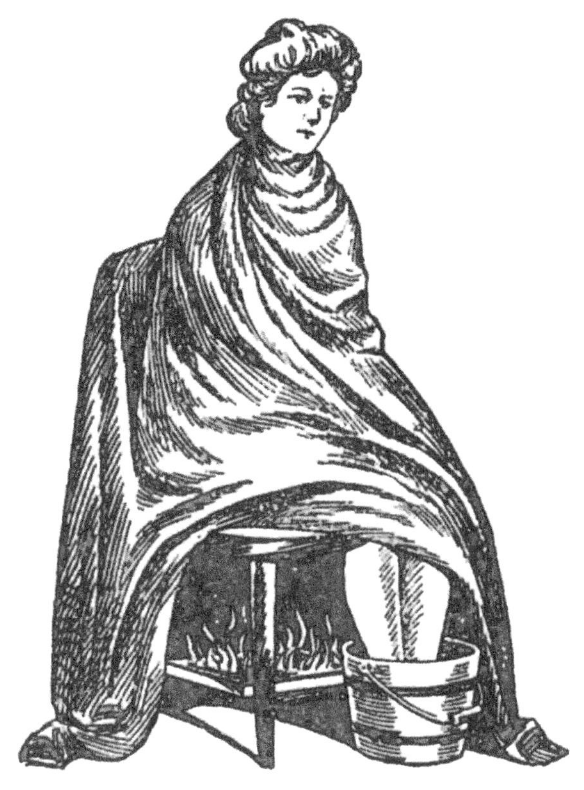

Figure 13 A vapor bath

aloes (*Aloe vera*) 'healeth especially the priuye members that haue a foras'. Testicular inflammation could be assuaged by the application of irio (wild cabbage) while cumin (*Cuminum cyminum*, antibacterial and a sexual stimulant) was recommended as the best remedy 'for swelling of the stones'. The term 'venereal' is derived from the Latin *venereus*, pertaining to Venus, the goddess of love.

TURNER'S *A BOOKE OF THE NATURES AND PROPERTIES... OF THE BATHES*

In this little book of 17 pages devoted to balneotherapy, William Turner (1568) wrote of immersion in spa water as a form of treatment. He quoted 25 ancient and contemporary authorities who agreed with his opinion that certain illnesses may be cured or alleviated by bathing in a medicinal spring and named eleven 'Bathes' of high repute in England, Germany, Italy and

Switzerland. Among other disorders he noted that baths were good for 'The casting of children out, before the dewe tyme appoynted by nature; The strangling or falling of the mother (eclampsia/or epilepsy); The 'coldness' of the mother (uterine disease); The stopping of weomens fleures; and The isshue of a manis nature, or sede'.

GERARD'S *HERBALL*

John Gerard (1545–1612) was an Elizabethan physician who, like many of his contemporaries, traveled extensively in the major European countries before settling down in England. On his return he lived at Fetter Lane, London, where he cultivated a medicinal garden which contained over a thousand different herbs. Gerard wrote *The Herball or General Historie of Plantes* (1597) which became the most famous herbal of the era. His text was based on the 1554 *Herbal* of Rempert Dodoens (1517–1585). Gerard acknowledged Dodoens in his text and also referred to other authorities including Dioscorides, Galen, Matthiolus and Theophrastus. There are over 1800 illustrations in his *Herball* of which only 16 are originals by Gerard. One of these was the first published representation of the 'Virginian' potato. The potato shown was not, however, a native of Virginia but was imported from Quito in 1580. The first potatoes to reach Europe, around 1500, were of the sweet potato.

Gerard's *Herball* is a fascinating document which included references to contemporary plant folklore and sites of antiquarian interest. Gerard was an avid collector of local and exotic plants and he received herbs from around the known world from acquaintances, friends and ships' captains (he mentioned 122 persons by name). In 1633 Gerard's *Herball* was amended and enlarged by the apothecary Thomas Johnson, with a second edition published three years later. It was this altered text which became the standard work from then onwards. In 1927 Marcus Woodward published an edited version of the *Herball* which was re-issued in 1964 and is currently available as a paperback edition (Woodward, 1994).

Despite its size and complexity, Gerard's herbal offers little in the way of medications for women. This appears surprising at first glance as herbals of the era were awash with remedies to 'bring down the courses [periods]' and other 'cures' for women. The main difference between Gerard's book and contemporary texts is that Gerard's sections which deal with plant 'vertues' are very brief and contain relatively scant indications for treatments of any sort.

Gerard refers to the various parts of plants and notes that barrenwort (*Epimedium sagittatum*, or horny goatweed, an aphrodisiac) 'beareth his seed in very small cods'; that meadow-saffron (*Colchicum autumnale*, or naked lady, an anti-inflammatory agent) 'bringeth forth his long cods with seed'; and that in the Indian swallow-wort (*Chelidonium majus*, or greater celandine, a uterine stimulant) 'there come in places two cods'. Henry Bradley in his *A Middle-English Dictionary* (1891) defines 'cod' as a bag, husk or scrotum and Joseph Shipley in his *Dictionary of Early English* (1955) explained that a 'codpiece' was a bagged appendage in the front of the tight-fitting hose or breeches worn by men in the fifteenth to seventeenth centuries. The word was often used for the organs it did not conceal. Cupid was called 'the king of codpieces' in Shakespeare's *Loves Labor's Lost*.

William Turner's herbal contains an entry for the plant known as 'satyrion' (*Orchis* species) which he described as an aphrodisiac. The herb's Latin name was *satyrium*, but it was better known by its English synonym and described as 'whyte hairs coddes, or in more unmannerly speche, hares ballocks'. The dictionaries relate that 'ballok' was once a polite term and that 'ballok-wirt' (testicle root) was a common name for the orchid (*Orchis morio*; from the Greek *orchis*, testicle). Salep was a drug or nutritious drink obtained from orchid roots, used by witches in love philters. Salep was also sold as a beverage in London before coffee became available. Regarding the virtues of plants, Gerard quoted Ruellis who wrote that 'they commonly say in France, how hee needs neither Physition nor Surgeon, that had Bugle and Sanicle'. Bugle (*Ajuga reptans*) is an astringent while sanicle (*Sanicula europaea*) is an astringent which was much employed as a vulnerary (for the treatment of wounds, from the Latin *vulnus*, wound).

Gerard's materia medica for women

Betony (*Stachys officinalis*) for convulsions (non-specific)

Chequered daffodil (fritillary) to beautify the bosoms
Henbane (*Hyoscyamus niger*) aphrodisiac and for convulsions
Lettuce (*Lactuca sativa*) for heartburn (non-specific)
Mandrake (*Mandrogora officinalis*) for fertility
Shepherd's purse (*Capsella bursa pastoris*) for bleeding (non-specific)
Sow-bread (*Cyclamen* species) an aphrodisiac
Sweet william (*Armeria rubra latifolia*) to beautify the bosoms
Wine (*vinum*) an aphrodisiac, or for convulsions.

PARACELSUS: A CHANGE OF DIRECTION

Theophrastus Philippus Aureolus Bombastus von Hohenheim (1493–1541) was born at Maria Einsiedeln, a small town near Zurich in Switzerland, and followed his father into medicine. Said to be 'an erratic genius' who exercised a revolutionary influence on medicine and pharmacy, he assumed the name Paracelsus, so claiming higher rank than the ancient Roman physician Celsus, whose *De Medicina*, first printed in 1478, was popular at the time (Wootton, 1910). Educated at the University of Basel and later in the 'laboratory' of Abbot Trithemius at Würzburg, Paracelsus had great chemical skills and called his medicines 'catholicon's, 'elixirs' and 'panaceas', soon developing a huge reputation for his remedies. Paracelsus returned to become city physician at Basel in 1525 and professor of medicine and surgery at the local university. He began his course of lectures by burning the works of Avicenna and Galen, denouncing reliance on ancient authorities in medicine. Paracelsus readily made enemies, and three years later, he left Basel after a dispute with the legal profession. In spite of his tribulations, however, Paracelsus grew in stature and popularity.

Paracelsus replaced the Galenic humoral theory with a 'chemical' philosophy which held that disease was caused by localized natural (or chemical) abnormality and that it should be treated chemically. The 'chemicals' were substances transformed by mixing and separation accompanied by heat and included metallic compounds, many of which were new to the apothecary: Paracelsus was largely responsible for popularizing the use of mercury for the treatment of syphilis, introduced zinc, and made great use of antimony, arsenic, copper, iron and lead. He also prescribed essential oils of herbs (including hellebore, *Helleborus niger* or *Veratrum viride*, and aniseed, *Pimpinella anisum*), oil of eggs, oil of coral, and even oil of man's skull (as a treatment for epilepsy).

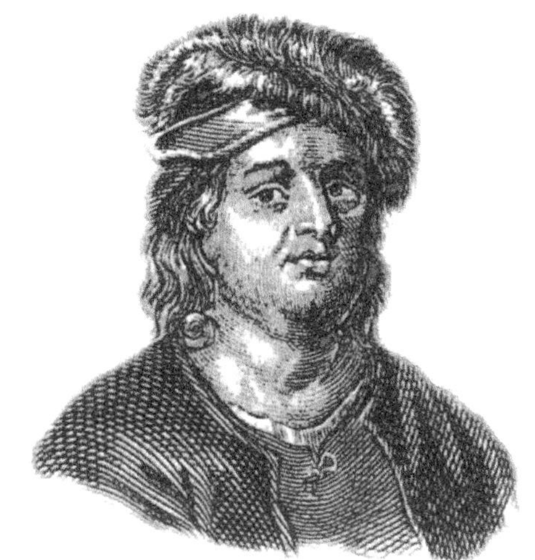

Figure 14 Paracelsus (1493–1541)

Paracelsus claimed to be able to obtain the 'magistery' (a term borrowed from Aristotle, meaning the essence) of a chemical or herb. He believed that substances were compounds of various elements, one of which (obtainable by chemical means) was the active principle. It was Paracelsus who coined the term 'laudanum' for opium and it is believed that he carried opium in the pommel of his sword, calling it the 'stone of immortality'.

Distillation techniques, evaporation, incineration, sublimation, metallurgical advances and the production of new compounds such as corrosive mercuric sublimate and calomel (mercurous chloride) were introduced by the Paracelsians. From that time onwards, the pharmacist, already a botanist and apothecary, also became a chemist. This new state of affairs gained a seal of approval when the College of Physicians included the new chemical remedies in their first *Pharmacopoeia Londinensis* of 1618, which they compiled in order to secure the compliance of local pharmacists (Cowen and Helfand, 1990). Similar recognition occurred throughout Europe and thus it was that Paracelsus, the great innovator, changed forever the art and practice of pharmacy. Although he was not particularly associated with obstetrics his innovations changed prescribing habits and inevitably had an impact on midwifery and gynecology.

Paracelsus died on 24th September 1541 and a monument was erected to his memory at Salzburg, with the inscription (here translated from Latin):

> Here lies Phillipus Theophrastus, The famous Doctor of Medicine, who by his wonderful art cured the worst wounds, leprosy, gout, dropsy, and other diseases deemed incurable and to his honor, shared his possessions with the poor.

A SELECTION OF MATERIA MEDICA FROM THE SIXTEENTH CENTURY

Acanthus

The acanthus (*Acanthus syriacus*) is named from the Greek *akanthos*: thorn or thistle, referring to the thorny dentate leaves of the plant, and *anthos* flowers. The acanthus is common in Mediterranean countries and is referred to in the Bible (Smit, 1990). The plant was also mentioned in Greek and Roman writings and the acanthus leaf (*A. spinosus*) was a commonly-used motif in architecture and design. Calimacus, the Greek architect of the fifth century BC, created the decorative foliage pattern for the capitols of Corinthian columns and his design, based on the acanthus leaf, was popular until the fall of the Roman Empire. The motif resurfaced during the Renaissance and appears as a decoration in some editions of Rösslin's *Der Schwangern Frauen und Hebammen Rosengarten*. *Acanthus mollis* is also known as brank ursine or bear's breeches and is one of the plants mentioned by Rösslin in his text of 1513. The herb contains mucilage and tannins which are useful in the treatment of inflamed tissues. Extract of the plant is also thought to be diuretic (Chevallier, 1996).

Aloe

Aloe (*Aloe vera*, or *Aloe barbadensis*) was mainly found in the subtropical zones of the Old and New Worlds. Although the use of aloes can be traced to Ancient Egypt and fourth century BC Greece, the plant was not available in Europe and China until after the tenth century AD. As time went by, aloe, originally only available from East Africa and Arabia, was imported from Zanzibar; from Barbados and the Dutch island of Curacao (c. 1650); from the Cape in Southern Africa (c. 1780) and from the island of Socotra (*Aloe perryi* Baker or cocotrine aloe). The thick sap from the leaves was the constituent most often employed and was simply referred to as 'aloe'. There was also an aloe wood (*Aquilaria agalocha*), also known as *lignum aloes* or 'paradise wood'. Noted for its aromatic scent, it was used in ancient times as a sacred incense.

The Sumerians and Egyptians used both aloe and aloe wood in ointments which were stored in shells and applied to treat the eye disease, trachoma. Aloe was used as an embalming agent and the body of Jesus was wrapped in aloe and myrrh 'as the manner of the Jews is to bury' (John, 19: 39–40). The Greeks and Romans introduced the use of aloe for women's disorders and it was helpful as an oral preparation for the treatment of the pica of pregnancy. Aloes were applied as a plaster to treat abnormal uterine bleeding and in later times a form of aloe tea was used as a fertility agent. Dorland's 1932 medical dictionary records that aloe is a strong purgative which may also be prescribed for amenorrhea. Extract of the plant is anti-inflammatory, controls fungal infections and stimulates the uterus (Bown, 1995). *Aloe vera* is now mainly used as a gel in cosmetics and toiletries for reputed moisturizing and anti-aging actions.

Lily

The name 'lily' is derived from the Latin *lilium*, similar to the Greek name for the plant, *lerion*. The lily (*Lilium candidum*) was the emblem of the goddess Juno and it is related in myth that the first lilies sprang from her breast milk. The Roman Christians adopted the story but in their version the lily grew from the milk of the Virgin Mary. Juno's northern counterpart was Eostre whose name gave us Easter and thus the Easter lily. Another story related that the first lily sprang from the tears shed by Eve as she was exiled from the Garden of Eden. The white or madonna lily has become closely associated with the Christian religion and represents the purity of the Virgin Mary while symbolizing the feminine principle. The 'lilies of the field' of the Bible may have been the martagon lily (*L. chalcedonicum*) which has brilliant scarlet flowers and grows in abundance on the plains of Galilee – and 'Solomon in all his royalty was not arrayed like one of these' (Matthew 6: 28–29).

Bernard de Gordon, professor at the famous French medical school of Montpellier, followed the fashion among medieval medical men and called his renowned book after a flower: Bernard's manuscript, the *Lilium Medicinae* of 1303, was one of the most highly-regarded medical treatises of the era and was eventually published at Naples in 1480. The lily has been part of the materia medica of women since antiquity, used in the treatment of menstrual and uterovaginal disorders. Over the centuries oil of lily (and oil of almonds) was an important ingredient of the pharmacopoeia for labor, used to lubricate the mother's vagina and the fingers of the probing midwives, and as an emollient to soothe the tissues of the birth canal. The lily-of-the-valley (*Convallaria majus*) contains cardiac glycosides similar to digoxin (Reynolds, 1996).

Mothers' milk

The word 'milk' derives from the Old English (Mercian) *milc* and the German *milch*. The goddess of milk was Lat, the pre-Roman deity also known as Latona, Leto or Leda and it is said that the Isle of Malta was sacred to her memory, the earlier form of its name being 'Ma Lata' (Walker, 1988). One myth recounts that the Greek god Zeus placed his mortal son at the breast of Hera so that the infant could gain immortality by suckling the breast of the queen of the goddesses. Hercules sucked so vigorously that he woke the sleeping Hera who drew her breast away with such force that milk spurted into the heavens to create the Milky Way. Hercules, however, had drunk Hera's milk and became an immortal god.

The 'river of stars' which forms the Milky Way was understood by the ancients to be a river of life-giving goddess milk. Egyptians believed that the milk came from the udder of the heavenly cow, Hathor, or Isis in her bovine form. The word 'galaxy' itself came from the Greek *gala*, which means 'milk'. The Milky Way was also known as the 'river of the divine lady' and also 'mother of the sky', the 'moonway' or the 'track of the white cow'. In one well-known European nursery rhyme, the white cow jumped over the moon, leaving a trail of her 'star-milk' across the sky.

In mythology, breasts have often been associated with mountains. In Sumerian myth, the 'mother mountain', Ninhursag, gave birth to the world. In ancient Greece the first 'owner' of Mount Olympus was the divine mother Gaea Olympia and she was known as 'the deep-breasted goddess'. The mountain was later taken over by her grandson Zeus. In India one of the oldest deities was Chomo-Lung-Ma or 'mother of the universe' and her mountain shrine is now known by its European name, Mount Everest. Another Himalayan peak, Annapurna, translates as 'great breast full of nourishment'. In County Kerry, in southern Ireland, there are twin mountain peaks known as the 'Paps of Anu', in memory of Anu or Aine, one of Ireland's ancient goddess queens.

In Ancient Egypt mothers 'baptized' their newborn with breast milk as they bestowed on the infants their *ren* (soul–name or milk-name) which gave us the word 'rennet', the milk-curdling enzyme. The Lesser Berlin and the Ebers Papyri (c. sixteenth century BC) contain spells, potions and incantations for increasing the milk supply and for protecting the mother's milk. A high value was placed on human milk particularly that of a woman who had borne a male child. The milk was included in many remedies, given either orally or by application, for conditions as diverse as cataract and eczema. 'Wet nursing' was well known at the time and in ancient Mesopotamia the code of laws of Hammurabi, King of Babylon (circa 1728–1686 BC), included a legal tract to safeguard against nurses illegally substituting babies for those who had died at the breast. In ancient Nineveh blindness was treated by application of a mixture of milk and saliva taken from the 'holy harlots' of the temples.

In the fifth century BC Hippocrates of Cos wrote that as soon as the embryo started to move the mother's milk made its appearance (although it did not flow until after the birth). He theorized on milk formation and lactation and was aware that menstruation would cease in the woman who was lactating but who was neither pregnant nor had given birth. To restrain menstruation he advocated the application of cupping glasses to the nipples. He also wrote of a special race of Scythian women warriors, known as the Sauronatae: the women had no right breast as their mothers had applied heated irons to the right side of the anterior chest wall of all female children. This prevented breast growth and allowed all the strength and tissue to grow into the right arm and shoulder. The Sauronatae women shot arrows and hurled javelins from horseback, but could only fight as long as they remained virgins.

Soranus of Ephesus in the second century AD wrote on the selection of wet-nurses; the testing of breast milk; methods to increase milk supply; and on how to treat milk which had become 'spoiled'. His writings were copied by all the great writers of the later Greco-Roman, Byzantine and Arabian periods. During the Middle Ages breast milk carried mystical connotations and, after the blood of Christ, the Virgin Mary's milk was considered the most holy and miraculous of fluids. Vials of the Virgin's milk were placed as relics in churches and were reputed to cure a wide assortment of ailments, including blindness and cancer. The relics were also used to protect pregnant women and nursing mothers. The theme of the nursing madonna, or *Maria lactans* became popular in art from the early fourteenth century and one famous work of art depicts 'The Lactation of St Bernard' in which he is seen to receive a stream of milk directly from the breast of the Virgin Mary (Yalom, 1997). The *Virgo lactans* image promoted breastfeeding as a sacred occupation.

Mother's milk was thought to have magical and potent medicinal properties and was used as a single agent or in various recipes for general medical use. Walter Cary (1560) wrote of mixing milk with onion, leek, and poppy to treat sore ears, lung disease and to promote sleep, respectively. A good supply of breast milk was essential and over the centuries various plants were administered to promote lactation. These included the *Asclepias* species of plant known as milkweed, and also *Asclepias syriaca* or milkwort.

Mother's milk was also part of the materia medica for women from ancient times until the eighteenth century and was commonly used to restrain excess menstruation, to reduce post delivery lochial loss and for inflammation of the uterus. Mixed with oil, milk was also used as an oxytocic. William Turner (1568) advised leek with milk for excess postnatal loss, and poppy with milk for the treatment of menorrhagia. He also wrote that if the poppy was mixed '[With] Weomans Milck it swageth the payn of the gout' and that '[If] it be put into the fundament after the manner of a suppositori it bringeth slepe'. Turner also indicated that if The Iuice of the Leke Take with Weomes Milke, [it] Stoppeth the isshue that commeth, when a woman hath had hyr byrth before hyr tyme'.

In modern times a product known as 'virgin's milk' was, in fact, rosewater lotion rendered milky by the addition of tincture of benzoin. Fresh milk from the cow (*Bos* sp.) was used to prepare *mistura scammonii* at the close of the nineteenth century and the mixture was prescribed as a cathartic to treat severe edema and cerebral congestion (Squire, 1890 p. 257). Currently, mothers are told that breastfeeding protects their infants against infections because of the antibodies contained in this marvelous *yin*, the 'milk of human kindness'.

Rose

The rose (from the Latin *rosa*) that inspired his own name of Eucharius Rösslin, and his son's pet name 'Rhodion', but also the title of Rösslin's book, *Der Schwangern Frauen und Hebammen Rosengarten*, with Soranus' *Gynecology*, one of the most famous book in obstetric history. The leaves, oil, sugar and water of red roses all found a place in the materia medica of *The Byrth of Mankynde*. Over a century later, Johan von Hoorn (1662–1724), a celebrated obstetrician, wrote the first Swedish handbook for midwives (its short title was *Jorde-Gumman*) which was also the first complete medical textbook published in Sweden (1697). On the title page there is an illustration of the Jericho rose, which was thought to facilitate childbirth.

The rose of Jericho (*Anastatica hierochuntica*), the rose of Sharon (possibly *Hyacinthus orientalis* or *Narcissus tazetta*), 'the rose that grows on the watercourse' (Ecclesasticus, 39: 13) and the rock rose (*Cistus incanus*) are all mentioned in the Bible. The rock rose secreted a sticky resin which adhered to the beards of

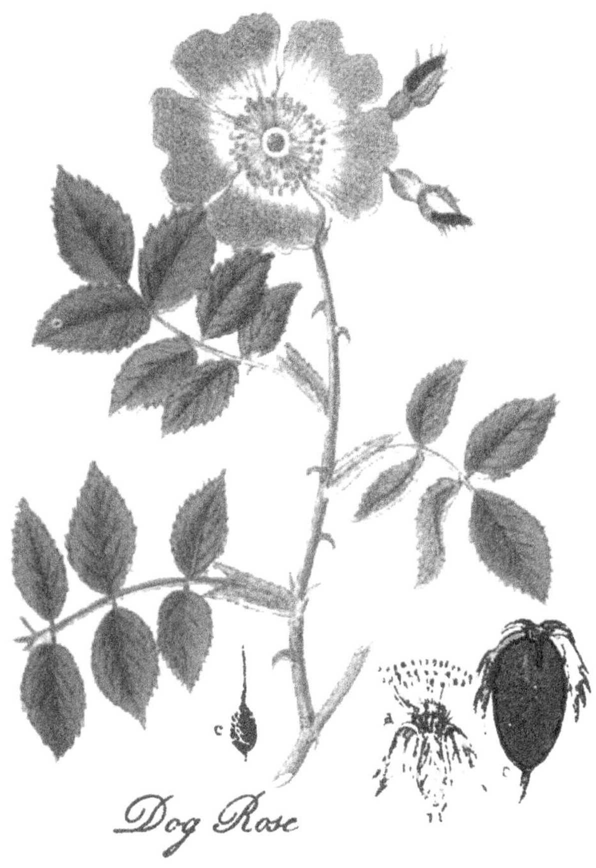

Figure 15 Rose (*Rosa* sp.)

grazing goats. Goatherds would remove the resin, knead it into balls and sell the product as labdanum or ladanum, known also as 'Arabic ladan'. Labdanum was used in the preparation of various medicines and is still used in perfumes. The roses of the Bible differ from roses of post-Biblical times which were usually *Rosa gallica* or *Rosa canina*.

The rose is of ancient origin and may initially have come from Iran. The Egyptians held it sacred and roses have been discovered in Egyptian tombs. The Greeks and Romans continued the tradition and the flower was popular at both weddings and funerals, and as a cure for hangovers. In Persia it was believed that every time a rose was plucked the nightingale sang mournfully for fear that the flower was hurt. Muslims believed that the rose was created from the tears or sweat of Mohammed. Roses of course have a long romantic tradition and Cleopatra seduced Anthony in a room that was knee-deep in rose petals. In Christian tradition, both red and white roses are considered sacred to the Virgin Mary: the white signifies purity; the red represents womanhood and also the blood of Christ. The rose symbolizes the love of Christ in its flower, and His sufferings, in its thorns. The rose window, whose intricate design was based on the flower, was first incorporated into Christian church architecture in the thirteenth century.

The Greek poet Sappho (born c. 650 BC) called the rose the 'the queen of flowers', and Pliny wrote of 32 remedies. Soranus of Ephesus used rose to treat venereal disease, to dry up breast milk and for a large number of female ailments. The *Rosa Anglica* (1314) was a popular book of medicine and pharmacy in England in the fourteenth century. It was written by John of Gaddesden, who claimed that his book was made up of five parts as the rose has five sepals, and that, just as the rose surpassed all other flowers, the *Rosa Anglica* was superior to all other books (Wootton, 1910). Gilbertus Anglicus, an Englishman who studied at Montpellier, published a medical book entitled *Compendium Medicinae* or the *Rosa Anglicana* at Lyon in 1510.

The red (and white rose) was adopted by alchemists as a symbol of the *vas spirituale*, the sacred womb from which the *filius philosophorum* (son of the philosophers) would be born. The apothecaries' rose (*Rosa gallica*) was prescribed as an essential oil (attar) or as dried petals to heal the heart and create a feeling of happiness. Nicholas Culpeper valued the apothecaries' rose for treatment of disorders of the head and alimentary tract. Walter Cary (1560) wrote that the red rose is cold in the first degree and dry in the second degree, and advised its use for 'melancolye' and also for 'bloody fluxe of the wombe [intestine]'. He described how to make sugar and syrup of roses and noted that even 'dry roses put to the nose to smell do comfort the brayne' (Cary, 1560). *Squire's Companion to the British Pharmacopoeia* (1908) devoted six pages to preparations of *Rosa gallica* and *Rosa damascena* noting that rose extract was mildly astringent with a pleasant odor and an agreeable vehicle for medicines. *Rosa centiflora* and other species were also used.

The rose contains carotenoids, fruit acids, rutin, tannins, vitamin C and a large number of other constituents. Medicinally, it is used as rose-hip syrup for its vitamin content. Rose extract acts as a diuretic, and is used in aromatherapy as a mildly sedative antidepressant. *Martindale the Extra Pharmacopoeia* includes red rose petal as an astringent and also lists rose oil, rosewater and rosewater ointment (Reynolds, 1996).

Saffron

Saffron is a species of crocus, in particular *Crocus sativus*, which flowers with blue blooms in the autumn. Its dried stigmas are the source of an orange-yellow substance used as a dye (long-used to color monks' robes) and as a flavoring in food. Up to 250,000 stigmas are required to produce a kilogram of dried saffron and, because of the labor-intensive harvesting techniques, saffron is an extremely expensive product. Five varieties of *Crocus sativus* are known in the wild state. In Ancient Egypt saffron was known as 'the blood of Thoth'. The Greeks and Romans called saffron ***krokos*** and ***karkom***, respectively, and saffron features in the Songs of Solomon 4: 13–14. The Arabs, who introduced the saffron crocus into Spain as an article of commerce, bequeathed to us its modern name, from *za'fan* meaning yellow.

Dioscorides mentioned saffron only as a perfume or a religious incense, but Soranus of Ephesus described its use for vaginal discharge and for drying up the milk supply (Temkin, 1956). Although William Turner (1568) advocated it as an aphrodisiac and an anticonvulsant for eclampsia, saffron was most often used for menstrual disorders. It was a constituent of ***emplastrum oxycroceum***, which also contained colophony, gum ammoniacum, mastic and vinegar. Saffron, sometimes sold as a cake known as 'saffron placenta', was included in all the major national pharmacopoeias until this century when it was demoted to the status of a coloring and flavoring agent.

The dried stigmas and the tops of the styles of *Crocus sativus* contain volatile oils including safranal which gives it its warm spicy odor and the glycosides, crocines (responsible for saffron's color), crocetins, picrocine, vitamins, fixed oils and carotenoids. Saffron is still used for menstrual problems in traditional Chinese medicine. The 1996 *Martindale, The Extra Pharmacopoeia* lists proprietary agents in which saffron is a constituent (Reynolds, 1996).

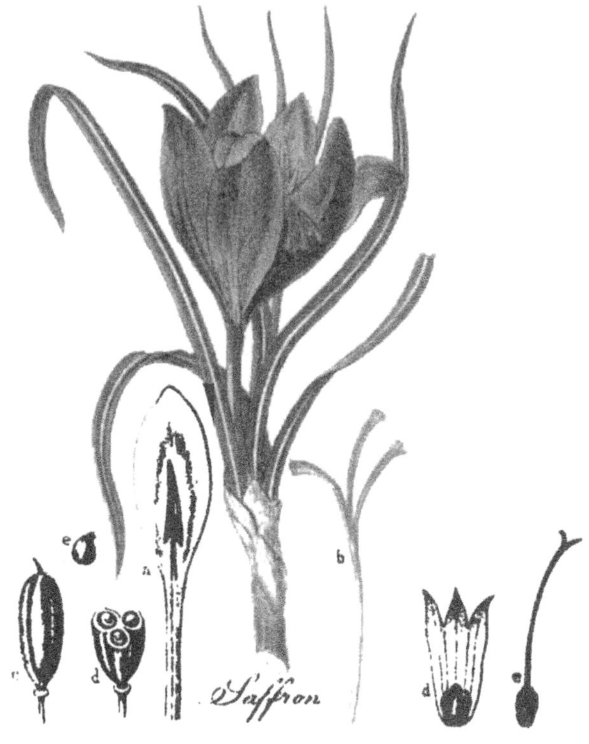

Figure 16 Saffron (*Crocus sativa*)

THE BYRTH OF MANKYNDE MATERIA MEDICA

Uses

Labor

Analgesia amber, *Aristolochia longa*, *Aristolochia rotunda*, bull's gall, canell, *Cassia lignea*, castoreum, cinnamon, diacinamomum, diagalanga, ducks grease, galbanum, hellebore, honey, lupins, madder, musk, myrrh, opopanax, opium, pepper, saffron, savin, storax, white bdellium, wine, yellow brimstone.

To induce/oxytocic ammoniacum, *Aristolochia rotuda*, asafetida, asarum, barley meal, bear's foot, benzoin, bothor martis, bran, *Cassia lignea*, castoreum, cicer, cicercula broth, cinnamon, colloquintida, colocinthis, conduit water, cyclaminus root, diachilon, dricroceu, fenugreek, galbanum, hollyhock, juniper, madder, maidenhair, mallow, malum terre root, melliot, myrrh, pennyroyal, petroleum, pyrethium, oil of blue flower de luce, oil of white lilies, rhubarb, rose, rue, savin, seraphinum, silver mountain, southernwood, wild gourd, wild nep, water, wine.

Puerperium

Postpartum bleeding acorn cups (*capsella*), bursa pastoris, bramble, lichen, myrtine oil, vine tops.

To cleanse after labor barbarris, baum, borage, bugloss, cloves, egg white, juice of berries, mace, marigold, muscadell, nightshade, oatmeal, oil of roses, plantain, purslane, rosemary, woman's milk.

Newborn navel

Bole armeniac powder, calf hoof (ashes of), cumin, egg white, myrrh, red lead powder, *sanguis draconis*, sarcocolla, snail shells (ashes of), white frankincense.

To increase mothers' milk

Aloe, bean meal, beet, bread, cardamom, cheese, crystal, hen broth, ladanum, lettuce, peas, oil of violets, sheep breast, sheep milk.

Menstruation

To induce aniseed, chervil, cinnamon, fennel seeds, juniper berries, motherwort, parsley, rue, savin, spikenard.

For excess acorns, bole ammoniac, cinkerfoil, daisies, frankincense, hematite, iron, mulberry, *sanguis draconis*, turpentine.

Selected remedies

The following list excludes the remedies used as beauty aids and treatments offered for children's disorders in Raynold's text.

Acorn cups, almond oil, aloe, alum, amber, aniseed, antimony, *Aristolochia*, asafetida, ass hoof

Basil, baum, bayberry, bean meal, benzoin, black hellebore, bole ammoniac, borage, branc ursine, brimstone, bursa pastoris

Cassia, castoreum, chervil, cicer, cinnamon, comfrey, coral (red), cumin, cyclaminus root, cypress nuts

Daisies, date stones, diachilon, diacinamomum, diagalanga, diamargariton, diatessaron, dill, dittany, duck grease

Eggs, eleborus, *electuarium* and wine, *electuarium athanasie*, eyes of salt fish

Fat, fennel seeds, fenugreek, fig, flinstones (burnt), fomentations, frankincense (white)

Galbanum, galingale, *Gallia muscata*, garlic, germander, goat's horn, goat's milk, goose grease, gourd, gum ammoniac

Hart's horn (burnt), hawk's dung, hellebore, hematites, hen's flesh, hollyhock, honey, horehound, horse hoof

Incense, iron, ivory (burnt)

Juniper berries

Kid

Lard, ladanum, laurel, leek, lettuce, lichen, lilies (white), lime, linseed, lupins

Maidenhair, mallow, marigold, medlars, melliot, mercury, mespilles, motherwort, musk, myrrh, myrtine oil

Nardine oil, nightshade leaves, nutmeg

Oatmeal, oil of blue flowers de luce, oil of violets, olive oil, onions, opium, opopanax, organine, ox gall, ox meat

Parsley, pears, peas, pennyroyal, pepper, plantain, policaria, pomegranate, purslane juice, pyrethium.

Quince

Red lead, rose, rhubarb, rice, rosemary, rue

Saffron, *sanguis draconis*, savin, sesame, silver mountain, southernwood, spikenard, squill, storax

Tamarind, tar, *terra sigillata*, thistle, thyme, tormentil, treacle, trifera magna, turpentine

Valerian, vergens, vine tops, vinegar, violets (oil of)

Water, in which red-hot steel was quenched, wax, wild nep, woman's hair (burnt), woman's milk, wool, wormwood

Zedoria

Raynold prescribed his remedies using the following measures' drachm, grain, 'handfull', ounce, quart, scruple, and 'spoonfull'.

References

Ballantyne, J. W. (1906). The Byrth of Mankynde, Its Author and Editions. *J. Obstet. Gynaecol. Br. Emp.*, 10(4), 297–325

Ballantyne, J. W. (1907). The Byrth of Mankynde. Its Contents. *J. Obstet. Gynaecol. Br. Emp.*, 12(3), 175–93

Bown, D. (1995). *The Royal Horticultural Society Encyclpaedia of Herbs and Their Uses*, p. 235. (London: Dorling Kindersley)

Bradley, H. (1891). *A Middle-English Dictionary*, pp. 42, 127. (Oxford: Clarendon Press)

Cary, W. (c. 1560). *A Boke of the Propertyes of Herbs*. (London: John Kynge for John Waley)

Chevallier, A. (1996). *The Encyclopedia of Medicinal Plants*, p. 157. (London: Dorling Kindersley)

Cowen, D. L. and Helfand, W. H. (1990). *Pharmacy. An Illustrated History*, pp. 59–62. (New York: Harry N. Abrams Inc.)

Crummer, LeRoy (1926). The Copper Plates in Raynalde and Geminus. *Proc. R. Soc. Med., Sect. Hist. Med.*, October, 53–6

Dodoens, R. (1554). *Kruydeboeck Ghedruckt*. (Antwerpen; Jan van der Lov)

Dorland, W. A. N. (1932). *The American Illustrated Medical Dictionary*, pp. 66–7. (Philadelphia: W. B. Saunders Co.)

Findley, P. (1939). *Priests of Lucina. The Story of Obstetrics*, pp. 78–98. (Austin: Little, Brown & Co.)

Fuchs, L. (1542). *De Historia Stirpium*. (Basileae, in officina Isingriniana)

Geminus, T. (1545). *Compendiosa Totius Anatomie delineatio, aera exarata*. (London: John Herford)

Gerard, J. (1597). *The Herball or Generall Historie of Plantes*. (London: E. Bollifant for B. and J. Norton)

Gordon, C. A. (1931). The Byrth of Mankynde. The 1540 edition. *Am. J. Surg.*, 13(1), 118–28

Hagelin, O. (1989) *The Byrth of Mankynde otherwise named The Womans Book*, pp. 18–23. (Stockholm: Svenska Lakaresallskapet)

Hellman, A. M. (1952). *A Collection of Early Obstetrical Books*, pp. 1–14. (New Haven, CT: Printed Privately)

Ingerslev, E. (1909). Rösslin's *Rosengarten*: Its relation to the past (The Muscio Manuscripts and Soranus), particularly with regard to Podalic Version. *J. Obstet. Gynaecol. Br. Emp.*, 25(1), 1–25

Ingerslev, E. (1909). Rösslin's *Rosengarten*: Its relation to the past (The Muscio Manuscripts and Soranus), particularly with regard to Podalic Version. *J. Obstet. Gynaecol. Br. Emp.*, 25(2), 6–92

Le Fanu, W. R. (1976). *Notable Medical Books, from the Lilly Library, Indiana University*, p. 35. (Indianapolis, Indiana: Eli Lilly & Co.)

Power, Sir D'Arcy (1927). The Birth of Mankynde or The Woman's Book a Bibliographical Study. *The Library*. 4th series, 8(1), 1–57

Raynold, T. (1545). *The Byrth of Mankynde*. (London: Tho. Ray)

Reynolds, J. E. F. (1996). *Martindale, The Extra Pharmacopoeia*, pp. 1002, 1749, 1694.2. (London: Royal Pharmaceutical Society)

Rohde, E. S. (1922). *The Old English Herbals*. (Longmans Green & Co.). Reprinted 1971, pp. 75–97. (New York: Dover Publication)

Rösslin, E. (1513). *Der Schwangern Frauen und Hebammen Rosengarten*. (Strasburg: M. Flkach Jr.)

Rösslin, E. Jr. (Rhodionis) (1532). *De Partu Hominis*. (Frankfurt: Christian Egenolph)

Rueff, J. (1554). *De Conceptu et Generatione Hominis*. (Tiguri: Christophorus Froschiuer)

Rueff, J. (1580). *Trostbuchle*. (Frankfort am Main; Sigmund Feyerabendt Buchhandler

Rueff, J. (1637). *The Expert Midwife or An Excellent and most necessary Treatise of the Generation on birth of Man*. (London: E. Griffin)

Shipley, J. (1955). *Dictionary of Early English*, p. 158. (New York: Philosophical Library Inc.)

Smit, D. (1990). *Plants of the Bible*, p. 29. (Oxford: Lion Books)

Squire, P. W. (1890). *Companion to the Latest Edition of the British Pharmacopoeia*, 15th ed., p. 257. (London: J. and A. Churchill)

Squire, P. W. (1908). *Squire's Companion to the British Pharmacopoeia*, 18th ed., pp. 257, 1021–6. (London: J. and A. Churchill)

Temkin, O. (1956). *Soranus' Gynecology*, p. 239. (Baltimore: The Johns Hopkins Press)

Turner, W. (1568). *A Booke of the Natures and Properties, as well of the Bathes in England as of other Bathes in Germanye and Atalye*. (Collen: Arnold Birkman)

Turner, W. (1568). *The First and The Seconde Parte of William Turner's Herbal*. (Collen: Arnold Birckman)

Turner, W. (1568). *The Third Parte of William Turner's Herbal*. (Collen: Arnold Birckman)

Vesalius, A. (1543). *De Humani Corporis Fabrica Libri Septem*. (Basileae: ex officina Ionnis Oporini)

von Bayerland, O. (1477). *Artzneibuch*. (Augsburg: G. Zainer)

von Bayerland, O. (c. 1495–1500). *Buechlein Der Schwangeren Frauen* (Augsburg) Facsimile (ed.) by Gustav Klein (1910). (Munich: C. Kuhn)

von Hoorn, J. (1697). *Den Swenska Wal-ofwade Jorde Gumman*. (Stockholm: Nathanael Goldenau)

Walker, B. G. (1988). *The Woman's Dictionary of Symbols and Sacred Objects*, p. 489. (New York: Castle Books)

Woodward, M. (ed.) (1927). *Gerard's Herball*. The essence thereof distilled by Marcus Woodward from the edition of Thomas Johnson (1636), pp. 143–4. (London: Spring Books)

Woodward, M. (ed.) (1994). *Gerard's Herbal. The History of Plants*. (London: Studio Editions)

Wootton, A. C. (1910). *Chronicles of Pharmacy*, Vol. 1, pp. 230–51. (London: Macmillan and Co.)

Yalom, M. (1997). *A History of the Breast*, p. 46. (New York: Alfred A. Knopf)

The seventeenth century 14

INTRODUCTION

In seventeenth century Europe there was a genuine attempt to standardize the well-known local medications and those that were imported from the Levant. As a result, the first edition of the *Pharmacopoeia Londinensis* was published in 1618. Later in the century the *Dispensatory Brandenburgicum* (1698) and the *Pharmacopoeia Edinburgensis* (1699) were collated and printed (in Latin) for the use of physicians and apothecaries (Urdang, 1951). The apothecaries followed the example of the physicians and surgeons and formed learned societies that carried the royal seal of approval of the various European monarchs.

As far as obstetrics and gynecology and the materia medica for women were concerned, the seventeenth century, was merely a continuation of the Greco-Roman and Arab eras. However, despite the fact that little real change had occurred in maternity care in almost two millennia, some of the ancient obstetric theories began to be questioned by the leading European accoucheurs in the late 1600s. It was in this century that obstetric forceps were developed by the Chamberlen family although the 'secret instrument' did not come into general use until the eighteenth century. The era of 'man-midwifery' came into being towards the close of the 1600s and was a major source of public concern and outrage for the next 100 years (Wilson, 1995).

This chapter explores the works of three authors of the era, the first (chronologically) being Nicholas Culpeper of England. He translated many ancient and contemporary medical texts from the Latin into the 'vulgar' English tongue, incurring the wrath of the medical establishment but the love and admiration of the 'common people'. His achievements, in such a short lifespan, were truly monumental and now, over three centuries later, various combinations of his translations remain in print as a deserved memorial to this oft-forgotten man of medical history.

The second author, James Wolveridge, wrote the *Speculum Matricis*, a book for midwives that is considered to be among the rarest of obstetric and gynecological texts. The book was plagiarized at a later date, becoming the anonymous *English Midwife, Enlarged* (1682). Wolveridge, a graduate of Trinity College, Dublin, wrote his book 'for the worthy matrons' of Ireland and England and desired that pregnant women and their midwives would follow his advice closely throughout pregnancy and during confinement.

The text *Traite des Maladies des Femmes Grosses, et de Celles qui sont nouvellement Accouchees* was written by François Mauriceau, of Paris in 1668 and his book was said to have established the 'science' of obstetrics. The text was translated into English in 1683 by Hugh Chamberlen (of the Chamberlen forceps family) under the title *The Diseases of Women with Child, And in Child-bed.*

CULPEPER'S *DIRECTORY FOR MIDWIVES*

Nicholas Culpeper's *Directory for Midwives* (1651) comprised 217 pages with an extra 25 leaves to the contents, errata non corrigenda, errata corrigenda and 'An Interpretation of certain crabbed Names which you shall meet with unexplained in this Treatise'. The book was so popular that a second edition followed in 1652. Culpeper, 'Gent. Student in Physick and Astrologie' corrected and enlarged the text prior to his death in 1654. The amended version was printed by John Streeter and sold by George Sawbridge in 1671. The larger format edition of 1684 contains a preface of six pages, 161 pages of text, 14 pages devoted to contents and other matters as noted above, and a three page testimony written by Alice Culpeper. The amended version quoted in this text was printed for H. Sawbridge (1684). The book continued to be published until 1777 and was reprinted 17 times.

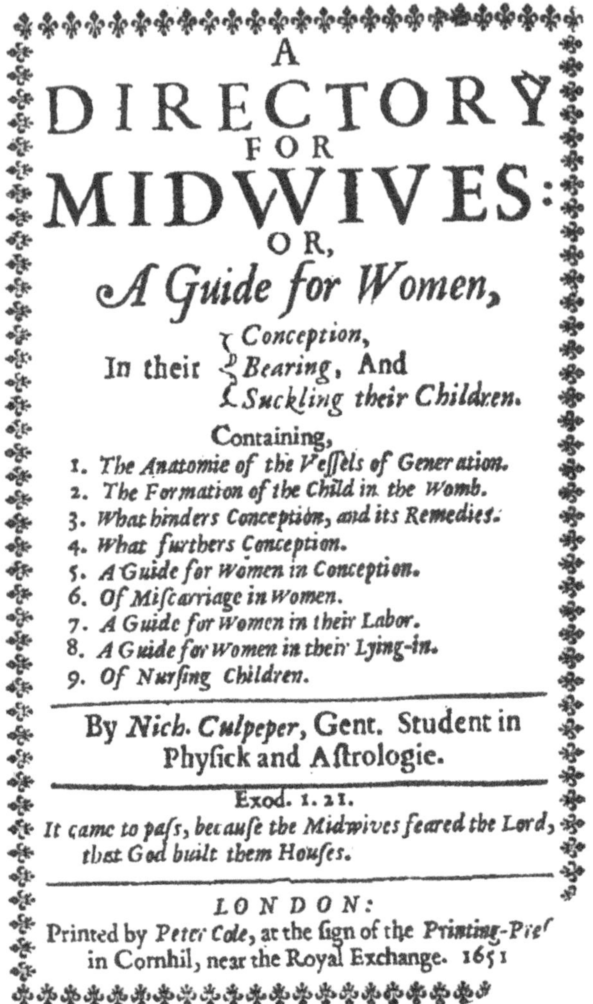

A

DIRECTORY

FOR

MIDWIVES:

OR,

A Guide for Women,

In their { *Conception,* *Bearing,* And *Suckling their Children.*

Containing,

1. *The Anatomie of the Veſſels of Generation.*
2. *The Formation of the Child in the Womb.*
3. *What hinders Conception, and its Remedies.*
4. *What furthers Conception.*
5. *A Guide for Women in Conception.*
6. *Of Miſcarriage in Women.*
7. *A Guide for Women in their Labor.*
8. *A Guide for Women in their Lying-in.*
9. *Of Nurſing Children.*

By *Nich. Culpeper*, Gent. Student in Phyſick and Aſtrologie.

Exod. 1. 21.

It came to paſs, becauſe the Midwives feared the Lord, that God built them Houſes.

LONDON:

Printed by *Peter Cole*, at the ſign of the *Printing-Preſs* in Cornhil, near the Royal Exchange. 1651

Figure 1 Frontispiece from Culpeper's *Directory for Midwives*

Culpeper's *Directory for Midwives* of 1651 was based on his own translations of the obstetric works of ancient and more recent authors, and he wrote: 'Such as would be skillful Physitians, let them read those Books of mine, viz. Platerus, Sennertus, Riverius, Riolanus, Bartholinus, Johnston, Veslingus, Rulandus, Fernalius, Sanctor, Cole etc.'. Culpeper added some personal observations on astrology, numerology and herbal lore as they related to women's disorders. He argued (often correctly) against many long-held obstetric theories, and he wrote from his own experience as a husband and father. Culpeper's *Directory for Midwives* was written in order to educate midwives so that they could function effectively without medical intervention. He also wished to highlight the many low-cost medicinal herbs available in England, as distinct from the expensive imported herbs and spices prescribed by physicians and remarked: *Praesentem narrat quaelibet herba Deum*, 'Every grass shows God is present with it'.

Culpeper opposed the involvement of men-midwives in obstetrics and peppered his text with jibes at his arch-enemies, the wealthy physicians, whose services the poor could not afford. He referred the reader to his translations of *Galen's Art of Physick* (1654) and to his own translations of the *London Pharmacopoeia* (1650, 1653, 1654) and wrote in positive terms of 'Doctors Experience and Reason' while denouncing, 'Doctor Conceit', 'Doctor Dunce', 'Doctor Ignorance' and 'Doctor Death'. 'Why', wrote Culpeper, 'do I talk to a learned Colledge of Physitians … they shall raise their Fees from ten shillings to twenty.' Culpeper's anatomical writings were relatively accurate for his time, probably because he dissected animals (he described experimentation with uterine vessels) and he was present during the postmortem examination of a pregnant woman. Apart from herbal remedies he offered little help for the woman in labor as he accepted that midwives were already 'well versed' in that area.

The *Directory for Midwives* contains nine books that are subdivided into sections and chapters.

Book 1 'Of the Vessels dedicated to Generation'

'Above all things, I hold it most fitting, that Women (especially Midwives) should be well skil'd in the exact knowledge of the anatomy of these Parts.'

'The Genitals of Men'

Culpeper detailed the male organs of generation and apologized for any offense caused to the 'good women' who would read his text. He wrote that the male seed was 'concocted by the Stones … called in Latine, Testes'. The seeds passed to a 'small body like a silk-worm, which is called Epididymis' and thence by 'Vasa Deferentia' to the 'Glandulae Prostatae' and then along the 'Conduit of the Yard'. Culpeper wrote: '[the] Latins have invented many names for the Yard,

I suppose done by venerious people (which Rome it seems was full of them, since which time vices have encreased there faster than vertues)'. He went on to detail the anatomy of the 'yard', with its outward skin and those 'parts of the Yard particular to itself ... Two Nervous Bodies, The Septum, The Urethra, The Glans, The Four Muscles and The Vessels'.

'Of the Genitals in Women'

'Having served my own Sex', wrote Culpeper, 'I shall see now if I can please the Women ... who have no more cause than Men (that I know of) to be ashamed of what they have'. Culpeper described '[the] Privy passage, the Lips, the Nymphae, the Clytoris, the Womb, the Stones and the Spermatic Vessels'. He agonized about the hymen: 'I confess much controversy hath been amongst Anatomists concerning this, some holding there is no such thing at all, others that it is, but is very rare, the truth is, most virgins have it, some hold all, I must suspend my own judgment till more yeers bring me more experience ... The Caruncula or fleshy Knobs, together with this, resemble the form of a Rose half blown; and therefore anciently called a Flower, and thence came the word [to deflower a virgin]'.

Culpeper was of the view that '[the vagina] in women of reasonable stature, it is eight Inches in length'. The uterus contained a 'Magnetick Vertue' that '[draws] the Seed to it, as the Loadstone draws Iron, or the fire the light of the Candle'. He disposed of Mundinus' and Galen's theory that the uterus contained seven cavities or cells within it – 'this is just as true as the moon is made of a Green Cheese'. With regard to the ovaries he wrote: 'The Stones of women (they have such kind of toys aswel as men) differ from the Stones of men ... [but] the use of the Stones in women, is the same that they are in men, viz. to concoct seed.' He referred to the fallopian tubes as 'Deferentia, or Carrying Vessels'.

Book 2 'Of the Forming of the Child in the Womb'

Culpeper wrote of 'the Parts proper to the Child in the Womb', dividing them in two: 'The Umbelicars, or Navel-Vessels and The Secundine', the first to nourish the fetus while the second 'Cloaths it, and defends it from wrong'. He informed the reader that the placenta was named after the Latin word for a sugar-cake. He discussed whether an 'Allontois' was present, and the function of the 'Urachos'. Culpeper made the important observation that 'in Holland all men are present at their Wives Labors: they are delivered upon their husband's laps and not upon a stool'. The presence of husbands at childbirth was obviously more common at this time than is usually acknowledged. Regarding copulation, he noted that 'the woman spends her Seed as well as the man; and both are united to make the conception', disagreeing with the ancient Greek philosophy that only the male seed was responsible.

In relation to fetal nutrition *in utero*, Culpeper wrote that 'the child is nourished in the womb by a very pure blood, conveyed into the liver by the navel-vein'. He discussed the theories of Hippocrates and the ancient authors who believed that the fetus sucked its nourishment 'at its mouth' from specially sited uterine nipples. Culpeper disagreed with this concept, pointing out that the ancient authorities had never dissected the human uterus.

Astrology

A portion of the second book contains an important tract entitled 'The formation of the Child in the Womb Astrologically handled'. This allowed Culpeper to write on one of his favorite topics: 'There must needs be Microcosmical Stars in the Body of Man, because he is an exact Epitome of the Creation'. This 'Microcosmical Sun, Moon and Stars' he believed to have played a part in human creation, every planet ruling particular parts of the body. Culpeper deduced that 'the womb of a woman is under Scorpio ... a fruitful Sign' and he explained that the other planetary signs were 'unfruitful' and did not 'rule the womb'. The evolving pregnancy was also said to be under planetary guidance:

> The first month of conception they give to Saturn;
> The second month they attribute to Jupiter;
> The third month they give to Mars;
> The Sun challengeth the fourth month they say
> Then came Venus ... in the fifth month;
> Mercury, he hath the sixth month appropriated to him

The Moon … she must have the seventh month bestowed upon her, in which they say, she compleats the child.

Astrology played an important role in medicine and therapeutics until the late seventeenth century. It was thought that astrological science related broadly to a person's character and illnesses and that the signs of the zodiac related to specific parts of the body. There are numerous drawings and paintings that illustrate the 'Zodiac man' and a good example from the fifteenth century is from the Guild Book of Barber–Surgeons of York. Zodiacal symbols number 12 and we currently recognize ten planetary symbols compared to Culpeper's seven.

Zodiac symbols Aries, Taurus, Gemini, Cancer, Leo, Virgo, Libra, Scorpio, Sagittarius, Capricorn, Aquarius, Pisces.

Planetary symbols Sun, Moon, Mercury, Venus, Mars, Jupiter, Saturn, Uranus, Neptune, Pluto.

The moon still shines bright in the labor wards of Dublin's National Maternity Hospital but according to a recent paper entitled 'Labour ward activity and the lunar cycle', research failed to find any influence of the moon on overall labor ward activity, instrumental delivery rates and prematurity, although cesarean sections were less likely to occur at the time of the full moon (Ong, Wingfield and McQuillan, 1998).

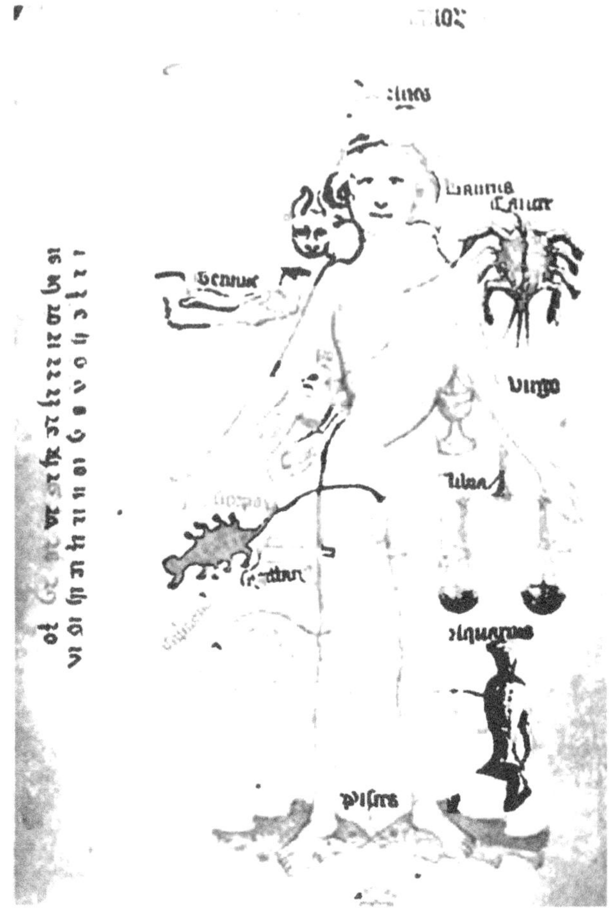

Figure 2 Fifteenth century depiction of the zodiac man

Numerology

Referring to the ancient art of numerology, Culpeper wrote: 'tis not the Compliment of Seven Planets that makes a child live, born at the seventh month, but the perfection of the number (Seven) which if I were but writing Divinity, I could prove by scripture to be the perfect number that is.' The power of the number seven was very important in numerology and was based on the seven days of creation, the seven planets, the seven sages, the seven seas and so on. The ancient Greeks were responsible for the notion that a fetus born at seven months gestation could survive but that one born at eight months would die as it was weakened by its failed exertions of the previous month. In regard to estimation of gestational age, Culpeper noted that there were solar months of 30 or 31 days while lunar months 'consisteth of twenty seven days some odd hours, and some odd minutes' and he advised that some women could be mistaken in their dates just as 'a woman can mistake one shooe for another in the dark'.

Book 3 'Of what Hinders Conception, together with its Remedies'

In the third book there are sections devoted to 'natural' and 'accidental' infertility. One cause of 'natural barrenness' was thought to be 'the letting of Virgin's blood in the arm before their courses come down'. This was sometimes done when a 13-year-old failed to menstruate: her mother 'takes the daughter's piss, and away to Doctor Dunce runs she'– diagnosing a 'fullness of blood', the doctor would then prescribe bloodletting, emetics and purging. Culpeper advised that if blood was taken from the foot (rather that from the arm, the more usual site) it provoked the blood to move downwards and therefore would bring on menstruation. Cures for 'natural barrenness' included 'the stones of a fox dried to powder, and a dram taken every morning in muscadel' or cock-stones as '[the] virtue procreative lives in the testicle'. Various herbs were also prescribed and there was a special fertility diet.

If a couple suffered from 'accidental barrenness' a barley or corn test was used. The seeds were steeped in separate pots of urine from each partner. If the seeds failed to grow, a natural barrenness was deemed to be present. 'The chief cause of barrenness in a woman, lies in her womb, and its infirmities', wrote Culpeper, who went on to list them: 'Stopping of the Menstruis; Overflowing of the Menstruis; Flux of the Womb; Falling out of the Womb; Inflammation of the Womb; Windiness of the Womb or Heat and Dryness of the Womb.' Remedies were offered in the form of herbal potions administered 'a little before the full moon'. Medicinal plants were applied by anointing or by injection into the vagina. Clysters (enemas) were administered to purge the body of 'the peccant [offending] humor'. Culpeper cautioned, however, against 'giving out any of those [medications] to any that is with child, lest you turn Murderers'. Bloodletting was another form of treatment.

'For the overflowing of the Menstruis' Culpeper recommended that the woman take 'Cinnamon, Cassia, Lignea, Opium, of each two drams; Myrrh, White Pepper, Galbanum, of each one dram, dissolve the Gum and Opium in White-Wine, beat the rest into Powder; then make them into Pills by mixing of them together exactly, and let the party diseased take two Pills every night going to bed: let not both the Pills contain above the weight of fifteen grains'.

Another cause of barrenness was 'Flux of the Womb': the flux was a red, white, or pale yellow discharge, thought to be uterine 'dregs' or refuse matter. Culpeper wrote that one form of treatment was particularly valuable: 'Of Dead Nettles (of which our blasphemous Physicians call Archangel, whereas the word Michael who is the Archangel, signifies as God) there are three sorts, white, red and yellow, viz. their Flowers are of that colour; the white flowers help the white, the red helps the red and the yellow helps the Flux in woman: you may use them which way you please'.

Prolapse of the womb was considered to be due to 'unskillful drawing out of the child by mother-careless when she turns midwife'. As it was thought that the womb fled from 'stinking things', medications of asafetida, oil of amber, burnt hair and other malodorous substances were applied to encourage the uterus to dash back into the pelvis. Alternatively Culpeper's 'Magnetick Cure' of sweet smells, wafted under the nose, was used to draw the womb into normal position. Inflammation of the womb, caused by abortion, ulceration, immoderate lechery and other factors, could be cured by a sympathetic diet or by vaginal injection of the juice of various herbs including 'Plantane'.

Regarding women and diets, Culpeper cautioned: 'I seldom prescribe diets to women, because they have gotten such a trick they will keep none ... excellent and true was the speech of Galen *Pleures gula periere quam gladio*, The throat destroys more than the Sword.' Bloodletting from the 'ankle vein' was employed or a wool pessary dipped in juice of plantane, purslane or sengreen was 'put up the Privities ... I confess I could have prescribed many more Medicines, as other Authors have done before me, as Pessaries, Baths, Fomentations, etc., but these if rightly used, are enough, for I write to help you not to trouble you'.

One form of 'barrenness against nature' was thought to be caused by the diabolical practice of self-pollution: 'the man can never [before it was remedied] have to do carnally with his wife ... and cannot give his wife due benevolence'. To prevent such mischief Culpeper noted that various authors had advised St John's wort, the well-known *fuga daemonum* or 'driver away of devils'. Lodestone or a whole squill, hung over the bed were lesser alternatives. However, '[if] the mischief be already done' wrote Culpeper, 'the cure is easy, and was done by the man making water through his Wife's wedding-ring, so there was one superstition helped another'.

Book 4 'Of What Furthers Conception'

The first section of this book deals with how a woman should 'order her body' if she wished to have children.

Culpeper believed in exercise: 'idleness is hateful to God, and destructive to the Creation; and that's the reason such women that live idly (as most of our City Dames do) have so few children ... whereas poor men and women that labor hard have many children usually, and they are strong and lusty.' He was also of the opinion 'as A Physitian and As a Divine [that] discontent wonderfully hinders conception, and content furthers it as much'. He advised women not to 'whine for lack of Children'. Culpeper wrote that exercise and enjoyment of music led to contentment of mind, which led to regular menstruation and encouraged conception.

On a cautionary note, Culpeper advised that overuse of the act of copulation 'makes the womb slippery ... and thats the reason Whores have seldom children; and also the reason why women after long absence of their husbands, when they come again, usually soon conceive'. The most suitable time for conception was shortly after menstruation. The timing of intercourse was vital as 'fear of surprise hindered conception'. He also warned that 'Apish ways and manners of copulation hindered conception'. Various herbal and animal products were advised to promote conception and could be applied as pessaries or plasters: 'Hold sweet Things to the place of conception, before the act of Copulation, because they draw the womb down; But after the act, to the Nose, to draw the Matrix up.'

Book 5 'A Guide for Women in Conception'

This book deals with the symptoms and signs of pregnancy; the sex of the unborn, and the conception of twins and 'of imperfect children'. Culpeper described the lack of menstruation; the loss of appetite; changes 'in the veins of the eye'; hardness and swelling of the breasts; and the prominent veins and red nipples of early pregnancy. The pregnant woman's urine was left for three days and, when strained, should reveal small living creatures in it. In another test, a green nettle placed in the woman's urine 'will be full of red spots on the morrow'.

The opinions of various authors regarding the sex of the unborn were discussed but Culpeper claimed that there was only one indicator of gender that never failed: '[let] her milk a drop of her Milk into a Bason of fair water, if its sinks to the bottom as it drops in, round in a drop, tis a Girl that goes withal, for if it be a boy it will spread and swim at top.'

Book 6 'Of Miscarriage in Women'

Culpeper believed that women were most likely to suffer miscarriage in the first two months of their conception and that many were delivered at the end of seven months 'because of the compleatness of the time, seven being of a Note of perfection'. A favorite treatment was syrup of tansie, 'a most excellent medicine, though it is not in the Colledges Worm-eaten Dispensatory; for the herb by a magnetick vertue draws the Child in the womb anyway, or retains it in its proper place'. Another well-known nostrum was the Ætites (or eagle-stone) which was hung around the neck of the pregnant woman.

Book 7 'A Guide for Women in their Labour'

'I do not here intend to teach Midwives how to perform their office, for that they know already, or least should' – Culpeper's tract on childbirth did not include any reference to the various modes of delivery but dealt with drug treatments in livebirth and stillbirth labors. Intrauterine fetal death was diagnosed when 'no motion of the child is perceived, ... though you put your hand in warm water and lay it upon her belly, for that's the way to make the Child stir'. Once intrauterine fetal demise was proven he offered seven different prescriptions as 'means to bring it away'. A remedy containing burnt cinnamon with white wine, which 'refresheth the child in the womb', was used if the fetus was sickly rather than dead. Culpeper advised that medications should not be given to hasten labor before the true time of birth except in those instances when the woman suffered ... 'an immoderate flux of blood, or have convulsions'.

If the newborn was weak, he advised that blood be milked from the placenta, along the 'navel string', to the infant. An alternative remedy was to 'six or seven drops of blood [crushed] out of the part of the Navel string which is cut off, and [given to] the child inwardly'. The 'distance the umbilical cord should be cut off from the child's body' was a contentious issue among both ancient and contemporary authors. Some believed that if the severed cord was long the infant's 'yard' would be of such a size that 'they may not be Cowards in the Schools of Venus. But [in] the females they cut it shorter, and they think forsooth, [that it] makes them modest, and their privities narrower'. The general consensus was that the cord should be cut four inches from the child's belly. Powder of bole armeniack was then applied, with a little cotton, as a drying agent, and the redundant navel string fell off unaided some days later.

Culpeper was aware that retention of the placenta could cause grave problems as 'it putrifies and thence come scurvy Diseases, Fevers, Apostumes, Convulsions and other the like diseases'. If midwives were to force it away he advised them to pare their nails first, for 'Musicians and Midwives must not wear their Nails too long'. If his directions were followed, there would be no need to 'give a Doctor ten shillings to guide you with an *ignis fatuus*' (Jack-o-lantern, or will o'the wisp). 'The womb is quick, the after-birth is dead. Let the quick expel the dead': Culpeper advised that the expulsive medicines used in labor could help to deliver the retained placenta. Other remedies included '[A] little white Hellebore in powder [sneezing powder] ... and the smoak of Mary Gold flowers received up a womans privities by a Funnel'.

Culpeper's materia medica for labor

Preparation for labor
Burnt-wine, cinnamon, eggs, mother-of-time, oatmeal caudle, oil of poppy, oil of violets, oil of waterlilies, penides, plantain, spermaceti, sugar, vervain
To induce labor
Stone aetites
Oxytocic
Ætites, ass hoof, betony, castoreum, cinnamon, date stones, dittany, featherfew, horse hoof, juice of leek, juice of parsley, juniper berries, lode stone, mugwort, myrrh, peony, stone parsley, pears, pennyroyal, red coral, savory in white wine, silver weed, snake skin, tansy, woman's milk
Analgesia
Swallow's nest, woman's milk
To cleanse after labor
Featherfew, mother-of-time, mugwort, pennyroyal, parsley juice, white wine.

Book 8 'A Guide for Women in their Lying-in'

This book dealt with the dietary requirements for the lying-in woman: 'For though the remedies of the Colledge of Physitians grow in the East Indies and you must give money for them, the remedies of God are near at hand, and to be had for gathering, or else he was mistaken, who said, His tender mercies are over all his works.' Culpeper advised the woman to rest for seven days after her delivery. During that time her diet was designed to restore her strength and to combat the potential peril of retention of the lochia, when 'grim Death usually looks his captives pale in the face'. Foul discharge from the uterus was treated with featherfew and other plant medications: '[you] need not ask in what quantity these herbs must be used; they are so harmless, you cannot offend in the use of them.'

Regarding 'The accidents a Woman was subject to in her Lying-in', Culpeper described the etiology and treatment of 'The After Pains; Retention of the Menstruis [and] Overflowing of the Menstruis'. He believed that retention of the menstruis was a mortal danger if not remedied while overflowing of the menstruis was easily cured by comfrey and other herbs.

Book 9 'Of Nursing Children'

Culpeper had a particular interest in the welfare of young children:

> 'My self having buried many of my children young, caused me to fix my thoughts intently upon this business ... I considered the multitude of children which died in London at the time of their suckling; how many got such insparable Diseases by ill Milk, that it could never be clawed off before Dr Death came and cured them ... I read authors such as I had, and such as I could get, [who] gave me such bold and contradictory reasons ... then I set myself to study; the result of which I bestowed upon you as freely as God bestowed upon me.'

There was no 'punctual time' for weaning but Culpeper advised that 'a year is enough [of breast feeding], if the child be strong and lusty'. Breastfeeding beyond that time was thought unnatural: 'unnatural food in their infancy and cockering in their youth will (if it were possible) make a Devil of a Saint'. He also believed that if children were breastfed for too long they were more prone to general debility and rickets.

Materia medica of Culpeper's *Directory For Midwives*

Acorn cups, aetites, agrimony, alexanders (horse parsley), almond, aloe, amber, ambergris, angelica, asafetida

Basil, bayberry, betony, birthwort, bole armeniac, borage, brains of pigeons, briony water, bugloss, burnet

Cassia (*Cinnamomum cassia*), castoreum, centaury, chicory, cinquefoil, colewort, comfrey, cow's hoof, crabs

Date stones, deadnettle, dittany

Eggs, emeralds, endive, eringo

Featherfew, fennel, fenugreek, fish

Galangal, galbanum, garden tansy, garlic, gentian, goat's milk, golden rod, gourd

Hart's tongue, heart of a male quail, honey, horse hoof, hystericum

Ivory powder, ivy

Jet burnet, juniper berries

Knot grass

Labdanum, leek, lettuce, linseed, liquorice, loosestrife, lovage

Mallows, mandrake, marigold, masterwort, mistletoe, mithridate, mother-of-time, mugwort, muskadel, myrrh

Oatmeal caudle, onions, opium

Parsley, pennyroyal, peony, pizzle of bull, plantain, polipodium, purslane

Raisins, red wine, rhubarb, runnet of hare

Sage, satyrion, savory in white wine, shepherd's purse, solomon's seal, spermaceti, stones of a boar, *Styrax calamitis*, succory, swallow's nest, sweet chervil

Tansy, tar grease, thistle, thyme, tormentil, turtledove

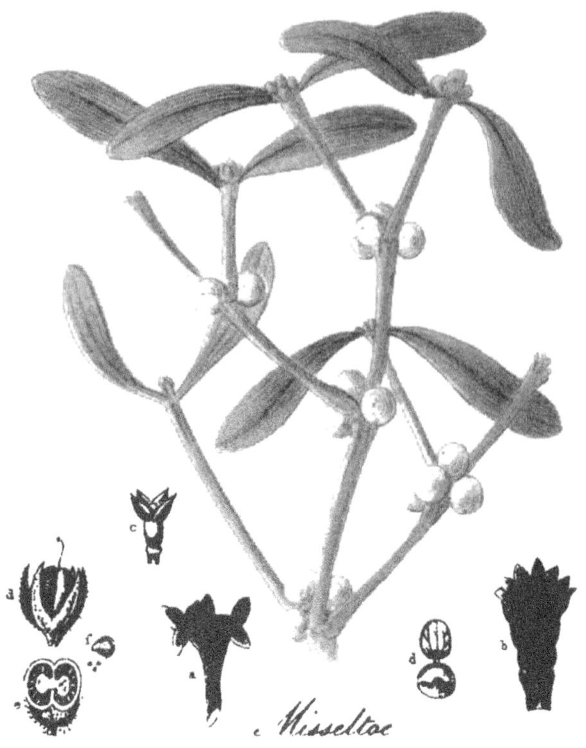

Figure 3 Mistletoe

Venice treacle, vervain, vine leaves, vinegar of roses, violet

White hellebore, white poppy seeds, willow leaves, woman's milk, womb of hare, woundwort.

CULPEPER'S *PHARMACOPOEIA LONDINENSIS: OR THE LONDON DISPENSATORIE*

Culpeper's *Physicall Directory* (1650), was a translation of the first London Pharmacopoeia. His *London Dispensatorie* (1654), a translation from Latin into English of the second London Pharmacopoeia was, like the *Physicall Directory*, an unauthorized translation but proved to be one of the most popular medical textbooks of the era. It was pirated in 1654 and reprinted 14 times before 1718. Culpeper's *London Dispensatorie* comprised 370 pages preceded by 12 Introductory leaves and a contents list of 20 pages. Culpeper added corrections to the College of Physicians Pharmacopoeia, noted that they had deleted many products unnecessarily, and derided their text in caustic terms. It was obvious that relations between Culpeper and the 'Colledge of Physitians' were very poor. The ***London Dispensatorie*** began with 'The Epistle Dedicatory', followed by 'A Premonitory Epistle to the Reader' and then a tract on 'Weights and Measures'. Culpeper took issue with the College's outmoded scheme of weights and measures because, although ancient Greco-Roman terms were used, the quantities actually dispensed differed from the original measures. Other methods of mensuration, including 'handfuls' and 'pugils' ('both ridiculous and contradictive') had been added to the 'New Dispensatory'. Pointing out that the weights and measures were borrowed from Arabia, France, Greece, Italy, ancient Rome and Spain, Culpeper wrote: 'O brave! should a man that borrowed his cloathes from so many Broakers in Lorg-lane be proud of them?'

Weights and measures

Of the 'Old Dispensatory':
Twenty grains make a scruple:
Three scruples make a Drachm:
Eight drachms make an ounce:
Twelve ounces make a pound.
Cochlearum, half ounce of syrup, or three drachms in water,
Canthus holds an ounce and a half,
Hemina (also called Cotyla) contains nine ounces.
Libra holds twelve ounces.
Sextary contains eighteen ounces.
Congie is six sextaries.

Of the 'New Dispensatory':
A spoon, half an ounce of syrup, three drachms of water.
A Taster, an ounce and a half.
A Congie, eight pounds.
A Handful is as much as you can gripe in one Hand.
A pugil as much as you can take up with your Thumb and two fingers.

'A Catalogue of the Simples conducing to the Dispensatory'

Culpeper included a detailed list of medications from the 'Old Dispensatory' with personal comments on their use. The main headings in the catalogue of medications were: 'Roots, Barks, Woods and their Chips or Raspings, Herbs and their Leaves, Flowers, Frvits and their Bvds, Seeds or Grains, Tears, Liquors, and Rozins, Jvyces, Things bred of plants, Living Creatures, Parts of Living Creatures and Excrements, Belonging to the Sea, and Mettals, Minerals, and Stones'. Culpeper advised his countrymen to cure themselves 'and never be beholding to such Physitians as the inequity of these times affords'.

'A Catalogue of the Simples in the New Dispensatory'

The catalog began with roots:

> '[these] be the Roots the Colledge hath made, and but only named, and in this order as I have set them down. It seems the Colledge hold a strange opinion, viz. That it would do an Englishman a mischiefe to know what the Herbs in his Garden are good for ... I do [know] and shal impartially reveal to them what The Lord hath revealed to me in Physick: I see my first labors were so well accepted, that I shal not now give over till I have given my country that which is called the whol body of Physik, in their owne Mother-Tongue'.

Culpeper then proceeded with a catalog of 'The Temperature of the Roots' and other parts of plants. Roots for instance, could be hot in the first, second, third or fourth degree; temperate in respect of heat, cold in the first, second, third or fourth degree, or moist. He went on to detail how plant and other medications should be 'appropriated to the several parts of the body', the properties of each part of a plant, and what each was useful for. In the same way he dealt with barks, woods, herbs, flowers, fruits and seeds. For example:

'*Roots appropriated to the Womb*' Birthwort long and round, galanga greater and lesser, hog's fennel, peony, male and female

'*To provoke the Menses*' Aromaticus, aron, asarabacca, asphodel, birthwort, calamus, capers, carrots, centaury the less, costus, cyperus long and round, dittany of Crete, elicampane, eringo, fennel, garlick, grass,

knee-holly, parsley, peony, smallage, valerian, waterflag, white dittany, etc.
'*To Stop the Menses*' Bistort, comfrey, tormentil, etc.

'Rerum Natura, as these, Gums, Rozins, Balsalms, Juices made thick'

Culpeper added: 'That my country may receive more benefit than ever the Colledge of Physitians intended from these, I shall treat of them severally'.

Ammoniacum ... gives speedy delivery to women in travail.
Asafetida ... [to] repress fits of the mother, [and] provokes lust.
Bdellium ... provokes the menses, softens the hardness of the womb, and expels the dead child.
Bitumen jadaicum ... for fits of the mother, provokes the menses,
Frankincense ... in an ointment for inflammations in women's breasts.
Labdanum ... provokes menses and helps hardness or stiffness of the womb.
Mastich ... stays fluxes.
Myrrh ... [is] dangerous for pregnant women, provokes the menses, brings away both the birth and after-birth, [and] softens hardness of the womb.
Opopanax ... provokes the menses, and helps all the cold afflictions of the womb; have a care you giveth not to any pregnant woman.
Sagapen ... expels the dead child and after-birth, [and] treats fits of the mother.
Styrax calamitis ... helps the hardness of the womb, and provokes the menses.

Following the same format Culpeper dealt with the medications derived from: 'Living Creatures, Mettels, Stones, Salts and other Minerals, Simple Distilled Waters, Simple Waters, Compound Spirits and Compound Distilled Waters, Tinctvres, Physical Wines, Physical Vinegers, Decoctions, Syrvps, Syrups made with Vineger and Honey, Rob or Sapa and Juyces, Lohoch or Eclegmata, Conserves and Sugars, Sugars, Species or Pouders, Electvaries, Purging Electuaries, Pills, Troches, Oyls, Simple Oyls by Infvsion and Decoction, Compvnd Oyls by Infvsion and Decoction, Oyntments more simple, Oyntments more compvnd, Cerecloaths, Plaisters, Chymical Oyls, Chymical Preparations, The General Way of making Extracts and The Way of making Salts'.

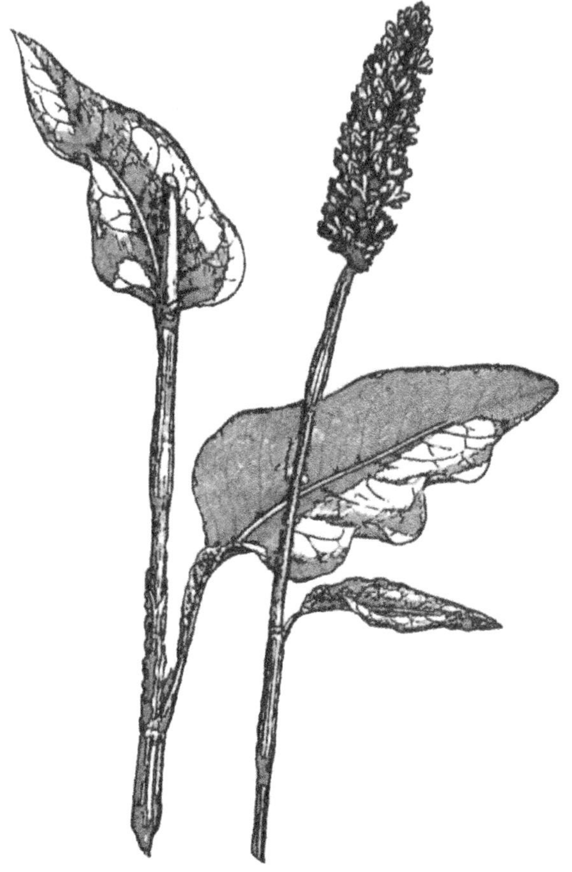

Figure 4 Bistort (*Polygonum* sp.)

CULPEPER'S *A KEY TO GALEN'S METHOD OF PHYSICK*

Appended to the 1654 version of Culpeper's *London Dispensatorie* was another of Culpeper's well-known works, *A Key to Galen's Method of Physick*, in which he laid out the rules for the general treatment of disease.

'Of the Temperature of Medicines'

'Herbs, Plants, and other Medicines manifestly Operate, either by Heat, Coldness, Dryness or Moisture: For the world being composed of many qualities, they and only they can be found in the world, and the mixture of them one with another'. Culpeper explained the Greco-Roman belief regarding the temperatures of medicines: all remedies could be classified as either hot or cold, dry or moist, in the first, second, third or fourth degrees.

'Of the Apropriation of Medicines to several Parts of the Body'

Culpeper wrote that the medicines appropriated to the womb were known as 'Hystericals:' 'Take notice that such medicines as provoke the Terms or stop them when they flow immoderately, are properly Hystericals, but shall bee spoken to by and by in a Chapter by themselves.' Recalling the works of the ancients he noted that the womb, in common with the brain and stomach 'is delighted with sweet and aromatical medicines, and flyes from their contraries ... sometimes the womb of a woman falls out, in such cases, sweet scents applied to the Nose, and stinking things to the privy passage reduces it to its proper place again, and this made some Physitians of opinion that the Womb of a woman was capable of the sense of smelling. For my part I believe nothing less.'

'Of the Properties or Operations of Medicines'

In this section of twelve chapters Culpeper dealt with the qualities and actions of medicines. Included are tracts on remedies to induce menstruation: ' for such as provoke the Terms, provoke also Urine, their Nature is almost the same viz. hot and thin essence ... Things provoking the Terms ought to be hot in the third Degree, and not very dry ... If the Body be full of ill humours, purge them out first ... retaining of them breeds Dropsies, Falling-Sickness and other cruel Diseases, yea sometimes Madness ... Hippocrates denyes any Women have the Gout so long as they have the Terms.'

'Medicines breeding, or taking away Milk'

'Seeing Milk is bred of Bloud, there is no question to be made but the way to encrease Milk, is to encrease the Bloud ... such things as bred Milk are hot and of thin parts, yet differ from those that provoke Urin or Terms ... those which breed Milk [are] temperately hot ... such things as lessen Milk must needs be contrary to such things as encrease it.'

'Of Medicines Regarding the Seed'

'As Milk, so also Seed takes it Original from Bloud ... such Medicines are temperately hot and moyst ... that being heat with spirits it may cause the Yard to stand ... also to provoke one to the sports of Venus, we use such things as stir to the venerial faculty ... These are hotter than those that increase seed ... For the time when seed should be increased, I need say nothing, unless I should say when a Man hath got a pretty Wench ... The Use of these Medicines is the propagation of Mankind, for the desire of Children, incites many to Copulation, but the pleasure that is in the act, ten times more.'

CULPEPER'S *THE ENGLISH PHYSICIAN ENLARGED*

In the original 'Epistle to the Reader' Culpeper wrote:

> '[all other authors] that have written on the nature of herbs, give not a reason why such a Herb was appropriated to such a part of the body, nor why it cured such a disease ... Then to find out the reason of the operation of Herbs, Plants, etc., and, by the stars went I; and herein I could find but a few authors, but those as full of nonsense and contradiction as an egg is full of meat. This not being pleasing, and less profitable to me, I consulted with my two brothers, Dr Reason and Dr Experience, and took a voyage to visit my mother Nature, by whose advice, together with the help of Dr Diligence, I at last obtained my desire; and, being warned by Mr Honesty, a stranger in our days, to publish it to the world, I have done it.'

The 1792 edition began with 'An Alphabetical TABLE of all the Herbs and Plants in this BOOK; as also what Planet governeth every one of them'. Culpeper then dealt with herbal medications using the following format: the name of the medication and any alternative title in English; a detailed description of the plant; the place of growth and the time of year suitable for harvesting; the 'government' and 'virtues' of each plant stating which planet ruled it and what the medicinal herb was used for; how it was prepared; and how the medication should be used. Culpeper devoted a separate section of his book to the methods 'of gathering, drying, and keeping Simples and their Juices' under the headings: leaves, flowers, seeds, roots, barks and juices. Finally he detailed the various forms of medicines and how they were to be compounded and stored. Troches, electuaries and some of the other types of medicines detailed below may sound strange to those in modern medical practice but the formulas for the compounds are almost all of great antiquity and date at least from the early days of Greek medical culture. The various medicinal compounds survived intact to the mid-twentieth century in conventional medicine and are still used in herbal medicine and some other forms of complementary and traditional medical practice.

Distilled waters The water was distilled in a pewter pot in which were placed herbs, flowers, fruits and roots. Culpeper reckoned that these distilled waters were the weakest of artificial medicines, and good for little but as mixtures with other medicines. Distilled waters differed from 'strong waters' which were alcoholic liquors.

Syrups 'A syrup is a medicine of a liquid form, composed of infusion, decoction, and juice ... [to which is added] honey or sugar for the more grateful taste and for the better keeping of it ... boiled to the thickness of new honey.'

Juleps 'Juleps were first invented, as I suppose, in Arabia; and my reason is, because the word Julep is an Arabian word. It signifies only a pleasant potion, as is vulgarly used by such as are sick, and want help, or such as are in health and want no money to quench thirst. Nowadays it is commonly used to prepare the body for purgation, to open up obstructions and pores, to digest tough humours, and to qualify hot distempers etc.' The julep was made by adding two ounces of syrup to a pint of distilled water. If a tart taste was desired then ten drops of oil of vitriol was added per pint of julep. All juleps were to be made fresh – 'It is in vain to speak of their duration'.

Decoctions 'All the difference between decoctions and syrups made by decoction, is this; syrups are made to keep, decoctions only for present use; for you can hardly keep a decoction a week at any time ... Decoctions made with wine last longer than such as are made with water.' The decoction was prepared by boiling the various parts of the medicinal herbs in water and then cooling and decanting the fluid.

Oil 'Oil olive, which is commonly known by the name of sallad oil, I suppose, because it is usually eaten with salads by them that love it, if it be pressed out of ripe olives, according to Galen, is temperate, and exceeds in no one quality.' Culpeper explained that simple oils were obtained by expressing fruits or seeds, while compound oils were made from oil of olives in which other simples had been immersed.

Electuaries 'Physitians make more a quoil than needs, by half, about Electuaries.' To make an electuary, the herbs, roots, seeds, flowers etc. were to be kept ready dried until required. The dried herbs were beaten down to powder, and one ounce of powder was added to three ounces of clarified honey and mixed well with a mortar. The medicine was stored in a pot.

Conserves Culpeper explained that there were two ways in which conserves were made, 'one of herbs and flowers, and the other of fruits'. The leaves and tender tops of the herbs or flowers were beaten down and weighed: 'To every pound of them add three pound of sugar, beat them well together in a mortar.' The fruits were pulped, pressed through a sieve, and an equal weight of sugar added. The mixture was beaten in a pewter vessel and placed over a charcoal fire until all the sugar had melted. Conserves were thought to keep for many years.

Preserves Culpeper wrote that barks, flowers, fruits and roots could all be preserved with sugar. The part to be preserved was first boiled in water and then pulped through a sieve. A pound of sugar was added to the boiled water and a syrup made. To every pound of the syrup was added four ounces of the pulp. Methods for making preserves varied among authors, and Culpeper noted that 'this art was plainly and first invented for delicacy, yet came afterwards to be of excellent use in physick'.

Lohochs 'That which the Arabians call Lohoch and the Greeks Elegma, the Latins call Linctus, and in plain English signifies nothing else, but a thing to be licked up.' Culpeper explained that 'they are in body thicker than a syrup, and not so thick as an electuary'.

A decoction of the medicinal plant was prepared, to the strained water was added twice its weight of honey or sugar and it was then boiled to a lohoch.

Ointments 'Various are the ways of making ointments, which authors have left to posterity, which I shall omit, and quote one which is easiest to be made ... Bruise those herbs, flowers, or roots you will make an ointment of, and to two handfuls of your bruised herbs add a pound of Hog's grease dried ... beat them very well together in a stone mortar with a wooden pestle and put it in a stone pot ... that it may melt; then take it out and boil it and strain it while hot. To this grease add as many more herbs bruised as before, let them stand in like manner, and boil as you did the former.'

Plaisters 'The Greeks made their plaisters of divers simples, and put metals into most of them, if not all; for having reduced their metals into powder, they mixed them with that fatty substance whereof the rest of the plaister constituted, while it was yet hot ... then they made it up in rolls, which when they needed for use, they could melt by fire again.'

Poultices 'Poultices are those kind of things which the Latins call Cataplasmata, and our Learned Fellows, that if they can read English, that's all, call them cataplasms, because it is a very crabbed word few understand.' The herbs or roots suitable to the ailment, were chopped small and boiled in water until a jelly formed. To the jelly was added a little oil, sweet suet and barley meal. Once mixed, the constituents were spread upon a cloth and applied.

Troches 'The Latins called them Placentula, or Little Cakes ... usually little round flat cakes, or you may make them square if you will ... They are made thus. At night when you go to bed take two drachms of fine gum-tragacanth; put it in a galli-pot, and put half a quarter of a pint of any distilled water ... [The] next morning you shall find in it such a jelly as the physicians call mucilage: with this you may make a powder into paste, and that paste into cakes called troches.'

Pills 'They are called Pilulae, because they resemble little balls; the Greeks called them Catapotia ... The way to make pills is very easy, for with the help of a pestle and mortar, and a little diligence, you may make any powder into pills, either with syrup, or the jelly I told you before.'

NICHOLAS CULPEPER: A BIOGRAPHY

Culpeper was born on 18 October 1616 at Ockley in Surrey, 19 days after the death of his father, Rector Nicholas Culpeper. His mother, Mary Attersoll, daughter of Rev. William Attersoll of Isfield in Sussex, returned with her baby to live with her father. Culpeper was educated at a free school in Sussex and went up to Cambridge in 1632, to continue his studies in Latin and Greek. It was hoped that he would study divinity but Culpeper was more interested in astrology and occult philosophy. He also had an interest in medicinal herbs and the 'practice of physick' from an early age. In 1634, while still in Cambridge, he planned to elope with the daughter of one of Sussex's noblest families. On her way to meet him, however, she was thrown from her carriage and died soon afterwards. The grieving Culpeper left Cambridge and failed to take a degree.

At the instigation of his grandfather, Culpeper was apprenticed as an apothecary in Temple Bar, London, where he met Samuel Leadbetter, a licensee of the Society of Apothecaries. At that time the apothecaries were dominated by the Royal College of Physicians which had received its charter in 1518. In 1617 the Worshipful Society of Apothecaries was created. One year later the College of Physicians published their official pharmacopoeia. It set out the drugs that apothecaries were allowed to dispense. Many apothecaries rebelled at the unwarranted interference in their affairs and continued to sell 'unauthorized' medications. A high state of disagreement and tension developed between the apothecaries and the College of Physicians.

Nicholas Culpeper remained as an apprentice with Samuel Leadbetter for a number of years but failed to complete his training and never became a 'Master of the Mortar and Pestle'. He began to practice illegally as an apothecary and physician. He was reprimanded by the Society of Apothecaries and incurred the wrath of the College of Physicians, thus sowing the seeds of a lifelong dispute. In 1642 he was accused of dabbling in witchcraft, an offense which carried the death sentence, but fortunately was found not guilty.

Culpeper married Alice Field and with her dowry they built their own home in Spittlefields on Red Lion Street, outside the walls of London. From 1644 until his death in January 1654 he practiced as an astrologer and herbal medical practitioner. He gained a high reputation for his practice among the poor and disadvantaged of society. He railed against the high costs of treatment by English physicians, who charged an angel (ten shillings) as their fee. Medical books of the time were published in Latin but Culpeper decided to translate them into English so that the general public would become more aware of the secret remedies possessed by the medical profession. His translation of the *London Dispensatorie* was published in 1649 and caused controversy, condemnation and dismay among the members of the Royal College. The physicians set up a barrage of abuse and ridicule and one even wrote that the paper (of Culpeper's books) was only 'fit to wipe one's breech withal' (Tobyn, 1997). The opposition to his translation of the *London Dispensatorie* spurred Culpeper on and the remainder of his life was spent in the study and translation into English of well-known ancient and contemporary European medical texts.

Culpeper developed consumption, which was aggravated by his excessive tobacco habit and moderate drinking of bad wine. He went into a decline and died on 10 January 1654 at the early age of 38 years. He was buried in the New Churchyard of Bethlehem, London. After his death, Culpeper's translations continued to be reprinted over the centuries. His 1720 *Pharmacopoeia Londinensis* and an edition of his *English Physitian* of 1708 were the first medical books printed in North America. Culpeper's *Herbal* was originally entitled *The English Physitian, or an Astrologo-Physical discourse on the Vulgar Herbs of this Nation* and was published in 1652. It remains popular and is published under many guises (Culpeper, 1983, 1992a and b, 1995). The story of the life and times of Nicholas Culpeper is well told by Olav Thulesius (1992) and Graeme Tobyn (1997).

JAMES WOLVERIDGE'S *SPECULUM MATRICIS: OR THE EXPERT MIDWIVES HANDMAID*

Speculum Matricis: or The Expert Midwives Handmaid (1671) is 'one of the rarest books on midwifery ... and one of the earliest ... to appear in English' (Spencer, 1927a). The first original work on obstetrics published in England by an Englishman was a translation from the Latin of William Harvey's 1651 *Exercitationes De Generatione Animalium* (Young, 1653). His work included a chapter on labor entitled 'De Partu'. This prompted the great medical historian James Hobson Aveling, Consultant Librarian to the Royal College of Obstetricians and Gynaecologists, London, to designate Harvey as the 'father of British midwifery'.

An Irish edition of the *Speculum Matricis* ('Mirror of the Womb') entitled *Speculum Matricis Hybernicum; or The Irish Midwives Handmaid* (1671) was described by Professor Elis Essen-Moller of Lund, Sweden (Essen-Moller, 1932). There is a second copy of the Irish edition in the Bodleian Library at Oxford. Kirkpatrick (1938) described a personal copy which he later donated to the Royal College of Physicians, Dublin. There is also a copy of the *Speculum Matricis* in the Library of the Royal College of Obstetricians and Gynaecologists, London (RCOG, 1968). The text is annotated in Herbert R. Spencer's *The History of British Midwifery from 1650 to 1800* (1927b) but does not feature in Garrison and Morton's medical bibliography (Norman, 1991).

Little is known of the author James Wolveridge. It appears that he was of English origin but graduated from Trinity College, Dublin, in 1664 (Cameron, 1916). Soon afterwards he settled in Cork and married Brigitt Fisher. He wrote the text 'from his study in Cork in 1669/70' and the book was printed by E. Okes, London, to 'be sold by Rowland Reynolds at the Kings-Arms in the Poultrey'. In the introduction to his book Wolveridge commended his work to 'The Patronage of the most Grave and Serious Matrons of England and Ireland, the first being the kingdom of his nativity and the latter his country whilst obliged to it'. The book was completed on 12 January 1670 and contains messages from the author to the reader; commendations from colleagues; an index containing the contents; a preface and 35 subsections of text.

The copy of the *Speculum Matricis* in the library of the Royal College of Physicians, Dublin, is hardcover and bound in leather: the pages are small, measuring five and seven-eighth inches by three and five-eighth inches. There are 27 leaves followed by 166 pages. The book has 8 plates and 21 engravings which bear the signature 'Cross'. Thomas Cross (1632–1682), a renowned engraver, was a busy artist who etched portraits of numerous authors and celebrities for the frontispieces of books that were published in the middle of the seventeenth century. His style was thought to be rather dry and stiff in manner but his portraits were a valuable contribution to the history of the period. Cross executed the portrait of Nicholas Culpeper that adorns the original and some of the later editions of *Culpeper's Herbal*. Thomas' son shared his great interest of engraving music notation on copper plates.

Although Herbert Spencer (1927b) was of the opinion that the *Speculum Matricis* was probably plagiarized from *The Expert Midwife* (the English translation of Jacob Rueff's *De Generatione Hominis*, published in 1637), James Wolveridge quoted a number of sources in his text: Aristotle, Bartholinus, Galen, Hippocrates, Ovid, Plato, Pythagoras, Synefius, Theoprastus, Tully (Cicero), The Bible, Harvey and Rodrigo de Castro (1546–1627), a native of Portugal, and one of the first Jewish immigrants to land in Antwerp where he became permanently domiciled. He penned a number of medical books including *De Universa Muliebrium Morborum Medicina* (1628), a text devoted to medical therapy and gynecology.

Although Spencer had misgivings about the originality of the *Speculum Matricis* he failed to mention that most obstetric texts of the era quoted extensively from Greco-Roman and contemporary authors on midwifery. There is no doubt that Wolveridge's text gave 'a good indication of Irish midwifery practice in the late seventeenth century' (Campbell-Ross, 1986). There were some innovations in the book, most of which is a manual of materia medica for women. It contained prescriptions using various permutations of 160 plant, 25 animal and 7 mineral medicinal substances. The *Speculum Matricis* was, in turn, quoted by the famous English obstetrician Percivall Willughby in his *Observations in Midwifery* (c. 1670, but first printed in England in 1863), by Hugh Chamberlen in his translation of François Mauriceau's *Diseases of Women* ... (1683), and by later authors. The text of the *Speculum Matricis* was plagiarized to become *The English Midwife Enlarged* of 1682 (Spencer, 1927b).

The opening pages dealt with the 'Anatomy of Generation' and was followed (in the usual layout for the era) by descriptions of pregnancy problems, labor and delivery and disorders of the puerperium. On page 26 Wolveridge introduced a dialogue between Eutrapelia, a midwife, and Philadelphos, her teacher and an expert doctor. The remainder of the text is in the form of a catechism with Philadelphos questioning the knowledge of the midwife while offering advice for many of the ills that were thought to befall women. This approach reflected the teaching methods used in ancient Greece and it is known that Soranus of Ephesus also wrote a short catechism for midwives. The name 'Eutrapelia' may derive from Euterpe, one of the nine Muses; patroness of flute players, and of joy and pleasure (from the Greek *euterpes* delightful). 'Philadelphos' may be derived from the Greek *phil*, lover of, and 'delphic' (relating to the oracle of Apollo at Delphi, one of the great authorities of ancient Greece).

Doctor Philadelphos described the attributes of a good midwife:

> '[the] best Midwife is she that is ingenius, that knoweth letters, and having a good memory, is studious, neat and cleanly over the whole body, healthful, strong and laborious, and well instructed in women's conditions, not so angry, nor turbulent, or hasty, unsober, unchaste; not unpleasant, quiet, prudent; not covetous but like the Hebrew Midwives, such as fear of God, that God may deal with them, and that the people may multiply and increase after their hands, and that the Lord may build them houses'.

Doctor Philadelphos also informed Eutrapelia that the midwives furniture should consist of '[A] fit stool, a sharp knife, astringent powder, a sponge, swathes, warm oyle of Lilies (and almonds), with which she may aptly anoint but the womb of the woman and her own hands'. He also gave detailed instructions for choosing a wet-nurse and discoursed on nurses' breasts, nipples, milk, general behavior and how the infant should be fed. The latter half of the book is almost entirely devoted to the therapeutics of female disorders. The weights and measures he used were: drachm, draught, drop, gallon, grain, handful, nut, ounce, pint, pugil, quart, scruple, and top.

Wolveridge's materia medica for breast conditions

To induce lactation Ale, alum, aniseed, barley, broth of calve's feet, broth of hen or capon, cinnamon, cumin, dill, egg, fennel, flax, lilies, mace, myrrh, myrtle, parsley, parsnip, smallage, sugar, wool, worms

For inflammation Alum, camphor, flax, frankincense, galbanum, groundsel, lead, olibanum, opium, rice, saffron, sheep's head, sugar, vinegar, water, wax-salve, willow

For milk quality Calf, 'herbs', hermesias, hog, rice, trotters, wheat, wine

Sore nipples Almonds (sweet), capon fat, duck fat, egg, goat fat, goose fat, henbane, lead, litharge, marrow, oil of egg yolk, oil of henbane, oil of poppy, oil of Saint John's wort, oil of sweet almonds, oil of yolk of eggs, pompholyx, poppy, red rose water, silver, stag fat, wax salve

To stop the milk Alum, camphor, cumin, flax, frankincense, groundsel, lead, myrrh, myrtle, olibanum, opium, rose, saffron, smallage, sugar, vinegar.

Oral preparations in the *Speculum Matricis*

Ale, brandy, caudle, cordial, decoction, diet, draught, drink, gruel, honey, infusion, julep, junkets, mead, milk, panada, panatelle, pill, posset, potion, syrup, tincture, water, wine.

Applied treatments in the *Speculum Matricis*

Bag, balm, bezoar, bleeding, cataplasme, cloth, clyster, cupping, embrocation, emplaster, fomentation, liniments, manchet, oils, powder, purge, suppository, swathes, tutia, ungent, wool.

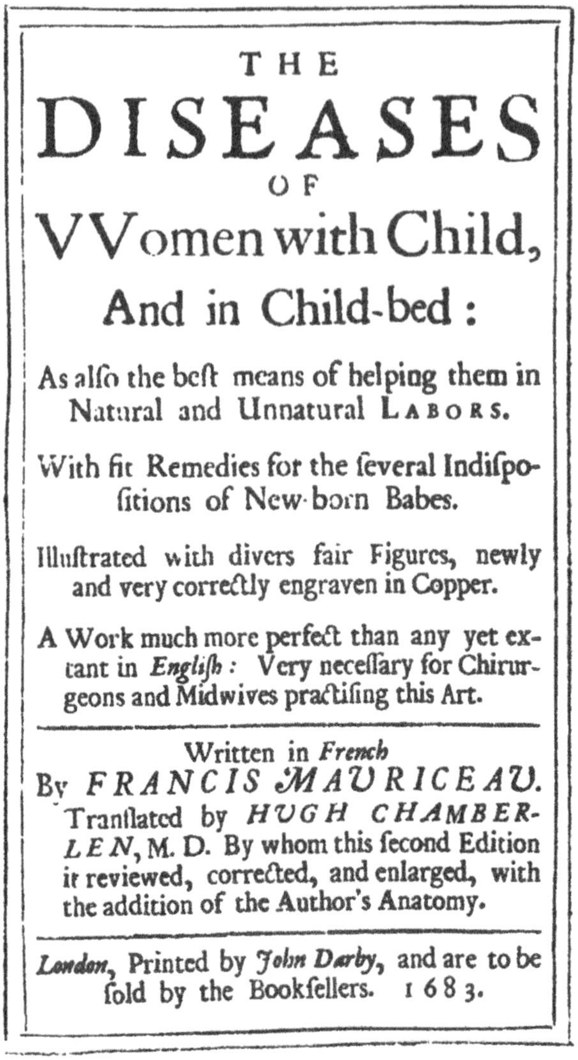

THE
DISEASES
OF
VVomen with Child,
And in Child-bed:

As alſo the beſt means of helping them in Natural and Unnatural LABORS.

With fit Remedies for the ſeveral Indiſpoſitions of New-born Babes.

Illuſtrated with divers fair Figures, newly and very correctly engraven in Copper.

A Work much more perfect than any yet extant in *Engliſh*: Very neceſſary for Chirurgeons and Midwives practiſing this Art.

Written in *French*
By *FRANCIS MAURICEAU.*
Tranſlated by *HUGH CHAMBERLEN*, M. D. By whom this ſecond Edition is reviewed, corrected, and enlarged, with the addition of the Author's Anatomy.

London, Printed by *John Darby*, and are to be ſold by the Bookſellers. 1683.

Figure 5 Frontispiece from Mauriceau *The Diseases of Women with Child*

FRANÇOIS MAURICEAU AND *THE DISEASES OF WOMEN WITH CHILD*

François Mauriceau (1637–1709), a Parisian master-surgeon and accoucheur, was the leading obstetrician of his day. His *Traite des Maladies des Femmes Grosses, et de Celles qui sont Nouvellement Accouchées* of 1668 was translated into English in 1683 by Hugh Chamberlen under the title *The Diseases of Women with Child, And in Child-bed.* It is claimed that Mauriceau's book established obstetrics as a science, based in part on hisoriginal observations on the role of the maternal pelvis in the labor process. He embraced the teachings of the ancients and quoted liberally from Hippocrates throughout his text. It was to Mauriceau that Hugh Chamberlen wished to sell the secret of his obstetric forceps but, after an unsuccessful attempt at forceps delivery of a deformed woman, the deal fell through. In this section I have used quotations extracted from a 1682 edition of Mauriceau's *Traite* ... and Chamberlen's English translation of the following year, which began with this title page:

'The Author's Epistle Dedicatorie'

> To all my Dear Brethern, the Sworn Master-Chirurgeons of the City of Paris, Gentlemen, Wanting a firm and solid Prop for the weakness of my Conceptions, I will imitate the generality of Authors, who choose the protection of some credible Persons, under whose Names to publish their Works to the World ... this obligeth me to address myself to you (as to the only fit judges of it) and to offer you the first Fruits of my Labors.'

The Book received the 'Approbation of the Four Sworn Provosts and Wardens of the Master-Chirurgeons of Paris' on 15 March 1668. The Grace and Privilege of the King was given at St. Germains on 10 June 1668 and allowed copyright on the book for ten years. Hugh Chamberlen translated the book into English.

'An Anatomical Treatise of the Parts of a Woman destined to Generation'

This tract on anatomy was omitted from the first edition of Mauriceau's book but Hugh Chamberlen included it in the translation 'for the benefit of our midwives'. The text dealt with the 'Preparing Vessels ... the Spermatic Vessels in women, called preparing, because they prepare and convey to the Testicles [ovaries], the Blood, of which seed is engendered, [and] differ not from those in men'. Chamberlen went on to describe the 'deferent' or 'ejaculatory vessels' which joined the 'Horn of the Womb' and served to discharge the female seed into the uterus. He gave a detailed description of the uterus, noting that it differed in size according to the age and 'disposition' of the woman. Mauriceau wrote that the pregnant uterus dilated and that its walls became thin, comparing it to the bladder – 'towards the last month of Reckoning, it was ... extream thin'.

In his discussion on the external genitalia Mauriceau noted: '[the] Clitoris hardly appears in dead Corps, being very small; but it is much greater in the living ... some have called it the Woman's Yard ... some women have this clitoris very long, so, that ... 'tis said, some abuse it with other Women'. The vagina was written of as an 'ante-Chamber to lodg the Man's Yard, as in a Sheath, which it conducts even to the inward orifice'. He compared the 'inward orifice' or cervix to 'the Muzzle of a Puppy newly pupp'd': towards the last months of pregnancy 'tis indued with a slippery and viscous Humor not unlike Snot ... The Body of the Womb resembles [as already said] a great Pear', wrote Mauriceau, who declared that, contrary to ancient opinion, it contained a single and not a seven-celled cavity.

The First Book 'Of Diseases, and different Dispositions, of Women with Childe, from the time of Conception to the full time of Reckoning'

Mauriceau wrote that his design was 'to enquire into the principal and most usual Maladies accompanying Great-Bellies, and having during their Course, particular Indications for their Cure'. In this book he dealt with the symptoms and signs of fertility and sterility; of conception and the conditions necessary for it; of the signs of conception; of pregnancy and its disorders including miscarriage, floodings (antepartum hemorrhage) and venereal disease. In a section about diagnosing the sex of the unborn infant, Mauriceau debunked the idea that males were conceived from sperm that came from the right testicle and wrote that it was not possible to foretell the sex of the infant *in utero*.

Regarding superfetation, Mauriceau wrote that 'there is great dispute, whether a Woman (who hath two or more Children at once) conceived them at once, or at several Coitions'.

Writing on how the pregnant woman 'ought to govern herself', Mauriceau advised: 'She should in this case resemble a good Pilot, who being imbarqed on a rough Sea, and full of Rocks, shuns the danger, if she steers with prudence; if not, tis by chance, if she escapes Shipwrack.' When writing about 'Accidents which happen to a Woman during the whole time of her being with Child', he included the nausea and vomiting of early pregnancy, which he thought originated from a 'sympathy between the Stomach and the Womb, because of this similitude of their Substance, and by means of the Nerves inserted in the upper Orifice of the Stomach, which have communication by continuity with those that passed to the Womb'. For the woman who was bothered with 'Pains of the Back, Reins [renal area] and Hips' he advised bleeding and laudanum (opium) in egg yolk with a strengthening cordial. Mauriceau also dealt with breast tenderness, urinary disorders, and swelling and discomfort of the legs. For hemorrhoids he advised diet, bleeding, the application of anodyne remedies and if necessary 'opening' with a lancet. His preference was treatment by application of leeches.

In the section called 'Of Floodings', Mauriceau wrote that placental separation caused the blood-loss and that in the maternal interest the infant should be delivered by version and breech extraction. In an emotional piece he related the story of his own sister 'whom I tenderly loved'. She presented with a severe antepartum hemorrhage. Her own surgeon abandoned her but Mauriceau arrived on the scene and, after much ethical self-deliberation, delivered the baby by breech extraction. Unfortunately his beloved sister died shortly afterwards.

Mauriceau prescribed mercurial ointment for venereal disease in pregnancy and told the case history of 'a young wench not above 20 Years old ... that hath the Pox ... miscarried of a dead child, rotten with the Pox'. The mother was subsequently treated by the mercurial 'salivation' cure and some time later became pregnant and gave birth to a healthy infant in the Hôtel Dieu.

The Second Book 'Of Labors, Natural and Unnatural, with the way how to help Women in the First, and the right means of remedying the rest'

Mauriceau disagreed with the ancient teaching that the infant initiated labor when it punctured the amniotic membranes with its fingers. He was of the opinion that 'the membranes are broken by the strong impulsion of the Waters'. Mauriceau described the role of the pelvis in childbirth and wrote that pelvic stricture could hinder the passage of the infant. At the famed Hôtel Dieu in Paris, where Mauriceau worked, parturient women were brought to a little room called 'the Stove' where they were delivered on 'a little low bed made for the purpose'. Alternatively, the patient was 'at Stool' and he indicated that a midwife's stool or 'a palate-bed' was to be used during the actual delivery. The woman was advised to 'lie on her back having her body in a convenient figure that is, her head and breasts a little raised, so that she is neither lying not sitting'. If the midwife should find that 'the Child come wrong, and that she is not able to deliver the woman as she ought to be ... let her send speedily for an expert and dexterous Chirurgeon in the practice'. (It was the chirurgeons, or surgeons, who practiced man-midwifery in France at that time.)

For floodings or convulsions in labor he thought that '[The] best Expedient and safest Remedy for Mother and Child in this case ... [is] fetching the Child away by the Feet'. Shoulder dystocia was a known complication of delivery and Mauriceau wrote that it was due to 'bigness and largeness of the Shoulders'. Mauriceau described the various forms of 'unnatural Labors, where Manual operation is absolutely necessary'. In the third edition of his book Mauriceau explained his method of delivery of the after-coming head in a breech birth. In recognition of his contribution to this art, his name was lent to the Mauriceau–Smellie–Veit maneuver for fetal head delivery in breech presentation. He argued against the 'Cruelty and barbarousness of the Caesarean Section' if carried out for fetal indications, and stated that 'we ought always to prefer the Mother's life before the Childs'. For infants who were born weak, he advised that 'the best and speediest Remedy is immediately to separate it, and open the Childs Mouth, cleaning and unstopping all the Nose, if there be any Filth, to help it so to breathe freely ... spouting some Wine into the Nose and Mouth of it'.

In the section on 'Unnatural Labors', where a 'manual operation' was absolutely necessary, Mauriceau wrote about the 'conditions ... requisite in a Chirurgeon' who practiced the art of midwifery:

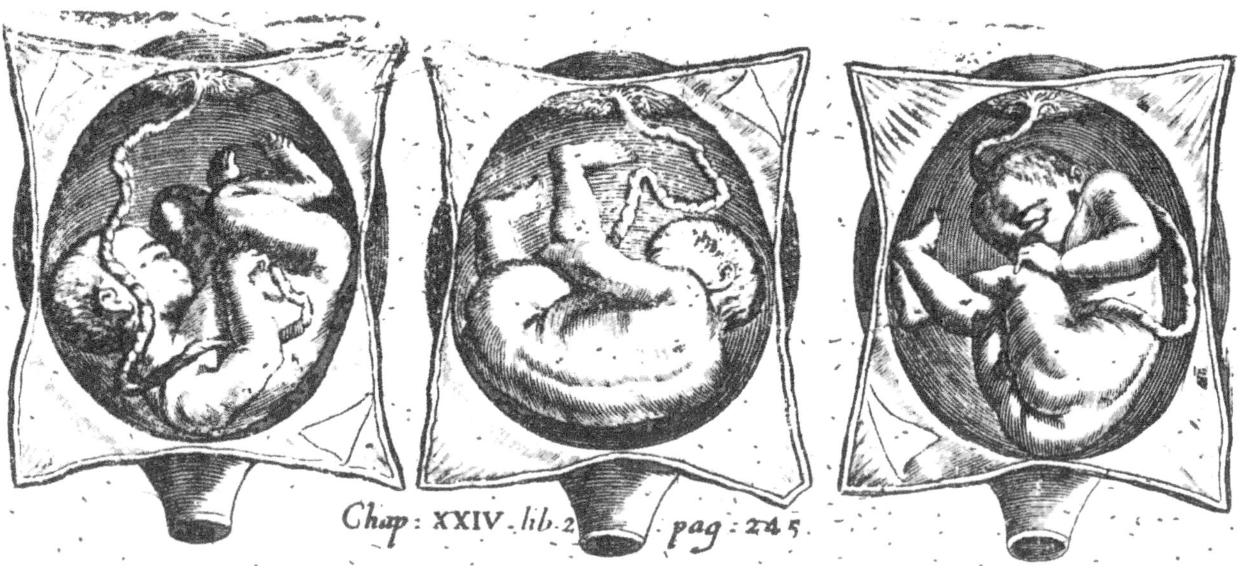

Figure 6 Fetal positions from Mauriceau

'He must be helpful, strong and robust; because this is the most laborious and painful of all the Operations of Chirurgery; for it will make one sometimes sweat, that he shall not have a dry Thread, though it were the coldest day in Winter ... He ought to be well shaped, at least outward appearance; but above all, to have small hands ... yet strong, with the Fingers long, especially the Fore-Finger, the better to reach and touch the inner Orifice: He must have no rings on his Fingers, and his Nails well pared, when he goes about the work, for fear of hurting the Womb. He ought to have a pleasant Countenance, and be as neat in his Clothes as in his Person, that the poor Women who have need of him, be not afrighted of him ... above all, he must be sober, no Tipler, that so he may at all times have his Wits about him; he must be discreet, modest, and secret, never discovering to Strangers those Incommodities and Diseases of Women which come to his Knowledge. He must be sage, prudent, and judicious ... He must be pitiful ... He must not be angry with the poor Woman ... of a well regulated Conscience ... He must deliver poor Women gratis, and treat them as tenderly and with as much humanity as the Rich ... A Chirurgeon indued with all these good Qualities, must be for his accomplishment and intire perfection, very knowing and expert in his Art, and chiefly in these'.

The Third Book 'Treating of Women in Child-bed, and of the Diseases and Symptoms befalling them at that time; Of Children new-born, and their ordinary Distempers; together with necessary Directions to chuse a Nurse'

When the delivery was completed Mauriceau prescribed anodyne and soothing potions or syrups. He wrote: 'All Authors do appoint, immediately after Delivery, the Skin of a black Sheep flaid alive, for this purpose, to be laid all over her Belly, and to lie on, four or five Hours'. He opposed the custom as it caused 'cooling and moistness of the mother which would make her chill' and considered it to be a 'Remedy of too much trouble; for there must always be a Butcher ready for every Woman that is laid'. Mauriceau gave dietary advice for 'the woman in childbed, ... [that was designed] to drive back the Milk in those Women who were not willing to give suck'. He described the process of perineal repair, the application of medications and pessaries for uterine prolapse, and many other conditions of the puerperium.

Mauriceau devoted the remainder of his text to the newborn and the choice and requirements of a good wet-nurse. |Finally, he addressed the reader: 'I believe I have acquitted myself to the Publick ... concerning the Diseases of Women with child, and in Child-bed ... I pray God ... that he will teach you the right way ... and that all may be for ever to his greater Glory.'

Materia medica for the puerperium

After birth pain Maidenhair, oil of sweet almonds, St John's wort, oil of walnuts
Infection Barley water, honey of roses, linimentum arcei
To cleanse the uterus after childbirth Acorns, barley, chervil, cypress nuts, eggs, honey of roses, linseed, lukewarm milk, marshmallow, oil of sweet almonds, plantain, pomegranate, province-roses, red wine, roch allum, *terra sigillata*, violet leaves, water, water in which iron was quenched, wine
To 'fix' uterus Civet, galbanum
To heal perineal tears Barley water, egg yolk, egg white, honey of roses, oil of roses, St John's wort
To nourish after delivery Anise, chicken, fig, jelly broth, liquorice, mutton, new-laid eggs, white wine
To purge Cassia, mallow, manna, oil of sweet almonds, rhubarb, senna, succory, syrup of succory, tamarind, water and wine
To treat the umbilical cord Alum, *desiccativum rubrum, diapompholigos*, lime-water, oil of roses, plantane-water, *unguentum refrigerans galeni (& populeon), unguentum rosatum*
Urinary retention Oil of sweet almonds, olive oil/old olive oil
Uterine abscess Agrimony, barley, oil of roses, wine, wormwood syrup.

A SELECTION OF SEVENTEENTH CENTURY MATERIA MEDICA

Almond

The almond, *Prunus dulcis*, (sometimes known as *Prunus amygdalus*) may be of the *dulcis*, sweet or *amara*, bitter varieties. The plant is named from the Old French *almande; amygdala* is the Latin equivalent.

The almond and the almond tree were mentioned several times in the Bible and it is known that the plant grew in Canaan. Genesis 43: 11 reads: 'Carry down the man a present, a little balm and a little honey, spices, and myrrh, nuts and almonds.' During a famine c. 1707 BC, Jacob requested a shipment of corn from Egypt and sent this gift of almonds in anticipation of a friendly response. The rod or stick of Aaron was an almond tree branch which was taken from Egypt during the Exodus (Moldenke and Moldenke, 1952). In the second century AD the great Greek herbalist Dioscorides wrote: 'Being layd to, they drive out the menstrua' (Gunther, 1959). Over the following centuries almonds and almond milk were used to treat excess menstruation, urinary retention and painful discharge of urine.

Oil of sweet almonds was part of the midwives 'furniture' and was used with hog's grease or other animal fat, fresh butter and oil of lilies to anoint the midwives fingers, and the female 'parts', as an aid to vaginal examinations and as an emollient for the laboring mother. Nicholas Culpeper, in his *Directory for Midwives* (1651), advised medication with almonds to prevent miscarriage. James Wolveridge (1671) applied almond oil to the birth canal during labor and advised both almond milk and almond oil as a soothing remedy for painful nipples in breastfeeding mothers. François Mauriceau (1683) applied oil of sweet almonds to the vulva and vagina after difficult births.

Almond oil was still used in maternity care in the twentieth century, externally as an emollient and internally as a demulcent and laxative. Oil of sweet almonds is a constituent of skincare preparations, and is present in an emulsion in some medicines. Bitter almond oil is used in commercial food flavoring and gives marzipan its distinctive taste (Bown, 1995).

St Valentine and the almond tree

St Valentine lived in Rome in the third century AD during the rule of the oppressive Roman emperor Claudius the Second. The Emperor had decreed that all Romans should worship the twelve gods of the Roman Pantheon – Valentine was a Christian and, in remaining true to his religion, he was sentenced to death. While Valentine languished in prison awaiting execution, his jailer, discovering that the Christian was a man of great learning, requested that his beautiful daughter Julia, who had been blind from birth, might be brought to Valentine for lessons. Valentine read Julia the stories of Rome's history and taught her arithmetic and religion. They prayed that one day God would grant her the gift of sight, and as they knelt together a brilliant light shone from heaven and Julia cried out, 'I can see!' On the eve of his death (c. AD 270), Valentine wrote to Julia urging her to stay close to God, and signed his letter: 'from your Valentine'. Julia planted a pink-blossomed almond tree beside his grave and, to this very day, messages of love are exchanged around the world on St Valentine's Day, and the almond tree remains a symbol of abiding fidelity and love.

The almond, may be a sign of pure love, but the *amara* variety was once used to make a paste, which was prescribed for gonorrhea in men – so much for fidelity. Also obtained from bitter almonds is prussic acid, one drop of which will kill a cat, 17 drops have been known to kill a man (Hare, 1901) – the ultimate in retribution? Those who have an interest in physiology will remember the amygdala, part of the limbic system of the brain, named after the almond. Electrical stimulation of the amygdala results in prolonged erections and intense sexual behavior in monkeys. Lesions of the amygdala cause placidity following by hypersexuality and, to quote from Starling Lovatt-Evans (Davson and Grace Eggleton, 1962), affected cats 'were as likely to mount a monkey, a dog even an old hen' or would exhibit a sexual mode known as 'copulation in tandem' – Move over, sildenafil (Viagra).

Amber

Amber, although long regarded as a stone, is a yellowish fossil resin from an extinct pine tree. Amber occurs in Tertiary deposits and often contains trapped insects. Its name is derived from the Arabic *anbar*, and the French *ambre*. The Old Latin word for the substance was *electrum* (*elektron* in Greek). When rubbed, amber develops a static charge sufficient to pick up small pieces of paper, and so amber, through *electrum*, gave us our name for electricity. The term for amber in ancient Greece and Rome was *lyncurium* or 'lynx stone', derived from the widespread belief that amber was the solidified urine of the lynx. In mythology, amber was believed to be formed from the tears of the Heliads (the sun nymphs) who wept bitter tears for their brother, Phaethon, who came to grief while driving the chariot of his father, Helios the sun god.

During the Middle Ages amber was used as an amulet: 'the stone amber, if carried promotes chastity' (Rowland, 1981). Perhaps this was an easier treatment than anointing the testicles with 'henbane juice to extinguish heat, erection and lust'. Nicholas Culpeper advised in his *Directory for Midwives*: 'let her, if she please, purge her body with Pills of amber' (the resin was mixed with other cleansing medications). The formula for Culpeper's amber pills was contained in his *London Dispensatorie*: 'amber and Mastich of each two drachms, Aloes five drachms, Agarac a drachm and a half, long Birthwort half a drachm with Syrup of Wormwood made into a mass ... it amends the evil state of a woman's body, and strengthen conception, and takes away what hinders it.'

Among other uses for the fossil resin, James Wolveridge advised 'Oil of amber in posset-ale to facilitate the birth, drive out the secundine, false conception, or dead child'. He also prescribed powdered amber, in poached egg, to strengthen the early pregnancy, and prevent miscarriage. Some confusion existed between amber and ambergris (also known as 'spermaceti'), the latter being an ash-gray substance cast up from the intestines of the sperm whale. Ambergris is from the French, *ambre, gris*, gray. Ambergris was used by Wolveridge to prevent miscarriage and pregnancy sickness.

Bezoar

The bezoar was a stony concretion found in the alimentary organs of ruminants, and known in the nineteenth century as *lapis bezoar orientalis* (Adams, 1847). The bezoar was a calculus formed by deposits of phosphates of lime accumulated around a nucleus such as hair or fruit stones. A bezoar stone could vary in size from that of a small nut to a mass large enough to be made into a goblet. Some interesting examples of bezoar stones are to be found in the collection of the Archduke Ferdinand at the Schloss Ambras, Kunsthistorisches Museum, Vienna.

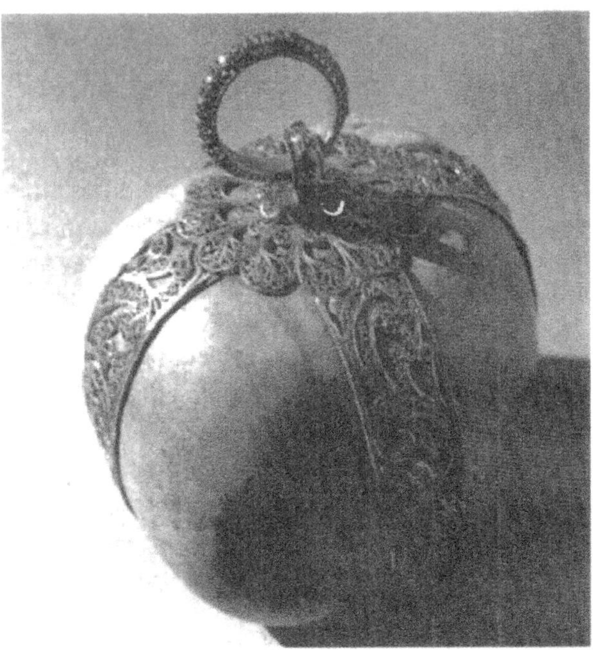

Figure 7 Bezoar (Courtesy of the Kunsthistorisches Museum, Innsbruck)

According to Wootton (1910), bezoar was first referred to as a medication by Avenzoar, an Arab physician of Seville in Spain, who practiced c. AD 1000. The bezoar gained its name through the Spanish *bezoar*, and Arabic *bazahr*, or Persian *padzahr*, for an antidote, and *zahr*, poison. Thus bezoar was thought to be alexipharmic (from the Greek *alexein*, to ward off; and *pharmakon*, poison). Many kinds of bezoar stones were sold but the most famous of all came from the intestines of the Persian wild goat. In the early eighteenth century bezoar cost up to five guineas per ounce in London. Only one bezoar stone was found per seven slaughtered goats and 12 stones weighed about one ounce. Alchemists prepared a synthetic bezoar, by treating 'butter' of antimony with nitric acid, from which they derived antimonious acid. Sicilian earth was sometimes called 'mineral bezoar'.

Although the bezoar was originally prescribed as an antidote to poisons it was also a valued remedy for fevers. Bezoar was availed of in obstetrics to prevent abortion for which Wolveridge advised 'a powder to be taken in broth ... of bezoar stone, four grains'. He was aware of the stone's antipyretic activity and administered 'bezoardical medicines such as provokes sweat ... where there have be vomitings, thirst, and want of sleep, occasioned by the great perturbations of the blood, and stopping of the Lochia [puerperal fever]'. Bezoar stones were included in the *London Pharmacopoeia* until 1746, and they are still used in Eastern medicine.

Coral

Coral is a hard substance of various colors and is the calcified skeleton of Anthozoa and of some Hydrozoa. It takes its name from the Greek *korallion*, the Latin *corallum*, and the Old French *coral*, but the word may originally have been derived from the Semitic. Until the seventeenth century the word 'coral' was applied exclusively to the red variety. In Greek legend, red coral was said to have grown from the blood of the fabled female monster, the Gorgon, Medusa. It was the Roman goddess of wisdom, Minerva (Athena in Greek mythology) who imbued coral with its special medicinal properties.

In general medicine coral was thought to be a potent anticonvulsant, much availed of by Paracelsus and his followers. Powdered coral in milk was fed to the newborn to prevent the 'falling sickness' (epilepsy). For many years coral was used as a young child's toy for biting during teething and coral necklaces were worn to protect children from the 'evil eye'. Powdered coral was an ingredient of materia medica for women and was considered a cure for sterility. During the Middle Ages coral was prescribed 'for a young girl's flux'; to prevent vomiting, and as an oxytocic – when placed near the 'privy party' it was thought to 'draw out the child and afterburden (Rowland, 1981). In the seventeenth century Nicholas Culpeper advised red coral for 'over-flowing of the menstruis', while in Ireland his contemporary, James Wolveridge, offered powdered coral in medications for menorrhagia; to prevent miscarriage, and as a purge in the 'consummated child'.

Pompholyx

Pompholyx is impure zinc oxide and is named from the Greek *pompholyx*, the slag of ore. Dioscorides described pompholyx as a deposit in smelting furnaces, and '[the] scraping and shaving of ye floors and hearths in the brass-finer's shops [and from] cadmia purposely blown with ye bellows for ye making of it ... It hath a binding, cooling, filling, purging and something of a drying faculty'.

Pompholyx became an ingredient of an ointment known as '*ungentum diapompholigos nichili* [after Nicholaus]' the formula for which was given by Culpeper in his *London Dispensatorie*: 'Take of oyl of Roses sixteen ounces, juice of Nightshade six ounces; let them boil to the consumption of the juice, then ad white Wax, five ounces, Ceruss washed two ounces, lead burnt and washed, pompholyx prepared, pure Frankincense, of each an ounce let them brought into the form of an ointment according to art ... [the ointment] cools and binds, dries and staies fluxes ... and fils hollow ulcers with flesh'. Wolveridge detailed the ingredients for an unguent which contained pompholyx, applied 'if the nipples be sore with fissures and clefts' and he also used pompholyx to prevent inflammation of the breasts during nursing. In his *The Diseases of Women* François Mauriceau included a tract entitled 'Of the Smartings, Redness and Inflammation of the Groin, Buttocks and Thighs of the Infant'. His treatment was *'Unguentum Diapompholigos*, spread upon a small Rag in form of a Plaister'.

Various unguents containing zinc oxide and other compounds of zinc remain in the national Pharmacopoeias to the present day. Zinc is employed in proprietary skin preparations as a mild astringent, as a soothing and protective application, and as a protective agent for skin excoriations. A cream preparation for diaper rash containing zinc oxide with wool fat, benzyl benzoate, benzyl cinnamate and benzyl alcohol is known as Sudocrem (Reynolds, 1982).

Vervain

The vervain plant, *Verbena officinalis*, takes its name from the Latin *verbena*, and the Old French *verveine*. The plant was long believed to have great aphrodisiac, magical and medicinal powers and was hung around the necks of children as an amulet to ward off infections (Vickery, 1995). The ancient Egyptians knew vervain by it's symbolic name 'tears of Isis'. In the first century AD Cornelius Celsus described vervain in his

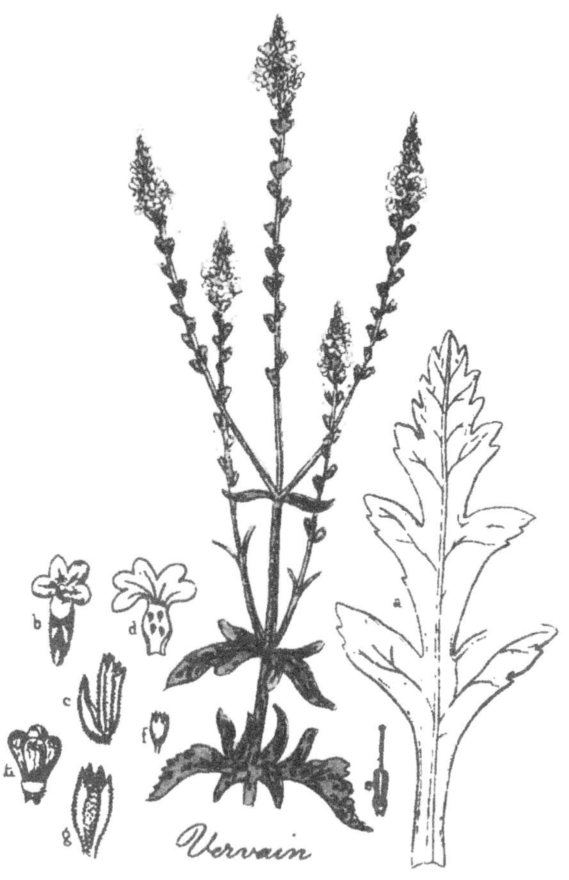

Figure 8 Vervain

De medicina relating how the leaves and twigs of the plant were commonly used in ceremonial processions (Spencer, 1871). Verbena was the classical name for altar plants. Dioscorides described two species of vervain, *Verbena supina* and *Verbena recta* (the latter was also known as *Sacra herba* or *Herba sanguinalis*). He reported that 'ye leaves applied as a Pessum with Rosaceum or New Swine's Grease, do cause a sensation of ye womb pains' (Gunther, 1959). During Saxon times in England (fifth and sixth centuries AD) it was thought that if a person wore a sprig of vervain they would not be barked at by dogs.

Vervain was used during the Middle Ages as a uterine stimulant for labor. At that time the plant also had a reputation as an antiaphrodisiac: 'vervain, carried or drunk, will not permit the penis to go stiff, until it is laid aside, and vervain placed under the pillow makes an erection impossible for seven days, which prescription, if you wish to test, give to a cock mixed with bran, and the cock will not mount the hen.' According to the *Medieval Woman's Guide for Health*, 'Columbine, extinguishes lust in the testicle ... Brimstone carried in the left hand will take away an erection. Likewise, the testicles of a cock with its blood placed on the bed cause a man to suppress intercourse' (Rowland, 1981).

Rembert Dodoens (1517–1585), the eminent Belgian botanist, wrote that 'vervain pound[ed] with swine's grease, or oil of roses, doth mitigate and appease the pains of the matrix being applied thereto' and named Dioscorides as the source of his information (Dodoens, 1619, English Translation). In his *Directory for Midwives* Nicholas Culpeper advised the plant as a medication during the puerperium to relieve general debility and for the woman whose milk was 'accidentally corrupted'. James Wolveridge (1671) prescribed vervain for 'after-pains'. In a late edition of *The English Physician*, Culpeper waxed poetic about vervain: 'This is an herb of Venus, and excellent for the womb to strengthen and remedy all to the cold grief's of it ... it helpeth the swellings and pains of the secret parts in man or woman, also for the piles or haemorrhoids' (Culpeper, 1792).

The 1991 *British Herbal Pharmacopoeia* describes vervain as a sedative and spasmolytic with reputed galactagogue effects. Vervain is a popular plant medication for menstrual disorders in Chinese medicine. In Western herbal medicine vervain is mainly prescribed for nervous complaints and to promote lactation but as it is a uterine stimulant it is not recommended for use during pregnancy (Bown, 1995).

References

Adams, F. (1847). *The Seven Books of Paulus Ægineta.* Translated from the Greek. Vol. 3, pp. 426–7. (London: The Sydenham Society)

Bown, D. (1995). *The Royal Horticultural Society Encyclopaedia of Herbs and Their Uses*, pp. 336, 368. (London: Dorling Kindersley)

British Pharmacopoeia (1864). *The British Pharmacopoeia*, p. 108. (London: Spottiswoode & Co.)

British Pharmacopoeia (1867). *The British Pharmacopoeia*, p. 228. (London: Spottiswoode & Co.)

The British Herbal Medicine Association (1991). *British Herbal Pharmacopoeia*, pp. 227–8. (Bournemouth UK)

Cameron, Sir, C. (1916). *History of the Royal College of Surgeons in Ireland.* (Dublin: Fannin and Co.)

Campbell-Ross, I. (1986). *Public Virtue, Public Love. The Early Years of the Dublin Lying-In Hospital*, p. 128. (Dublin: The O'Brien Press)

Culpeper, N. (1650). *A Physicall Directory: or a translation of the Dispensatorie made by the Colledge of Physitians of London.* (London: Peter Cole)

Culpeper, N. (1651). *A Directory for Midwives: or, A Guide for Women, in their Conception, Bearing, And Suckling their Children*, pp. 115, 82, 80, 145, 157. (London: Peter Cole)

Culpeper, N. (1652). *The English Physitian: or an Astrologo-Physical Discourse of the Vulgar Herbs of this Nation. Being a Complete Method of Physick, whereby a Man may preserve his Body in Health; or Cure himself, being sick, for three pence charge, with such things only as grow in England, they being most fit for English Bodies.* (London: Peter Cole)

Culpeper, N. (1653). *Pharmacopoeia Londinensis: or the London Dispensatorie. Further adorned by the Studies and Collections of the Fellows now living of the said Colledge*, pp. 252, 314. (London: Peter Cole)

Culpeper, N. (1654). *A Key to Galen's Method of Physic.* (London: Peter Cole)

Culpeper, N. (1654). *Pharmacopoeia Londinensis: or the London Dispensatorie. Further adorned by the Studies and Collections of the Fellows, now living of the said Colledge.* (London: Peter Cole)

Culpeper, N. (1684). *Directory for Midwives: Or, A Guide for Women, in their Conception, Bearing, and Suckling their Children. Newly corrected from many gross Errors.* (London: H. Sawbridge)

Culpeper, N. (1708). *The English Physitian.* (Boston: Nicholas Boone)

Culpeper, N. (1720). *Pharmacopoeia. Londinensis: or the London Dispensatorie.* (Boston: Nicholas Boone)

Culpeper, N. (1792). *The English Physitian Enlarged with 369 medicines made of English herbs that were not in any impression until This*, pp. 307–8. (London: A. Law, W. Millar & R. Cater)

Culpeper, N. (1983). *Culpeper's Colour Herbal.* Edited by David Potterton. Illustrated by Michael Stringer. (London: W. Foulsham & Co.)

Culpeper, N. (1992a). *Culpeper's Complete Herbal.* (London: Bloomsbury Books)

Culpeper, N. (1992b). *Culpeper's Complete Herbal and English Physitian. A 20th Century Guide to the Discoveries and Remedies of England's Greatest Herbalist.* (Leicester, UK: Magna Books)

Culpeper, N. (1995). *Culpeper's Complete Herbal.* (Hertfordshire UK: Wordsworth Editions)

Davson, H. and Grace Eggleton, M. (1962). *Starling and Lovatt Evans Principles of Physiology*, p. 1163. (London: J. and A. Churchill Ltd.)

de Castro, Rodrigo (1628). *De Universa Muliebrium Morborum Medicina.* (Hamburg: Froben)

Dodoens, R. (1619). *A New Herbal or History of Plants. First set forth in the Dutch Almaigne Tongue, by that Learned Rembert Dodens, Physician to the Emperor, and now first translated out of French into English by Henry Lytte Esquire. Corrected and amended*, pp. 88–9. (London: Edward Griffin)

Essen-Moller, E. (1932). A Rare Old Irish Medical Book. *Ir. J. Med. Sci.*, 6th series, 78, 312–14

Gunther, R. T. (1959). *The Greek Herbal of Dioscorides*, pp. 86–7, 451–2. (New York: Hafner Publishing Co.)

Hare, H. A. (1901). *Text-Book of Practical Therapeutics*, p. 60. (London: Henry Kimpton)

Harris, R. (1783). *Collectanea Hibernica Medica. being A Collection of, Repositorie for, Papers of Advice, Discussion, and Research, in all Departments of Medicine.* (Dublin: J. Exshaw)

Harvey, W. (1651). *Exercitationes De Generatione Animalium. Quibus Accedunt Quaedam de Partu: De Membranas ac Humoribus Uteri: et De Conceptione.* (London: William Dugard for Octavian Pulleyn)

Kirkpatrick, T. P. C. (1938). A Note of the Speculum Matricis of James Wolveridge, M. D. *Ir. J. Med. Sci.* 12

Mauriceau, F. (1668). *Traite des Maladies des Femmes Grosses, et de Celles Qui sont nouvellement Accouchees.* (Paris: chez l'Auteur)

Mauriceau, F. (1683). *The Diseases of Women with Child, And in Child-bed: Translated by Hugh Chamberlen, M. D.* pp. 319; 396–7. (London: John Darby)

Mauriceau, F. (1682). *Traite des Maladies des Femmes Grosses, Et De Celles Qui Sont Nouvellement Accouchees.* (Paris: Derniere Edition)

Moldenke, H. N. and Moldenke, A. L. (1952). *Plants of The Bible*, pp. 35–8. (Waltham, Massachusetts: Chronica Botanica Co.)

Norman, J. M. (1991). *Morton's Medical Bibliography*, 5th edition. An annotated checklist of texts illustrating the history of medicine. (Cambridge, UK: Cambridge University Press)

Ong, S., Wingfield, M. and McQuillan, K. (1998). Labor ward activity and the lunar cycle. *J. Obstet. Gynaecol.*, 18(6), 538–9

RCOG (1968). *Short-Title Catalogue of Books Printed before 1851 in the Library of the Royal College of Obstetricians and Gynaecologists*, 2nd edition, p. 85. (London: Headley Brothers Ltd.)

Reynolds, E. F. (1982). *Martindale. The Extra Pharmacopoeia*, pp. 509–10. (London: The Pharmaceutical Press)

Rowland, B. (1981). *Medieval Woman's Guide to Health. The First English Gynecological Handbook.* Modern English Translation, pp. 33, 79, 83, 85, 159, 163, 157. (London: Croom Helm)

Rueff, J. (1637). *De Generatione Hominis.* Latin translation of the *Trostbuechle* of 1554. (Tiguri: Froschouer)

Spencer, W. G. (1871). *Celsus' De Medicina.* An English Translation, Vol. 1, p. 493. (London: Heinemann Ltd.)

Spencer, H. R. (1927a). Wolveridge's *Speculum Matricis* (1671) with Notes on Two Copies in the Society's Library. *Proc. R. Soc. Med.*, 20, 1080–6

Spencer, H. R. (1927b). *The History of British Midwifery 1650–1800*, Appx 1, pp. 14, 15. (London: John Bale, Sons & Danielsson Ltd.)

Thulesius, O. (1992). *Nicholas Culpeper: English Physician and Astrologer.* (London: MacMillan Press)

Tobyn, G. (1997). *Culpeper's Medicine. A Practice of Western Holistic Medicine*, pp. 3–39. (Shaftesbury, UK: Element Books Ltd.)

Urdang, G. (1951). The Development of Pharmacopoeias. *Bull. WHO*, pp. 577–603

Vickery, R. (1995). *A Dictionary of Plant-Lore*, p. 381. (Oxford: Oxford University Press)

Willughby, P. (1863). *Observations in Midwifery*, p. 213. (London: Shakespeare Printing Press)

Wilson, A. (1995). *The Making of Man-Midwifery. Childbirth in England 1660–1770.* (London: UCL Press)

Wolveridge, J. (1671a). *Speculum Matricis Hybernicum: or The Irish Midwives Handmaid.* (London: E. Okes)

Wolveridge, J. (1671b). *Speculum Matricis or The Expert Midwives Handmaid*, pp. 28, 41, 74, 125, 126, 128, 129, 130–1, 134, 136, 138–9. (London: E. Okes)

Wootton, A. C. (1910). *Chronicles of Pharmacy*, 1, p. 111. (London: MacMillan & Co. Ltd.)

Young, J. (1653). *Exercitationes de Generatione Animalum*, Translation of William Harvey 1651. (London: Pulleyn)

The eighteenth century 15

INTRODUCTION

The eighteenth century is often referred to as 'The Age of Reason' because accepted ideas and beliefs were questioned, and new theories were based on what was considered to be rational thinking. The art of midwifery slowly evolved into the early glimmerings of science and the terms obstetrics and gynecology were generally used for the first time. Knowledge of botany, materia medica and therapeutics increased and the pharmacopoeias were stripped of many ancient and unproved medications.

Among the many notables of the eighteenth century were two accoucheurs who played a pivotal role in the transition from medieval midwifery to 'modern' obstetrics and also a physician who brought order to botanical science. All three men were embroiled in controversy as a result of the advances they made but their detractors are now long forgotten. They were among the most famous personalities of the era and their works, with their materia medicae for women are explored in this chapter.

Chronologically, the first was Fielding Ould who, in his *A Treatise of Midwifery* (1742), established midwifery as an area subject to scientific investigation. Ould was the first to elucidate a mechanism of labor and to advise a conservative approach to placental delivery. He is also remembered for his description of episiotomy and the use of opiates as analgesics and sedatives in labor. The so-called Dublin school of midwifery began with Fielding Ould's seminal work.

The botanical 'filling' for this eighteenth century 'sandwich' is the Swedish physician–botanist, Carl Linnaeus, professor of medicine at Uppsala University. Linnaeus introduced the binomial method of identifying plants and animals, the first system of botanical classification. His *Materia Medica* of 1749 was the most important medico-botanical work of the era.

Across the sea from Ireland, Fielding Ould's contemporary in England, William Smellie, was the author of a massive three-volume treatise on midwifery. Among many other accomplishments Smellie laid down rules and regulations for the correct use of the newly-available obstetric forceps, and he became known as the 'master of British midwifery'.

OBSTETRICS, GYNECOLOGY AND MATERIA MEDICA IN THE EIGHTEENTH CENTURY

The man-midwife controversy

The following quotation from Stephen Brody's *The Life and Times of Sir Fielding Ould* (1978) sets the scene remarkably well:

> 'By the end of Renaissance the process of birth itself, shrouded in religious and ethnic superstition, was still being neglected by the foremost medical thinkers of the Age. Similarly, the practice of midwifery was held in contempt by the established medical community, even as late as the mid-eighteenth century. With advances in medical knowledge, however, it was inevitable that the care of the lying-in patient would ultimately progress from the hands of the unskilled sixteenth-century midwife to those of the trained accoucheur or man-midwife and finally to those of the accoucheur–physician, skilled in the art of healing.

The apothecaries, barber-surgeons and physicians were the three classes of medical practitioners in the early eighteenth century. Maternity care was in the hands of the midwives. When in difficulties the midwives sought the help of surgeons or apothecaries. Midwifery was considered a disreputable field of endeavor for the skilled physician but despite that many became involved in the care of women. Although reviled by midwives, causing the outrage of clerics, physicians and the public in general, man-midwives made important contributions to midwifery and with the advent of the obstetric forceps their future was in no doubt. Although

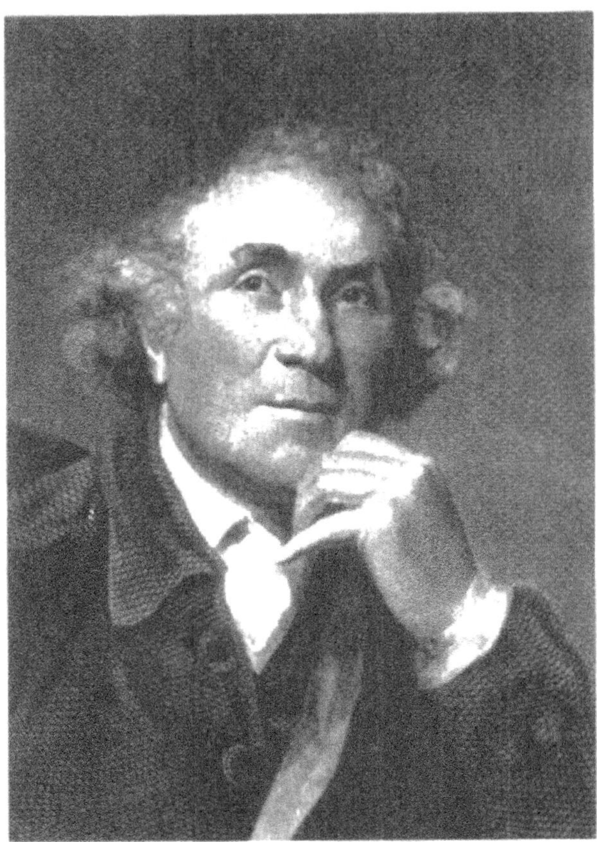

Figure 1 William Hunter (1718–1783)

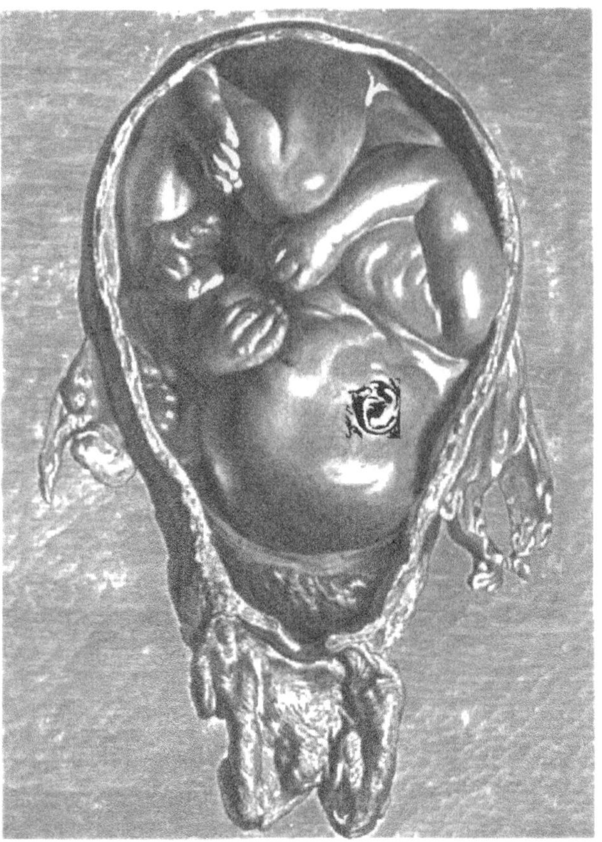

Figure 2 Hunter's *Anatomy of the Human Gravid Uterus*

barred from taking medical degrees in the early eighteenth century in Europe, by the end of the era most men-midwives also held the rank of physician.'

Both Fielding Ould and William Smellie became involved in the man-midwife controversy, as will be recounted later. The anatomists, men-midwives, physicians and surgeons of the era became interested in maternal and fetal anatomy and in the technicalities of the mechanisms of labor and the art of midwifery developed gradually during the eighteenth century.

William Hunter (1718–1783), one of the great names of anatomy, obstetrics, and gynecology, trained as William Smellie's assistant. Hunter's *The Anatomy of the Human Gravid Uterus* (1774) provided a major impetus to the understanding of the pregnant uterus and of the fetus. William Hunter's brother John assisted with the dissections and the artists were Robert Strange and Jan Van Rymsdyk.

The obstetric forceps

At the beginning of the eighteenth century the obstetric instruments available to the accoucheurs, apothecaries and surgeons included the crochet, fillet, scissors and the vectis. Onto the midwifery scene at this time came Edmund Chapman, an accoucheur and surgeon of Halstead in Essex. In his *An Essay on the Improvement of Midwifery* (1733) Chapman gave an account of his experience as a man-midwife and his use of the obstetric forceps (from as early as 1723). Chapman's was the first published account of obstetric forceps which had been developed but kept secret by the Chamberlen family. An illustration of obstetric forceps was included in the second edition of Chapman's book (1735).

The use of the obstetric forceps meant that in difficult cases the man-midwife no longer had to conduct version and breech extraction, or delivery with instruments which would critically injure or kill the fetus. Many types of forceps were introduced throughout the century and the modified instruments offered greater ease of use and safety for both mother and infant. Midwives, however, did not convert to using the obstetric forceps, so contributing to the rapid development of a separate class of 'instrumentalist' man-midwives. The story of the evolution of obstetric forceps was provided by Kedarnath Das (1929) and by Walter Radcliffe (1947).

General improvements

The Rotunda Hospital Dublin, originally known as the Lying-in Hospital, was set up and similar facilities flourished throughout Europe. Obstetric diagnosis was improved, the contracted pelvis was studied, and pelvimetry was introduced. Some advances were made in the area of gynecology, mainly in the knowledge of anatomy and physiology of reproduction. Towards the end of the eighteenth century Alexander Gordon and Charles White were among the first to proclaim the doctrine of aseptic obstetrics (Chapter 14).

Materia medica

In previous eras materia medica for women comprised at least 50% of obstetric volumes; in the eighteenth century medications contributed less than 5%. Authors referred the reader to apothecaries or physicians better versed in the art of prescribing, or to textbooks of therapeutics. Obstetric textbooks became volumes describing reproductive anatomy, unusual cases and the mechanics of delivery in difficult labors.

In pharmacy there was a standardization of drug treatments and some of the ancient but revered remedies were deleted from formularies. Cowen and Helfand (1990) related the story of the cleansing of the pharmacopoeias of the eighteenth century. The event was portended by the publication of William Heberden's *Antitheriaka: an Essay on Mithridiatum and Theriaca* (1745), a 19-page monograph denying the efficacy of such polypharmaceuticals and resulted in their removal from the pharmacopoeia and, as a result, other remedies in use through established custom being cleansed from the pharmacopoeias.

Another innovation was the awakening of interest in drug testing with, in essence, the beginning of modern pharmacology. In Europe Gerhard van Swieten began to experiment with native plants in an effort to replace old imported (and expensive) drugs, many of which were of doubtful efficacy. The Swedish botanist and naturalist Carl Linnaeus classified plants and much duplication was eliminated from the pharmacopoeias which became increasingly scientific. The pharmacopoeias became merely lists of drugs and formulas with directions for compounding. Companion publications, known as 'dispensatories', described the drugs and gave indications for their use in medicine. The dispensatories, based on Nicholas Culpeper's classic *London Dispensatorie* (1654), became popular as textbooks of therapeutics.

The emergence of American obstetrics

In America, William Shippen Jr. (1736–1808) returned to Philadelphia in 1762 with an MD obtained from Edinburgh and began courses on anatomy and midwifery at the State House. In 1765 John Morgan (1735–1789) and William Shippen Jr. were involved in setting up the first medical school in the New World, based at Philadelphia, and modeled on the Edinburgh school. The Pennsylvania Hospital was opened in 1751 by Benjamin Franklin and Thomas Bond. In 1742 Samuel Bard was born in Pennsylvania and in the following century his treatise on midwifery (Chapter 16) was the first American book on the subject. The story of the evolution of American obstetrics and gynecology has been told by Theodore Cianfrani (1960), associate professor of obstetrics and gynecology at the Graduate School of Medicine, at the University of Pennsylvania, Philadelphia, and by Herbert Thoms (1935), Palmer Findley (1939), James Ricci (1945 and 1949) and Harold Speert (1980, 1994).

FIELDING OULD'S *A TREATISE OF MIDWIFERY*

The Preface

Ould began by praising the 'great Author of our Being [who] has contrived the human Body with surprising

A

TREATISE

OF

MIDWIFRY.

IN

THREE PARTS.

BY

FIELDING OULD, Man-Midwife.

DUBLIN:

Printed by and for OLI. NELSON at *Milton's* Head in *Skinner-Row*;

And for CHARLES CONNOR at *Pope's* Head at *Effex-Gate*, M DCC XLII.

Figure 3 Frontispiece from Ould's *A Treatise of Midwifery*

Accuracy'. He went on: 'the Wisdom of Providence is very fully displayed in the whole Scene of Procreation; and the Concurring circumstances which contribute to Parturition are surprisingly beautiful, as will plainly appear to the curious Reader through the Whole Theory and Practice of natural Deliveries.' Ould advised that well-meaning men should be encouraged to contribute their knowledge to the common good for the perfection of the art of midwifery but cautioned against the use of instruments 'contrived [by previous authors] for the Performance of their Operations: For many of their Schemes are like those of Navigators and Geographers, who never make use of a Compass, but in their Closet'.

The Treatise, Part I

In olden times it was women alone who practiced midwifery and their skill was never called into question but, wrote Ould 'as medicinal Knowledge increased, it became very apparent that there was more Learning and Dexterity required ... And then it was, that Men, who were well acquainted with Operations in general, applied themselves to the Improvement of this Art'. Ould apologized for his direct style of writing English – 'the candid Reader must not expect to find, either Purity of Stile, or Elegance of Expression, in this Undertaking ... I spent that Time which others employ in their Improvement in polite Literature, in a more laborious Manner; namely, in the Dissection of human Bodies, and a constant Application to Practice.'

As a preface to his discussion on the anatomy of the genital tract, Ould stated that 'I suppose the Reader already an Anatomist' and restrained himself from engaging in a long treatise. He was particularly interested in the anatomy of the vagina and 'the prodigious Distension it must undergo, in giving Passage to a Foetus of almost any size'. He described the vagina and its enclosing muscle layers as resembling 'a loose knit stocking'. The placental anatomy was well described but Ould was of the opinion that blood would flow from the mother via the umbilical vein, if cut. In his piece on the fetal cranial bones he related how they 'slip over each other to contract the Size of the Head, in its passage through the Perforation of the Pelvis'.

Ould wrote a detailed description of 'touching', the term used for vaginal examination of the pregnant woman. He described the various postures in which women were to be delivered: in France, for instance, 'the patient always lies on her back, with her Head raised, her Heels approaching to her Thighs, and Knees extended from each other'. Ould considered that this posture 'may answere well enough in natural and easy labors' but that it was not suitable in difficult cases or when instrumental delivery was required: 'the Side [left lateral position] is certainly the most advantagious Posture for natural Labors.' Ould was a proponent of coccygeal pressure as an aid to delivery and used rectal examination in labor to check cervical dilatation and descent of the presenting part. From his close observations of childbirth Ould was aware that 'in the most favourable Labors, poor Women endure as much Pain as Mortals are well able to undergo'. Ould was one of the first of the era to prescribe opiates, finding them to be 'of surprising service'.

The materia medica of Part I

'Costiveness' (constipation) 'This Evil must be removed by a Clyster ... the Intestinum Rectum must be much stuffed with Faeces, which certainly hinders the Exit of the Child.'

'Dryness and Constriction of the Parts' 'In this Case emollient Clysters, and injections into the vagina are of great Use; I have found great Advantage from a Decoction of Linseed and Oil of Almonds, injected frequently into the vagina.'

Early labor 'At this Time she must take no solid Food except Bread; Broth or Jelly being the most proper Nourishment; her Drink should be so as will promote a small Degree of Warmth, and at the same Time not very heating; such as Sack-Whey made strong or small as there is Occasion; giving now and then some Spoonfuls of cold Cinnamon or Pennyroyal-Water, by Way of Cordial when the Pain seems to grow languid.'

Tedious labor 'Strengthening Broths, heating Cordials ... then an Opiate is of surprising Service'.

Vaginal examination 'The Operator ... must put his Hand well greased with Fresh Butter or Oil, under the Bed-cloaths, without uncovering any Part of the Patient; and introducing his fore-finger into the Vagina, must find out the Orifice of the Womb.'

Puerperal infection 'When the Discharge of the Lochia ceased ... it was followed by that of a foetid, sanious, black Ichor ... she was cured, by the Help of anodine detersive [cleansing] injections, and taking some few Medicines of the hysterical Tribe, by the Advice of her Physician.'

The Treatise, Part II

Fielding Ould advised the young practitioner that he should be 'well acquainted with Chirurgical Operations of all Kinds' before becoming a man-midwife and pointed out the contrast between surgery and midwifery in surgical cases: 'you have the Assistance of your Eye' in midwifery 'you must not only operate in the Dark, but even use cutting Instruments'. Ould was indebted to his experience of midwifery in France as there was no opportunity for training in Dublin. In Paris he had experienced 'occular Demonstration of Women being delivered, both in natural and praeternatural Labours'. Being aware that labors occurred at unexpected hours his advice to the budding man-midwife was that he should 'always observe an exact Regularity in the general Conduct of his Life, keeping up the strictest Rules of Sobriety; for he knows not the Instant he may be called'.

The materia medica of Part II

Uterine discharge in pregnancy 'The illegitimate and dangerous Flux, is out of the usual Time, and the Consequence of some external Hurt, some extraordinary Passion of the Mind, as Fright, Anger, excessive Joy, Grief, etc., taking Medicines improperly ... the Patient is in great Danger of being lost, if not timely assisted, by the Extraction of all the then Contents of the Womb.'

Mole or 'false-conception' 'As soon as the Existence of this extraneous Mass can be certainly discovered, it is necessary by some Means to procure the Discharge of it; which must be done by the Help of such Emenagogues as the Physician shall think proper, and by the Surgeon's Hand ... [and] the Help of Medicine ...' Ould described how, in one case, '[We] went on for twelve Hours, at the End of which Time, I gave her a quieting Draught, which composed her for an Hour and a half, and intirely removed that terrible Complaint'.

Intrapartum bleeding 'We both examined her alternately several Times, and could make no Discovery of Particulars therefrom; however the first Indication of all Accounts, was that we should contrive Means to give her some Respite from her Pain, in order to recover in some Measure, her Strength and Spirits; to which End we gave her twenty Drops of Liquid Laudanum [opium], in a Draught of Cold Cinnamon-water, whereby she soon fell asleep, which gave us Time to consider what was to be done.'

Extraction of a child by the feet 'Having given the Patient a Draught of some Cordial Liquor, such as Sack-Whey, Cinnamon-Water or the like, and being placed on her Knees as before directed, the right Hand must be introduced into the Womb, being well greased either with Oil or Fresh Butter, take hold of [the feet] ... and draw forth with Care and Caution.'

Uterine prolapse 'It must be remedied by a skillful Physician; at the same Time using Pessaries such as are described in all Books of Midwifery. The Application of strengthening and astringent Plasters ... is likewise of great Use in this Case. The Part must be fomented with the most emollient mucilaginous Decoctions than can be contrived, and all possible Means must be used by the Hands, to restore it to its natural Situation.'

The Treatise, Part III

'The remaining Part of This Treatise shall be wholly taken up in the Illustration of that Part of Midwifery, where the Mother's Life is not to be saved, but by bringing away the Child, either whole or separately by the Help of Instruments'.

In emotional language Ould wrote of the 'most dreadful Apprehensions' of the laboring woman '[with] sharp Hooks, Knives of various Kinds, Forceps, etc. thrust into the Womb ... here we have not only the Mother's Danger to fear, but even the Murder of an innocent Babe ... A Murderer of this Kind, is next in Guilt to the Mother who murders her own child ... yet it is not to be denied, but that such Operations are very useful and necessary, when undertaken with Caution, Skill and Prudence'.

Ould advised episiotomy with 'a Pair of crooked-probe Sizars when ... by Reason of the extraordinary Constriction of the external Orifice of the Vagina' the fetus could not emerge. If expulsion of the fetus was impeded by either maternal weakness or by disproportion of the size of the fetal head and the maternal pelvis, Ould suggested that the large obstetric forceps 'which is in general Use all over Europe' could be used. For forceps delivery Ould advised that the patient should be placed on her knees with her head on the lap of an attendant. He included directions for the application of the obstetric forceps and the contraindications to their use.

To achieve an easier delivery in those cases with a dead fetus *in utero*, where breech extraction was not possible, Ould advised against the application of the crochet (a metal hook) 'thrust into the Eye, Ear, behind the head or into some of the sutures' or the fillet (a linen cloth to be fixed around the head 'as a stone in a Sling'). In his view the use of sharp knives or the bistoury (a surgical knife) applied vaginally could not possibly 'secure the patient from destruction, when used to decompress the hydropic infant prior to attempted vaginal delivery'. In consequence of his experiences in these terrible cases Ould invented an instrument, the *terebra occulta* to decompress the fetal head safely. There are two illustrations and detailed comments on the instrument in his book. An example of the *terebra occulta* may be viewed in the Royal College of Physicians, Dublin.

The materia medica of Part III

Application of the obstetric forceps 'Being warmed and oiled.'

Treatment to the vulva and vagina prior to a destructive operation on the fetus '[With] The Help of a Fomentation of Bran and Water boiled, which was the most expeditious Remedy that could be then got, I obtained a Passage for my Hand, so as to lessen the size of the Head by evacuating the Brain, and brought forth a Child almost rotten; immediately after the Delivery, the Patient made four Quarts of Urine; having had no Evacuation, either this Way or by Stool for four Days before.'

Delivery of a woman 'of Low Stature and Distorted Shape' 'With exceeding great Difficulty, I put my Hand very well oiled, through this narrow Passage, and with as much difficulty turned the Child so as to bring it by the Feet; after two Hours excessive hard Toil, I brought the Body and Arms into the World; but had it been to save my own Life, I could not have brought away the Head.' Fielding Ould then used his *terebra occulta* to perforate the infants head and evacuate the brain and finally achieved the delivery: 'This patient recovered, and is still living and well, which in my Opinion could not have happened were it not for the Assistance of the *Terebra Occulta*. This was the most laborious Operation I ever performed; though it was in the midst of the great Frost, yet I sweated through all my Cloaths; and my Left Hand was so swelled, that I could not make use of it rightly in ten Days after.'

Care of the episiotomy wound Ould was the first to describe episiotomy and advised: 'The Wound must be united by a Stitch, at the same Time leaving some of it open at the Orifice of the Vagina, which must be preserved so, by keeping some Lint between the Lips ... this Lint must be dipt in some vulnerary [wound] Ointment, and a Compress dipt in Brandy over it, which must be often changed on Account of the Discharge of the Lochia.'

Treatment of a 'Scirrhous' cervix due to previous injury 'First taking Care that the Rectum and Bladder, may be emptied of their Contents; [both] may be brought to pass by the Help of a Clyster, as going to stool will excite the Discharge of Urine'. Ould described the incision of the cervix and delivery of the child. After the birth 'there must be anodine emollient Injections immediately made use of, while the Physician does his Part, by ordering such internal Medicines as he shall think proper'.

FIELDING OULD (1710–1789): A BIOGRAPHY

Fielding Ould, Ireland's most renowned man-midwife, was born in Galway (Cameron, 1916). He and his brother Abraham were children of Captain Ould of the Welsh Fusiliers and Lettice Shawe, the daughter of Reverend Fielding Shawe, Canon of Tagh Saxon. Ould's father fought at the battles of the Boyne and of Aughrim and was later assassinated in London. In 1729 Ould moved to Trinity College, Dublin, where he became a dissector in the anatomy department. He also attended courses in botany, chemistry and natural philosophy but failed to sit for his matriculation (Kirkpatrick, 1912).

Ould traveled to Paris where he studied midwifery with Gregoire the Elder, the first Frenchman to give private lessons in midwifery. During his two years of study in Paris Ould carefully examined every laboring woman in his care and he observed that in normal labor the fetal head entered the pelvis in the lateral position and rotated prior to delivery. This was to be his greatest (but not his only) contribution to the art of obstetrics. Much of Ould's French experience formed the basis for his *Treatise of Midwifery* (1742). In 1733 Ould married Gracia Walker who was related by marriage to the Chamberlen family who introduced the obstetric forceps into midwifery practice.

From 1736, Ould began work as a man-midwife and soon developed a large private and public practice in Golden Lane, Dublin. He applied for, and was granted a license to practice midwifery by the College of Physicians in Ireland in 1738 as he was found by examination to be 'singularly well qualified' in the art of obstetrics (Widdess, 1963). Four years later his *Treatise of Midwifery. In Three Parts* was published and he dedicated it to the Fellows of the College of Physicians who gave it their imprimatur. In 1745 Ould became assistant master of the Dublin Lying-in Hospital (later known as The Rotunda Hospital). The hospital was the first maternity institution in Ireland and Great Britain and provided much-needed facilities for the women of Dublin. In 1759, after the untimely death of its founder, Bartholomew Mosse (1712–1759), Fielding Ould became the new Master and during his term of office 3800 women were delivered. He was responsible for the building of the 'Round Rooms', a building for entertainment and fund-raising, later known as the 'Rotunda', which gave the Lying-in Hospital its name from about 1767. Ould was knighted in 1760 by John Russell, the 4th Duke of Bedford, Lord Lieutenant of Ireland and President of the Board of Governors and Guardians of the Rotunda. On this occasion a poem appeared in the 'Medical Review'

> 'Sir Fielding Ould, the sword of Knighthood gained, For saving Ladies' lives in child-bed pained'

The short poem prompted a Dublin wit to write the following epigram:

> Sir Fielding Ould is made a Knight,
> He should have been a Lord by right;
> For then each Lady's prayer would be
> Lord, Good Lord, deliver me!
>
> (O'Donel Browne, 1947)

Ould had a long professional career which extended from 1736 to 1788. He had an extensive practice and was obstetrician to the destitute as well as to the nobility. He attended the Countess of Wellesley at the birth of Arthur, the Duke of Wellington. According to McClintock (1858), the literary reputation of the Dublin School of Midwifery commenced with Fielding Ould who took an active and leading part in the management of the affairs of the Rotunda for 28 years. Ould died on the 29th November 1789 from a stroke, shortly after delivering a patient, and was buried at the cemetery adjoining St Anne's Church, Dawson Street, Dublin.

Fielding Ould and the man-midwifery controversy

The practice of man-midwifery gave rise to heated debate both among the professionals and the general public. The story of the trials and tribulations of Fielding Ould and his wish for advancement and recognition is but one of many played out in the eighteenth century. Abused by midwives, husbands and physicians alike, the man-midwives brought 'scientific' knowledge and new skills to the practice of the art of obstetrics. As with all innovations, however, the new practice of midwifery brought some negative aspects in its train.

Fielding Ould left Trinity College without a degree, a fact that was to have very serious consequences for himself and for the relationship between the College of Physicians in Ireland and the University, two bodies that were closely connected academically for over sixty years (Coakley, 1992). Despite the fact that Ould was granted a license to practice midwifery in 1738 and that he had dedicated his *Treatise* to the 'President, Censors, and Fellows of the College of Physicians', a rift developed between Ould and the College. A warning shot was fired in 1746 when the College of Physicians decreed: 'It has been found that several persons [no names were given] licensed to practice midwifery only have notwithstanding presumed to practice Physic in general ... we will not for the future consult with any of them as Physicians, nor with any other person, who is not a graduate or a licensed Physician of this College.'

At that time Ould had a large obstetric practice but wished to improve his professional prospects by obtaining a medical degree. In 1753 he was conferred with the degree of B.A. *speciala gratia* from Trinity College Dublin. In 1756 he applied to be examined for a Bachelors of medicine degree by the College of Physicians, who at that time were responsible for the final medical examinations at Trinity College. The Physicians refused to examine him and pointed out that in 1701 the Boards of both institutions had agreed that the Fellows of the College of Physicians would be the examiners for a degree in medicine at Trinity College, and that only those who had graduated (properly) from Trinity would be admitted to the License of Physic and eventual Fellowship of the College of Physicians (Coakley, 1992). The College of Physicians also refused Ould's request because it was contrary to their 1736 bylaw which stated that 'no man for the future shall have a license to practice mid-wifery and physic together'. In 1757 the College of Physicians demanded that all their graduates sign a resolution forbidding consultation with man-midwives.

By this time, however, Ould had become a powerful figure in Dublin and Trinity College considered it could not continue to ignore such a distinguished candidate. In 1758 Francis Andrews became the new Provost at Trinity College and he was of the opinion that Ould should be allowed to proceed to a medical degree. Through Andrews' influence Ould was granted a Bachelors Degree in Physic in 1760 by Trinity College. The College of Physicians refused to examine him as a candidate for an M.D. degree whereupon Trinity College conducted their own qualifying examination and Ould finally received his doctorate of medicine in 1761. Shortly afterwards the College of Physicians resolved that recipients of such medical degrees would not be licensed by their College and they severed their links with Trinity (Widdess, 1963). The College of Physician's estimation and limitation of the practice of men-midwives was not universally approved and in 1775 Gilborne wrote:

> Why may not any doctor that would chuse
> For a man's relief his total knowledge use?
> Or does one portion of Apollo's trade
> More than the rest his votaries degrade?
>
> (Spencer, 1927 p. 32)

The attitude of the College of Physicians softened and on 3 October 1785, when Ould was aged 75, he was admitted as a Licentiate in Medicine by the College of Physicians with a group of leading obstetricians, although he was never granted his fellowship (Fleetwood, 1983). In the same year the physicians elected Francis Hopkins, physician–midwife, as their president.

CARL LINNAEUS' MATERIA MEDICA

The observations in this section are taken from *Materia Medica, Liber 1. De Plantis* (1749), a Latin text which detailed some of the important medicinal plants known to Linnaeus. In his bibliography, Linnaeus included the works of fifteen authors, including Dioscorides, whom he held in high esteem. The introduction contained a section on weights and measures, chemists signatures for various oils, tinctures etc., and the correct dosages of a large number of medications. He included details on the preparation and composition of various well-known medications, many of which were similar in content to those contained in Nicholas Culpeper's 1654 *Pharmacopoeia Londinensis: or the London Dispensatorie.* The 30 introductory pages were followed by 188 pages of text, a further 43 pages of indices of the 'official' medicinal drugs and their composition, and a list of the official/botanical names for the plants mentioned in the book (e.g. official name, *Agnus Castus;* botanical name, *Vitex*). The *Index Morborum* contained a summary of general medical complaints and the plant medications used to treat them. Under the heading *Pharmacopoeorum* Linnaeus included simples (the important parts of the medicinal herbs such as roots, flowers, etc.) and *Praeparata* (the forms in which herbal medication could be administered, such as oil or syrup, etc.):

Simplicia

Radix	*Succus*
Lignum	*Flos*
Cortex	*Fructus*
Folia	*Semina*

Praeparata

Aqua Distillata	*Conserva*
Oleum Stillatitium	*Syrupus*
Oleum Embryeumat	*Rob*
Oleum Coctum	*Conditum*
Oleum Expressum Spiritus	*Confecti*
Essentia	
Extractum	
Sal	

Under the heading *Vires* (the nature or strength) Linnaeus explained that medications may be liquid, solid or solid–liquid mixtures. He further subdivided them into *alternatives, evacuantia, muscalaria, nervines, topica* and *visceralia.* The *Evacuantia* heading contained those medicinal plants thought to be abortives and emmenagogues. The *Visceralia* included a subgroup entitled *Venerea* which dealt with aphrodisiacs, *uterina* and *lactifera.* Drugs that affected sterility were included under the *Topica* heading. Linnaeus' entry for the ginger plant is typical:

Classis 1

MONANDRIA

MONOGYNIA

1. AMOMUM scapo radicato, spica ovata.

Inschi, Rheed. Mal. 11. P. 21. t. 12
Locus: India Orientalis Nunc Jamaica. Perennis, sera.

Pharm: ZINGIBERIS COMMUNIS Radix Zj. Condita cum Vel Sine Brodio.

ALBI Radix Zj, optima, Condita cum vel sine Brodio.

QUALITAS: Fervida, Servida, Acris, Aromatica, Subfragrans.
VIS: Calefaciens, (recens eccoprotica), Stomachica, stimulans.
USUS: Colica, Diarrhoea, Hysteria.
COMPOSITA: Andromach. Mithridat. Diascord. Benediot. Hamech. Diasatyrium, Alhandal, Troch. Agaric.

Reaction to *Materia Medica*

Although Carl Linnaeus is now highly regarded for his contributions to materia medica and botany, he did not always command such admiration and respect: *uva amara* (sour grapes) was evidenced from an unexpected quarter, a 'Society of Gentlemen in Edinburgh' in Scotland, the unnamed editors of the *Encyclopaedia Britannica* (1771). In the section on botany and its relationship to medicine, the editors firstly emphasized the importance of the knowledge of medicinal plants to the practice of physic. The reader, thus lulled into a false sense security, could not have expected the ensuing onslaught on Linnaeus in which he was likened to 'the most obscene romance-writer'! The core issue was Linnaeus' 'sexual system' of classifying plants into major groups which was based primarily on the number of their pistils and stamens.

The Society of Gentlemen further stated that 'Apart from introducing the Binomial System Linnaeus also introduced a method of reducing plants to classes, genera and species founded upon the supposition that vegetables propagate their species in a manner similar to that of animals ... it is from this circumstance that Linnaeus's system of botany has got the name of the sexual system ... he calls the stamina of flowers the males, or the male parts of generation; and the pistils females, or the female parts of generation, plants whose flowers contain both male and female parts, are said to be hermaphrodites, etc.... His classes, orders, and genera, are all derived from the number, situation, proportion, and other circumstances attending these parts.'

The authors finished their botanical section with a treatise entitled 'Of the Sexes of Plants' (saving their vitriol for the conclusion). In a historical review they outlined the many famous authors of antiquity who had propagated the theory of plant sexuality, and put forward arguments for and against the notion. Reverting to the Latin so as not to offend common delicacy the editors quoted Linnaeus and his description of the plant 'love scene': 'the calix is the bride-chamber in which the stamina and pistilla solemnize their nuptials, *Vel, si mavis Cunnus, feu Labia ejusdem, inter quae organa genitalia masculina & femina delicatissimae istae partes, foventur & ab externis injuriis muniuntur.'* The editors deduced in strident fashion that Linnaeus' works were flawed: 'In many parts of this Treatise, there is such a degree of indelicacy in the expression as can not be exceeded by the most obscene romance-writer ... It is a certain fact that obscenity is the very basis of the Linnaean system ... But the bad tendency upon morals is not the only evil produced by the sexual theory. It has loaded the best system of botany that has hitherto been invented, with a profusion of foolish and often unintelligible terms, which throw an obscurity upon the science, obstruct the progress of the learner, and deter him from ever entering upon the study.'

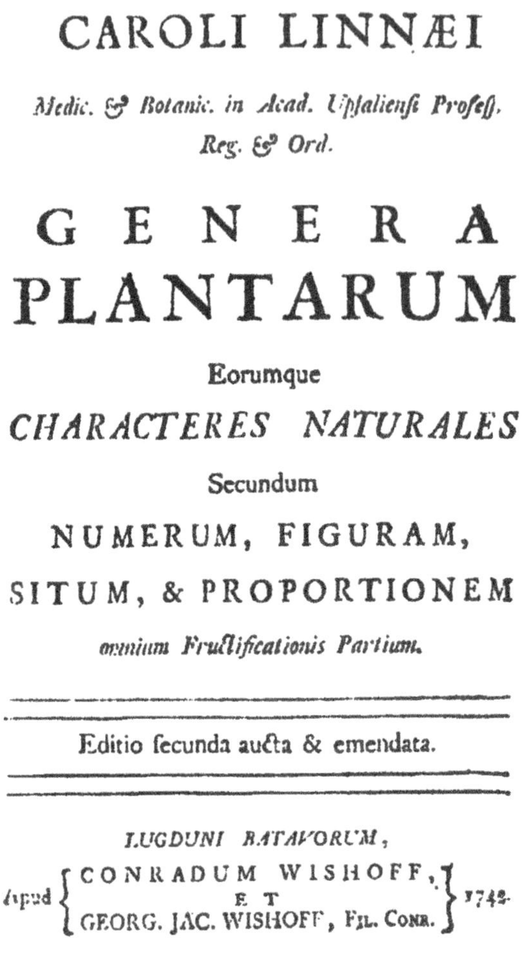

CAROLI LINNÆI

Medic. & Botanic. in Acad. Upſalienſi Profeſſ.
Reg. & Ord.

G E N E R A
PLANTARUM

Eorumque

CHARACTERES NATURALES

Secundum

NUMERUM, FIGURAM,
SITUM, & PROPORTIONEM

omnium Fructificationis Partium.

Editio ſecunda aucta & emendata.

LUGDUNI BATAVORUM,

Apud { CONRADUM WISHOFF, ET GEORG. JAC. WISHOFF, FIL. CONR. } 1742.

Figure 4 Frontispiece from *Genera Plantarum* by Carl Linnaeus (1707–1778)

CARL LINNAEUS (1707–1778): A BIOGRAPHY

Carl Linnaeus (Karl von Linné) was born in Råshult, Kristianstad, Sweden. His father, a parish curate, encouraged him to study for the ministry. However, the youth was so interested in botany and physic that his father relented and Carl was enrolled in the medical school at Uppsala University. As a student, he supervised the botanical physic garden there (founded in 1655) and kept careful notes on all the medicinal plants in his care. In 1732 he traveled extensively throughout Lapland, collecting plants. From there he moved to The Netherlands where he received his medical degree. In 1738 he returned to Sweden and practiced as a physician in Stockholm, becoming professor of medicine and botany at the University of Uppsala in 1741.

It was during this part of his career that Linnaeus formalized the Greek-rooted Latin nomenclature of plants. Many previous writers, including those of ancient Greece and Rome and the great Chinese herbalists, had designated plants by generic and specific binomials, but little attempt had been made at categorization. According to Jeremy Norman, editor of *Garrison and Morton's Bibliography* (1991), binomial nomenclature was probably devised in the first place by Joachim Jung, c. 1640, but Linnaeus advanced the system and developed formal classification. In Linnaeus' system, each plant was allocated two Latin names, the first of which was for the genus (or group) while the second for the species (or kind). Although amended later, this system is still used worldwide to identify plants. Linnaeus' success in developing a system of botanical classification led to similar but unsuccessful attempts to classify diseases.

Linnaeus wrote in Latin under the name Carolus Linnaeus or Caroli Linnaei. He developed the theory of his plant classification in his *Systema Naturae* (1735), the most important edition of which was the 10th, published in two volumes (1758–1759). His *Materia Medica* (1749) laid out the important medicinal plants, some of which are mentioned below. In his *Species Plantarum* (1753) Linnaeus described almost 8000 plants using the binomial system, clearly demonstrating its value. Linnaeus was an avid reader and writer and mentioned many authors in his texts. He was of the opinion that John Bartram, a pioneer of America's earliest botanical garden at Philadelphia, and the first native born American botanist, was the greatest naturalist and botanist of the era.

Linnaeus gave ginseng its first systematic description, calling the genus to which the plant belongs, *Panax*. *Panax* comes from the Greek *pan,* meaning all, and *akos,* meaning cure, that is 'all-healing' or a panacea. The name ginseng is the sound of two Chinese characters, *gin* (man) and *seng* (essence). In Chinese medicine ginseng was thought to vitalize the five organs; increase the intellect; prolong life; relax the agitated nervous and cardiovascular systems; and keep one young. *Linnaea borealis* is a plant named for and by Carl Linnaeus (Bown, 1995). His own description of *Linnaea* was 'a plant of Lapland, lowly, insignificant, disregarded but for a brief space – from Linnaeus who resembles it'. Linnaeus was ennobled, and styled 'Carl von Linnaeus' in recognition of his medical and botanical achievements, and his epitaph on a monument in Uppsala cathedral describes him as *Princeps Botanicorum* (Stearn, 1992).

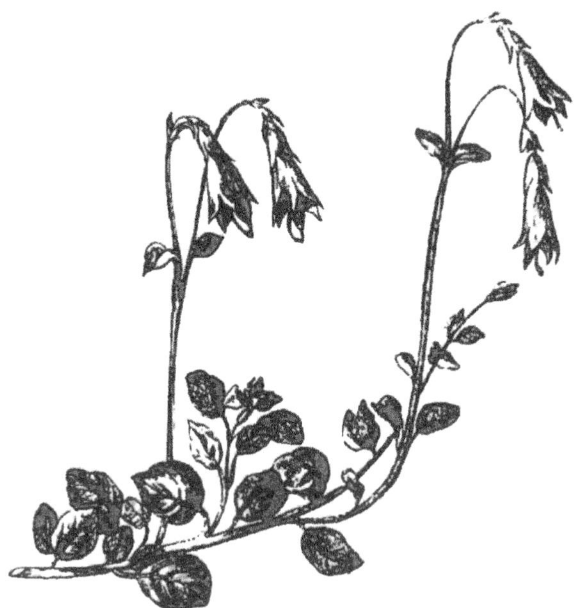

Figure 5 *Linnaea borealis*

WILLIAM SMELLIE'S *TREATISE ON THE THEORY AND PRACTICE OF MIDWIFERY*

This was the first volume of the three-part series that was William Smellie's celebrated contribution to the works on obstetrics and gynecology. The second and third volumes appeared in print in 1754 and (posthumously) in 1764, respectively. The *Treatise of the Theory and Practice of Midwifery* (1752) contained an introduction of 72 pages followed by 454 pages of text. An extra nine pages of advertising were included for his volume of anatomical drawings and illustrations of obstetric instruments.

A

TREATISE

ON THE

Theory and Practice

OF

MIDWIFERY.

By W. SMELLIE, M.D.

LONDON:

Printed for D. Wilson, at Plato's Head, near Round-Court, in the Strand.

MDCCLII.

Figure 6 Frontispiece from Smellie's *Treatise on ..... Midwifery*

The Preface

William Smellie wrote that he had intended to publish his treatise as a set of lectures, as delivered in a midwifery course. The treatise '[was not] cooked up in a hurry ... above six years ago I began to commit my lectures to paper, for publication: and from that period, have from time to time altered, amended and digested what I had written, according to the new lights I received from study and experience'. Over a ten-year period in London, he had instructed over 900 pupils, in almost 280 courses on midwifery, and during that time 1150 poor women had been delivered in the presence of his pupils. Smellie also ran a private practice 'which hath been pretty extensive' at the same time.

The Introduction

Smellie treated the reader to an outline of the history of obstetrics and gynecology with the opening words: 'It must be a satisfaction to those who begin the study of any art or science, to be made acquainted with the rise and progress of it.' Seventy-two pages later he reminded the reader that ... 'we find among the ancients, several valuable jewels, buried under the rubbish of ignorance and superstition because the assistance of men was seldom solicited in cases of Midwifery, till the last extremity'.

Book I

In this portion of the treatise Smellie dealt with '[the] structure and form of the pelvis ... the external and internal parts of generation proper to women ... of the Catamenia and Flour Albus ... [and] conception'. He also included observations on the changes of pregnancy, multiple gestation, abortion and the structure and function of the placenta.

Smellie defined the stages of miscarriage, now obsolete but worth recording: 'A miscarriage that happens before the tenth day, was formerly called an efflux, because the Embrio and secundines are not then formed, and nothing but the liquid conception, or Genitura is discharged. From the tenth day to the third month, it was known by the term expulsion ... betwixt that period and the seventh month, she was said to suffer an abortion ... when delivery happens between the seventh month and full time, the woman is said to be in labor ... but instead of these distinctions, if she loses her burden at any time from conception to the seventh or eighth, or even in the nineth month, we now say indiscriminately, she has miscarried, or parted with the child'.

The materia medica of Book I

Amenorrhea If the menses were retained Smellie was of the opinion that the woman became plethoric and that she should be treated by exercise, fumigation, plentiful bleedings, repeated purges, and warm baths. His materia medica included 'chalybeat and mercurial medicines, together with warm, bitter and stomachic ingredients, assisted with proper diet and exercise, according to the prescriptions to be found in Hoffman, Friend's *Emmenologia*, and Shaw's *Practise of Physick*.

Flour albus Smellie described the flour albus as a profuse discharge of mucus from the canal of the 'neck of the uterus'. His therapy included cathartics, emetics, purging and venesection and he also believed that exercise was beneficial. Anodynes were prescribed if the flour albus was thought to be of cancerous nature. He again advised that prescriptions be obtained from Hoffman.

Book II

The main topics discussed in this book were 'the diseases incident to pregnant women' and there were chapters devoted to nausea and vomiting; hemorrhoids, leg edema, dypsnea, incontinence of urine, and venereal disease. Other subjects explored were miscarriage, intrauterine fetal death, delivery of the placenta and 'flooding'.

The materia medica of Book II

'Flooding' (antepartum hemorrhage) 'On the first appearance of flooding, the patient ought immediately to be blooded to the amount of eight to twelve ounces ... if costive [constipated], an emollient clyster must be injected ... and mixtures of the tincture of roses and rhubarb acidulated with spirit of vitriol ... shall seem to be indicated.'

Gonorrhea and lues venerea (syphilis) The treatment consisted of 'bleeding, repeated doses of gentle cathartics mixed with Mercurials, a low diet, emulsions impregnated with Nitre, and lastly, balsamic, strengthening, and astringent medicines.'

Hemorrhoids Bothersome piles were treated by applying leeches 'to the parts'.

Leg swelling and dypsnea The woman was generally relieved 'by bleeding at the arm or ancle to the amount of eight or ten ounces'. Emollient glysters and laxative medicines were offered and oil of almonds and syrup of violets were taken nightly with rhubarb and 'opening pills'. Women with resistant edema were treated with 'Confect. Cardiac' in strong wine, to which warm spices were added.

Nausea and vomiting of early pregnancy 'A light, nutrative and spare diet' were advised and 'if she is costive, emollient clysters and opening medicines'.

Book III

This part of the volume dealt with 'the Child's situation in the Uterus' and had portions devoted to 'touching', 'the signs of conception', true and false labor and 'The division of Labours'. Smellie informed the reader that in natural labor the head presented, while in praeternatural labor 'the child is brought by the feet, or the body delivered before the head'. Smellie wrote that the left lateral position was known as the 'London method' although it was described by Fielding Ould in his *Treatise of Midwifery* (1742) as being the 'Dublin method'.

The materia medica of Book III

'Touching' 'Touching is performed by introducing the forefinger lubricated with pomatum into the vagina.' Pomatum was a medicated ointment or cream, normally used on the hair or as an application for beautifying the face. The name is the Latinized form of the French *pommade*, originally derived from the Latin *pomum*, an apple, as apples made up a considerable part of the original formulation of apple pulp, lard and rosewater (Wootton, 1910 vol. 2, p. 298).

'Lingering labor' 'It will be convenient to prescribe some innocent Placemus ... but if she is actually weak and exhausted it will be necessary to order something that will quicken the circulating fluids, such as preparations of amber, castor, myrrh, volatile spirits, the pulv. myrrh composit. of the *London*, or pulv. ad partum of the *Edinburgh Pharmacopoeia*, with everything in point of diet and drink that nourishes and strengthens the body.' The intriguing *pulvis ad partum*, later used to describe ergot (the sclerotium of *Claviceps purpurea*) does not, however, appear in my copy of the *Edinburgh Pharmacopoeia* (1817).

Instrumental delivery In his section 'Of laborious labours' Smellie wrote of the causes and management of difficult and prolonged labor. He detailed the use of fillets, forceps and of Amand's net. Smellie also described the extraction of the infant with a crochet when the child could be 'neither delivered by turning, nor extracted with the forceps, and it is absolutely necessary to deliver the woman to save her life'. The woman meanwhile would be supported by 'frequent draughts of broth, jelly, caudle, weak cordial and anodyne medicines'. Smellie's text on midwifery contains the first set of rules for the safe use of the obstetric forceps.

Resuscitation of the newborn In his tract 'How to manage the Child after Delivery' Smellie noted '[sometimes] the child, if alive, is not easily recovered: sometimes a great many minutes are elapsed before it begins to breathe.' In that situation he advised that 'the child be kept warm, moved, shaken, whipt; the head, temples, and breast, rubbed with spirits, garlic, onion, or mustard applied to the mouth and nose'. Smellie also advised that 'the child has been sometimes recovered by blowing into the mouth with a silver Canula, so as to expand the lungs'. This was the first reference to the 'modern' approach to resuscitation of the newborn in an obstetric text.

Cesarean section The author gave detailed instructions for the performance of cesarean section and wrote that 'the apparatus consists of a bistory [surgical knife], probe, scissars, large needles threaded, spunges, warm water, pledgets, a large tent or dossil [a plug or cloth dressing], compresses, and a bandage for the belly'. At the completion of the operation the uterus was not repaired but the anterior abdominal wall was stitched with interrupted sutures. The wound was 'dressed with dry pledgets or dossils dipped in some liquid balsam, warmed, covered with compresses moistened with wine and bandaged to keep on the dressings and sustain the belly'. If the woman was seen to be in great danger of death, she was offered 'broths, caudles, and wine ... the Cort. Peruvian. administered in powder, decoction, or extract, is frequently of great service in this case'. Cort. Peruvian, or cinchona, contains quinine and other alkaloids known to be antiseptic, to reduce fevers and to slow the heart rate (as well as their antimalarial effects).

Book IV

Here William Smellie used his wide experience to advise on 'The Management of Women from the Time of their Delivery to the End of the Month, with the several Diseases to which they are subject during that Period'.

The materia medica of Book IV

After-care On the completion of childbirth the woman was cleansed and pomatum applied to the external parts to relieve the discomfort. A nourishing drink of warm wine or caudle laced with 'nutmeg and sugar grated together in a spoon' was offered to the exhausted parturient.

Infection Genital infection was treated by venesection and 'warm fomentations, cataplasms and emollient glysters ... in order to avoid this mischance [sloughing of the vagina] emollient injections ought frequently to be thrown up into the Uterus, and large tents or dossils dipt in vulnerary balsams, applied in the Vagina Os Externum'.

Lacerations The tears and lacerations resulting from childbirth were treated with 'Lunar caustick: and if the opening is large ... with a double stitch'.

Milk fever Cort. Peruvian, confect. cardiac, subastringents and opiates were all advised for the fever accompanying breast infection in the puerperium. Confect. cardiac, a tonic, contained up to 60 ingredients. The compound has a long history, beginning with Sir Walter Raleigh and ending with pulvis cretae aromaticus BP in the late nineteenth century.

Retention of lochia with fever The potentially fatal childbed fever was treated with absinthe, castor, cinnamon water, lemon juice, opiates and syrup of crocus.

Suppression of lactation If the woman wished not to breastfeed, 'in order to prevent too great a turgency in the vessels in the breasts, and the secretion of milk', the breasts were covered with emplaster di minio, diaplama or emplastrum simple, or with cloths dipped in camphorated spirits. Sudorifics (agents that promote sweating) were prescribed if the other remedies were not helpful.

Prolapse Smellie used pessaries 'of a flat form, with a little hole in the middle, and made of cork waxed over, ivory, box, ebony, [or] lignum vitae, of a triangular, quadrangular, oval or circular shape'.

Uterine inflammation Fomentations and poultices were applied.

Uterine purge Clysters, laxatives and venesection were prescribed to induce uterine bleeding 20 days post-delivery in the woman who was not breast feeding or who had insufficient lochia.

Smellie included a section on the diet of the parturient woman and the treatment of constipation. He concluded his first volume with chapters on 'the Management of New-Born Children with the Diseases to which they are Subject'; 'the requisite Qualifications of Accoucheurs, Midwives, Nurses, who attend lying-in women'; and 'wet and dry Nurses for Children'.

WILLIAM SMELLIE'S *A COLLECTION OF CASES AND OBSERVATIONS IN MIDWIFERY*

In the preface to this, his second great volume on obstetrics, William Smellie wrote that between 1722 and 1739 he took notes of all 'the remarkable cases that occurred in midwifery; and that in London since the year 1740, to the present time I have been more careful and minute in forming a collection with a view to make it public'. This book contains a collection of unusual cases undertaken by Smellie in his midwifery practice, laid out in 30 chapters and comprising 512 pages. Only a small number of medications are mentioned.

WILLIAM SMELLIE'S *A COLLECTION OF PRETERNATURAL CASES AND OBSERVATIONS IN MIDWIFERY*

This volume was printed after Smellie's death, and so instead of the usual introduction there was an 'Advertisement' from the publishers:

> 'It may be necessary to inform the public, that this volume of Preternatural Cases in Midwifery, compleats the plan of Dr Smellie's work, and fulfills a promise which he made in the preface prefixed to the preceding volume ... This, with the two former volumes, we may venture to call a Compleat System of Midwifery. It is the fruit of forty years experience, enriched with an incredible variety of practice.'

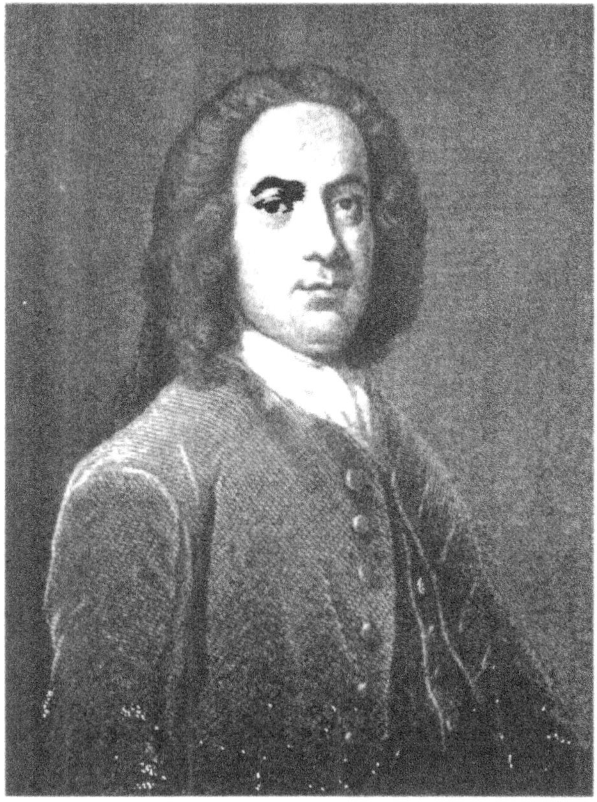

Figure 7 William Smellie (1697–1763)

This third volume of 544 pages contained collections of Smellie's interesting and unusual cases. Details of medications form only a minute portion of the text.

WILLIAM SMELLIE (1697–1763): A BIOGRAPHY

William Smellie was born in the village of Lanark in Scotland. Accounts vary somewhat but it appears that Smellie was apprenticed to William Inglis, a local apothecary, and thereafter went to sea and qualified as a surgeon's mate. It is also related that Smellie served a medical apprenticeship with a Dr Gordon. Smellie studied medicine at Glasgow and in 1720, at the age of 23, began his practice of medicine in Lanark. He served the community as a family doctor, physician, surgeon and accoucheur for the following 19 years. The eminent English historian Herbert Spencer, professor of obstetric medicine at University College, London, told the story that Smellie 'used to carry in his pocket spirits of Hartshorn, tincture of Castor and liquid Laudanum in separate bottles, and from these he compounded his medicines' (1927 pp. 43–60).

Smellie was distressed by the results of local midwifery practice and thus began his avid interest in obstetrics. Palmer Findley (1939) wrote that Smellie observed at first hand the brutal management of difficult labors 'in the hands of midwives whose blunt hook and crochet were ever ready at hand when nature's forces failed'. He continued: 'Midwives and local practitioners never employed version and so mutilating operations were freely resorted to in obstructed labors.' Smellie made notes of his experiences in maternity care and studied all the well-known obstetric texts. At the age of 42 he went to London in search of further obstetric expertise but was disappointed by the state of midwifery there and went to Paris to study under Gregoire the Elder in 1739. On his return, he began a midwifery practice, first in Pall Mall, London, then at Gerrard Street and later at Wardour Street. As soon as he was well established he began to teach the art of obstetrics.

Smellie constructed ingenious models for instruction which he used in the process of childbirth, described here by a pupil (Findley, 1939):

> 'they are composed of real bones mounted and covered with artificial Ligaments, Muscles and Cuticle to give them the true Motion, Shape and Beauty of natural Bodies and the contents of the Abdomen are imitated with great exactness ... Besides his large machines (which are three in number) he has finished six artificial Children with the same minute Proportions in all their Parts, so that with the apparatus he can perform and demonstrate all the different kinds of Delivery with more Deliberation, Perspicuity, and Fulness that can be expected on real Subjects.'

James Hobson Aveling, the English historian and obstetrician, told the story of how Smellie fell foul of the midwives in London, particularly a Mrs Elizabeth Nihell, an ardent critic of 'he-practisers' and 'instrumentarians'. Mrs Nihell trained as a midwife at the Hôtel Dieu, Paris, and practiced with her surgeon–apothecary in the Haymarket, London. As the acknowledged leader of the midwives she strongly opposed the new man-midwives and the obstetric forceps they had introduced. Nihell put pen to paper and wrote: '[the] disciples of Dr Smellie ... in short those broken barbers, tailors, or even pork butchers ... [are] turned [into] an intrepid physician and man-midwife ... to arms! to arms! is the word; and what are those arms by which they maintain themselves, but those instruments [the obstetric forceps], those weapons of death' (Aveling, 1872). Medical practitioners also became embroiled in the man-midwifery controversy (see above). Despite discrimination and intimidation, however, Smellie continued on his chosen career.

Until the introduction of the obstetric forceps, Smellie's obstetric equipment consisted of a blunt hook, a noose, a straight crochet and a perforator – all instruments designed for the destruction of the undelivered dead child. Only his own hands were at his command in delivering the living child. Smellie experimented with the obstetric forceps and designed a long curved forceps which was a big improvement on those already available. He used a wooden forceps for a time so that women would not be frightened by the clanking sounds of the metal variety.

Some aspects of Smellie's obstetric practice, particularly his conservative approach to placental delivery, were very similar to the methods of Fielding Ould, but he made no reference to Ould in his text. Smellie was the first to apply forceps to the after-coming head in breech presentations and he is eponymously remembered in the Mauriceau–Smellie–Veit maneuver in breech deliveries. (This consisted of exerting traction on the fetus with one hand over the fetal shoulders and the fingers of the other hand in either the mouth or on each side of the infant's nose.) Smellie gained his MD from the University of Glasgow in 1745. He was a prolific writer and his most outstanding contribution, his three volume set, including *A Treatise on the Theory and Practice of Midwifery*, ensured Smellie's influence throughout England, Europe and America.

At the age of 62 Smellie retired to his native village of Lanark with his wife Eupham, whom he had married in 1724 (the couple were childless). In Lanark Smellie put the finishing touches to the third volume of his work but he died before it was published. He was interred on 5 March 1763, near the wall of St Kentigern's Kirk in Lanark. Eupham died six years later at the age of 79 at a time when William Smellie's *Treatise on Midwifery* had achieved 'worldwide' fame. William Smellie was honored by being accorded the appellation, the 'master of British midwifery'.

A SELECTION OF EIGHTEENTH CENTURY MATERIA MEDICA

Medications whose names bore the prefix *dia* are of great antiquity and were popular from ancient Greco-Roman times until the late nineteenth century. They include a large number of compounded medicines, and many were used in the materia medica of women, such as diachylon, diabolanum, diagrydium and dia-sulphuris. Information about dia medicines is difficult to obtain and so this section of the chapter is entirely devoted to them. The Greek preposition *dia* means through or from, and appears in many English words. In relation to therapeutics, it denotes a compound medication, usually an electuary or a confection.

To make matters confusing, when the dia went out of fashion the dia compounds had their names changed, e.g. diascordium (an electuary) became known as 'electuarium diascordium'. The dia medications were available as powders, electuaries and plasters. Nicholas Culpeper, in his *London Dispensatorie* of 1654, included the lists of ingredients and the formulation method for dia medications and their indications in the seventeenth century. The dia medications reached their peak popularity in the nineteenth century. Perusal of *The Works of Aristotle* (Pseudo-Aristotle, 1830) revealed 25 different dia formulations which were used for fertility treatment, menstrual problems, uterine inflammation, vaginal discharge, pregnancy sickness and for skin complaints. Remnants of the 'dia fashion' were to be found in therapeutics until late in the twentieth century, e.g. diamorphine (diacetylmorphine), the addictive analgesic and potent respiratory depressant, heroin.

Diachylon

Diachylon is the Greek for 'with juices' and the original prescription contained litharge (lead oxide) and plant sap. In ancient Greco-Roman times Soranus of Ephesus, second century AD, advised diachylon suppositories for 'hysteria', menstrual disorders and urethritis, and a diachylon cataplasm or plaster was available for the treatment of molar pregnancy (Temkin, 1956; Wootton, 1910 vol. 1). It is claimed that the original formula for diachylon plaster was compiled by Claudius Menecrates, physician to Emperor Tiberius. Menecrates is also credited with a work on remedies *Autocrator Hologrammatos,* which translates as 'The Emperor, whose words are written in full'. The *Autocrator* was so-named because it was dedicated to Tiberius.

The renowned Galen of Pergamum (AD 131–201) altered the formula for diachylon by including the mucilage of fenugreek, of linseed, and of marshmallow, and old oil of golden litharge (mucilage was obtained by boiling the seeds and roots in water). Almost five centuries later diachylon was prescribed by Paul of Aegina (AD 620–690) for inflammation of the uterus secondary to injury or to 'retention of the menses'. If the uterine inflammation was very painful he also applied poppy juice per vagina. He offered the medication after miscarriage or childbirth. Paul instructed that the diachylon plaster should be melted in a double vessel with rose oil and the juice of plantain, of endive, or of succory (Adams, 1844 vol. 1).

The Arabian physician, Mesue the Elder (AD 777–837), wrote at length about the diachylon plaster and further complicated its formula by the addition of extra herbs mixed with lanolin and wax. Mesue was a Christian who became director of the hospital at Baghdad and he was one of the principal Arabic translators of the era. From Thomas Raynold's *The Byrth of Mankynde* we learn that diachylon plaster was 'layde over all the bottome of the bellye & the pryuie passage, to provoke and drawe furth the latter or hynder byrthe if nede be' (1545, Folio 105).

In 1746 The London College of Physicians altered the name of diachylon to 'emplastrum commune' but the old name refused to die. In the nineteenth and twentieth centuries diachylon was commonly known as 'emplastrum plumbi' (lead oleate). At that time diachylon ointment was formed (in another revised formula) by melting together equal parts of lead plaster and soft paraffin, and mixing this with an equal quantity of zinc and mercuric oleate ointments. Diachylon was recommended for sweaty feet by Hobart Amory Hare, professor of therapeutics and materia medica at Jefferson Medical College, Philadelphia (Hare, 1901). On a more serious note, however, J.W. Ballantyne (1906) of London recalled that diachylon pills were used to provoke abortion.

Diamargariton

Diamargariton was a remedy used to help deliver the placenta (Raynold, 1545 Folio 74):

> 'and if in this meane whyle the woman faynte or sowne by reason of great payne ensuynge of the takynge awaye of this secondyne, then must ye ministyre suche thynges to her they which comforte the head and the harte, as be electuaries which are conficte with Muske, Ambre and the confection of precious stones: as Diamargariton, and such other. Also such thynges the which comfort the stomacke: as Diagalanga, Diacinamomum, and suche lyke whiche are alwaye in a readinesse at the Apothecaries, the whiche also she shall receaue with wine.'

'Diarmargariton', wrote Culpeper, quoting the Arab physician, Avicenna, 'is appropriate to women, and in them to diseases incident to their matrix, but his reasons I know not.' Diamargariton frigidum was known to 'restore such as have labored long'. Diarmagariton, a medicine which 'cherasheth the Animal Vital Spirits' was thought to be 'special good for women' (Culpeper, 1654). It was employed for the pregnant woman who had fainted, by James Wolveridge (1671).

Diascordium

Diascordium was a compound medicine devised to prevent the ravages of the plague by Frascatorius, a physician and poet of high repute in the early sixteenth century, who wrote the famous poem *Syphilis, sive morbus Gallicus.* The poem, published in 1530, described the skin lesions of syphilis and their treatment with mercury (Wootton, 1910 vol. 1). Diascordium became so popular that it was used for many ailments, rivaling the famous 'Venus treacle' invented by Andromachus during the reign of the tyrannical emperor, Nero (AD 54–68). The original formula for diascordium was a complex mixture of bistort, bole armeniac, cassia wood, cinnamon, clarified honey, Cretan dittany, galbanum, gentian, ginger, gum arabic, Lemnian earth, long pepper, opium, scordium (water germander), sorrel seeds and storax made into an electuary (Wootton, 1910 vol. 2).

In his *London Dispensatorie,* Culpeper had this to say about the compound: 'It is a well composed Electuary, a something appropriate to the nature of women, for it Provokes the Terms, hastens their Labor, helps their usual sickness at the time of their Lying-in, I know nothing better.' His seventeenth century contemporary, the Irish accoucheur–physician James Wolveridge, offered diascordium in a caudle if 'the child is costive' (1671). In 1746 two forms of diascordium were available, either with or without opium. The compound was a popular household opiate and was frequently given to children for soothing purposes. As was the case with most dia medicines, its composition was altered over the years by deleting a number of the components. Eventually, in a formula that contained canary wine, diascordium evolved into what became known as 'pulvis catechu compositus' in the British pharmacopoeia.

Diatessaron

This compound was composed of equal parts of *Aristolochia rotunda* (birthwort root), centaury, gentian root, the tops and leaves of germander and ground pine. Variants of the compound are to be found in the works of the great Byzantine medical encyclopedists Aetius of Amida, Alexander of Tralles and Paul of Aegina. During the Middle Ages, treacle of diatessaron with bull's gall, cockle flour, myrrh, rue and savin was included in a suppository used to induce menstruation (Rowland, 1981). Diatessaron was advised in *The Byrth of Mankynde* to induce labor in the presence of intrauterine death: 'take the treacle Diatessaron: and geue of it to the women for to drynke, and it will expel this dead byrthe' (Raynold, 1545 Folio 99).

Nicholas Culpeper gave a formula for diatessaron in his *London Dispensatorie* (1654): 'Take Gentian, Bayberries, Mirrh, Round Birthwort, of each two ounces, Honey 2 lb, make them into a electuary according to Art.' The name and constituents of the compound altered from time to time and other names included antidotos podagrica and tetrapharmacum. Diatessaron medication had to be taken for up to a year and was therefore also called *medicamentum ad annum*. Diatessaron was a popular treatment until well into the nineteenth century. It was used by the Duke of Portland to treat gout and was eventually available as the 'Duke of Portland's Gout Powder' (Wootton, 1910 vol. 1).

A brief review of some other dia medications

Diacalamentha 'This seems to be ... appropriate to the feminine gender ... viz. To bring down the Terms in women, to bring away the birth and the after-birth, to Purge them after Labor, yet it is dangerous for women with child. ...Diacalamentha compound [and] Diacalamentha simple ... provokes Urin and the Terms in Women ... [The compound contains] Mountain Calaminth, Pennyroyal, Origanum, the seeds of Macedonion Parsley, Common Parsley, and Hartwort, the seed of Smallage, the tops of Time, the seeds of Lovage, black Pepper, make them into Pouder according to the Art' (Culpeper, 1654).

Diacaloythios An emplaster of diacaloythios was applied 'between the hips', to prevent abortion (Wolveridge, 1671).

Diacinnamomum 'Or in plain English, a composition of Cinnamon, heats the stomach...Provokes the Terms in Women' (Culpeper, 1654). Diacinnamomum was one of the remedies advised to help expel the placenta in *The Byrthe of Mankynde* (Raynold, 1545 Folio 74).

Diacitonicon This medicinal syrup was prescribed as a uterine purge in the Middle Ages (Rowland, 1981).

Diacodion This was a medieval compound medicine used to purge the uterus of blood (Rowland, 1981). Diacodion (also referred to as diacodium) and another compound, diagredium (or diagrydium) were first introduced by Themison, a physician who lived during the reign of Augustus Caesar (31 BC–AD 14), the era of classical Roman literature (Wootton, 1910 vol. 1).

Diacolocynthidos Nicholas Culpeper (1654) wrote: 'It helps the falling sickness, madness ... pains in the breasts and stomach ... hardness of women's breasts.'

Diaconiton This syrup was used to prevent vomiting in women (Rowland, 1981).

Diacorallion 'It stops the Terms and Whites in Women, if administered by one whose wits are not a wool gathering' (Culpeper, 1654).

Diacydonium 'Stop fluxes and the Terms in Women' (Culpeper, 1654).

Diagalanga 'such thynges the whiche comforte the stomacke: as Diagalanga, Diacinnamomum, and suche lyke whiche are alwaye in a readinesse at the apothecaries, the whiche also she shall receaue with wyne ... yf the secondyne [placental] tarye or stycke' (Raynold, 1545 Folio 74).

Dialacca This compound contained gum lacca and a large number of herbs including rhubarb: 'let women with child forebear it', wrote Culpeper (1654).

Diapompholigos François Mauriceau, in his *The Diseases of Women with Child, and in Child Bed* (1683), wrote a tract on inflammation of the umbilical region in the newborn. Among a large number of treatments he included the application of diapompholigos 'with a Swathe to keep them fast, until the navel be ciccatrized and preferably healed'.

Diasatyron This medication contained upwards of 30 components including aniseed, cinnamon, cloves, erigno, garden parsnips, ginger, Indian nuts, pine nuts, rocket, satyrion and other botanicals, mixed with musk and sugar, dissolved in malaga wine, and made into an electuary. Culpeper (1654) noted that 'it provokes lust exceedingly and speedily helps such as are impotent in the acts of Venus; you make take two drachms, or more at a time'.

Diaspermaton This was thought to be one of the best cordials for inducing uterine bleeding during the Middle Ages (Rowland, 1981). Nicholas Culpeper (1654) was in agreement: 'Diaspermaton Provoked the Urine – and by inference – the Terms'.

A selection of remedies for women in the eighteenth century

Absynth, aceto syr. asafetida, agnus castus, amber, amygdala dulcet, angelica, anise, *Aristolochia*, artemisia

Balsam, bole armeniack, brandy, Brasilian rubr. lign., bryonia, burnt feathers

Calendula, calomel, camphor, castor, chalybeate waters, confectio cardiaca, coriandum, coris, cort. Peruvian, cyclamen (sow bread), cynoglossum

Damocrat, diambra, *Dictamnus creticus*, dossils of lint

Elaterium, elect. mithridat., emollient clyster, emollient decoctions, emollient herbs, emulsions in nitre, enulae herb, epithemes, eryngium, exil.vitrioli

Foeniculum, fragaria, frankincense, French claret, fresh butter, Fuller's earth

Galanga, galbanum, garlic, gentian root, geranium robert., Glauber's salt, glysters, guajacum, gum olibanum, gum plant

Helleborus niger, hirundinaria, hyssop, hyoscyamus

Imperatoria, indigo, ipecacuanha, iris

Jasminum, jelly broth, julep cordial

Lactuca, laudanum, laxative glyster, leeches, ligusticum, lilium, linaria, lunar caustic

Magnesia, mandragora, manna, mastich, matricaria, mel rosarum, *Mentha sylvestris*, mercury, mulled wine, myrrh

Nigella, nitre, nitrous medicines, nutmeg, nymphaea

Oil, oil of sweet almonds, oleum hyosciami, olibanum, onions, opening clysters, opium, opobalsamum, opopanax, oxycrate

Paeony, papaver, paragorick draught, petroselinum, pilul. gummos, *Piper nigrum*, pulv. castor, pulv. ipecacuan, pulv. myrrh, pulv. rhababari

Rapa, red wine, rhubarb, rice, roman vitriol, rose

Sabina, sal ammoniac, saline draughts, sanguis draconis, sarsaparilla, sassafras, satyrium, sesamum, siler mont., solanum, spermaceti draughts

Tabacum, tartari vitrioli, theriac.venet., tincture of castor, tincture of roses, tincture thebaic, tolu balsamnum, tormentil

Valerian, vanilla, vin.rubr., vinegar, viola, vitriol, vomica nux, vulnerary balsams

Warm fomentations, warm milk, warm water, warm wine, water in which red hot iron was quenched, whey, white caudle, white wine, wine

Zedoaria longa, zingiber.

References

Adams, F. (1844). *The Seven Books of Paulus Ægineta*, translated from the Greek. Vol. 1, pp. 620–1. (London: The Sydenham Society)

Aveling, J. H. (1872). *English Midwives. Their History and Prospects*, pp. 118–26. (London: J. and A. Churchill)

Ballantyne, J. W. (1906). *Green's Encyclopedia and Dictionary of Medicine and Surgery*, Vol. 2, p. 337. (Edinburgh and London: William Green & Sons)

Bown, D. (1995). *The Royal Horticultural Society Encyclopedia of Herbs and their Uses*. (London: Dorling Kindersley)

Brody, S. A. (1978). The Life and Times of Sir Fielding Ould: Man-Midwife and Master Physician. *Bull. Hist. Med.*, 52, 228–50

Cameron, Charles A. (1916). *A History of the Royal College of Surgeons in Ireland*, pp. 32–3. (Dublin: Fannin & Co.)

Chapman, E. (1733). *An Essay on the Improvements of Midwifery*. (London: A. Bettersworth)

Cianfrani, T. (1960). *A Short History of Obstetrics and Gynecology*, pp. 223–71. (Springfield, IL: Charles C. Thomas)

Coakley, D. (1992). *Irish Masters of Medicine*, pp. 27–32. (Dublin: Townhouse)

Cowen, D. L. and Helfand, W. H. (1990). *Pharmacy. An Illustrated History*. (New York: Harry N. Abrams Inc.)

Culpeper, N. (1654). *Pharmacopoeia Londinensis or the London Dispensatorie*, pp. 198–222, 237. (London: Peter Cole)

Das, Sir K. (1929). *Obstetric Forceps. Its History and Evolution*, pp. 143–52. (Calcutta: The Art Press)

Encyclopaedia Britannica (1771). *Encyclopaedia Britannica or a Dictionary of Arts and Sciences, Compiled upon a new plan*, pp. 627–53. (Edinburgh: A. Bell and C. Macfarquhar)

Findley, L. P. (1939). *Priests of Lucina. The Story of Obstetrics*, pp. 169–77. (Austin: Little, Brown & Co.)

Fleetwood, J. F. (1983). *The History of Medicine in Ireland*, pp. 117–18. (Dublin: Skellig Press)

Hare, H. A. (1901). *A Text-Book of Practical Therapeutics*, p. 266. (London: Henry Kimpton)

Heberden, W. Snr (1745). *Antitheriaka: An Essay on Mithridiatum and Theriaca*. (London)

Hunter, W. (1774). *The Anatomy of the Human Gravid Uterus exhibited in Figures.* (Birmingham: John Baskerville)

Kirkpatrick, T. P. C. (1912). *History of the Medical Teaching in Trinity College Dublin and of the School of Physic in Ireland,* pp. 117, 123–5. (Dublin: Hanna & Neale)

Linnaei, C. (1749). *Materia Medica, Liber I. De Plantis.* (Holmiae: Laurentii Salvii)

Linnaei, C. (1753). *Species Plantarum.* (Stockholm: Salvius)

Linnaei, C. (1735). *Systema Naturae.* (Lugduni Batavorum, Apud Theodorum Haak)

Mauriceau, F. (1683). *The Diseases of Women with Child and in Child Bed. Translated by Hugh Chamberlen, M. D.,* p. 394. (London: John Darby)

McClintock, A. H. (1858). On the Rise of the Dublin School of Midwifery; with Memoirs of Sir Fielding Ould, and Dr J. C. Fleury. *Dublin Quart. J. Med. Sci.* XXV(49), 1–20

Norman, J. M. (1991). *Garrison and Morton. Morton's Medical Bibliography,* 5th ed. p. 20. (Vermont: Gower Publishing Co.)

O'Donel Browne, T. D. (1947). *The Rotunda Hospital 1745–1945,* pp. 21–2. (Edinburgh: E. & S. Livingstone Ltd.)

Ould, F. (1742). *A Treatise of Midwifery. In Three Parts.* (Dublin: Oli. Nelson & Charles Connor)

Pharmacopoeia Edinburgensis (1817). *Pharmacopoeia Collegii Medicorum Edimburgensis.* (Edinburgh: Bell & Bradfute; D. Brown & A. Black)

Pseudo-Aristotle (1830). *The Works of Aristotle. The Famous Philosopher.* (London: Miller, Law and Cater)

Radcliffe, R. (1947). *The Secret Instrument. (The Birth of the Midwifery Forceps),* pp. 38–40. (London: William Heinemann Medical Books Ltd.)

Raynold, T. (1544). *The Byrth of Mankynde,* English translation, Folios 74, 105. (London: Tho. Ray)

Ricci, J. V. (1945). *One Hundred Years of Gynaecology.* (Philadelphia: Blakiston Co.)

Ricci, J. V. (1949). *The Development of Gynaecological Surgery and Instruments.* (Philadelphia: Blakiston Co.)

Rowland, B. (1981). *Medieval Woman's Guide to Health. The First English Gynaecological Handbook,* pp. 69, 79, 163. (London: Croom Helm)

Smellie, W. (1752). *A Treatise on the Theory and Practice of Midwifery.* (London: D. W. Wilson)

Smellie, W. (1754). *A Collection of Cases and Observations in Midwifery.* (London: D. W. Wilson and T. D. Durham)

Smellie, W. (1764). *A Collection of Preternatural Cases and Observations in Midwifery.* (London: D. W. Wilson and T. D. Durham)

Speert, H. (1980). *Obstetrics and Gynecology in America: A History.* (Chicago: The American College of Obstetricians and Gynecologsts)

Speert, H. (1994). *Obstetrics and Gynecology: A History and Iconography.* Revised Second Edition of *Iconographia Gyniatrica.* (San Francisco: Norman Publishing)

Spencer, H. (1927). *The History of British Midwifery from 1650 to 1800,* pp. 32, 43–60. (London: John Bale, Sons & Danielsson)

Stearn, W. T. (1992). *Stearn's Dictionary of Plant Names for Gardeners,* pp. 191–2. (London: Cassell)

Temkin, O. (1956). *Soranus' Gynecology,* pp. 141, 160. (Baltimore & London: The Johns Hopkins University Press)

Thoms, H. (1935). *Classical Contributions to Obstetrics and Gynecology.* (Springfield, IL: Charles C. Thomas)

Widdess, J. D. H. (1963). *A History of the Royal College of Physicians of Ireland. 1654–1963,* pp. 65, 66, 104–5. (Edinburgh and London: E & S Livingstone Ltd.)

Wolveridge, J. (1671). *Speculum Matricis or The Expert Midwives Handmaid,* pp. 112, 132, 137. (London: E. Okes)

Wootton, A. C. (1910). *Chronicles of Pharmacy,* Vol. 1, 91, 309, 406; Vol. 2, 127–9, 286–7, 298. (London: MacMillan & Co.)

The nineteenth century 16

INTRODUCTION

During the nineteenth century major changes occurred in medicine. The art of midwifery slowly developed into early 'scientific' obstetrics and gynecology. A plethora of books were produced on obstetrics and gynecology and many advances were made in the understanding of anatomy and physiology, and the pathology and therapeutics of women's diseases. Samuel Bard's *A Compendium of the Theory and Practice of Midwifery* (1807) was the first of many American texts on midwifery and severed the reliance of his countrymen and women on European publications. Ergot was introduced into mainstream medicine by John Stearns of New York in 1807. Amidst a medical, religious and social furor, James Young Simpson championed the use of anesthetics in midwifery from 1847. The scourge of puerperal sepsis was addressed and the era of antisepsis and chemotherapy in midwifery began in the latter part of the century.

The best work of the century on botanical medicine was the *Flora Medica* (1838) a worldwide survey of medicinal plants by John Lindley professor of botany in University College, London. In America Samuel Thompson detailed the North American medicinal herbs in 1835 and 1841 publications, while Albert Coffin's *Botanic Guide to Health* of 1866 proved to be another important text. Francis Adams' publications on Paul of Aegina and Arabian medicine in the 1840s (Chapter 11) are an important repository of information on the available materia medica for women.

From the early nineteenth century the chemical laboratory began to supplant mother nature as a source of medicines. Narcotic alkaloids were isolated from the opium poppy (*Papaver somniferum*) in 1804 by the German pharmacist, Friedrich Wilhelm Sertürner, who discovered morphine as the active agent of opium. He was a pioneer of the pharmacological experiments that introduced the vegetable alkaloids. The other important alkaloids, atropine, cocaine, hyoscyamine and quinine were introduced

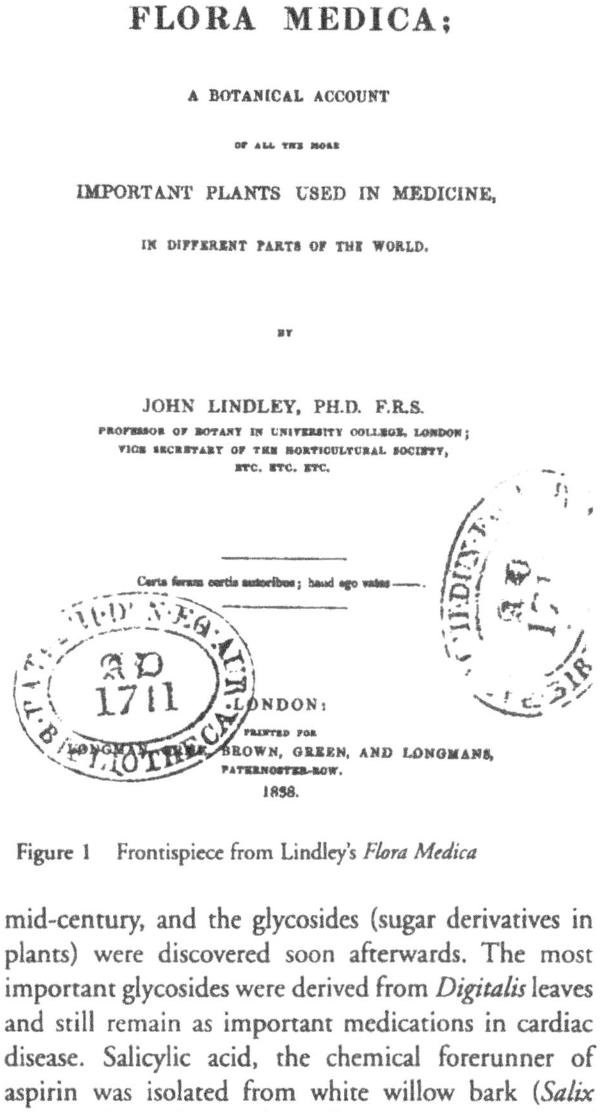

FLORA MEDICA;

A BOTANICAL ACCOUNT

OF ALL THE MORE

IMPORTANT PLANTS USED IN MEDICINE,

IN DIFFERENT PARTS OF THE WORLD.

BY

JOHN LINDLEY, PH.D. F.R.S.

PROFESSOR OF BOTANY IN UNIVERSITY COLLEGE, LONDON;
VICE SECRETARY OF THE HORTICULTURAL SOCIETY,
ETC. ETC. ETC.

Certa ferens certis auctoribus; haud ego vates.—

LONDON:
PRINTED FOR
LONGMAN, [illegible] BROWN, GREEN, AND LONGMANS,
PATERNOSTER-ROW.
1838.

Figure 1 Frontispiece from Lindley's *Flora Medica*

mid-century, and the glycosides (sugar derivatives in plants) were discovered soon afterwards. The most important glycosides were derived from *Digitalis* leaves and still remain as important medications in cardiac disease. Salicylic acid, the chemical forerunner of aspirin was isolated from white willow bark (*Salix alba*) and was first synthesized in 1859. Aspirin itself was first developed in Germany in 1899.

So-called 'herbal medicine', practiced by physicians since antiquity, and the newly evolved 'bio-medicine' began to drift apart. The new Western medicine came into conflict with traditional medical practice in Asia, Europe, and America, and it became illegal to practice 'complementary' medicine without an orthodox qualification. As a result, the National Institute of Medical Herbalists was formed in England in 1864 and, in time, the example was followed in most countries. This unfortunate schism between allopathic and other forms of medicine continued into and throughout the twentieth century. Many chemical substances were substituted for the tried and trusted medicinal herbs and new therapies such as electrotherapy came on stream.

Against this briefly-outlined background of tumultuous change in medicine, midwifery, science and therapeutics first the American and then the European materia medica for women is explored in this chapter.

SAMUEL BARD'S *A COMPENDIUM OF THE THEORY AND PRACTICE OF MIDWIFERY*

In 1955, Philip Williams of Philadelphia based his presidential address to the 78th Annual Meeting of American Gynecological Society, held in Quebec, on a book review of Samuel Bard's *A Compendium of the Theory and Practice of Midwifery* (1807) adding details about Bard's personal and professional lives. In his address, Williams wrote that he had selected Bard's *Compendium of Midwifery*, 'the first obstetrical text written by an American author published in the United States' as a matter of historical priority. Bard's text gains pride of place in this chapter for the same reason. The life and times of Samuel Bard were also related by Herbert Thoms, professor emeritus, obstetrics and gynecology and curator of Yale Medical Memorabilia, at Yale University, in his book, *Chapters in American Obstetrics* (1933).

The Introduction

> 'Having frequently in the course of my practice, and particularly since my residence in the country, had occasion to observe how much our midwives stand in need of instruction, ... I have thought that a concise, cheap book, containing a set of plain but correct directions for their practice in natural labors, and for the relief of such complaints, as frequently accompany pregnancy and labor, or which follow after delivery, would in the present state of this country prove a useful work. In a work of this nature, all claim to originality must necessarily be relinquished ... A little more has been added ... with copies of the most useful plates ... copied from the best works that could be met with, chiefly from Smellie, Hamilton and Bell.'

A

COMPENDIUM

OF THE THEORY AND PRACTICE

OF

MIDWIFERY,

Containing

PRACTICAL INSTRUCTIONS FOR THE MANAGEMENT OF

WOMEN

DURING PREGNANCY, IN LABOUR, AND IN CHILD-BED;

Calculated

To correct the Errors, and to improve the Practice, of

MIDWIVES;

As well as to serve as an Introduction to the

STUDY OF THIS ART,

For

STUDENTS AND YOUNG PRACTITIONERS.

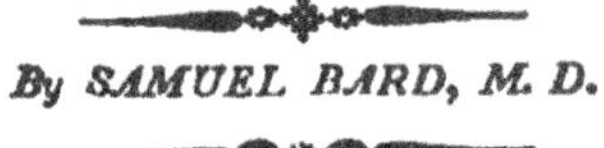

NEW-YORK:

PRINTED AND SOLD BY COLLINS AND PERKINS,

NO. 189, PEARL-STREET.

1807.

Figure 2 Frontispiece from Samuel Bard's *A Compendium ... of Midwifery*

Bard went on to recommend the obstetric writings of European practitioners but confessed that he had not 'mentioned Smellie, whose works are in the hands of almost every practitioner in this country'.

The main part of the book is divided into five chapters. Not included in the contents list was a historically important appendix of 22 pages that Bard devoted to the materia medica of midwifery, details of which appear below.

Chapter I

Concentrating on the skeletal aspects of the female pelvis, Bard provided anatomical descriptions illustrated by four etchings of the pelvis, one of the fetal skull, one of a cephalic presentation of a fetus *in utero* with the vertex descending into mid pelvis, and a lateral section of the pelvis illustrating the soft tissues. Bard's discourse on 'the Womb and its Appendages' had five illustrations that depicted the uterus, ovaries and early pregnancy.

Chapter II

Bard remarked that in regard to the regularity of the monthly discharge '[There] occurs great variety in this respect between different women'.

Delayed onset of menstruation 'Relaxed and feeble young women ... should make use of such remedies as tend to strengthen the habit in general, such as bitters, a glass of good wine, constant exercise in the open air ... the cold bath ... [they] should drink chalybeate water ... should take some mild preparation of iron, this remedy should be preceded by a vomit, and a cathartic ... having by these means strengthened the habit, they may take aloetic medicines, a dose or two of rhubarb and calomel, have sparks drawn from them at an electric machine, or employ warm bathing, by sitting in a warm bath, so that the water may rise above the hips.'

Painful menstruation Women were advised to observe the rules of good general health but 'when the pain is very severe to allay it with opium'.

Profuse flow of the menses Among the remedies prescribed were 'an infusion of rose leaves, or oak bark, and acidulated with the acid of vitriol'.

Menopause Bard gave general directions for women entering the menopause including 'this general observation: that every kind of excess, particularly that of spirituous liquors should be avoided'.

Sickness and vomiting of the early months For the hyperemesis of early pregnancy Bard advised 'a simple and light diet to correct acidity, to keep the bowels open by Magnesia, and to strengthen the stomach by a cup of cold Chamomile Tea or a light infusion of Gentian or Columbo'.

Hemorrhage before the fifth or sixth month Bard advised bloodletting, 'and copious in proportion to the strength of the patient ... [the] bowels should be immediately opened by salts ... saline draughts may be given every four or six hours, and five or six drops of Laudanum may be added to each.' He also advised intravaginal medication with 'a piece of spunge or lint, dipped in cold port wine, vinegar or brandy ... or cold astringent liquors, such as a decoction of oak bark, or a solution of alum'.

Chapter III

Natural labor Bard wrote: 'We may fairly conclude that the frequent interference of art, in so essential and natural a process as labor, cannot be necessary.' In early labor patients were assessed for 'costiveness', and mild laxatives were administered. If the perineum was resistant he advised that it should be anointed and lubricated with pomatum, hog's lard or oil.

Tedious labor Bard advised against the practice of 'giving strong, heating aromatic teas, cordials and spirituous liquors, with a view to strengthen the pains'. In prolonged labor he was of the opinion that there were no remedies to promote uterine contractions but did concede: 'It was formerly the practice to endeavor to excite the action of the womb by hot and stimulating medicines: prescriptions for this purpose [the ***pulvis ad partum***] are to be found in pharmacopoeias of no very early date.' The ***pulvis ad partum*** must have been ***pulvis parturiens***, or ergot, introduced into clinical obstetrics by John Stearns of New York in January 1807. Bard's book, although dated 1807, was published in the following year so his mention of ***pulvis ad partum*** was right up to date.

Premature labor Venesection was advised as well as 'emptying the bowels by an injection, resting and horizontal posture, and opiates so as to procure ease'.

Analgesia Although he was against the routine use of analgesia Bard was of the opinion that in protracted labor 'rest must be procured by moderate anodynes' (specifically Laudanum, Opium), but he inferred that analgesics interfered with the contractions.

Eclampsia If convulsions occurred during labor Bard advised: 'let the midwife empty the bowels by a stimulating clyster ... Let her attend to the evacuation of urine ... and promote perspiration by tepid drinks.' Other treatments included blistering, application of emetics and venesection from the jugular vein or temporal artery. When the fits were ... 'attended with frothing of the mouth and laborious breathing ... delivery, then is the only remedy'. He was aware that any obstetric manipulations would increase the number and intensity of the convulsions and advised that 'solid opium, to the quantity of a grain in every hour, or thirty drops of Laudanum, as far as three doses, or powerful anodyne clysters, consisting each of one hundred drops of Laudanum, may be repeated at like intervals, until the convulsions are suspended'.

Antepartum hemorrhage Bard wrote of flooding (hemorrhage) as being either accidental or necessary. His first remedy was bloodletting, followed by absolute rest, the application of cold to external parts and ice or snow introduced into the vagina. Bard wrote of the technique of stuffing the vagina with soft linen to stop the flow of blood and promote clotting. He objected to the remedy as he believed it would only conceal and not control the hemorrhage. He advised 'the introduction of the hand and ... turning the child, it is the only remedy ... the membranes ... must not be broken, until it is determined to proceed to immediate delivery'.

Preternatural labor Bard explained that preternatural labors were 'all those in which the body of the child is delivered before the head: in which the feet, knees, or breech of the child presents; or in which the child, lying across, presents with the arm, shoulder, thigh, back or belly'. In all such cases he advised that the help of a skillful and experienced practitioner should be sought.

Retained placenta In such cases Bard advocated the process of manual removal.

For flooding after the birth Postpartum hemorrhage cases 'generally arise from an atony (or total inactivity) of the womb' wrote Bard, who advised friction of the abdomen and the introduction of cold water, ice, snow spirits or vinegar, into the vagina, in an effort to stimulate uterine contraction.

Acute uterine inversion Bard wrote about the 'terrible disease ... [of] the inverted womb', how to avoid it and how to treat it: 'The means by which these alarming, and too frequently fatal accidents may very generally be prevented [is to] suffith the labor to proceed with as little interference as possible.'

Chapter IV

The puerperium Bard advised: 'After one or two days, women should rise from their beds ... it is not now so general among the higher classes of society, to be confined for eight or ten days.'

After pains These were treated by laudanum and the 'braided, swollen and inflamed' external parts were bathed with warm milk and water, and anointed with fresh hog's lard.

Milk fever This dreaded problem could be prevented by 'putting the child early to the breast, emptying the bowels by an emollient injection, restricting the patient to a low diet ... [with] tepid drink, aided by the *spiritus mindereri*.' If the symptoms were preceded by ague (fever) then venesection, application of fresh lard, butter or simple cerate to the breast with a little good oil were prescribed. Bard added: 'it is likewise common with some nurses, to cover them [the breasts] with cabbage leaves, softened in warm vinegar ... any other broad leaf, particularly those of the button-wood or burdock, are to be preferred, as they are not so apt to become offensive.'

Breast lumps Breast lumps led to abscesses and so were treated with fomentations, poultices and diachylon or mercurial plaster.

Sore nipples 'This painful and ... sometimes a very obstinate disease' was treated with simple cerate: a wax ring was placed on the nipple to defend it from 'the friction of the clothes'. Other treatments were applications of lead solution, alum in brandy, borax or rum.

Puerperal (child-bed) fever Bard advised antimonial solutions, drinks, laudanum, Peruvian bark, purgation and venesection, and referred the reader to 'the admirable writings of Mr. White of Manchester, and Dr Denman'. Bard concluded this section of the book with tracts on 'Swelled Leg' and 'Mania', (advising opium and camphor for the latter) and on the problems of the newborn infant.

The Appendix

> 'In this appendix are given, not only all the remedies referred to in the foregoing essay, but receipts for their preparation, their proper doses and directions for their general use. Some few, are added with a view to render it more complete, as a domestic pharmacopoeia, for the use of families at a distance from medical advice; or on slight occasions, it may not be necessary to call in a physician.'

Sudorific drinks Balm, catnip, sage tea, water

Mucilaginous drinks Barley water, flax seed tea, gum arabic, marshmallow tea, quince seeds

Astringent drinks Infusion of galls, oak bark, roses

Glysters, simple and emollient Barley water, flax seed tea, infusion of quince seeds, mallow tea, milk and water, solution of gum arabic, thin starch with water, warm water

Purgative and stimulating clysters Any of the above with the addition of brown sugar, chamomile flowers, common salt, common soap, molasses, vinegar

Anodyne clyster New milk or mucilaginous substances with the addition of laudanum

Nourishing clyster A strong soup made of brandy, laudanum (may be added), meat, new milk

Mild laxatives Brimstone, brown sugar, castor oil, cream of tartar, Glauber's salts, ipecacuanha, magnesia, molasses, rhubarb, saltpeter, syrup

Active purges Calomel, Glauber's salts, jalap, rhubarb, vitriolated tartar

Aloetics Anderson's pills, gum guaiacum, myrrh, socotrine aloes, tartar emetic

Emetics Ipecacuanha with tartar emetic, ipecacuanha, tartar emetic

Sudorifics Mindererus' spirits (salt of hartshorn with vinegar)

Sudorific anodyne Laudanum with Mindererus' spirits

Effervescing draught Ipecacuanha, lemon juice, lime juice, pearl ash, salt of hartshorn, salt of wormwood, saltpeter, tartar emetic, vinegar, water

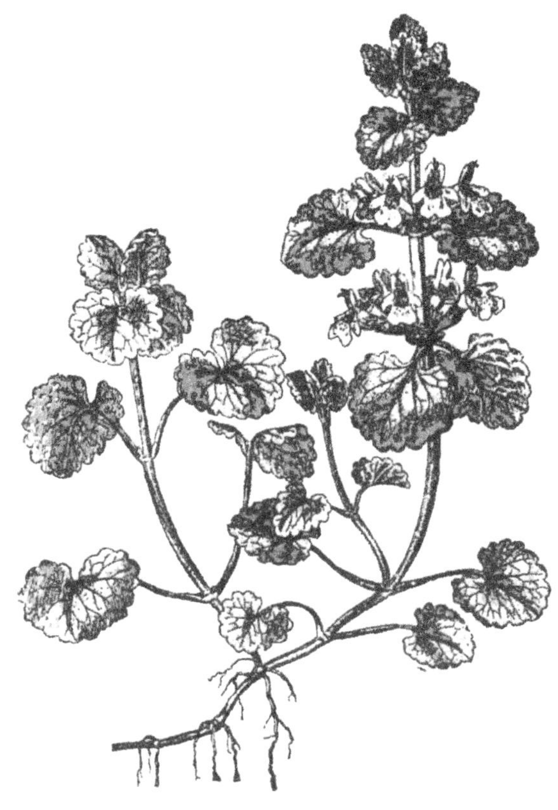

Figure 3 Catnip (*Nepeta* sp.)

Diuretics and alternatives Chamomile, gum of arabic mucilage, melon seeds, pumpkin seeds, saltpeter, squills, sweet almonds, sweet spirits of niter

Alternative diet drink Figs, lignum vitae, liquorice, parsley, raisins, sarsaparilla, water

Anodynes and antispasmodics Asafetida, camphor, gum pills, gum ammoniac, laudanum, sweet spirit of niter, sweet spirit of vitriol

Absorbents and correctors of acidity Fine washed chalk, fossil alkali, gum arabic, lime water, magnesia, magnesia with rhubarb, pearl ashes, salt of wormwood, water

Bitters and strengthening remedies Chamomile tea, columba, gentian, iron filings, orange peel, Peruvian bark, vitrolic acid

Cordials A little brandy toddy or a glass of wine, compound spirits of lavender, essence of peppermint, oil of cinnamon

Local applications Bread and milk poultice, cerate with galls, saturnine cerate, white mercurial ointment

Warm and discutient liniments Camphor, liniment of camphor dissolved in oil or strong spirits; opodeldoc liniment of camphor, hard soap and strong spirits; volatile liniment of fresh butter, hartshorn, hogs lard, and sweet oil; Mindererus spirits; warm plaster; aether

Astringent and antiseptic lotions and injections Alum, borax, chamomile tea, galls, green tea, oak bark, red rose leaves, spirits, sugar of lead, vinegar, water, white vitriol.

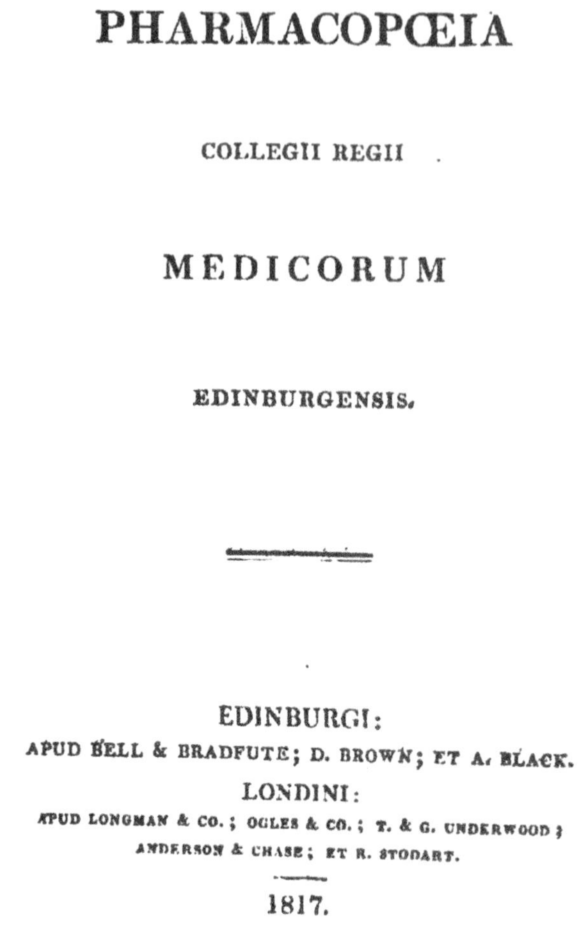

SAMUEL BARD (1742–1821): A BIOGRAPHY

Samuel Bard was born in Philadelphia and four years later his family moved to New York City. Bard entered King's College where he pursued classical studies. His decision to embark on a career in medicine meant that he had to choose between the two great centers of learning of the era, Leiden and Edinburgh. He decided on the latter and departed from New York in September 1761. England and France were at war at the time and Bard's vessel was captured on the high seas by a French privateer. Bard was held as a prisoner of war at a castle in Bayonne but was released after Benjamin Franklin, who was residing in London at the time, intervened on the young New Yorker's behalf.

In London Samuel Bard became assistant to Alexander Russell at St Thomas' Hospital. Some six months later he moved to Edinburgh where William Cullen and his colleagues were among the world's foremost medical teachers. Bard graduated from Edinburgh in 1765 after defending his thesis, *De Viribus Opii*. On leaving Edinburgh he returned to New York where he entered medical practice with his father John Bard, who was the first in the New World to report a case of extra-uterine pregnancy, and a close friend of both Benjamin Franklin and George Washington.

Influenced by his memories of the Edinburgh medical teaching system Samuel Bard decided to open a medical school and with Jones, Middleton, Tennent and Clossy, he founded the Medical School of Kings College, and the New York Hospital (Findley, 1939).

PHARMACOPŒIA

COLLEGII REGII

MEDICORUM

EDINBURGENSIS.

EDINBURGI:
APUD BELL & BRADFUTE; D. BROWN; ET A. BLACK.
LONDINI:
APUD LONGMAN & CO.; OGLES & CO.; T. & G. UNDERWOOD; ANDERSON & CHASE; ET R. STODART.

1817.

Figure 4 Frontispiece of the *Pharmacopaeia Edinburgensis* (1817)

Bard was the first professor of physic and later held the chairs of materia medica and midwifery. Medical degrees were first conferred by the New York School of Medicine in 1769. King's College became Columbia College and Bard became professor of chemistry and natural philosophy in the new school. In 1792 he became dean of the Medical School of Columbia College and finally president of the College of Physicians and Surgeons in the University of the State of New York. He retired from his practice to his estate at Hyde Park in 1799 and wrote his ***Compendium of the Theory and Practice of Midwifery***. The first edition was aimed at improving the practice of midwives but subsequent editions were to serve as an introduction to the study of midwifery for medical students and young medical practitioners. The first printing was incorrectly dated 1807 – the text was first published in 1808. The

Compendium was reprinted several times, subsequent editions appearing in 1812, 1814, 1817 and 1819. Samuel Bard died on May 25 1821, aged 79, within 24 hours of the death of his wife of 56 years (Thoms, 1933).

CHARLES MEIGS' *THE PHILADELPHIA PRACTICE OF MIDWIFERY*

In *The Philadelphia Practice of Midwifery*, Charles D. Meigs, professor of obstetrics and the diseases of women and children, at Jefferson Medical College, Philadelphia, included a special chapter entitled 'Of Milk Fever' (pp. 397–408). He detailed the anatomy of the breast and how it altered during pregnancy and also the postpartum changes in the breast:

> 'After the child is born she deserves no change in them until the second, or more commonly the third day, so that until forty-eight or seventy-two hours have elapsed we have no reason to look for any movement in that direction. But about this time the breasts commence swelling, they ache, and suffer shooting pains throughout their substance: swelling goes on until the skin of the mamma fairly shines with the tension; blue veins that are very broad are seen creeping in every direction over the superficies of the hemisphere, and even the nipple partakes of the engorgement.'

On milk fever

Meigs wrote:

> 'In this state the breast may be compared to two great phlegmons upon the most sensitive part of the body, and we need feel no surprise at finding such a state of the glands accompanied with fever, … ushered in with rigors, headache, and pains in the back and limbs … as soon as the milk fever begins, the patient ought to take some aperient medicine, such as castor oil, salts, Seidlitz powders [magnesium citrate] or salts and magnesia: it is always cooling and calming for a feverish patient to have the bowels moved freely … for my own part … I rarely fail to let blood from the arm … To take eight or ten ounces of blood, then, and to give a smart purge, is a very safe and commendable proceeding in all cases of milk fever that are a little severe.'

In regard to sore and excoriated nipples Meigs wrote: 'for my own part I do not believe in the cucumber ointment so praised by Velpeau, nor the ungentum populeum, nor the lead-water, nor the castor oil, nor the borax and brandy of Sir Astley [Cooper], nor the infusion of green tea, nor the slippery elm bark'. He went on:

> 'I advise on blood to be drawn by a circle of leeches set on a white part of the breast just beyond the areola. This leeching, followed by the emollient poultice of flax seed mixed with crumbs of bread and milk to cover the whole nipple and areola is soon followed by a reduction of the inflammation … after this the cucumber ointment, or a true pomade made with scraped pippins stewed in prepared lard … [and] the gentle stimulation of weak solution of nitrate of silver … causes the cure to be soon affected.'

During the treatment of sore nipples the patient could use a pewter nipple shield, or the nipple of a heifer as an artificial nipple.

Breast abscess

Treatment consisted of a purgative followed by bloodletting, after which a poultice of milk and bread was applied. He recommenced 50 or 60 leeches be applied near to the painful part and that 'great care should be taken … in proceeding to puncture the breast'. Meigs advised that a student who intended to practice obstetrics should dissect the breast after having carefully studied Sir Astley Paston Cooper's *The Anatomy of the Breast* (1840).

THE PSEUDO-ARISTOTLE SERIES

The Pseudo-Aristotle hand-books on obstetrics and gynecology ran to numerous editions spanning the eighteenth, nineteenth and early twentieth centuries. The handbooks (for example, those of 1776, c. 1830 and c. 1900) were composite works of ancient medical texts, supplemented with tracts on obstetrics and gynecology written by contemporary authors. The

Works of Aristotle were manuals on sex and pregnancy, in the tradition of Culpeper, and played a very important role in educating the public. Each manual contains large tracts of text devoted to medications for women. These were mainly of herbal origin, and there were few references to the newer 'chemical' remedies.

Materia medica from the works of Aristotle

Medications to avoid when pregnant Aloes, brimstone, castor, coloquintida, fennel, garlic, mint, mustard, olives, onions, pennyroyal, pepper, rue, scammony, spices, turbith, white wine.

Medications for uterine inflammation
Agnus castus, aniseed
Barley meal or water, bay leaves, bean meal, betony, bugloss
Calamint, chamomile, cassia, cinnamon
Deer suet, diacimium, diagalangal, dill
Egg white, endive, eringo
Fenugreek, feverfew, fig
Goat's milk
Honey of roses, horehound, hyssop
Keir (bleach), knotgrass
Lily, linseed
Mallow, melilot, mercury, milk, mugwort
Oil of aniseed, oil of roses, opium
Pennyroyal, plantain, poppyheads, purslane
Quinces
Rhubarb, rosewater, rosemary, rue
Sage, senna, sorrel, spa waters, succory
Thyme, turpentine
Violets
Water lilies, white wine, wormwood.

CHARLES WEST'S *DISEASES OF WOMEN*

In the latter part of the nineteenth century a large number of books were printed in both Europe and America relating to obstetrics and gynecology, many of which were vast tomes. Charles West, physician accoucheur to St Bartholomew's and the Middlesex Hospitals wrote a treatise entitled *Lectures on the Diseases of Women.* There are only scattered references to materia medica in the 687 pages of text which contains 16 formulas. The compound medications came under the headings of: Anodyne (analgesic), antiphlogistic (anti-inflammatory), aperient (gentle purgative), astringent (arresting discharges), chalybeate (iron containing), mucilaginous (viscid paste or gum), sedative (allays anxiety), and stimulant. One example, an aperient chalybeate prescription contained: ferri sulphatis, magnesiae sulphatis, acid sulph. dil., syrupi aurantii, and aquae carui.

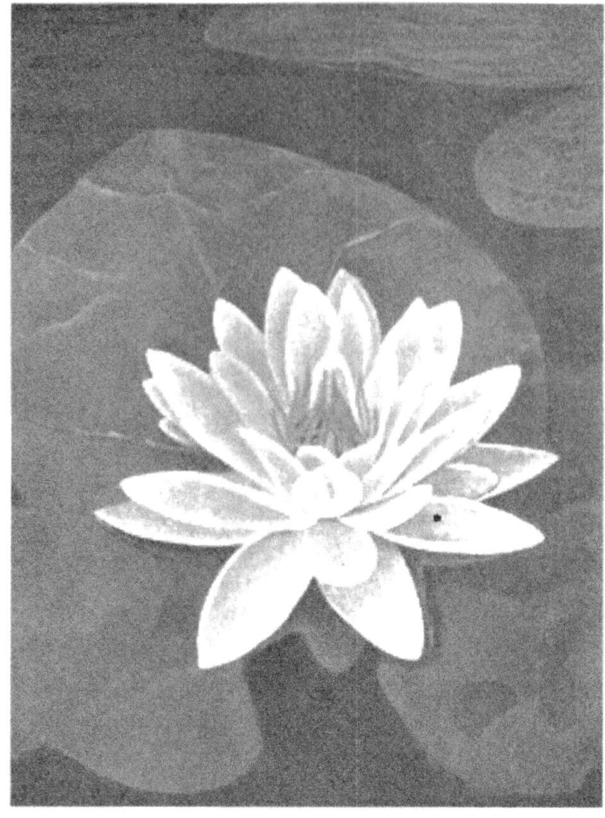

Figure 5 White water lily (*Nymphea odorata*)

HENRY MACNAUGHTON JONES AND *UTERINE THERAPEUTICS*

Professor MacNaughton Jones of the Queen's University Cork, devoted his *Practical Manual of Diseases of Women and Uterine Therapeutics for Students and Practitioners* (1885) entirely to gynecology. He also included a section on spa waters and their uses in gynecology (pp. 441–4).

PRACTICAL MANUAL
OF
DISEASES OF WOMEN
AND
UTERINE THERAPEUTICS.

For Students and Practitioners.

BY

H. MACNAUGHTON-JONES, M.D., M.CH., M.A.O. (HON. CAUS.),
FELLOW OF THE ROYAL COLLEGES OF SURGEONS OF IRELAND AND EDINBURGH;
FORMERLY
UNIVERSITY PROFESSOR OF MIDWIFERY AND DISEASES OF WOMEN AND CHILDREN IN THE QUEEN'S UNIVERSITY,
EXAMINER IN MIDWIFERY AND DISEASES OF WOMEN AND CHILDREN IN THE ROYAL UNIVERSITY OF IRELAND,
AND
LECTURER ON SURGICAL AND DESCRIPTIVE ANATOMY, QUEEN'S COLLEGE,
CONSULTING SURGEON TO THE MATERNITY AND TO THE WOMEN AND CHILDREN'S HOSPITAL, CORK.

SIXTH EDITION,
REVISED AND ENLARGED.

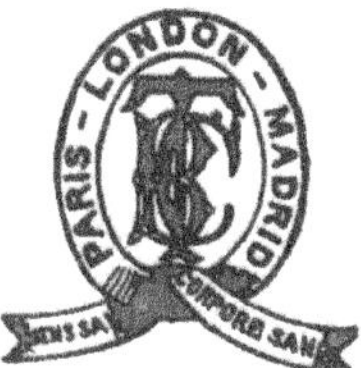

LONDON:
BAILLIÈRE, TINDALL AND COX,
20 & 21, KING WILLIAM STREET, STRAND.
1894.

Figure 6 Frontispiece from MacNaughton-Jones' A *Practical Manual of Disease of Women and Uterine Therapeutics* (1894)

Spas and health resorts

Spas and health resorts have been important in the healing process since antiquity. William Turner helped to popularize the European spas in his *Booke of the Natures and Properties, as well of the Bathes in England, as of other Bathes in Germanye and Italye* (1568) and balneotherapy was a favorite remedy for many diseases until the mid-twentieth century. According to MacNaughton Jones, spa waters were '[helpful for] Affections of the Skin; Liver; Urinary organs; Glandular organs; Special for Impoverished Blood; for Special Affections of Women; for Joints and Rheumatism, and for the Lungs'. There were spas for women in Bavaria, Northwest Germany, and Lincolnshire, England. The spa waters contained alkalis, sulfates and saline solutions of arsenic, bromine, chlorides, iodine and iron.

Vaginismus

MacNaughton Jones offered dilator therapy (Sims' vaginal rest) for this 'state of extreme irritability of the nerves supplying the vulvar orifice and the vagina'. Locally applied treatments included atropine, belladonna, chloral, iodoform, morphine, and nitrate of silver (the fused stick lightly touched to the sensitive spots). Atropine and belladona, isolated from the *Atropa belladonna* plant (deadly nightshade) were also used in the Middle Ages for diseases of the vulva. 'But the proposition of Gaillard Thomas is not to be lost sight of, viz., in those cases where the marital act is impossible from the attendant pain, to thoroughly anaesthetize the woman, in the hope that complete connection [intercourse], under these circumstances, may result in pregnancy', wrote MacNaughton Jones. The problem of vaginismus had been addressed by Marion J. Sims some years previously: the patient was etherized and placed on her left side, the hymen was stretched and clipped with scissors, and the resultant hemorrhage was treated with liq. ferri persulphatis. The perineum was incised in a Y-shape and a glass dilator inserted which the patient wore for five hours each day for three weeks or longer (Sims, 1866 pp. 335–7).

Uterine discharges

'In gynaecological practice the treatment of uterine discharges by the topical application of agents to the uterine canal, both of cervix and body, is of every day occurrence. In the commonly occurring troubles – subinvolution, endometritis, ... cervical and corporeal, granular conditions of the canal, after removal of polypi, those conditions consequent upon gonorrhoea – we have to apply caustics, astringents, and absorbents to the interior of the uterus'. The following were the most important intrauterine medications employed: acetate of lead, belladonna, carbolic acid, chloride of zinc, chloro-acetic acid, chromic acid, hazeline, iodine and carbolic acid, iodine, iodoform, mercury, morphia, nitrate of silver, nitric acid, perchloride of iron, sulfate of zinc, and tannin.

SIDNEY RINGER'S *HANDBOOK OF THERAPEUTICS*

At the close of the nineteenth century Sidney Ringer, professor of the principles and practices of medicine at University College Hospital, London, summarized the materia medica for women in his 'Index to Diseases'. Of interest is the new reliance on chemicals and the reduced number of plant medications, in contrast to previous centuries. Limewater, mentioned by both Samuel Bard and Sidney Ringer, referred to a suspension of calcium hydroxide in water. The lime was obtained from slaked limestone (calcium carbonate).

Ringer's remedies for women

Amenorrhea Aconite, *Actaea racemosa*, aloes, ammonium chloride, cold sponging, ergot, hot sitz-bath, iron, mustard, permanganate, santonin, spinal icebag

Barrenness Iodide of potassium (when due to syphilis)

Breasts, inflammation of Belladonna, digitalis

Change of life *Actaea*, ammonia, bromide of potassium, calabar bean, camphor, change of air and scene, eucalyptol, hot sponging, iron, nitrite of amyl, valerianate of zinc, vinegar and water sponging, warm bath

Convulsions Bitartrate of potash, sulfate of soda, tartrate of potash, bromide of potassium, chloral, chloroform, ice, morphia, spinal icebag, *Veratrum viride*

Dysmenorrhea *Actaea*, antipyrin, arsenic, cajeput, *Cannabis indica*, croton chloryl, gelsemium, hammamelis, hot sitz-bath, nitrite of amyl

Flushing heats Bromide of potassium, eucalyptol, nitrite of amyl, nux vomica, valerianate of zinc

Gonorrhea Aconite, alkalis, avoidance of alcohol, bismuth, blistering, *Cannabis indica*, cantharides, cocaine, copaiba, copper sulfate, cubebs, glycerin of tannin, iron, lead, oil of sandalwood, silver nitrate, sulfo-carbolate of zinc, turpentine, zinc

Hemorrhage postpartum Compression of aorta, ice, ipecacuanha, iron, mechanical excitation of vomiting, opium with brandy

Hysteria Aconite, actaea, alcohol, apomorphia, asafetida, bromide of potassium, *Cannabis indica*, chloroform, cod liver oil, iron, morphia, musk, nux vomica, opium, paraldehyde, phosphorus, valerianate of zinc, volatile oils, zinc

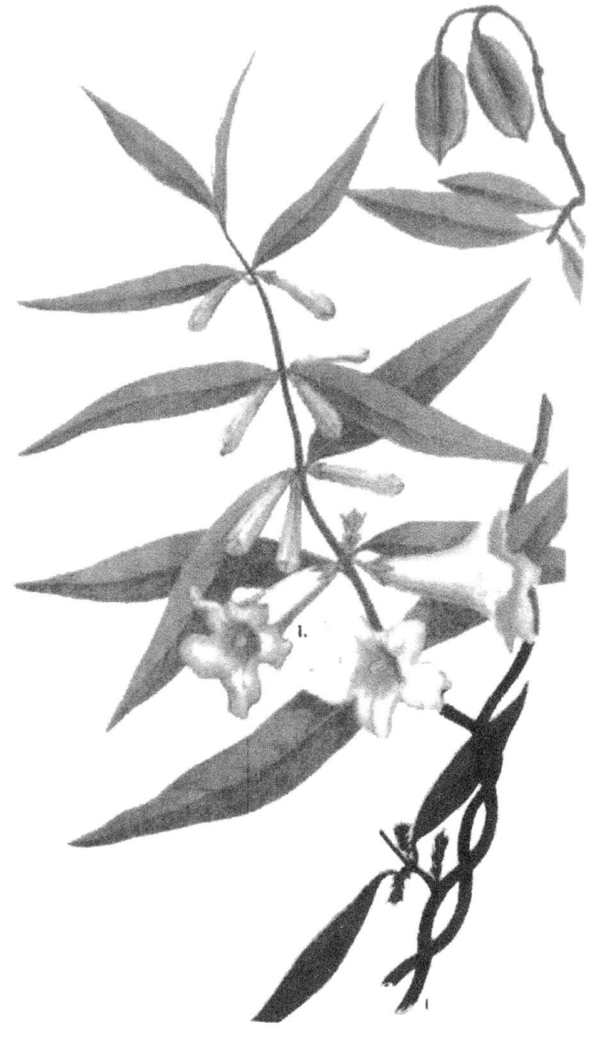

Figure 7 Gelsemium

Impotence Cantharides, strychnia

Leukorrhea Alkalis, alum, belladonna, bicarbonate of potash or soda, boracic acid, carbolic acid, cold sponging, copper, ergot, iron, lead, limewater, phosphate of lime, spinal icebag, tannin, zinc sulfate

Mammary abscess Belladonna, mercury and morphia (oleate of), sulfide of calcium, tobacco

Menorrhagia *Actaea*, bromide of potassium, *Cannabis indica*, chloride of ammonium, digitalis, ergot, hammamelis, lemons, oil of cinnamon, phosphate of lime, quinia, spinal hot water bag, tannin and gallic acid

Nipples, sore Arnica, brandy and water, collodion, glycerin, limewater, sulfurous acid, zinc shield

Nymphomania Bromide of potassium, camphor

Ovarian neuralgia Gelsemium

Ovarian tumors Iodine

Pregnancy *Actaea* (to prevent miscarriage), bromide of potassium (for frightening delusions in later months), cocaine (internally for vomiting), ipecacuanha (for acidity), sea-bathing

Prolapse alum, ergotin, ice, nux vomica, strychnia, sulfur, tannin

Puerperal fever Antimony, bromide of potassium, chloral, morphia, permanganate, turpentine

Puerperal peritonitis Antimony, chlorine solution

Sexual desire (inordinate) Camphor

Spermatorrhea Belladonna, bladder to be emptied after first deep sleep, bromide of potassium, cantharides, cold douche, cold sponging, digitalis, hypophosphates, phosphorus, quinia, spinal icebag, strychnia

Suspended animation at birth Cold water smartly sprinkled on face

Syphilis Cod liver oil, iodide of iron, iodide of potassium, iodol, lamp bath, mercury, nitric acid, oils of mezereon and sassafras, soft soap, zinc

Thrush Borax, copper sulfate, glycerin, glycerin of borax, salicylic acid, sulfurous acid

Uterine diseases *Actaea racemosa*, belladonna, camphor, carbolic acid, carbonic acid gas, caustic lime, chloroform, ergot, glycerin, glycerin of tannin, iodoform, iron, lead, opium

Vagina, diseases of Boroglyceride, cocaine, glycerin of tannin

Vulvitis Alum, glycerin of tannin, lead, limewater.

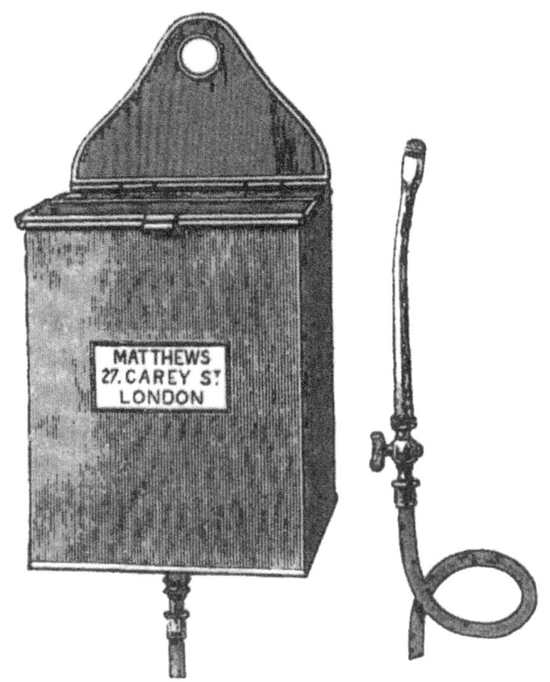

Figure 8 Vaginal douche (MacNaughton-Jones, *Diseases of Women*)

A SELECTION OF NINETEENTH CENTURY MATERIA MEDICA

Castor oil

Castor oil is a medicinal and lubricating oil obtained from the seeds of the tropical castor oil plant, *Ricinus communis*, also known as 'palma Christi'. The Latin *ricinus* was the name for the dog tick, *Ixodes ricinus*, and was used for the palma Christi seeds because of their resemblance to the insect. In Greek, the insect was called *kroton* and Dioscorides described the palma Christi seeds as 'kroton seeds'.

There are two theories as to how the plant became known as the castor oil plant. In the West Indies there was a mistaken notion that the agnus castus plant (chaste tree) yielded the castor seeds and so for a time that plant was incorrectly known as the castor oil plant. A second theory concerned the very popular medicinal compounded 'oil of castor', obtained from castoreum (secretion from the preputial follicles of the beaver, *Castor fiber*) and mixed with aromatic gums, spices and wine. The taste of the oil of castoreum was somewhat similar to that expressed from palma Christi seeds and so the latter became known as 'castor oil'. The leaves of the palma Christi are large and deeply divided into segments, appearing rather like a hand. The plant contains ricin and is exceedingly toxic.

The castor oil plant has been cultivated for over 6000 years and was once the source of oil for lamps.

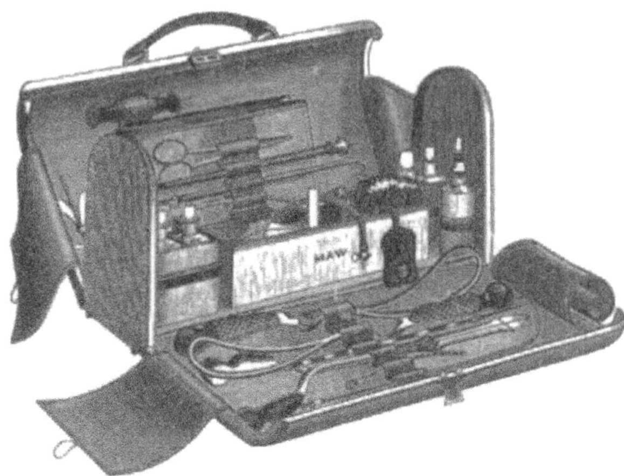

Figure 9 Nineteenth century obstetric bags from *Surgeon's Instruments* catalogue

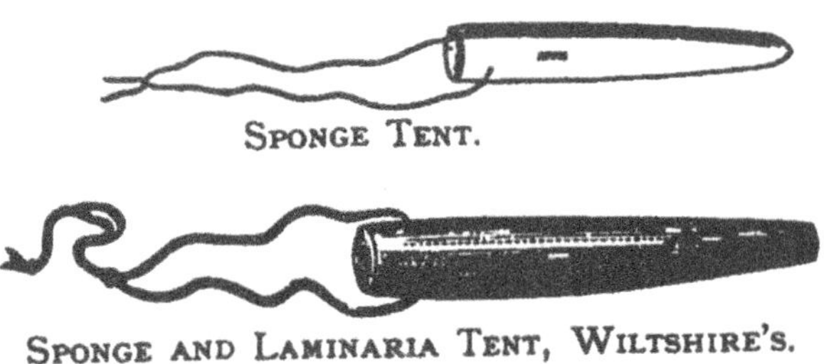

Figure 10 Nineteenth century sponge and tents from *Surgeon's Instruments* catalogue

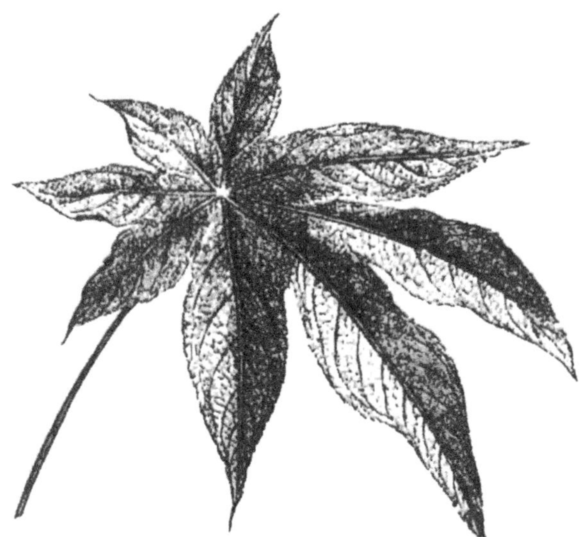

Figure 11 Castor oil plant (*Ricinus* sp.)

Seeds of the plant were found in the sarcophagi of the Ancient Egyptian pharaohs. The Ancient Egyptians referred to the castor oil plant as the 'Sillicyprian plant' from which they extracted 'kiki' or castor oil. The ancients were aware that the seeds were extremely toxic and Greek physicians believed the oil was mainly suitable as an external application. *Cicinum oleum* (castor oil) was mentioned as an emollient and an ingredient of medicated plasters by Cornelius Celsus of the early first century AD (Spencer, 1989). The Roman encyclopedist, Pliny the Elder (AD 23–79) wrote in his *Historia Naturalis* that: 'Castor oil is taken with an equal quantity of warm water to open the bowels ... Fresh leaves [of the plant] by themselves [are useful for] for diseases of the breast' (Jones, 1951).

In the following century Pedianus Dioscorides referred to castor oil as 'kroton aekiki', or 'crotona', from which the pressed oil called cicinum was obtained. The oil was not to be taken by mouth but was useful for candlemaking or inclusion in medicated plasters for breast problems. Ingestion of the oil led to 'ye purging ... [which] is harsh and extremely laborsome ... Ye leaves be imbruised with ye flour of Polenta doe Assuage ye Oedemata and inflammations of ye eyes, and do abate milk-swollen breasts' (Gunther, 1959). Castor oil was not referred to by Soranus of Ephesus, the great gynecologist–physician of the second century AD.

The castor oil plant appears to have been forgotten until it was reintroduced in 1764 by Dr Peter Canvane, of Bath, who had practiced for some years in the West Indies. He wrote a treatise on castor oil and advised it as a gentle purgative in cases of 'dry belly-ache'. So popular did the plant become that it was admitted to the *London Pharmacopoeia* in 1788 and shortly thereafter to the Continental pharmacopoeias (Wootton, 1910). Carl Linnaeus (1749) included ricinus in his materia medica and wrote that the bitter oil was used for inflammation, as an antihelminthic, and as a purge. John Lindley, professor of botany at University College, London wrote of the ricinus in his *Flora Medica*: 'The seeds of this plant yield by expression the well-known valuable cathartic substance called castor oil' (1838 pp. 183–4).

Castor oil was routinely used in the induction of labor during the mid-twentieth century. Alfred Beck, professor of obstetrics and gynecology at Long Island College of Medicine, New York advised: 'The routine usually followed in the medical induction of labor is as follows:- 6.00 a.m. one ounce of castor oil, 7.00 a.m. Quinine ten grains followed by a warm enema. 8.00 a.m. Pituitary extract three minim. and repeated at half hour intervals until labor is established or until six doses have been given' (Beck, 1942).

The castor oil–quinine–pituitrin method of inducing labor was popular in Europe, although the pituitrin was withheld until the effects of the castor oil and quinine were known. The 'European method' was to give castor oil at 7 a.m. followed by a hot bath and an enema. Three hours later, quinine bi-hydrochloride five grains was administered, and repeated at two-hourly intervals to a maximum of four doses. If contractions had not begun two units of pituitrin were given at 9 p.m. and repeated every 30 minutes, to a maximum of eight doses, until pains became regular. If the method was not successful, the drugs were repeated on the following two or three days. Eden and Holland (1940) wrote that the fourth dose of quinine might not be tolerable, and reported that it may have been quinine that was responsible for fetal death in 1% of the cases in which the castor oil–quinine–pituitrin method of induction had been used. Castor oil was also commonly given to women in early labor, followed by a bath and an enema (a regime known as 'OBE').

The treatment of constipation

From ancient times until well into the twentieth century enemas and purgatives were important forms of treatment for many medical, obstetric and gynecological conditions. The clyster/glyster (enema) was a primary treatment for everything from amenorrhea to vulvitis. In 1622 Mindererus published a treatise on the use of a special 'compound of aloes'. The nine ingredients he prescribed (agaric, aloes, ammoniacum, costus, lignum aloes, mastich, myrrh, rhubarb, saffron) were eventually contained in the compound 'Rhubarb Pill' of the early twentieth century (Wooton, 1910 vol. 2, p. 89).

Howard A. Kelly of Johns Hopkins University, devoted almost a full chapter to constipation in his book *Medical Gynecology* (1909): '[Constipation] is one of the commonest abnormal conditions with which the physician has to deal with, and is the cause of much ill health and discomfort in women ... In constipation, nutrition and metabolism are interfered with and a series of circulatory disturbances arise ... caused by absorption of the poisonous retained products ... [patients] habitually constipated are apt to show it in their faces ... In a word, so long as pronounced constipation is the habit of the body, all the organs are bathed daily in blood rendered impure by the absorption of faecal products, and the consequences are usually those which might be legitimately expected'. Kelly's prescription for constipation comprised: belladonna, cascara, exercise, gentian, magnesium sulfate, mint, roughage, strychnine, sulfur, water. He also described and illustrated the correct posture for defecation.

Peter Wyatt Squire, in his *Companion to the British Pharmacopoeia* (1908), detailed the 94 medicines which promoted intestinal evacuations (cathartics). Included among them were 39 aperients (laxatives), 23 purgatives, 21 'drastics' (hydragogues), and 11 mineral waters. In contrast, he could only list 23 emmenagogues.

Electrical treatment

The story of electricity began when the Greek natural philosopher Thales (c. 624–545 BC) observed that amber, upon being rubbed with cloth, attracted small bits of straw. Two millennia later, Jerome Cardan, an Italian mathematician, contrasted the properties of amber and lodestone, the magnetic black rock in 1551. William Gilbert, physician to Queen Elizabeth I of England, discovered in c. 1600 that some other materials, such as diamond, glass, sulfur and wax, also behaved like amber. Gilbert called these materials 'electrics', a term based on *electrum*, the Latin for amber. Another English physician, Sir Thomas Brown, devised the word 'electricity' in 1646. Many famous physicians, including Benjamin Franklin, experimented with electricity and it was he who developed the theory of positive and negative charge. It was shown at a later date that positive electricity resulted from a deficiency of electrons and negative electricity had an excess.

ENEMAS, etc.

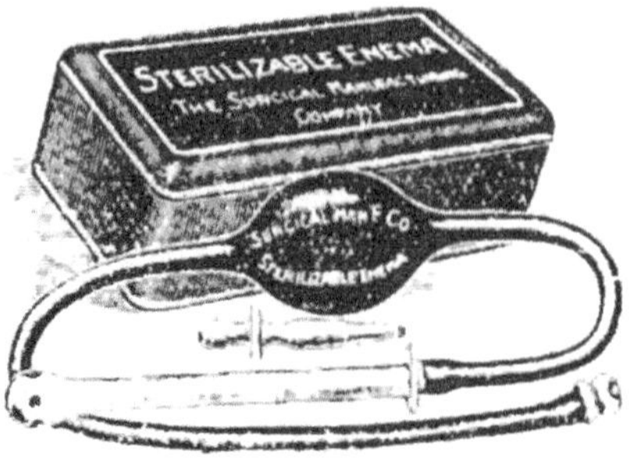

6920 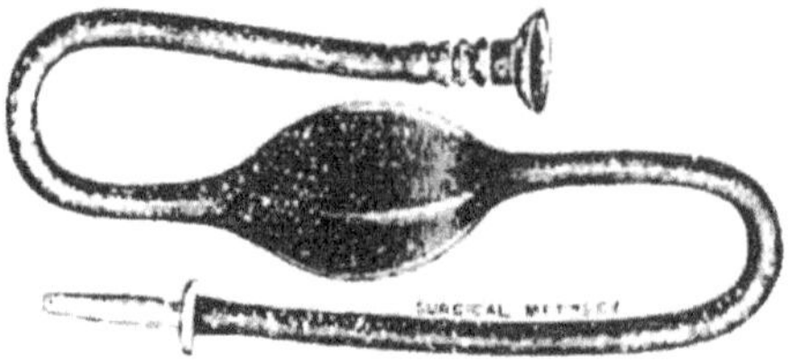 6921

6920 **THE "SURGMAN" RED STERILIZABLE ENEMAS.** Complete with glass or rubber vaginal and rectal pipes, in metal cases, as illustrated ... each 3/6 per doz. **36/0**
6921 **RED STERILIZABLE HOLDFAST ENEMAS.** Special make for hard wear, complete with bone pipes and holdfast ends, in metal case ... each 3/6 per doz. **36/0**

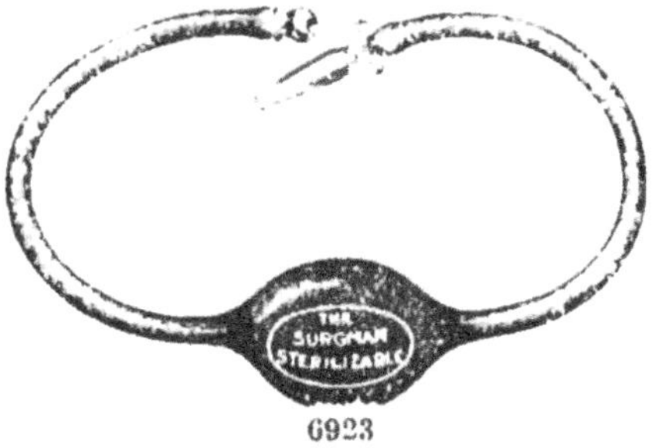

6923 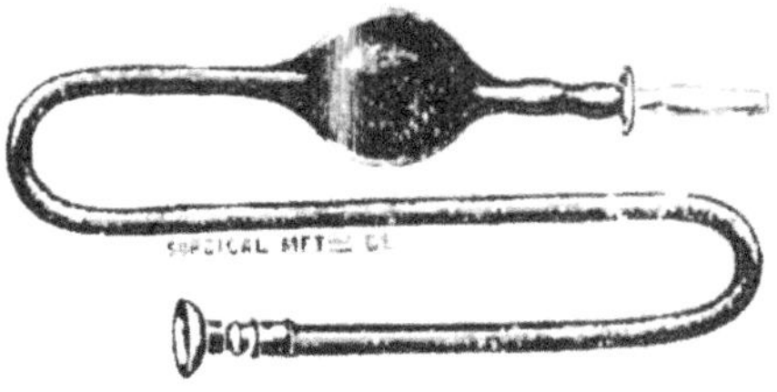 6924

6923 **RED STERILIZABLE ENEMAS,** without holdfast ... ... each 2/0 per doz. **21/0**
6924 **THE "AUTO" STERILIZABLE ENEMAS,** with short discharge and long suction and holdfast end, and with bone pipes ... ... each 2/6 per doz. **27/0**
Can be used by patient without assistance.

6925 **ENEMAS,** for Hospital out-patients' use, in black, red or green rubber, complete in card boxes, with vaginal and rectal pipe ... ... each **2/0** per doz. **21/0**

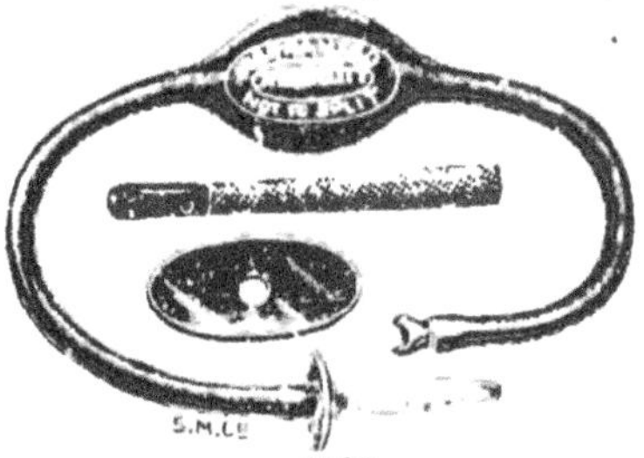

6925

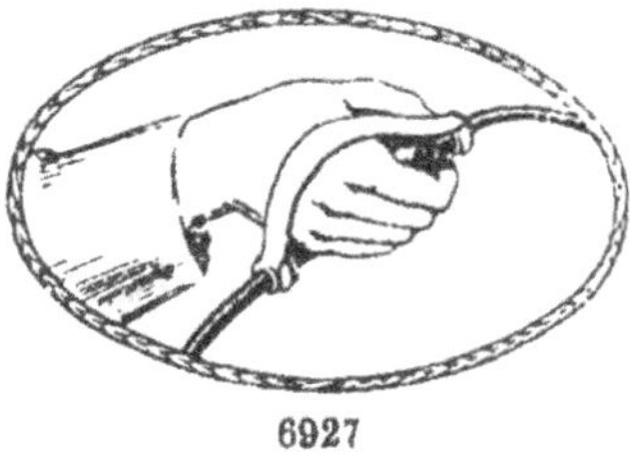

6927 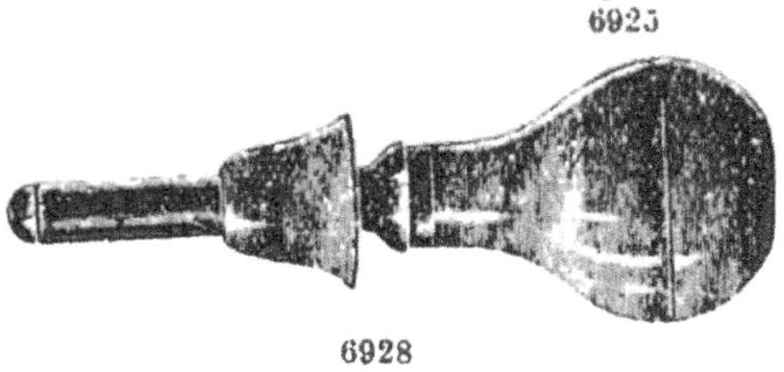 6928

6927 **THE "SAFETY GRIP" ENEMAS,** sterilizable rubber, complete in box with rubber vaginal pipe, etc. ... ... each **4/0**
6928 **FOUNTAIN SYRINGE OR WHIRLING SPRAYS,** in best red rubber **6/6**

The Surgical Manufacturing Co., Ltd., 83/85, Mortimer Street, London, W. 1.

Figure 12 Enemas from *Catalogue of Surgical Instruments*

BRITISH PHARMACOPŒIA

PUBLISHED UNDER THE DIRECTION OF THE

GENERAL COUNCIL

OF

MEDICAL EDUCATION AND REGISTRATION

OF THE UNITED KINGDOM

PURSUANT TO

THE MEDICAL ACT, 1858.

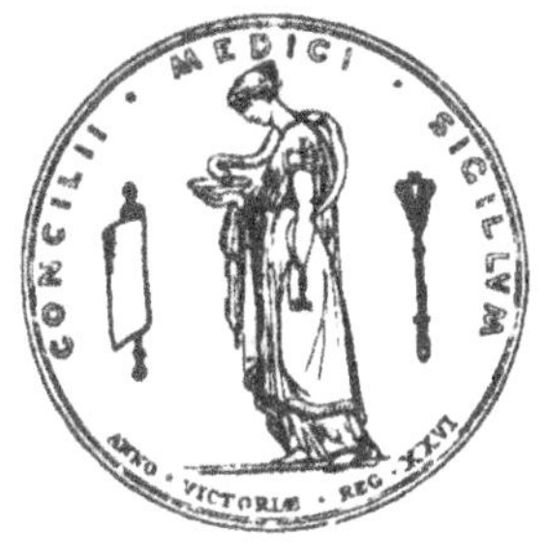

LONDON:

PRINTED FOR THE GENERAL MEDICAL COUNCIL BY

SPOTTISWOODE & CO., NEW-STREET SQUARE, E.C.

1864.

Figure 13 Frontispiece from the first official *British Pharmacopaeia* (1864)

Luigi Galvani, (1737–1798), an Italian professor of anatomy and obstetrics at Bologna, performed one of the first animal experiments with electric current in 1786. A dead frog was suspended by its legs on a copper hook and the hook was hung over an iron railing: the frog's legs twitched when they touched the iron railing. Galvani deduced that the twitching was due to 'animal electricity'. Other investigators involved in the early research of electricity included Alessandro Volta, Hans C. Oersted, André Marie Ampere and George S. Ohm. In 1831 Michael Faraday (1791–1867) studied the effects of electromagnetism and found that a moving magnet induced an electric current in a coil of wire. Electric generators and transformers work by means of the induction principles formulated by Faraday and the American physicist, Joseph Henry (1797–1878).

Faradism and galvanism involved the treatment of disease with an electric current. Both forms of therapy were very popular in the nineteenth century and both were applied to obstetrics and gynecology. Samuel Bard, in his *Compendium of the Theory and Practice of Midwifery* (1807), was one of the first to write on the use of electricity in gynecology, advocating its use in the treatment of amenorrhea. He wrote: 'having … strengthened the habit, they may take Aloetic medicines, a dose or two of Rhubarb and Calomel, [and] have sparks drawn from them at an electric machine'.

MacNaughton Jones of Cork wrote of the use of 'galvanization and the employment of the galvanic stem and pessary'; He advised: 'If electricity is likely to do good, perhaps the safest mode of applying it is directly to the cervix, by means of such a Rheopore as that of Maw … the current is not completed until the sponge of the Rheopore is passed inside the cervix.' MacNaughton Jones included illustrations of various 'galvanic stems' for insertion into the cervix and an illustration of Leclanché's 20-cell constant current battery. He was of the opinion: 'Good is … effected by wearing one of the many varieties of electrical apparatus now so elegantly contrived for female use' (MacNaughton Jones, 1885 pp. 113, 125).

In the 6th edition of his book MacNaughton Jones devoted an entire chapter to gynecological electrotherapeutics: 'During the comparatively short period that has elapsed since the last edition of this work was passing through the press, a large number of gynaecologists … have given the treatment of various uterine affections by electro-therapy an impartial trial, and have reported favourably of this conservative therapeutical step.' He was aware that in 1873 Routh and Althus had used continuous currents of high intensity in the treatment of uterine fibroids, and of Cutter of America, and Apostoli, who were other major contributors. MacNaughton Jones described the indications

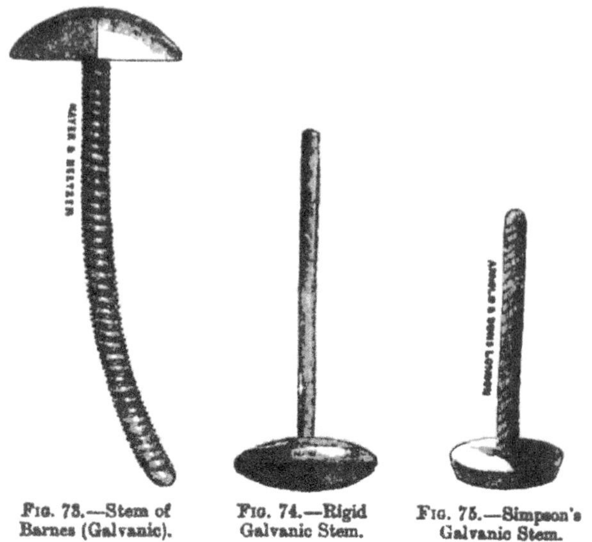

Fig. 73.—Stem of Barnes (Galvanic).
Fig. 74.—Rigid Galvanic Stem.
Fig. 75.—Simpson's Galvanic Stem.

Figure 14 Galvanic stems from MacNaughton Jones, *Diseases of Women*

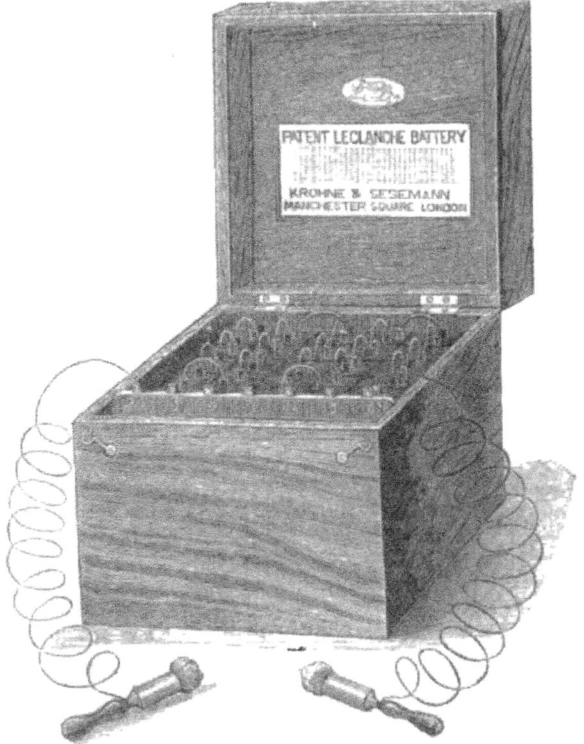

Figure 15 A battery from MacNaughton Jones, *Diseases of Women*

and appliances for faradic treatment and galvano-caustic treatment (see table) and included illustrations of various batteries and appliances in his text (MacNaughton Jones, 1894 pp. 463–82).

J.M. Baldy, professor of gynecology at the Philadelphia Polyclinic, was enthusiastic about the use of electricity and included it as a treatment for seven gynecological conditions in his *American Text-Book of Gynecology* (1894). The electrical treatment of gynecological complaints remained in vogue in the early twentieth century and Howard Kelly enumerated 14 indications for its use, including constipation (1909). John Whitridge Williams of Johns Hopkins University, however, reflected a growing disenchantment with the use of electrotherapy in some situations in obstetrics and gynecology: 'The use of electricity ... and all methods of treatment which aim at destroying the fetus and thus terminating pregnancy without operation [in ectopic pregnancy] are absolutely unjustifiable' (Williams, 1903). As time went by electrotherapy fell totally out of favor and Comyns Berkeley and Victor Bonney in *A Textbook of Gynaecological Surgery* (1935) relegated the use of electricity to diathermy and electric cautery. Nowadays electricity is used for the same purposes but faradic stimulation still plays a role in the treatment of female urinary incontinence.

Iodine

The word 'iodine' was derived from the Greek *ioeides*, violet-colored, (in turn from *ion*, a violet, and *eidos*, form). Iodine is a halogen element (atomic number 53), discovered by Bernard Courtois of France in 1811. At the time he was experimenting with the extraction of alkali from seaweed, while manufacturing artificial niter. He accidentally added a little too much sulfuric acid to the crystallized soda and '[he] was surprised to see beautiful violet vapours disengaged, and from these, scales of grayish-black colour, and of metallic lustre were deposited' (Wootton, 1910 vol. pp. 351–3). Joseph Gay-Lussac and Humphry Davy began experimenting with the new substance and in 1813 Davy recognized iodine as a simple element, and named it. Thomas Prosser (1769) was the first to record the use of powdered sponge for the cure of bronchocele or Derby neck (goiter). Jean François Coindet of Geneva,

Table 1 Indications for electrotherapy (MacNaughton Jones, 1894)

Faradization	
Low-tension current	*High-tension current*
Amenorrhea	Coccygodynia
Arrested involution	Oophoralgia
Chronic metritis	Perimetritis
Dysmenorrhea	Salpingo-ovaritis
Menorrhagia	Vaginismus
Secondary postpartum hemorrhage	Various manifestations of hysteria
Sub-involution	
Acute stages of perimetritis and ovaritis	
Galvanization	
Galvano-chemical cauterization	*Galvano-chemical puncture*
Acute and chronic metritis-endometritis	Cellulitis
Atresia	Fibroids
Fibroid of the uterus – polypi	Perimetritis
Hematocele	Pyosalpinx
Hypertrophy of the uterus	Salpingitis
Malignant disease	
Oophoralgia	
Ovarian and tubular cysts	
Ovaritis and periovaritis	
Peri-uterine inflammation	
Salpingitis	
Sub-involution	
Ulceration of the neck of the uterus	

an Edinburgh graduate, suspected that iodine was the active constituent of burnt sponge, much prescribed empirically in the treatment of goiter. He proved his theory and became the first physician to use iodine in treatment (Coindet, 1820). Further studies on the value of iodine in the treatment of goiter were carried out between 1895 and 1923.

Tincture of iodine was used as an antiseptic in French surgery in 1839 and was employed in treating battle wounds during the US Civil War. Iodoform was first prepared by Georges Simon Serullas (1822). An antiseptic and local anesthetic with a saffron like odor, it was a yellow crystalline substance (triiodomethane) and contained about 97% iodine (Ringer, 1888 pp. 341–4). It was first used in medicine by Bouchardat in 1836 but only came into general use as an 'iodoform dressing' in surgery in the late 1870s. Iodoform was particularly useful for syphilitic sores, soft chancres and orchitis. It was employed as a vaginal bolus, in a compound with cocoa-nut fat, in cases of uterine cancer. In high dosage it could have serious side-effects including death. Iodol (tetraiodopyrol) contained 80% iodine and was prescribed in place of iodoform, having a great advantage in being free from smell. Iodol prevented suppuration and was highly useful in syphilis and as a general antiseptic.

James Marion Sims was instrumental in developing the specialty of gynecology and founded the Women's Hospital in the State of New York, the first institution of its kind. In his *Clinical notes on Uterine Surgery* (1866) Sims wrote:

'The most successful treatment of (uterine) haemorrhages from fibroids is that of Doctor Savage, of the Samaritin Hospital. He dilates the canal of the cervix with a sponge tent, and injects the cavity of the uterus with a solution of iodine, which has been so far both harmless and efficient. His formula is this:

> Rx.
> Iodine
> Iodide-Potassium.
> Rect. Spt. Wine
> Water'.

Sims wrote that Professor Fleetwood Churchill's iodine treatment for induration of the cervix 'produced a greater amelioration in these cases than anything else'. Iodide of silver was also found useful in the treatment of granular erosion of the uterus. MacNaughton Jones offered iodine paint treatment for pelvic inflammation, and in chronic stages of the disease used iodide of potassium (1885 p. 269). Hobart Amory Hare wrote of the use of iodide of potassium in the treatment of tertiary syphilis and related that up to ten ounces of tincture of iodine might be injected into ovarian tumors in an effort to treat them conservatively (Hare, 1901).

The use of iodine and iodoform grew in popularity and Howard A. Kelly of Johns Hopkins University found tincture of iodine to be a successful treatment for membranous dysmenorrhea, gonorrheal infection, bone syphilis and cancer of the cervix, while iodoform with gelatin was used as an injection in septic abortion. Iodoform bougies were used in the treatment of cancer; iodoform gauze was added to tampons for various infections and inflammations; and iodoform powder was used after 'artificial abortion', after catheterization in the puerperium; and in the 'dry treatment' of gonorrhea (Kelly, 1909 pp. 632–3).

According to the editors of Goodman and Gilman's *Pharmacological Basis of Therapeutics*, iodine is still among the most valuable antiseptic agents. The iodophors, loose complexes of elemental iodine with carrier-molecules, serve as sustained-release reservoirs of iodine. The iodophors are currently used in surgical scrubs, generally in the form of povidone–iodine (Betadine), although the effects of povidone–iodine on skin flora are not as marked as those of 1% iodine tincture or with chlorhexidine (Goodman Gilman *et al.*, 1985).

Peruvian bark

Peruvian bark, *Cinchona officinalis*, also known as 'cinchona bark', 'Jesuits' bark', 'Cardinal's bark', 'red bark' (*Cinchona pubescens*), 'bark' and eventually as 'Peruvian Cort.', was the bark of an evergreen tree from Peru, *Cinchona succirubra*. Peruvian bark was introduced into Europe in 1640 and was first advertised for sale in England by James Thompson in 1658. It was made official in the *London Pharmacopoeia* of 1677 as *cortex Peruanus* (also as *Cinchona officinalis*) and was prescribed as a febrifuge, tonic and astringent. Carl Linnaeus, in his *Materia Medica* (1749) named the Peruvian bark 'cinchona', noting that it came from Loxa, in Peru, and that it was used for critical fevers.

The name was taken from the Countess Anna del Chinchon, wife of the Viceroy of Peru. According to legend, the Countess became critically ill with malaria, and when other remedies failed the court physician suggested the use of a native remedy, quinina. Some quinina bark was procured from Loxa in Ecuador and successfully used to treat the ailing Countess, whereupon the bark was renamed cinchona bark. By 1639 cinchona bark was being imported into Spain for the treatment of ague (fever) related to malaria and other infections (Poser and Bruyn, 1999).

Apparently, the first account of Peruvian bark appeared in a religious book written in 1633 and published in Spain in 1639. The author, an Augustinian monk, wrote that powdered bark cured fevers. In Latin America the priests of the Society of Jesus (Jesuits) had become protectors and friends of the native Indians. The Jesuits were aware of the potential benefits of Peruvian bark and it was they who arranged the collection of the bark in Peru, Bolivia and Ecuador. After collection the bark was dried, powdered, and exported to Europe, where it was sold for the benefit of the Order. From 1650 the bark took on its new name, Jesuits' bark. In Rome, the medication was sponsored by the eminent philosopher, Cardinal de Lugo, and it then became known as Cardinal's bark. The bark could be used as a powder, extract or infusion. In 1820 Pelletier and Caventou isolated the alkaloids quinine and cinchonine from the cinchona plant (Poser and Bruyn, 1999). Quinine was the main treatment for malaria until synthetic antimalarials became available. Malaria, caused by a protozoan parasite transmitted by mosquitoes, derives it's name from the Italian *mal*, bad, and *aria*, air. The disease was known by various names including 'swamp fever' (Hobhouse, 1986; Poser and Bruyn, 1999).

Peruvian bark became popular in the eighteenth century in obstetrics and gynecology and Charles White in his *Treatise on the Management of Pregnant and Lying-in Women* (1773) used the bark in the treatment of puerperal fever ('the bark is an excellent remedy in these eruptive fevers') and mentioned it as a medication for use in the prevention of 'many disorders peculiarly incident to the pregnant state'.

Samuel Bard offered Peruvian bark as treatment for 'Flour Albus, the whites'; for pelvic pain after delivery; for uterine prolapse following childbirth and for 'the putrid symptoms ... of Puerperal or Child-bed Fever'. Bard also used the remedy to strengthen the constitution and as an antipyretic and anti-inflammatory (1807 pp. 186, 187, 189, 192–9). John Burns (1820), Regius professor of surgery at the University of Glasgow, suggested the use of 'the cold sea-bath, bark [Peruvian] combined with bitters, and mild injections of vegetable astringent' for uterine inflammation and

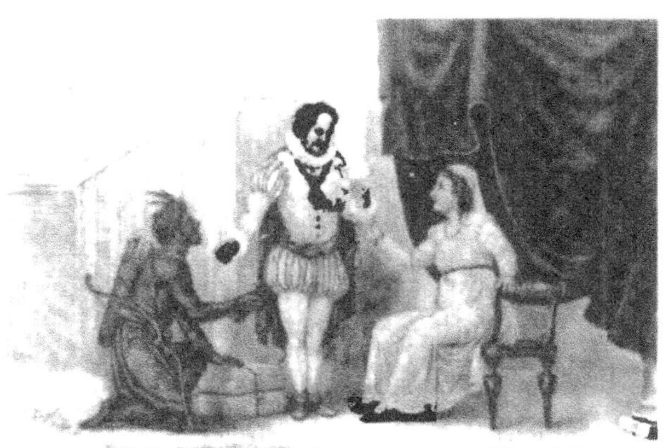
ÆGROTAT LIMÆ CONIUX CHINCONIA FEBRIM
CORTICE MIRANDO POCULA TINCTA FUGANT

Figure 16 The Countess of Chinon receiving quinine

also mentioned the use of bark with emetics, diaphoretics, laxatives and vitriolic acid in the treatment of puerperal sepsis. Charles Meigs opined: 'it is well known that the remedy for intermittent fever [of breast infection] is the Peruvian bark or its preparation' (1842 p. 402). MacNaughton Jones advised quinine in the treatment of peri-metritis and vaginal infection (1885 p. 266) and quinine sulfate with gentian and mercury for endometritis (1889 pp. 297, 346).

Howard Kelly reported that quinine gave 'excellent results as a uterine contractor; it should be given in solution every ten minutes, but not more than two or three doses in one day' (1909 p. 445). Whitridge Williams was of the opinion that 'five grains of the sulphate [of quinine] given in a freshly prepared pill or in solution, and repeated twice at intervals of one hour, may prove of great benefit' in prolonged labor due to secondary uterine inertia (1903 p. 565). F.J. Browne (1950), emeritus professor of obstetrics and gynaecology at the University of London, related: 'for induction of labor quinine has been much used, but opinion now is that it may harm the fetus, causing passage of meconium and even fetal death so it has largely lost favour. Certainly small doses only, not more than ten grains, should be used.' The oxytocic properties, never very well proven, were not sufficient to impact on the use of ergot, but quinine, in combination with stilbestrol, was commonly used to induce medical abortion until the early 1980s.

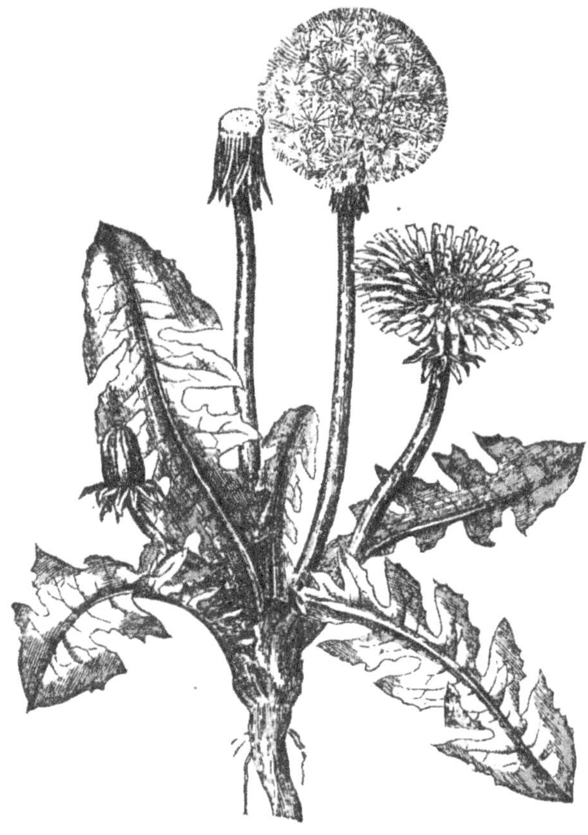

Figure 17 Dandelion (*Taraxacum officinale*)

Quinine was the first natural product to be used in sustained chemotherapy; it was also the first for which a substitute was sought in synthetic chemistry. Its use as an antipyretic was overtaken by acetyl salicylic acid (aspirin) and phenacetin in the late nineteenth century, but in recent times quinine has once again been used in the treatment of malaria.

Lydia E. Pinkham's Vegetable Compound

Lydia Pinkham's 'Vegetable Compound' was one of the most popular patent remedies for women's disorders in America. It contained alcohol, black cohosh, chamomile, dandelion root, Jamaica dogwood, life plant, liquorice, pleurisy root, and (eventually) vitamin B1. The label on the bottles claimed:

> '[A] cure for prolapsus uteri or falling of the womb and all female weaknesses including leucorrhoea, irregular and painful menstruation, inflammation

and ulceration of the womb, floodings etc., For all weaknesses of the generative organs of either sex. It is second to no remedy that has ever been before the public, and for all diseases of the kidneys it is the greatest remedy in the world. Prepared by Mrs Lydia E. Pinkham, Lynn, Massachusetts USA.'

Born Lydia Estes in Lynn, Massachusetts, in 1819, she married Isaac Pinkham in 1843. Isaac was offered a recipe for a 'cure for weaknesses of females' in settlement of a debt and he passed the recipe to Lydia. She added pleurisy root to the bitter brew of herbs and alcohol and offered it around among her family and friends. Due to unprecedented demand for the product it was decided in 1873 to bottle the formula and begin commercial sales. The nostrum became so successful that eventually a factory was built in Lynn where some 450 employees participated in the manufacture of 'Lydia Pinkham's Vegetable Compound'. Both Lydia and her compound were eulogized in song in the 1880s:

'Oh, we'll sing of Lydia Pinkham
And her love for the Human Race.
How she sells her Vegetable Compound,
The papers they publish,
They publish her face'.

The highest annual sales reached four million dollars in 1925 and the Lydia E. Pinkham Medicine Co. continued until 1941 when the Federal Trade Commission ordered it to cease trading. The company was eventually sold to Cooper Laboratories Inc. in 1968. Lydia Pinkham's Compound was still available in drug stores in 1978 (Speert, 1980).

Howard A. Kelly wrote: 'There is a strong tendency among the poorer classes to secretly use [for dysmenorrhea] either gin or whiskey, and this point should be especially borne in mind among dispensary patients. The various patent medicines taken for the relief of pain all contain a large percentage of alcohol and their use should be systematically discouraged' (1909). The percentage of alcohol by volume in some of these compounds, as given by the Massachusetts State Board Analyst is shown in Table 2.

Table 2 Percentage of alcohol in patent medicines, Massachusetts State Board Analyst (Kelly, 1909)

Patent medicine	*Alcohol percentage by volume*
Lydia Pinkham's Vegetable Compound	20.6
Peruna	28.5
Paine's Celery Compound	21.0
Jackson's Golden Seal Tonic	19.6
Schenk's Sea-weed Tonic	19.5
Ayer's Sarsaparilla	26.2
Hood's Sarsaparilla	18.8

James Harvey Young in *The Toadstool Millionaires* (1961), a social history of patent medicines in America before federal regulation, wrote that so famous was Lydia Pinkham that '[Many] small newspaper offices possessed no cut of a woman's face except that of Lydia's maternal countenance, which occasionally was shifted from an advertising to a news column to do double duty as Queen Victoria'. Lydia Pinkham was also immortalized in a popular European song of the late 1960s.

'We'll drink a drink a drink,
To Lily the Pink the Pink the Pink
The Saviour of the human race
She invented medicinal compound
Most efficacious, in every case'.

References

Baldy, J. M. (1894). *An American Text-Book of Gynaecology Medical and Surgical, for Practitioners and Students*, p. 695. (London: F. J. Repman)

Bard, S. (1807). *A Compendium of The Theory and Practice of Midwifery*, pp. 66, 186, 187, 189, 192–9. (New York: Collins and Perkins)

Beck, A. C. (1942). *Obstetrical Practice*, p. 764. (Baltimore: Williams & Wilkins Co.)

Berkeley, C. Sir and Bonney, V. (1935). *A Textbook of Gynaecological Surgery*, p. 18. (London: Cassell & Co.)

Browne, F. J. (1950). *Post-graduate Obstetrics and Gynaecology*, p. 469. (London: Butterworth & Co.)

Burns, J. (1820). *The Principles of Midwifery; including The Diseases of Women and Children*, p. 87. (London: Longman, Hurst, Rees, Orme & Brown)

Coindet, J. F. (1820). Decouverte d'un Nouveau Remede contre le Goitre. *Bibliotheque Universelle*, 14, 190–8

Cooper, Sir A. P. (1840). *On the Anatomy of the Breast*, 2 Volumes. (London: Longman)

Eden, T. W. and Holland, E. (1940). *A Manual of Obstetrics*, p. 654. (London: J. and A. Churchill Ltd.)

Findley, P. (1939). *Priests of Lucina. The Story Of Obstetrics*, pp. 197–202. (Boston: Little, Brown & Co.)

Goodman Gilman, A., Goodman, L. S., Rall, T. W. and Murad, F. (1985). *Goodman & Gilman's The Pharmacological Basis of Therapeutics*, 7th ed. pp. 964–6. (New York: MacMillan Co.)

Gunther, R. T. (1959). *The Greek Herbal of Dioscorides*, No. 164 pp. 558–9. (New York: Hafner Co.)

Hare, H. A. (1901). *A Textbook of Practical Therapeutics, with a special reference to the Application of Remedial Measures to Disease and their Employment upon Rational Basis*, pp. 238–45. (London: Henry Kimpton)

Hobhouse, H. (1986). *Seeds of Change – Five Plants That Transformed Mankind*, pp. 3–40. (New York: Harper & Row)

Jones, W. H. S. (1951). *Pliny. Natural History*, Book 23, pp. 471–2. (Harvard: Heinemann)

Kelly, H. A. (1909). *Medical Gynecology*, pp. 189–205, 622, 632–3. (London: Appleton and Co.)

Lindley, J. (1838). *Flora Medica; A Botanical Account of all the More Important Plants Used in Medicine, in Different Parts of the World*, pp. 183–4, 634. (London: Longman, Orme, Brown & Green)

Linnaeus, C. (1749). *Materia Medica, Liber 1. De Plantis*, pp. 24, 154. (Holmiae: Laurentii Salvii)

MacNaughton Jones, H. (1885). *Practical Manual of Diseases of Women and Uterine Therapeutics*, 2nd ed. pp. 113, 125, 269, 266, 441–4. (London: Bailliere, Tindall & Cox)

MacNaughton Jones, H. (1889). *Practical Manual of Diseases of Women and Uterine Therapeutics for Students*, 6th ed. pp. 463–82, 297, 346. (London: Balliere, Tindall & Cox)

Meigs, C. D. (1842). *The Philadelphia Practice of Midwifery*, 2nd ed. pp. 397–408, 402. (Philadelphia: James Kay, Jr. & Brother)

Poser, C. M. and Bruyn, G. W. (1999). *An Illustrated History of Malaria*. (New York & London: Parthenon Publishing)

Prosser, T. (1769). *An Account and Method of Cure of the Bronchocele or Derby Neck*. (London: W. Owen).

Pseudo-Aristotle (1776). *Aristotle's complete and experienced Midwife*, 13th ed. made English by William Samon M. D. (London)

Pseudo-Aristotle (c. 1830). *The Works of Aristotle, the Famous Philosopher. A New and Improved Edition*. (London: Miller, Law, and Cater)

Pseudo-Aristotle (c. 1900). *The Works of Aristotle, the Famous Philosopher, containing 1 His Complete Masterpiece 2 His Experienced Midwife. 3 His Book of Problems. 4 His Remarks on Physiognomy. 5 The Family Physician*. (London)

Ricci, J. (1950). *Aetios of Amida*, pp. 24–6. (Philadelphia: Blakiston & Co.)

Ringer, S. (1888). *A Handbook of Therapeutics*, pp. 341–4; 589–632. (London: H. K. Lewis)

Serullas, G. S. (1822). Memoire sur l'iodure de potassium, l'acide hydriodique et sur un Compose Nouveau de carbone, d'iode et d'hydrogene. *Ann. Chim. Phys.*, **20**, 163–8

Sims, J. Marion (1866). *Clinical Notes on Uterine Surgery. With Special Reference to the Management of the Sterile Condition*, pp. 121, 227, 396, 335–7. (London: Robert Hardwicke)

Speert, H. (1980). *Obstetrics and Gynecology in America: A History. Lydia Pinkham*, pp. 243–5. (Baltimore, MD: Waverly Press Inc.)

Spencer, W. G. (1989). *Celsus De Medicina*, English Translation. Vol. 2. pp. 42, 58. (London: Heinemann & Co.)

Squire (1908). *Squire's Companion to the British Pharmacapoeia*, 18th edition. (London: J. and A. Churchill)

Thoms, H. (1933). *Chapters in American Obstetrics*, pp. 26–34. (Springfield, IL: Charles C. Thomas)

Turner, W. (1568). *A Booke of the Natures and Properties, as well of the Bathes in England, as of other Bathes in Germanye and Italye*. (Collen: Arnold Birckman)

White, C. (1773). *A Treatise on the Management of Pregnant and Lying-In Women*, pp. 20, 30, 118, 112. (London: Edward & Charles Dilly)

Williams, P. F. (1955). A Book Review: Samuel Bard's 'A Compendium of the Theory and Practice of Midwifery'. *Am. J. Obstet. Gynecol.*, 70(4), 701–10

Williams, J. Whitridge (1903). *Obstetrics. Textbook for the Use of Students and Practitioners*, pp. 554, 565. (New York and London: D. Appleton & Co.)

Wootton, A. C. (1910). *Chronicles of Pharmacy*, Vol. 1, pp. 351–3; Vol. 2, pp. 89, 89–93. (London: Macmillan & Co.)

Young, J. H. (1961). *The Toadstool Millionaires. A Social History of Patent Medicines in America before Federal Regulation*, p. 104. (Princeton, NJ: Princeton University Press)

The twentieth century 17

INTRODUCTION

A glance at *Drugs in Pregnancy and Lactation* (1994) by Gerald Briggs and Roger Freeman of California and Sumner Yaffe of Maryland, reveals that there are in excess of 5000 well-referenced drug monographs in their book. The present diminutive chapter on the materia medica of women in the twentieth century – 'The David Chapter' – is not in competition with the aforementioned 'American Goliath' but aims its slingshot at some of the more important medications that have saved many mothers and their offspring in the past century. Not forgotten are the tragedies surrounding some drugs, originally hailed as marvelous innovations, that unintentionally killed or maimed women and their children.

This chapter deals with specific drugs (e.g. aspirin), with groups of drugs, and with conditions such as menorrhagia, where a number of therapeutic agents are described. While the principal thrust of this chapter involves allopathic medicine, herbal and complementary medicines are the only therapies available to millions of women worldwide. Herbal medications evolved from antiquity and prescribed until recent times by physicians, have not essentially altered over that time.

The modern medications for women, oftentimes abused, are readily available in the 'developed world', but not for the millions of women in disadvantaged societies who die for lack of the simple inexpensive 'new' drugs that we take for granted. The shocking maternal mortality and morbidity and perinatal mortality statistics of 'developing' nations are often worse than comparable rates for Europe and North America at the beginning of the twentieth century. There were ways then, and there are ways now, to alleviate much of the suffering. This chapter is dedicated to those underprivileged women, and to those who care.

Twentieth-century obstetrics and gynecology – source material

For those with an interest in the further study of the many changes that occurred in obstetrics and gynecology in this century, a number of useful references are appended. The obstetrics and gynecology for the period 1900–1950 were explored in depth in the *Historical Review of British Obstetrics and Gynaecology. 1800–1950* (Munro-Kerr, Johnstone and Phillips, 1954). John R. Brown (1964) of the School of Hygiene, Toronto, published a paper entitled 'A chronology of major events in obstetrics and gynecology' highlighting major achievements in the first 40 years of the twentieth century. T.L.T. Lewis (1964) of Guy's Hospital and Queen Charlotte's, London, included a very good 30-year history (from 1934) in his *Progress in Clinical Obstetrics and Gynaecology.*

Another source of note is the section 'Obstetrics in Broad Perspective' contained in the 14th edition of *Williams' Obstetrics* (Hellman and Pritchard, 1971) – also the updated versions in the 18th and 20th editions. Fritz Fuchs of New York related the history of obstetrics from 1956 to 1982 in his Presidential Address to the New York Obstetrical Society, reproduced as the most entertaining and innovative 'An Alphabet of Progress' in the *American Journal of Obstetrics and Gynecology* (1983). There is an historical overview of the many achievements from 1900 to 1992 by Michael O'Dowd and Elliot Philipp in their *The History of Obstetrics and Gynaecology* (1994 pp. 21–40).

OBSTETRICS AND GYNECOLOGY IN THE EARLY TWENTIETH CENTURY

At the beginning of the twentieth century maternal mortality rates, long used as an index of the effectiveness of midwifery care, varied between five and ten per thousand births in Europe and America. It became apparent that well-fed, parous, rural women were less likely to die as a result of pregnancy than city dwellers and those who delivered in institutions. Primigravidas and mothers of large families were at particularly high risk. Most of the deaths were preventable. Failure to provide adequate antenatal care and proper supervision and management of women in labor were indicted as major reasons for the high death rates.

Chemotherapy and antibiotics

With the introduction of the sulfonamide drugs there was a major reduction in the maternal mortality rates from 1930 onwards, because the primary cause of maternal mortality, puerperal sepsis, could now be treated effectively. The advent of penicillin in the early 1940s, combined with the adoption of aseptic techniques, dramatically reduced mortality and morbidity from sepsis and played a major role in the treatment of the killer venereal disease, syphilis. The introduction of treatment for eclampsia, for thromboembolism, and for heart disease, anemia and other undercurrent illnesses had a major role to play in safeguarding women's lives.

Antenatal care

The introduction of antenatal care, generally attributed to J.W. Ballantyne of Edinburgh, allowed professionals to assess the general health and welfare of pregnant women for the first time. Ballantyne's first antenatal bed was endowed at the Royal Maternity and Simpson Memorial Hospital in 1901. Home visits to antenatal patients began in the same year in Boston, USA, and the first antenatal clinic was opened there in 1911.

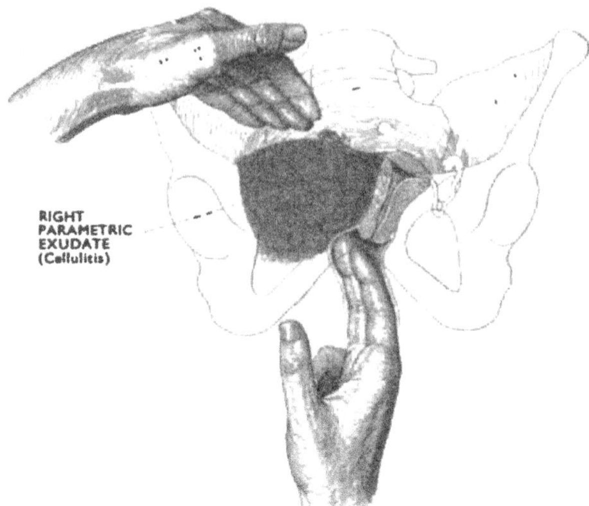

Figure 1 Depiction of puerperal sepsis from O'Donel Browne, *Manual of Practical Obstetrics*

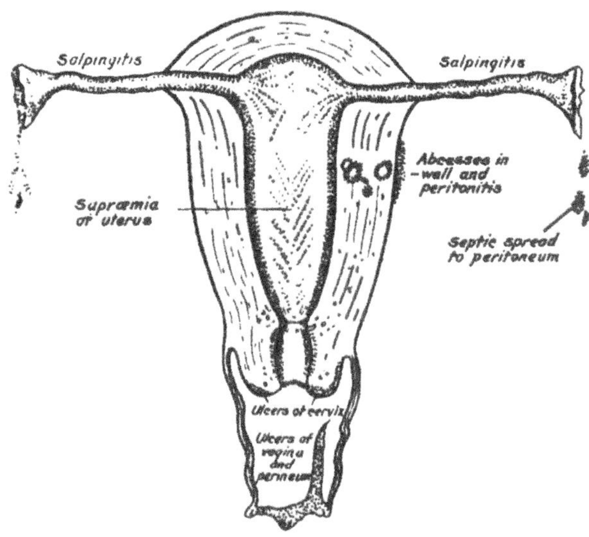

Figure 2 Uterine sepsis from O'Donel Browne, *Manual of Practical Obstetrics*

Eclampsia

The recognition of antenatal pathology, particularly the early diagnosis of pre-eclampsia, had a major impact on maternal mortality. The relationship between hypertension, proteinuria and edema, and pre-eclampsia was recognized at the beginning of the twentieth century. When Stroganoff introduced anti-eclamptic therapy at the end of the first decade it led to a remarkable fall in deaths from the disease. The combination of anticonvulsant and antihypertensive treatments introduced in the 1960s lowered death rates still further. In the 1990s magnesium sulfate, combined with antihypertensives became the treatment of choice.

Antepartum hemorrhage

In 1900 treatment of antepartum hemorrhage was by tamponade of the cervix and vagina to control the bleeding. The cervix was then manually dilated and internal version and fetal extraction were performed. Maternal mortality was close to 10% and perinatal mortality was over 50%. Macafee of Belfast introduced expectant management of antepartum hemorrhage and reduced maternal mortality to 0.7% and perinatal mortality to less than 25% during the years 1932 to 1944.

Cesarean section and blood transfusion

The cesarean section, considered a dangerous operation until about 1912, became more commonly used in the management of the low-implanted placenta and other complications of pregnancy and labor, reducing further the maternal and perinatal mortality rates. Obstetric flying squads were instituted in the late 1930s, allowing treatment of the woman in her own home before transfer to hospital. Blood transfusions became a possibility after Landsteiner showed in 1900 that there were different blood groups and that reactions did not occur when group-compatible blood was transfused.

Anesthesia

In the early part of the twentieth century many women died as a result of poor anesthetic technique, and the use of anesthetic gases that were dangerous for the pregnant woman. The development of safer anesthesia was a slow process but it had a major impact on obstetrics and gynecology, reducing maternal mortality and morbidity and leading eventually to satisfactory analgesia in labor.

TWENTIETH CENTURY ADVANCES IN OBSTETRICS AND GYNECOLOGY

Some of the advances which led to a reduction in maternal mortality and morbidity and perinatal mortality and morbidity are listed below. Some beneficial changes in the management of labor and the field of gynecology are also noted. These lists are fleshed-out and enlivened by the voices of experience that follow: the observations of two obstetricians, J.B. Greenhill and Stanley Hewitt, who practiced their art on opposite sides of the Atlantic.

Advances that reduced maternal and perinatal mortality and morbidity rates

Antenatal care, antenatal corticosteroids, antibiotics, anti-eclamptics, antithrombotics, avoidance of rhesus sensitization, avoidance of teratogenic influences, better education, blood transfusion and anti-d (rhogam), flying squads, improved health care services, improvements in medical and nursing techniques, less traumatic delivery, rubella immunization, safer anesthesia, sick care baby units, social changes, sulfonamides, surfactant, treatment of pregnancy-associated diseases.

Advances in the management of labor

Analgesia, beta-sympathomimetic agents, induction methods, maternal and fetal monitoring, methods of resuscitation, safer assisted vaginal delivery, safer cesarean section, syntometrine, syntocinon, training of medical, nursing and allied personnel.

Advances in the management of gynecological cancer

Anesthesia, antithrombotic agents, chemotherapy, earlier methods of detection, improvements in operative capabilities, radiotherapy.

Advances in the investigation and management of:

Endometriosis, endoscopy, family planning, gonadotropins, infertility, menstrual cycle disorders, hormones (estrogen, progesterone, prostaglandins, etc.), urology, venereal disease, DNA manipulation.

J.P. Greenhill, 'Progress in Obstetrics and Gynecology, 1921–1975'

J.P. Greenhill, professor of gynecology at Cook County Hospital, Chicago, and editor of the *Year Book of Obstetrics and Gynecology* (1975), detailed the progress in the specialty during the 50 years 1921–1975:

> 'In 1921, when I became the first resident at Chicago Lying-in Hospital, the practice of

obstetrics was rather primitive ... Relatively few pregnant women were given good prenatal care ...

The only routine laboratory tests we carried out were those for urine, blood counts, gonorrhea and syphilis (Wassermann reaction). We had no special clinics for physical illnesses such as heart disease, nephritis, diabetes, cardiovascular disease, hypertension and toxemia. The term 'high-risk patient' did not exist. We did not have the assistance of specialists except when we called them in consultation.

Most deliveries were spontaneous, but we performed many low- and mid-forceps deliveries and even high-forceps operations. Today a high forceps operation is almost a criminal act. We delivered nearly all breeches from below and we became extremely skillful in this art. We did extremely few cesarean sections for placenta previa, including total placenta previa.

It was difficult to get blood for transfusion in those days ... We had no antibiotics whatever ... Of course when an abscess was present it was incised and drained, but this complication is extremely rare today.

We did not know how to locate the placenta except by vaginal examination ...

Another disease in which fantastic progress has been made is erythroblastosis, a disease that caused innumerable deaths and fetal malformations ... We had no available pituitary extract until a few years later, even though it had been advocated by Hofbauer as early as 1918.

We saw many babies with congenital deformities. It was several years before we learned that a special group of malformations was due to rubella acquired by the mother in the 1st trimester of pregnancy.

We knew nothing about amniocentesis. Fetal monitoring formerly was done only by means of a stethoscope applied every 5–30 minutes during labor.

[*Gynecology:*] In the entire history of medicine, one of the foremost contributions made is the Papanicolaou smear for the detection of cancer of the cervix and *corpus uteri*. The Schiller test, which was described later, also became important for the detection of cancer ... Colposcopy, first described by Hinselmann, rapidly became popular and useful worldwide ... The improvements in gynecologic surgery during the past half century have been enormous.

Studies and tests of infertility have resulted in the birth of thousands of healthy babies who might not otherwise have been born. ... During the last few years there have been experiments to produce babies both in lower animals and in human females by starting fertilization *in vitro*. If applied to human beings, cloning may result in the development of individuals ... identical to whatever donor individuals had been chosen: boys genetically exactly like the father, girls like their mother or individuals like some true or false hero of art, science, or sports or like some demagogue or some saint.

The field of endocrinology has become awesome. A great contribution, to mention only one, is the induction of ovulation in women who do not produce ova spontaneously ... the introduction of radiotherapy, both intrauterine and external, has greatly improved the incidence of 5- and 10-year cures ... The diagnosis and treatment of cancer of the breast have changed considerably during the past few years.'

Stanley Hewitt, progress in obstetrics and gynecology, 1940–1981

Stanley Hewitt, past chairman of Ireland's 'Institute of Obstetricians', considered the many advances in the specialty during the previous 40 years.

'Neonatology, a relatively new specialty has developed over the last few years only, and is probably now one of the greatest advances in the prevention of mortality and morbidity, especially in premature babies. Virginia Apgar, one of America's foremost anesthesiologists ... introduced in 1953 the Scoring System which bears her name, and probably started the scientific basis for the careful assessment of the well-being of babies.

With regard to obstetrics, let us consider in a bit more detail the two great groups of maternal mortality and morbidity, and perinatal mortality and morbidity, which, after all is what it is all about, or rather their prevention is what it is all about ... In the past, the 3 major killers of mothers were hemorrhage, sepsis and toxemia (in which I include eclampsia); whilst a few mothers still unfortunately die of these conditions, to all intents and purposes all 3 have now moved down the table. ... With the ready availability of Epidural analgesia in our hospital, virtually no inhalation anesthetics are administered in our labor wards at all.

... mention must be made of the Obstetric Flying Squad first instituted by Farquahar Murray in Newcastle in 1937.

Obstetricians and gynecologists have to be wary of becoming over-confident in their ability to do better than Nature and thus intervene too much; we should also take stock of unnecessary operating.'

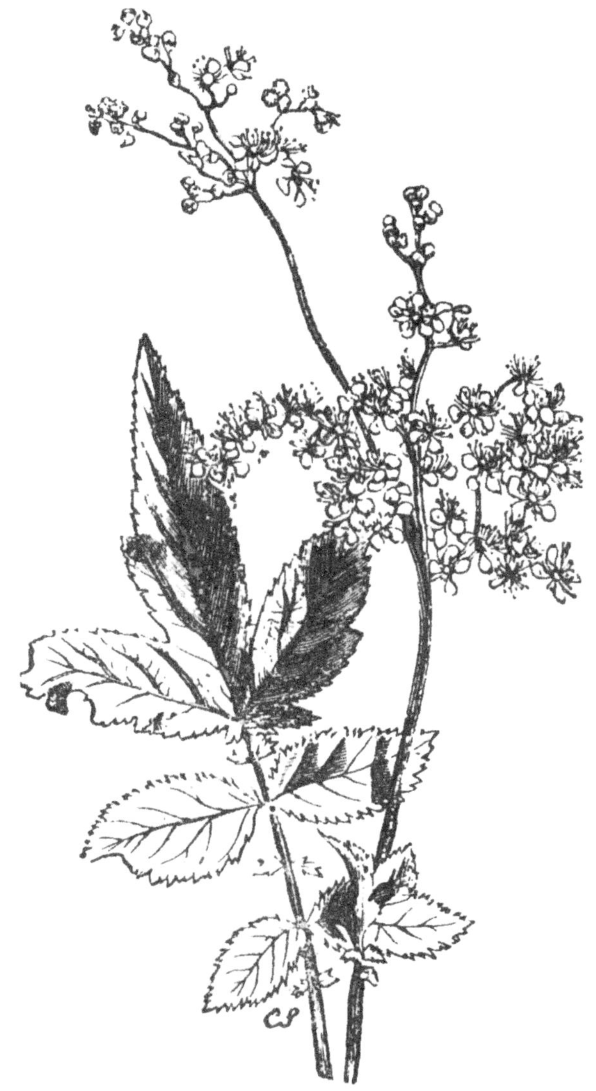

Figure 3 Meadowsweet (*Filipendula ulmaria*)

A SELECTION OF TWENTIETH CENTURY MATERIA MEDICA – INDIVIDUAL DRUGS

The following seven drugs had a major impact on women's health and on the welfare of their children and extended family units.

Aspirin

On 25 April 1763 the Rev. Edmund Stone reported to the Royal Society that willow bark had a bitter taste similar to Peruvian bark which was prescribed at that time for agues (fevers) and malaria. Rev. Stone treated 50 people who had symptoms of rheumatic fever and the willow bark gave satisfactory results in almost every case.

The active principle of the willow bark (from *Salix alba vulgaris*) is a bitter glycoside called salicin, first isolated in pure form by Leroux in 1829 who also demonstrated that salicin had antipyretic effects. On hydrolysis, salicin yielded salicylic acid (and glucose), a chemical that was originally produced in 1835 from salicylaldehyde as found in meadowsweet (*Spiraea ulmaria*, now known as *Filipendula ulmaria* in the Rosaceae). Salicin was also present in oil of wintergreen (*Gaultheria procumbens*), much used by native North American Indians and still listed in the US pharmacopoeia, and extracts of other plants (Flower, Moncada and Vane, 1985). In 1859 Kolbe of Leipzig, aided by Lautemann, made a synthetic form of salicylic acid, by the reaction of carbolic acid (derived from phenol, obtained from coal tar) and carbon dioxide in the presence of an alkali, and the commercial production of salicylic acid became practical in 1874 (Wootton, 1910). Dr Thomas Maclagan of Dundee treated acute rheumatic fever with salicin in 1876 with good results, and synthetic salicylic acid became popular in the treatment of rheumatic fever and other rheumatic disorders (Hollman, 1992 pp. 8–9).

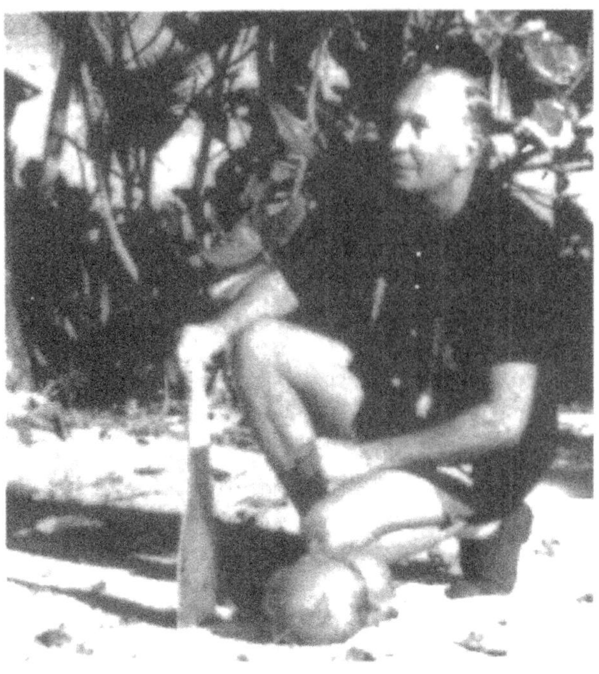

Figure 4 Ralph Douglas Reye (1912–1977)

The original formulation of salicylic acid caused gastric irritation and in 1899 Felix Hoffman developed the compound acetylsalicylic acid and called it aspirin (derived from 'A', from acetyl; 'spir', from spireae and 'in', a common ending for drug names) although acetylsalicylic acid had already been prepared by Charles Gerhard, a French chemist, in 1853 (Bayer, 1938). Its medicinal value was fully recognized in 1899 when Heinrich Dreser, a German scientist, wrote about its effectiveness. By the beginning of the twentieth century aspirin was found to be a valuable analgesic, anti-inflammatory and antipyretic. It soon became the fastest-selling drug in the world.

Aspirin rapidly found its way into the materia medica of women and was used for the relief of dysmenorrhea, although it had some competition from phenacetin (ethoxyphenylacetamide, originally derived from coal tar, or gaseous hydrocarbon). Aspirin and the aspirin-like drugs including indomethacin, acetaminophen (paracetamol) and a large number of other agents were introduced from the 1960s onwards for a similar purpose. During the 1970s many of the products were found to inhibit the biosynthesis and release of arachidonic acid, the precursor of prostaglandins.

In 1963 Ralph Reye, an Australian doctor, reported a syndrome that bears his name which comprised brain inflammation and liver disorders. This rare disease affected infants and children who had had viral infections such as chickenpox, gastroenteritis and influenza, and half of those involved died from the effects of the syndrome. In 1982 the American Surgeon-General became convinced that there was enough evidence to show a link between aspirin and Reye syndrome and ordered that the medication was not to be given to children or teenagers with influenza or chickenpox: within four years the incidence of Reye syndrome was halved.

Research proved that aspirin had a wide range of beneficial pharmacological actions, including its effects on coagulation which lead to prolongation of the bleeding time: aspirin was found to inhibit platelet adhesion and to have other effects on coagulation and fibrinolysis. It was postulated that inhibition of thromboxane synthesis by platelets was a mechanism through which aspirin might be used in the prophylaxis of pre-eclampsia and intrauterine growth retardation. Aspirin is currently the treatment of choice for women who have recurrent miscarriages related to the anti-phospholipid antibody (aPL) syndrome. Treatment with 75 mg acetylsalicylic acid daily was found to increase the live-birth rate in such patients (RCOG, 1998).

Diethylstilbestrol (DES)

Estrogenic preparations became commercially available during the 1930s, but the efforts to purify and standardize these products led to many errors. The first artificial estrogen was synthesized by Cook and associates (1933). At that time E.C. Dodds, who was involved in that first synthesis, was the Courtauld professor of biochemistry at the Middlesex Hospital, London. Following the 1933 publication there were many papers on synthetic estrogens from his unit. In 1938 Dodds, and Robinson of Oxford, prepared various combinations of substituted stilbenes and found that the diethyl derivative was the most effective. Unlike some other hormonal drugs, diethylstilbestrol (DES) was found to be effective when administered orally. The potency of the compound was five times that of estradiol. DES was easy to prepare in pure form and was cheap to produce. Dienestrol and hexestrol were two other compounds which showed only minor structural and therapeutic differences from DES and they also became available through the work of Dodds and co-workers (Dodds *et al.*, 1938 a–d).

The synthesis of diethylstilbestrol was a major scientific and commercial achievement. The therapeutic applications of DES included lactation suppression; control of menopausal symptoms; control of breast and prostate cancer; hormonal support in threatened miscarriage, and 'morning-after' contraception. During the decade 1945 to 1955 DES was frequently prescribed for threatened miscarriage and a conservative estimate claimed that more than two million women received the drug during pregnancy.

Soon after the introduction of DES toxic effects of the synthetic hormone were reported in laboratory animals. In 1969 Clinch and Tindall noted transitory liver function changes in postpartum women receiving DES to suppress lactation. Two very important studies were published in the early 1970s which demonstrated an association between maternal DES treatment in pregnancy with neoplasia in female offspring. Herbst and colleagues (1971) presented a case–control study which linked maternal DES treatment with vaginal clear-cell adenocarcinoma in daughters, the first human example of transplacental carcinogenesis. One year later Noller and associates (1972) found an association between maternal stilbestrol and cervical adenocarcinoma. These and other reports led to a rapid decline in the use of DES after 1975.

According to Lanier and associates (1973), it appeared that about 4 per 1000 women exposed to the drug *in utero* were likely to develop cancer. Abnormalities of the vagina and cervix were frequently found to be diagnostic of *in utero* DES exposure, vaginal adenosis being the most common abnormal finding. A cervical hood or 'cockscomb' appearance was described along with other abnormalities of the cervix and vagina, all of which varied in their frequency and severity. Abnormalities of the uterine cavity (in particular a T-shaped irregularity of the cavity) or of the Fallopian tubes were reported in up to two thirds of DES exposed women. There was general agreement that the frequency of late pregnancy complications, preterm delivery and perinatal death were increased in women who clearly exhibited changes due to *in utero* exposure to DES (O'Dowd and Philipp, 1994).

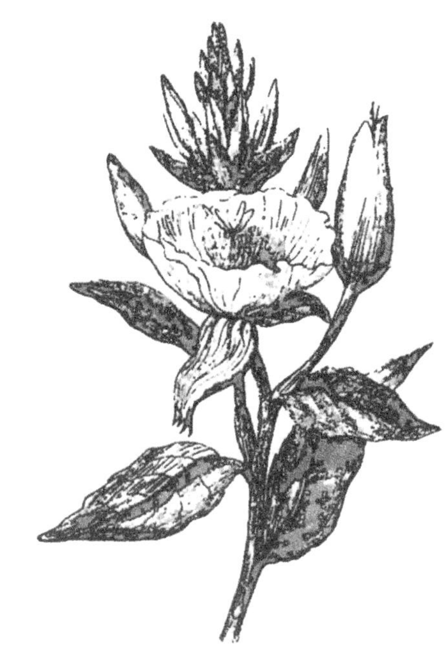

Figure 5 Evening primrose

Evening primrose oil

The evening, or tree, primrose, originally a native of North America, was imported into Italy and from there carried all over Europe. Maude Grieve in her *Modern Herbal* (1931 p. 658) related that the botanical name for evening primrose is *Oenothera biennis*; from Greek *oinos*, wine, and *thera*, a hunt, as it was once thought that the roots of evening primrose evoked a relish for wine, although others said that it dispelled the effects of alcohol. A medication was made from the leaves and stem peelings of Evening primrose to treat 'certain female complaints' such as pelvic fullness.

Judy Graham (1984) described the early history of the plant in her book *Evening Primrose Oil*. Plant enthusiasts brought the evening primrose from Virginia to Europe in 1614 as a botanical curiosity but most of the strains came to Europe during the eighteenth century in soil used as ballast for cotton cargo ships. In Europe the evening primrose became known by the appellation 'King's cure-all'. A German scientist named Unger (1917) examined the plant and determined that the seeds contained approximately 15% of oil. Two years later, a preliminary report appeared showing that the oil contained oleic and linolenic acids, and a new fatty acid that was named gammalinolenic acid (GLA) (Heiduschka and Luft, 1919).

Research on evening primrose and GLA began in earnest in the 1960s. John Williams, a research biochemist, manufactured capsules of evening primrose oil with the brand name Naudicelle. During the 1970s clinical research was carried out on the use of evening primrose oil in a number of medical conditions. Dr David Horrobin was instrumental in setting up the company Efamol Ltd. to develop, market and research evening primrose oil. The GLA of evening primrose oil was found to be a precursor of prostaglandin E1, which was responsible for many of the medicinal benefits.

David Horrobin (1983) discovered that in patients with a deficiency of essential fatty acids, prolactin had exaggerated effects and could cause premenstrual symptoms and Abraham (1983) postulated that the premenstrual syndrome was caused by prostaglandin E1 deficiency. Soon afterwards it was discovered that patients with premenstrual tension syndrome had lower levels of GLA when compared with controls. Brush (1984) suggested that there was a defect in the biosynthetic pathway of essential fatty acids in these women, and that evening primrose oil, a rich source of GLA, could be used as treatment. The physical symptoms of premenstrual tension syndrome, particularly breast tenderness, responded well to evening primrose oil at a dose of two or three 500 mg capsules twice daily, from three days prior to the onset of symptoms until menstruation.

Folic acid

The discovery

The discovery of folic acid is intertwined with that of vitamin B12 and their relationship to megaloblastic anemia. In the mid-nineteenth century, between 1824 and 1855, a number of cases of what was probably megaloblastic anemia were described by Combe and Addison. It was initially thought that the anemia was related to a gastric complaint. In 1860 Austin Flint described the severe gastric atrophy associated with the anemia and the term 'progressive pernicious anemia' was coined in 1872. It was discovered by Whipple in 1925 that liver was a potent treatment for iron deficiency anemia, in dogs. Minot and Murphy treated pernicious anemia in the same way with positive results. It became obvious that both an 'intrinsic' (or gastric) factor and an 'extrinsic' factor were involved in the causation of the anemia, and it was discovered that vitamin B12 was the extrinsic factor (Hillman, 1985).

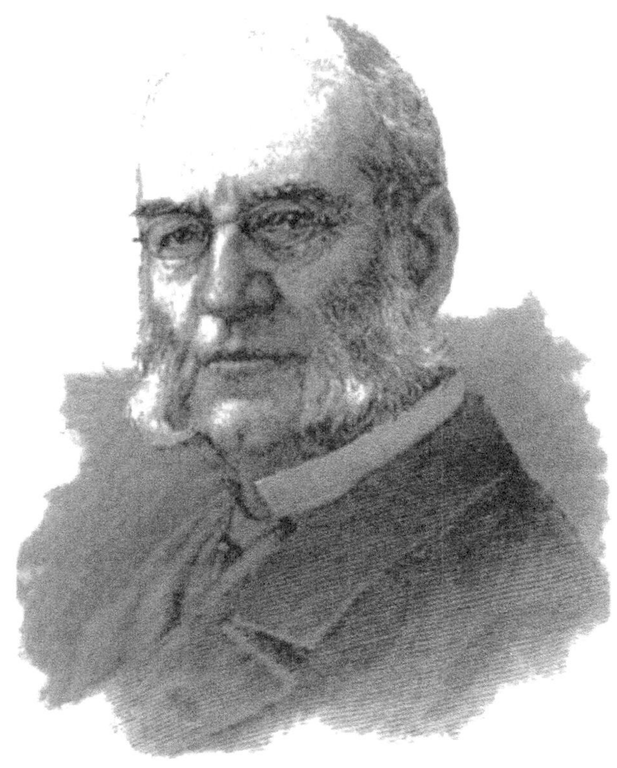

Figure 6 Austin Flint (1812–1886)

In 1932 Wills and Bilimoria described a macrocytic anemia in Indian women that responded to a crude liver extract but was unresponsive to the purified fractions known to be effective in pernicious anemia. The factor was known as 'Wills' factor' and later 'vitamin M', for which the term folic acid was introduced by Mitchell and co-workers (1941) following its isolation from leafy vegetables. The name was derived from the Latin *folio*, a leaf, and the Greek *phyllon*. It was discovered that lack of folic acid produced diarrhea, weight loss and megaloblastic anemia, the last two symptoms resembling those of vitamin B12 deficiency. The structure of the original vitamin-like material, isolated from spinach leaves, was elucidated in 1941 (Evans, 1996). Folic acid, the second-youngest vitamin, was synthesized in 1945. Folic acid (pteroylglutamic acid) is found in fresh green vegetables, liver, yeast and some fruits. Lengthy cooking can destroy up to 90% of the folate content of food.

Folic acid and pregnancy

Bryan M. Hibbard (1964) of the Department of Obstetrics and Gynaecology at the University of Liverpool, wrote in his The William Blair Bell Memorial Lecture on 'The Role of Folic Acid in Pregnancy': 'The formation and development of every human cell is dependent on an adequate supply of folic acid. Folic acid governs the synthesis of the precursors of DNA – the nucleic acid which gives each cell life and character ... [Comparison] of epidemiological factors in patients with folic acid deficiency and with abruptio placentae shows a close correlation ... those factors ... may also operate in certain cases of abortion or congenital malformation can be produced.'

Hibbard wrote of pregnant women who were prescribed the folic acid antagonist iminopterin as an abortifacient. In one series of twelve patients, nine aborted and one gave birth to an infant with major malformations. In summary he related that defective folic acid metabolism occurred in approximately one in ten pregnancies in his community. The defect was partially or wholly responsible for one third of cases of pregnancy anemia and there was a constant relationship between the occurrence of abruptio placentae and folic acid deficiency. Hibbard theorized that defective folic acid metabolism was responsible for some abortions and fetal malformations and he therefore advised that all pregnant mothers should have early and adequate prophylactic therapy.

Folic acid and fetal malformation

Elizabeth D. Hibbard and R.W. Smithells (1965) of the Department of Obstetrics and Gynaecology at the University of Liverpool and Alder Hey Children's Hospital, Liverpool, reported that there appeared to be a significant relationship between malformation of the fetus and defective folate metabolism in the mother. In 1964 they investigated 98 women who gave birth to infants with severe malformations, principally of the central nervous system. A formiminoglutamic acid (FIGLU) excretion test, to detect folic acid deficiency, was carried out as soon as the malformation was diagnosed prenatally, or within two to three days of delivery, in all 98 mothers. Results of FIGLU excretion tests in the mothers of malformed infants were compared with matched mothers with normal infants. Of 177 women attending one of the hospitals in the study, 11.4% had positive FIGLU tests. The women delivered of malformed infants showed an incidence approximately five times the normal for folate deficiency. Hibbard and Smithells concluded that 'the familial occurrence of serious nervous system malformations might be mediated, in some instances, through genetically determined defective folate metabolism'.

Prevention of malformations

The possible prevention of neural tube defects (NTD) by periconceptional vitamin supplementation was reported on by the researchers R.W. Smithells and colleagues (1980, 1983). They detailed the results of a trial on multivitamin supplementation where one of 178 (0.6%) infants of fully-supplemented mothers had an NTD; 13 of 260 (5%) infants of unsupplemented mothers, however, were affected. The 'study mothers' were prescribed Pregnavite forte F, a multivitamin and iron preparation that contained 0.36 mg folic acid with ascorbic acid, calcium phosphate, ferrous sulfate, iron, nicotinamide, riboflavin, thiamin, vitamin A and vitamin D. The research team concluded that vitamin supplementation had prevented some NTDs: 'This is the most straight-forward interpretation and is consistent with the circumstantial evidence linking nutrition with NTDs ... We hope that the data presented will encourage others to initiate similar and related studies.'

Laurence and associates (1981) conducted a double-blind, randomized controlled trial of folate treatment in women who had had one child with a neural tube defect. Sixty of the affected women were prescribed

4 mg of folic acid per day prior to conception, and 51 women had placebo. There were no recurrences of NTDs among compliant mothers in the first group, but two among the non-compliers, and four among the mothers in the placebo group. Laurence and co-workers concluded that 'folic acid supplementation might be a cheap, safe and effective method of primary prevention of neural tube defects ... this must be confirmed in a large, multicenter trial'.

A Medical Research Council vitamin Study Group (1991) collated results of 1000 pregnancies for which outcomes were known and demonstrated a 72% reduction in NTD recurrence with periconception supplementation using 4 mg folic acid per day. In 1992, immediately after the publication of the MRC findings, the Departments of Health in the United Kingdom and the Centers for Disease Control in the United States issued recommendations on the prevention of the recurrence of NTDs – women with a previously affected pregnancy were to be advised to take 4 mg folic acid daily from at least four weeks before conception until the third month of pregnancy (Department of Health, 1992).

In a major medical breakthrough, Czeizel and Dudas (1992) reported in the *New England Journal of Medicine* that the 'first occurrence' of NTD could be prevented in the majority of instances by periconception vitamin supplementation, demonstrating a highly significant protective effect of 0.8 mg of folic acid per day (with other vitamins). Recommendations for the prevention of occurrent NTDs were issued by the government of the United Kingdom and the United States in 1992 that *all* women capable of becoming pregnant should consume 400 µg of folic acid daily. Similar recommendations were issued in other countries (Department of Health, 1992; Centers for Disease Control, 1992).

On 1 January 1998 the US Food and Drug Administration (FDA) stipulated that folic acid should be added to certain cereal-grain products. It was the first amendment to the US Food fortification laws since the early 1940s. Despite the information and guidance, however, there was minimal compliance with the Department of Health (UK) recommendations for routine prophylaxis to prevent NTDs. Mathews, Yudkin and Neil (1998) reported the shocking statistic that an average of only 30% of women took folic acid before pregnancy. As a result, an intensive educational program was established both within the medical profession and in the general community, with the aim of folic acid supplementation in the majority of women at risk of pregnancy.

Conclusion

It is now known that the minimum daily non-pregnant requirement of folic acid is 50 µg while pregnant patients require 400 µg per day, the recommended dose for the prevention of 'first occurrence' NTD. Supplementation should begin prior to and be continued for the first 12 weeks, of pregnancy. The major neural tube defects are spinal bifida (51%), anencephalus (40%), encephalooele (8%) and iniencephaly (1%) and are due to failure of the embryonal neural tube to close normally. Folic acid supplementation can prevent up to 70% of NTDs but for the remaining 30% of women who seem to be folate-resistant there is no preventative therapy.

Rubella vaccine

Rubella was recognized as a distinct entity in the early nineteenth century and its German name *rotheln* was replaced in English by 'rubella' in the late 1860s, although the name 'German measles' still remains in common usage. Because of its mild clinical manifestations rubella received scant attention until Greg (1942) of Sydney, Australia, noted the association between intrauterine rubella infection and congenital cataract in 1941. Greg reported a series of 78 cases of congenital cataract in 44 of whom a congenital heart lesion co-existed. He drew attention to the fact that in 68 instances the mothers had suffered from an attack of rubella, the infection occurring in the first three months of pregnancy in 67 of the cases. Greg's suggestion of a link between rubella infection in pregnancy and subsequent fetal abnormality was greeted with caution and an editorial in *The Lancet* commented: 'The possibility remains that he [Greg] cannot yet be said to have proved his case' (*The Lancet*, 1991). We now know that there was indeed an association and that infection with the rubella virus appears to produce a sub-lethal interference with normal development. Virus particles cross the placenta and in some cases persist for many months into postnatal life – the 'continuing rubella syndrome'.

The 'congenital rubella syndrome' was studied in great detail by Dr Lou Cooper (1968) from St Luke's Roosevelt Hospital, Central New York, who conducted a long term follow-up of 20 000 children born with the syndrome in the USA during the rubella epidemic of 1964–1965. One-third of the patients were found to be profoundly handicapped and required institutional care. The typical syndrome comprised cataract, deaf mutism, congenital heart lesions, microcephaly, mental defects, pyloric stenosis and intestinal atresia. The risk of congenital defect after maternal rubella in the first trimester of pregnancy was 15–20%, being highest in the first month (about 50%) and lowest in the third month (about 8%). The infants born to mothers who had been infected during the second and third months of pregnancy had multiple handicaps and the majority of affected infants had degrees of deafness. Congenital defects were comparatively rare when rubella infection was contracted after the fourth month of pregnancy.

R.W. Smithells (1971), professor of paediatrics at Leeds University, wrote: 'Attempts to prevent rubella embryopathy in the past rested on three equally unsatisfactory approaches.' These three approaches consisted of deliberate attempts to spread rubella among schoolgirls; the administration of gammaglobulin to pregnant women exposed to rubella; and termination of pregnancy. Smithells continued: 'The main hope for the future lies in the active immunization of non-immune adolescent girls with rubella vaccine. A number of different vaccines have been developed since rubella virus was first cultured in 1964.' Rubella immunization was introduced in the UK in 1970 (*The Lancet*, 1991) and the congenital rubella syndrome became a rarity.

Thalidomide

Thalidomide, the sedative and hypnotic, was first synthesized in West Germany in 1954. Following extensive trials it was made available there in 1956–57, without prescription, as Contergan. In Great Britain it became available on prescription as Distaval. The chief merit of the drug was that overdose did not cause coma and it appeared that lethal doses could not be achieved, particularly by intending suicides. As thalidomide could be obtained without prescription, the sedative soon achieved huge popularity. It became a routine hypnotic for use in hospitals, it was recommended for children with coughs and fever, and was contained in a number of proprietary medications. According to Professor D.R. Laurence of London University, the sedative became known as 'West Germany's baby-sitter' (Laurence, 1973).

In 1959, the German chemical company Chemie Grunenthal received a letter from a Dr Voss warning that patients on treatment with the drug had developed peripheral neuritis, and it was also soon recorded that prolonged intake of Thalidomide could cause hypothyroidism. In July 1961 the company made their first settlement in recognition that thalidomide had caused damage. By 1960–61 it was reported that an outbreak of phocomelia had occurred in West Germany. Phocomelia is the medical term for 'seal extremities,' a term which arose because the rudimentary hands and/or feet that stemmed directly from the trunk resembling the flippers of a seal. In November 1961 William McBride, an Australian obstetrician–gynecologist, reported an association between thalidomide and birth defects in a letter to *The Lancet* (1961). The drug was taken off the market in December 1961.

The West German Health Ministry subsequently estimated that thalidomide had caused birth deformities in about 10 000 babies, of whom 5000 survived, 1600 of the children requiring artificial limbs. In Britain there were at least 600 live births of malformed children, of whom about 400 survived. In the USA the Food and Drug Administration had not approved the drug when the lethal effects were discovered and general distribution was avoided. However, thalidomide babies were born in the USA following indiscriminate clinical trials by over a thousand doctors who gave the drug to an estimated 20 000 patients of whom at least 207 were pregnant. It was claimed that in 1962 Japan had at least a thousand children with major deformities as a result of thalidomide, due to irresponsible and unrestricted over-the-counter selling of thalidomide, even though its effects were then known.

It was later demonstrated that those mothers who took thalidomide during the crucial period 37–44 days from the first day of the last period were most likely to deliver a child with fetal anomaly, with an estimated incidence of 20%. Thalidomide, like most drugs of the time, was not tested on pregnant animals before marketing. The discovery of the relationship between thalidomide ingestion in pregnancy and phocomelia, and other fetal malformations was only the start of the sad story for those who were involved: Martin and Karen Fido detailed the family problems, legal issues and survivors' stories in their book *The World's Worst Medical Mistakes* (1996).

Vitamin K

A fall in the neonatal prothrombin level is normal during the first few days of life. The decline is due to immaturity of the production mechanism within the liver. If this is severe enough it will result in hemorrhagic disease of the newborn (HDN), the worst manifestation of which is intracranial hemorrhage. The fall in the prothrombin level is likely to be greatest in premature infants. Other risk factors include maternal pre-eclampsia, prolonged labor, birth asphyxia, breastfeeding and surgical procedures. Estimates vary but the rate of HDN was around 4 per 100 000 (Slattery, 1994). The use of prophylactic vitamin K resulted in a significant and clinically important reduction in hemorrhage in treated babies (Lehman, 1944; Dam *et al.*, 1952).

Deficiency of vitamin K causes a bleeding tendency because the vitamin is necessary for the synthesis of prothrombin and factor VII by the liver. vitamin K1 is present in green foods and vegetables while vitamin K2 is produced in the intestinal canal. Vitamin K treatment was introduced to prevent HDN in 1935. In the 1950s synthetic vitamin K, menadione (Synkavit), was used in a dose of 30 mg or more, and was discovered to cause red cell hemolysis and kernicterus, a grave form of neonatal jaundice (Allison, 1955; Laurence, 1955; Meyer and Angus, 1956).

In the 1960s intramuscular phytomenadione (Konakion), 1 mg, became standard prophylaxis against HDN in Britain but argument raged as to whether it should be given selectively or to all babies. Debate also arose about whether oral vitamin K would give the same protection against HDN as the intramuscular preparation. The argument in favor of oral treatment was partly based on the fact that bottle-fed babies almost never suffered from vitamin K deficiency bleeding because they absorbed vitamin K from their supplemented milk formulas. Golding and associates (1990, 1992) reported that although vitamin K had been widely used for over 30 years, as prophylaxis against HDN the first case–controlled study of its long-term safety (in terms of the risk of cancer) was not published until August 1992. These researchers reported that the administration of intramuscular vitamin K was associated with a doubling of the risk of malignant disease in children. Other studies did not support this and proponents of intramuscular vitamin K argued that as about 1 in 600 children developed cancer in the first 15 years of life, it would be difficult to prove that the intramuscular vitamin was at fault (Draper and McNinch, 1994).

A SELECTION OF TWENTIETH CENTURY MATERIA MEDICA – DRUG GROUPS

Advances described in the twelve sections that follow were the main moving points in the twentieth century.

Menorrhagia

The early twentieth century – Kelly's medications

Howard A. Kelly (1909) of Johns Hopkins University held the prevailing view on menorrhagia at this time: 'There are various drugs which have considerable influence in controlling uterine hemorrhage, though there are none which can be depended on to effect permanent cure.' This remains true almost one hundred years later. Kelly advised a number of medications – these and his reasons for their prescription are quoted here:

Apiol 'Garden parsley [apiol] has recently been spoken of in the treatment of menorrhagia. I have seen a case in which it gave great relief.'

Calcium chloride 'This is occasionally of service, in doses of five grains after each meal during the intermenstrual period.'

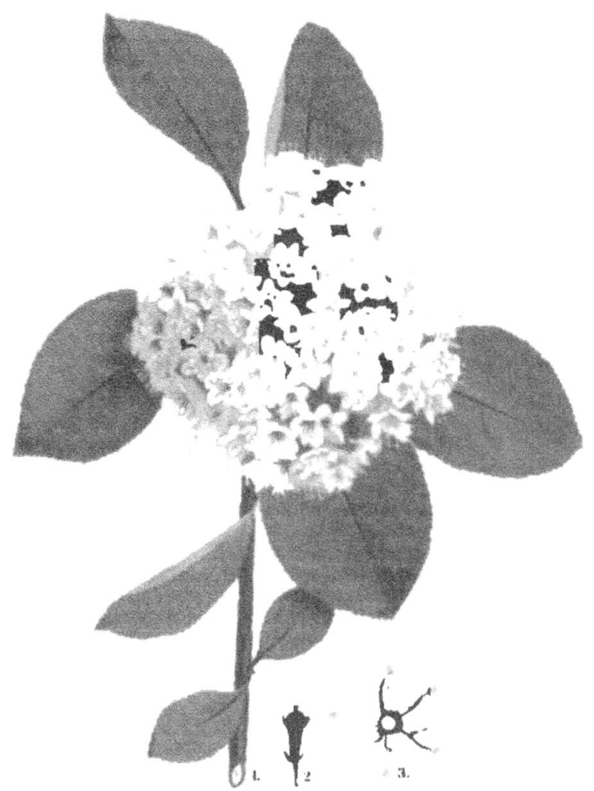

Figure 7 Viburnum

Epinephrine 'The extract of the adrenal glands has been given for the relief of menorrhagia with some success.'
Ergot 'Ergot is a remedy much in use formerly, but largely abandoned now.'
Gallic acid 'This is a remedy highly recommended by T.A. Emmet and, more recently, by W.L. Taylor. Both Emmet and Taylor advise combining the acid with cinnamon.'
Hydrastis canadensis 'This drug, commonly known as golden seal, has a direct action on the vaso-motor nerves and is therefore useful in cases of sub-involution, interstitial fibroids, and all forms of uterine congestion.'
Stypticin 'This is a drug which has found favor in the treatment of uterine hemorrhage within the last few years.'
Styptol 'Is recommended as being cheaper and more efficacious than stypticin.'

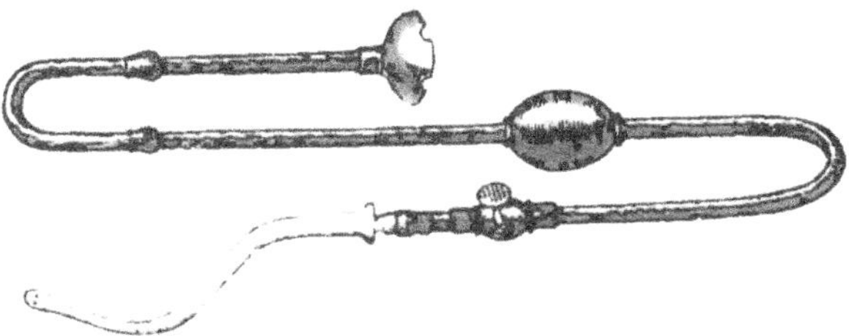

Figure 8 Vaginal douche from O'Donel Browne, *Manual of Practical Obstetrics*

Viburnum prunifolium 'This is a remedy highly recommended for use in the menorrhagia associated with constitutional conditions.'

Kelly also advised mechanical measures, including the applications of caustics, cold applications, dilatation and curettage, hot douches, intrauterine electricity, uterine tampons, and vaginal packs.

The 1950s

Little had changed when P.F.M. Bishop (1950), a London endocrinologist, wrote: 'To decide whether to treat a case of functional bleeding symptomatically with ergot and iron, rationally with endocrine preparations, or radically with surgery or radiotherapy, may be a matter of great difficulty and bitter controversy.' Bishop related that in 1938 Albright treated irregular bleeding with progesterone while in 1939 Karnaky used estrogen. In a note of caution, Bishop advised: 'Should the gynecologist choose to be conservative and resort to endocrine therapy, let him not over-estimate its possibilities ... he cannot cure the condition, he can only allay the symptoms, sometimes, until Nature mercifully calls a halt or decrees a remission.'

The 1970s and beyond

Over 20 years later it became apparent that anti-prostaglandin agents could reduce excess menstrual blood loss and in the 1980s mefenamic acid became a regular treatment for abnormal uterine hemorrhage. Westrom and Bengtsson (1970) and Nilsson and Rybo (1971) treated menorrhagia with tranexamic acid and reported a significant reduction in menstrual blood loss. The fibrinolytic inhibitors became the mainstay of therapy although the combined oral contraceptive and continuous or intermittent progesterone treatment were much used. In the late 1990s the Mirena intrauterine progesterone contraceptive was found helpful. Although it is not possible to compare directly the clinical studies of early and later anti-menorrhagic drugs, there is no doubt that drug treatment has not been entirely satisfactory at either end of the century and many women have had to endure operative intervention with endometrial ablation or hysterectomy.

Endometriosis

Endometriosis was first discovered by the Czech pathologist, Carl von Rokitansky (1860) who was working in Vienna. Following his initial observation there were many reports of the condition during the final two decades of the nineteenth century. The well-known description 'chocolate cyst' was coined by Sampson (1921) when he described 'perforating hemorrhagic chocolate cysts of the ovaries'. He also introduced the modern name for the condition, endometriosis. William Blair-Bell (1922), a founding member of the Royal College of Obstetricians and Gynaecologists in London, first used the term 'endometrioma'. For a good account of the chronology of the early events in the history of endometriosis, see the article by Bayard Carter of Duke University Medical Center, Durham, USA, 'Treatment of Endometriosis' (1962).

Stilbestrol

The medical treatment of endometriosis began with Karnaky in 1948: therapy consisted of stilbestrol in doses sufficient to achieve drug-induced amenorrhea with alleviation of endometriotic symptoms (O'Connor, 1987).

Pregnancy hormones

Based on Sampson's original observation that pregnancy had a beneficial effect on endometriosis, R.W. Kistner (1958) reported on 58 cases treated by inducing pseudopregnancy with ovarian hormones. (Endometriotic tissue may possess estrogen, progesterone and androgen receptors.) Symptomatic improvement was presumed to be due to the decidualization and atrophy of implanted endometrial tissue. Pseudopregnancy remained as a popular therapy for endometriosis throughout the 1970s and was effected by oral or injectable progesterones. Cyclical therapy with the combined oral contraceptive pill was also thought to be helpful.

Pseudomenopause

The next treatment of note was that of 'pseudomenopause'. Greenblatt and associates (1971) introduced danazol which brought about a hormonal state similar to chronic anovulation. As a result, the endometriosis implants atrophied. Danazol bound itself to the progestin, androgen and glucocorticoid receptors. Its net effect was the creation of a high-androgen, low-estrogen environment that was detrimental to endometrial growth. Unfortunately the side-effects of danazol were common and primarily due to its androgenic properties. Despite this, the patients who persisted with treatment reported that danazol was effective in alleviating endometriosis-associated pain. A number of other steroid and anti-steroid treatments have been used, including gestrinone, tamoxifen and the synthetic RU486.

Medical oophorectomy treatment using intranasal administration of luteinizing hormone-releasing hormone agonist was introduced in 1982 and showed immediate potential as a new and effective treatment for endometriosis (Meldrum *et al.*, 1982). The gonadotropin-releasing hormone (GnRH) agonists had demonstrable efficacy, becoming a valuable alternative to danazol, and were proposed as first-line hormonal therapy. It was suggested that for those patients who had severe menopausal symptoms in response to GnRH additional estrogen replacement therapy would be beneficial.

Surgical treatment

The surgical treatment of endometriosis was first mooted when J.R. Fraser (1925) suggested removal of the ovaries in an effort to halt the cyclical changes in the ectopic endometrial tissues and relieve symptoms. Various forms of hysterectomy, with or without ovarian conservation and removal or diathermy of endometriotic deposits, were also used. Eventually a laparoscopic approach became popular and allowed electrocoagulation and laser destruction therapy. Conservative surgery was the procedure of choice for patients who wished to retain their fertility and who failed to conceive following medical treatment. The well-known association between endometriosis and subfertility increased the demand for *in vitro* fertilization when other fertility measures had failed.

Cancer therapy

The alkylating agents

A highly toxic group of chemicals known as the alkylating agents were first synthesized in 1854. It was the effect of nitrogen mustards on transplanted lymphosarcoma in mice in 1942 that launched the era of modern cancer chemotherapy. They include the modified nitrogen mustard drug, cyclophosphamide, and busulphan, chorambucil and melphalan.

Methotrexate

In 1948 this antimetabolite was found to produce remissions in leukemia. Hertz (1963) determined that methotrexate achieved cures of choriocarcinoma and his discovery gave great impetus to the search for other chemotherapeutic agents. Single dose methotrexate has also been used to treat unruptured ectopic pregnancy.

Madagascar periwinkle

The beneficial properties of the periwinkle (*Vinca rosea*) were known in medicinal folklore for many years. This seemingly innocuous plant, was found to contain in excess of 70 alkaloids, of which the vinca alkaloids, vincristine and vinblastine, became well established in the treatment of cancer.

Progesterone

This post-ovulatory and pregnancy hormone has been used for a variety of gynecological complaints and as adjunct therapy in patients with endometrial carcinoma.

Cisplatin

The platinum coordination agents were first identified as antitumor agents in 1965 and cisplatin was introduced into clinical practice four years later. Cisplatin

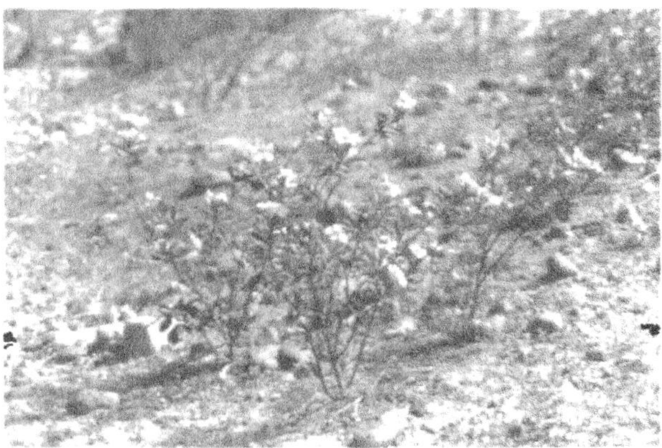

Figure 9 Madagascar periwinkle (*Vinca rosea*)

has played an important role in combination chemotherapy of metastatic ovarian carcinoma.

Taxanes

Paclitaxel (Taxol), an antineoplastic agent obtained from the bark of the Pacific yew (*Taxus brevifolia*) was introduced in 1989. The drug is of major benefit for secondary breast cancer and for patients with primary or secondary ovarian cancer (see Chapter 21). Docetaxel (Taxotere) is also used in the chemotherapy of breast cancer.

Topoisomerase I inhibitor

The topoisomerase I inhibitor, topotecan (Hycamtin was obtained from *Camptotheca acuminata*) was found to be as effective as paclitaxel in the treatment of metastatic ovarian cancer.

Radiotherapy

Radium, so-called because of its radiant quality, was discovered in 1899 by Marie and Pierre Curie in pitchblende, and was found to be a spontaneous source of radiation. As early as 1903, Margaret Cleaves wrote on the use of radium in cancer treatment. The three main centers, Manchester, Paris and Stockholm, developed their own techniques for administering radium between 1910 and 1933. Internal radium therapy was complemented by external-beam radiotherapy developed in the 1920s and 1930s. Supervoltage cobalt

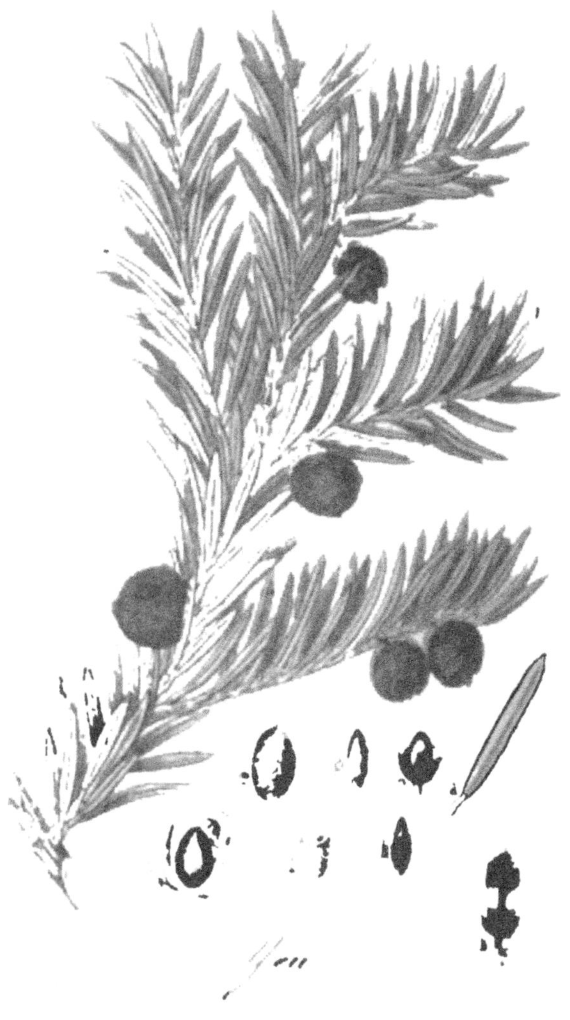

Figure 10 Yew (*Taxus* sp.)

units came on-stream in the late 1950s and linear accelerators were developed thereafter (O'Dowd and Philipp, 1994).

The history of surgery in gynecological cancers is beyond the scope of this book but may be found with the story of radium treatment in *The History of Obstetrics and Gynaecology* (O'Dowd and Philipp, 1994).

'Unstable Bladder'

Terence Millin and Charles Read (1950) of London, described this bladder condition: '[It] manifests itself with increased urinary frequency, chiefly, if not wholly, by day, with pain referred to the urethra or vagina ... the urine will usually be sterile ... formerly the condition was believed to be due to concomitant cervicitis ... the results of therapy have proved disappointing ... the modern view is that the condition is in reality a manifestation of a pelvic congestion ... unrelieved sexual desire is perhaps the commonest cause, and nothing short of the elimination of such basic causes will be rewarded by a complete cure.' Most of these patients were eventually classified as having detrusor instability or unstable bladder, a term first coined by Bates (1971).

Treatments for unstable bladder
Belladonna first used by Langworthy (1936)
Bladder distension
Bladder retraining techniques
Emepronium carrageenate an anticholinergic agent with peripheral effects similar to those of atropine introduced in the late 1960s.
Oxybutynin chloride, an antispasmodic drug, reported to be effective in the management of idiopathic detrusor instability by Paulson (1979) and still a popular drug.
Imipramine useful for nocturnal frequency.
Propantheline bromide introduced in the early 1950s, the drug of choice for many years.

Induction of ovulation

Over the centuries our ancestors used many herbal remedies to increase their fertility but history had to wait until the twentieth century for what Kenneth Bowes described as 'seminal studies' on the subject and the introduction of a novel infertility treatment using low-voltage X-ray irradiation 'either to the ovary alone, or to the pituitary gland ... to induce ovulation'. The technique was first advanced by Isidor Clinton Rubin, of New York, the inventor of the famous Rubin's test for tubal patency. (See Thomas Baskett's *On the Shoulders of Giants* (1996) for Rubin's biography.) Bowes accepted that 'the nature of X-ray treatment had not led to its universal acceptance' and that if a woman's gonadotropin levels were high it would be 'useless to flog the already tired horse' (Bowes, 1950).

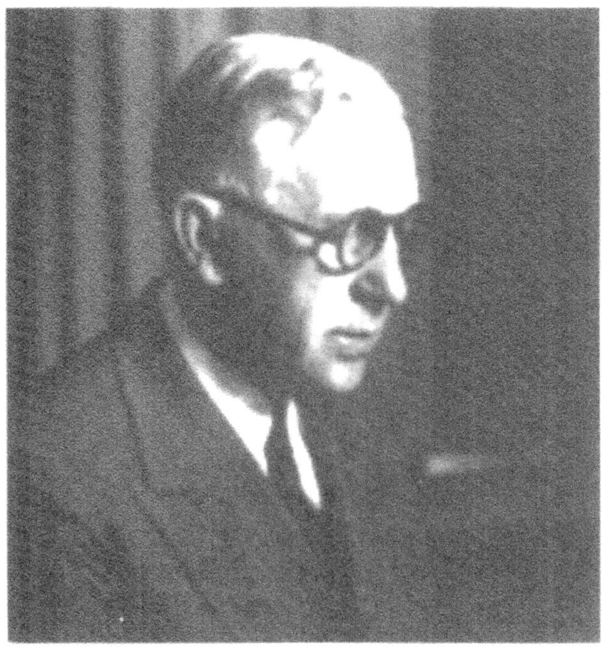

Figure 11 Isidor Clinton Rubin

Antiestrogens

It was known for some time that low potency estrogens such as chlorotrianisene could limit certain actions of estradiol in animals. In 1958 Lerner and associates developed the specific anti-estrogen, MER 25, but the compound was too toxic for use in humans. Further research led to the development of the orally active compound clomiphene. The drug was found to stimulate ovulation and although the twinning rate was increased somewhat by its use, clomiphene had few major side-effects. Clomiphene was introduced into clinical practice by Greenblatt and co-workers (1962) and remained as first-line therapy in ovulation stimulation to the close of the century.

Gonadotropins

In 1938 Davis and Koff reported the artificial stimulation of ovulation using pregnant mares' serum but therapeutic results were disappointing (Bowes, 1950). The first successful use of gonadotropins to induce ovulation in hypogonadotropic women was accomplished by the use of human pituitary extracts (Gemzell *et al.*, 1958). The first human pregnancy resulting from treatment with urinary gonadotropins was reported in France by Lunenfeld and associates (1962).

Gonadotropin releasing hormone

Gonadotropin releasing hormone was isolated in 1971 and work by Knobil (1980) showed that the drug should be administered in pulsed doses in order to be effective. The first report of a pregnancy in which luteinizing hormone-releasing hormone analogs were used to achieve pituitary 'down-regulation' came from Porter *et al.* (1984) in a paper in *The Lancet.*

Bromocriptine (Parlodel)

Women with high prolactin levels, either during breastfeeding or as a result of pathological hyperprolactinemia, developed failure of ovulation accompanied by secondary amenorrhea. It was observed centuries ago that lactation was inhibited in women suffering from ergotism and modern research showed that dopamine inhibits the release of prolactin. It was postulated, therefore, that dopaminergic agents might help to control excessive production of prolactin and so lead to resumption of ovulation. The theory proved correct and in 1971 the ergot-derived dopamine agonist, bromocriptine (Parlodel) was widely and successfully used in the treatment of such cases.

During the 1980s bromocriptine was used liberally to prevent lactation and breast engorgement in those mothers who chose not to breastfeed. Although the results of treatment were excellent there were some disturbing reports in the literature of side-effects, including myocardial infarction, hypertension, severe headache and seizures and routine use of the drug to prevent lactation was stopped, except in unusual circumstances such as stillbirth.

Impotence

Although erectile dysfunction is not a female problem its effects can have a devastating effect on sexual relationships. An estimated thirty million men in the USA suffer from the condition, which affects approximately 10% of the male population worldwide. Impotence remained untreated for the majority of those affected until the advent of effective remedies in the 1980s. Erectile dysfunction may be of vascular, neurogenic, hormonal, psychological, iatrogenic, or mixed etiology. Many drugs were known to be associated with erectile dysfunction including the major tranquilizers, antidepressants, anxiolytics, antihypertensives, alcohol and recreational drugs, and many others.

When the World Health Organization set out the fundamental rights for the individual they included the right to sexual health: each individual should have the capacity to enjoy and control their sexual and reproductive behavior in accordance with a social and personal ethic; they should have freedom from fear, shame, guilt, false belief, and other factors inhibiting sexual response and sexual relationships; and finally, there should be freedom from organic disorders, disease and deficiencies that interfere with sexual and reproductive function (WHO, 1970).

Intracavernosal therapy

Richard Lechtenberg of New Jersey, and Dana Ohl of Ann Arbor, Michigan described the early history of intracavernosal pharmacotherapy for impotence in their book *Sexual Dysfunction* (1994). They wrote: 'The first report of erection induced by penile injection of a pharmacologic agent was by Virag [1982]. He described the accidental injection of papaverine into the cavernosal body during a penile revascularization procedure. This resulted in an erection lasting approximately two hours.' Virag, from the Center for Study and Research on Impotence, Paris, gave credit for the technique to Michal and colleagues (1977) who had accidentally injected papaverine into the penile cavernous body (formerly known as 'the nervous body', possibly in anticipation) during a surgical shunting procedure – a prolonged fully rigid erection of two hours' duration was the result (Virag *et al.*, 1977).

Giles Brindley (1983) reported that the injection of phenoxybenzamine had relatively similar effects. Lechtenberg and Ohl (1994) wrote:

> 'The effectiveness of phenoxybenzamine in inducing erection was underscored by the same Doctor Brindley at the American Urological Association Meeting in 1983. At the end of his lecture on the physiology of erection he informed the audience that he had self-administered phenoxybenzamine just prior to his lecture and then proceeded to display the result of his injection. Following this spectacular demonstration of the effectiveness of phenoxybenzamine, Doctor Brindley retired to less public settings, where he tested several intracavernosal agents on himself to find out whether or not they would induce erection'.

Brindley reported these further experimentations to the *British Journal of Pharmacology* (1986).

Virag continued with intracavernosal injection of papaverine as a method for testing impotent men, and documented that erections were substantially improved in two-thirds of patients investigated in this way. In all, Virag reported that of 30 patients subjected to intracavernous injection of 80 mg papaverine, followed by an infusion of 1% heparin in normal saline via an infusion pump, 14 patients (7 of whom had diabetes) had two or more artificial erections. Of these 14, four reported a return to a normal sexual life; nine described a significant improvement in penile rigidity; and one experienced no effect on his sexual activity and was treated by arterial revascularization (Virag *et al.*, 1984).

Zorgniotti and Lefleur (1985) realized that combination therapy for inducing erections might prove to be even more effective and so papaverine and the alpha-blocker phentolamine were mixed in a single syringe for cavernosal injection. Of 62 patients, 59 were able to engage in intercourse after treatment and a third of the group were trained in self-injection therapy. Numerous studies that followed reported consistently good results for the technique.

Intracavernosal therapy with prostaglandin E1 was introduced by Ishii and associates (1986) and the new treatment was marketed by the aptly-named pharmaceutical company, Upjohn. Alprostadil (prostaglandin E1) gained its product license in 1994 and was available in four different doses. Marketed as Caverject, alprostadil caused burning penile pain or tension in 16.8% of users but was otherwise well received. Prostaglandin E1 had an 80% success rate with only a small risk of priapism or of the formation of painless penile fibrotic lesions (almost 10% after two years).

MUSE

The 'medicated urethral system for erection' (MUSE) consisted of a pellet of prostaglandin for intra-urethral treatment. Because of its ease of use it was a popular treatment with both patients and physicians, but in common with other prostaglandin treatments, it was associated with a relatively high incidence of penile pain which made patients less willing to continue the treatment. Alprostadil used intra-urethrally was successful in somewhat less than 50% of cases (Padma-Nathan *et al.*, 1997). Unfortunately for MUSE, however, the system was marketed just prior to the introduction of the 'rage of the age', sildenafil.

Viagra

By the end of the 1980s the drug armamentarium for the treatment of impotence included imipramine, naftidrofuryl, papaverine, phenoxybenzamine, phenotolamine, prostaglandin E1, thyroxamine, and verapamil. The mid-1990s saw the introduction of new drugs that worked by enhancing nitric oxide-mediated relaxation of the smooth muscle of the corpus cavernosal (Boolell *et al.*, 1996; Gingell *et al.*, 1996; Eardley *et al.*, 1996). Trials on one such drug, sildenafil (Viagra) showed a response rate of almost 90% in men with erectile dysfunction of no organic cause. Sildenafil is a type 5 phosphodiesterase inhibitor that causes the release of nitric oxide, an essential part of the erectile process. Early reports suggested that it could produce an effective response in almost 90% of patients who presented with psychological erectile dysfunction. Although there were a number of side-effects, priapism (a problem with intracavernosal injections) was not reported with Viagra. (Priapism, is penile erection sustained for more than six hours, and requires expert attention.)

Early reports revealed than sildenafil citrate was contraindicated in men on medication with organic nitrates, and there were a number of deaths among men at risk of heart disease. The main adverse effects of sildenafil were headache, flushing, dyspepsia, and visual disturbances (a blue tingeing of vision) and they were usually mild. Although Viagra was licensed for use in impotence it was said not to have aphrodisiac properties – it helped in the achievement and maintenance of erection in patients with erectile dysfunction, in the presence of sexual stimulation.

Abi Berger (1998) examined the massive media attention which surrounded the 'little blue pill' (the original 'blue pill' was mercury): 'It must surely be every drug company's dream: to have a product so sexy that the need for marketing and public relations has been obviated by a tidal wave of media hype. Since March 1998, when the little blue pills became available in the United States, we have had news stories, regular updates, features, television and radio programs, and even serious broadcast editorials on the myths and legends of what has been dubbed the "Pfizer Riser".' Unprecedented demand and the potential consequences to national drug budgets caused a number of governments to ban the prescription from their National Health Systems.

In April 1998, when that the news came through of the approval for Viagra by the Food and Drug Administration in the United States, Fred Charatan of Florida wrote: '[This has] caused Pfizer's shares to surge on the New York Stock Exchange ... Market analysts project that sales of sildenafil citrate could peak 2.5 billion dollars a year in the United States alone ... Viagra is the first in a new class of drugs known as phosphodiesterase type 5 inhibitors that work by improving blood flow to the penis ... In twenty-one clinical trials conducted on 4,000 men, sildenafil citrate was found to be effective in 70% of cases ... Sildenafil citrate was originally developed to treat angina. But patients in trials reported more erections as a side-effect ... [sildenafil] should not be taken by patients who are already taking nitrates in any form, including glyceryl trinitrate, because the combination may lower blood pressure ... During sexual stimulation, penile nerve endings release nitric oxide, which in turn causes the production of cyclic guanosine monophosphate (cGMP). This substance is a vasodilator so that the blood flow to the penis is enhanced, leading to an erection (Charatan, 1998).

Viagra became the fastest-selling drug in the USA with prescriptions running at an estimated 10 000 a day. Market analysts said that it was the most successful drug launch in history, outstripping the antidepressant drug Prozac and the anti-baldness remedy, Regaine. Aided by internet sales, Viagra became the most popular drug worldwide in the twentieth century, displacing aspirin from its number one position. Two years after the first clinical reports on sildenafil and its anti-impotence effect, three American pharmacologists were awarded the Nobel Prize for Medicine for their work on nitric acid as a signaling molecule in the cardiovascular system (although their work had not been on erectile dysfunction) (Mullner, 1998).

Yohimbine

This drug was touted as a cure for erectile dysfunction for many years. Reid and colleagues (1987) found that yohimbine had a modest effect on psychogenic impotence but no effect on organic erectile dysfunction. Pittler and Ernst (1998) carried out a meta-analysis on all the double-blind randomized placebo controlled trials of yohimbine for erectile dysfunction and claimed that yohimbine was an effective non-invasive option for initial drug treatment.

Other treatments

Mechanical treatments included vacuum devices and occlusive rings, which were usually not of much value. Surgery to correct venous leakage and microvascular techniques for revascularization of the corpora did not have good results. The only surgical treatment of any value was the insertion of penile prostheses, introduced in the 1970s.

Drug treatment of preterm labor

Progesterone

The hormone progesterone was known to preserve early pregnancy and prevent preterm labor in animals. Progesterone increased resting membrane-potential and propagation of impulses but despite that Fuchs and Stakemann (1960) found no effect in their double-blind controlled study of progesterone administration to patients in preterm labor.

Ethanol

This substance was found to inhibit the release of oxytocin from the neurohypophysis (Fuchs and Wagner, 1963). Contradictory results were obtained in controlled studies of its effect in preterm labor and Lauersen and colleagues (1977) reported that in a multi-center study ethanol did not compare favorably with ritodrine for postponement of delivery. Unwanted side-effects of the alcohol were common in both fetus and mother.

Prostaglandin synthetase inhibitors

As prostaglandins play an important role in the initiation of labor it was theorized that anti-prostaglandin agents could be used to prevent labor. Their use was restricted, however, by potential adverse effects on the fetus such as premature closure of the ductus arteriosus and primary pulmonary hypertension, and by their negative effect on the fetal and neonatal response to hypoxia.

Calcium antagonists

Ulmsten, Andersson and Wingerup (1980) tested calcium antagonists in a small clinical trial of patients with preterm labor. The drug was shown to inhibit myometrial activity. The calcium antagonist nifedipine was used for a time but did not retain its initial popularity.

Magnesium sulfate

The drug of choice in the treatment of pre-eclampsia, magnesium sulfate was thought by Steer and Petrie (1977) to be superior to ethanol.

Beta receptor agonists

Of the many drugs which have been used to inhibit uterine activity in premature labor, the beta-adrenergic agents such as Isoxsuprine, mesuprine and orciprenaline (derivatives of epinephrine) were the most widely studied. The modern beta-receptor agonists, fenoterol, ritodrine, salbutamol and terbutaline were found to be effective uterine relaxants. Wesselius de Casparis and associates (1971) demonstrated that ritodrine postponed premature labor for longer than either sedation or placebo. Ingemarsson (1984), in an article on the pharmacology of tocolytic agents, concluded that beta-receptor agonists were the drugs of choice in the treatment of preterm labor. Rare but serious side-effects of pulmonary edema, myocardial ischemia and possible adverse influences on carbohydrate metabolism, were reported when beta-agonists were combined with corticosteroids (RCOG, 1997).

Nitroglycerin

Graeme Smith and James Brien (1998) of Canada wrote on the use of nitroglycerin for uterine relaxation in preterm labor. They advised that more objective assessment with randomized multi-center trials comparing nitroglycerin with other methods of uterine relaxation, was required to elucidate properly the place of the agent in obstetric practice.

Antibiotics

Results of recent studies suggest that 25 to 50% of preterm births are caused by common genital tract infections and the subsequent maternal/fetal inflammatory response, and that prompt diagnosis and antibiotic treatment could prevent many preterm births.

Antenatal corticosteroids and respiratory distress syndrome

Respiratory distress syndrome (RDS), previously known as hyaline membrane disease, was known to affect 40–50% of neonates born before 32 weeks gestation. Mary Ellen Avery (1981) of Harvard Medical School, Boston, related: 'In the early 1960s we estimated the incidence of fatal hyaline membrane disease in the USA to be 3.8 per 100 births under 2500 g [birth weight], or a national figure of 12 000 deaths per year.' Following the introduction of better modes of treatment, 'in particular ventilators and the use of continuous distending airway pressure' Avery reported that neonatal mortality fell by almost a half. However, RDS continued to occur in about 10–15% of infants weighing under 2500 g, about 1% of live births. In 1967 a new syndrome of chronic pulmonary insufficiency, or 'bronchopulmonary dyplasia', was found to complicate treatment of RDS. Other major complications were intracranial hemorrhage and problems that resulted from the use of umbilical artery catheters.

Liggins and Howie (1972) reported on a novel treatment, using antepartum glucocorticoids to prevent the RDS in premature infants in a controlled trial. Their treatment (beta-methasone, 12 mg twice daily) reduced the incidence of RDS from 24% in controls to 9% in treated cases. Antenatal corticosteroid treatment dramatically reduced the incidence of RDS and bronchopulmonary dysplasia and the other untoward complications of therapy. The glucocorticoids induced the enzymes necessary to synthesize the phospholipid component of pulmonary surfactant, which is deficient in RDS. Betamethasone or dexamethasone were used in an interchangeable fashion in many studies. All the reported prospective controlled clinical trials showed a reduction in the incidence of RDS in infants whose mothers received glucocorticoids more than 24 hours, and less than seven days, before delivery (Avery, 1981).

Patricia Crowley (1995) of the Coombe Hospital, Dublin, performed a meta-analysis of 15 randomized controlled trials conducted between 1972 and 1994 and confirmed the benefits of antenatal corticosteroids in prematurity. Since then, antenatal corticosteroids have been more commonly used. It is now recommended that antenatal corticosteroid therapy is given to women between 24 and 36 weeks gestation for antepartum hemorrhage; preterm rupture of the membranes; threatened preterm labor; and any condition that may result in elective preterm delivery (RCOG, 1996).

Corticosteroid treatment was associated with a reduction in the risk of neonatal death from intraventricular hemorrhage. Corticosteroids also enhanced the efficacy of neonatal surfactant therapy by improving fetal lung maturation and increasing the production of endogenous surfactant. In research that was years ahead of its time, Enhorning and Robertson (1972) experimented with the tracheal deposition of surfactant in premature rabbits. Surfactant became commercially available for use in premature infants almost 20 years later.

The American College of Obstetricians and Gynecologists (ACOG) summarized the value of steroids:

> 'The benefits of antenatal administration of corticosteroids to fetuses at risk of pre-term delivery vastly outweighed the potential risks. These benefits included not only a reduction in the risk of RDS but also substantial reduction in mortality and IVH [intraventricular hemorrhage]. All women between 24 and 34 weeks of pregnancy at risk for pre-term delivery are candidates for antenatal corticosteroid therapy ... treatment should consist of either two doses of 12 mg of betamethasone, intramuscularly, given 24 hours apart or four doses of 6 mg of dexamethasone, intramuscularly, given 12 hours apart. Optimal benefits begin 24 hours after initiation of therapy and lasts seven days' (ACOG, 1994).

Diabetes and insulin

The story of insulin has been related by Victor Cornelius Medvei (1993). The word 'insulin' was first used by J. de Meyer in 1907 and popularized later by Sir Edward Albert Sharpey-Schafer in 1916. It was derived from the Latin *insula* meaning island, an allusion to the fact that it was obtained from the islets of Langerhans in the pancreas. J.B. Collip published a description of 'the original method ... used for the isolation of insulin ... for the treatment process employed to produce the first clinical cases' (1923).

Diabetes and pregnancy

John Whitridge Williams (1903) found that in diabetic patients 'gestation sometimes exerts a very deleterious influence upon the course of the disease', but he was somewhat wide of the mark when he concluded: 'the so-called diabetes of pregnancy is merely a lactosuria which is not likely to be attended by serious symptoms, the patients being spontaneously delivered of healthy children at term.' He was presumably writing about glycosuric patients with normal blood sugars and not about true diabetics. At the beginning of the century it was demonstrated at autopsies that women with established diabetes had uterine atrophy and lacked ovarian follicles.

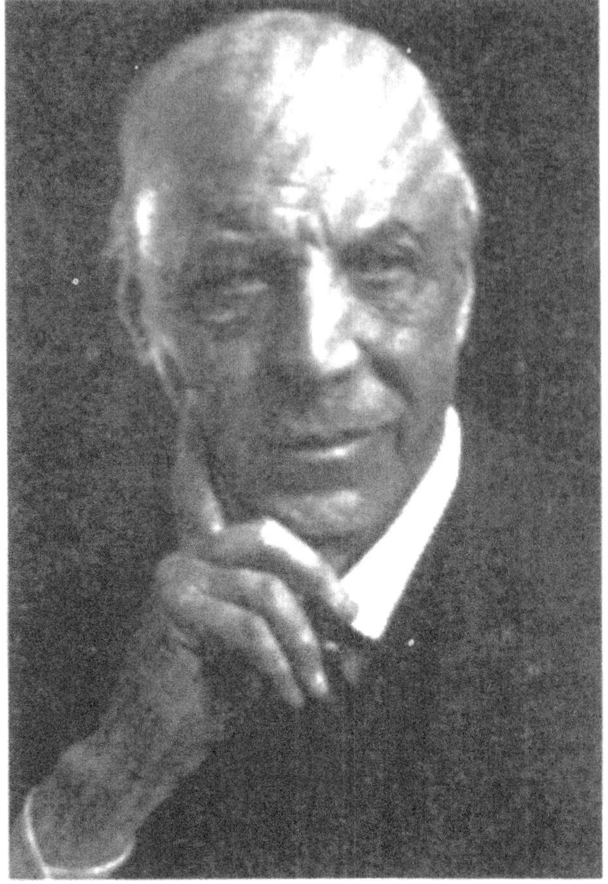

Figure 12 Edward Sharpey-Schafer (1850–1935)

Diabetes and its effects on women were described in textbooks of the 1940s: 'Untreated diabetics seldom become pregnant ... juvenile cases, when not treated with insulin ... usually die before they reach marriageable age' (wrote A.C. Beck in 1942) or they were sterile due to amenorrhea, probably due to low body mass. Even 30 years after the introduction of insulin the complications of pregnancy diabetes were only just beginning to be understood. It was only in the late 1970s that tight control of blood sugar levels during pregnancy led to better outcomes for pregnant mothers and their offspring.

The story of the impact of the discovery of insulin on pregnancy in women with diabetes was related by

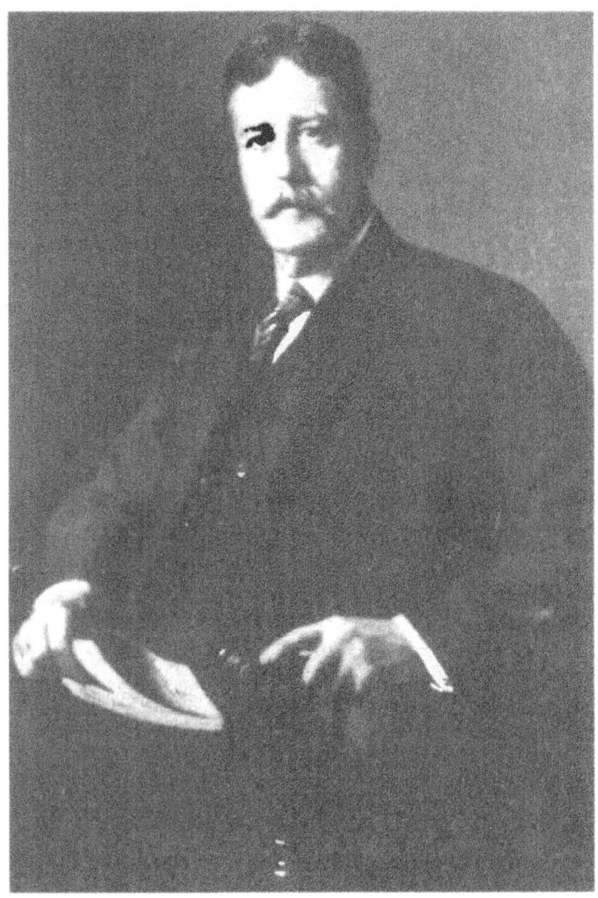

Figure 13 John Williams

Steven Gabbe of Columbus, Ohio. In a fascinating paper in the 'After Office Hours' section of the journal *Obstetrics and Gynecology* (1992) Gabbe related:

> 'Before the discovery of insulin in 1921, pregnancies in women with diabetes mellitus were a rarity because most reproductive-aged patients died soon after diagnosis of this illness. In the limited number of pregnancies reported in the pre-insulin era, both perinatal and maternal mortality were approximately 50%, with stillbirths being the primary cause of perinatal deaths. Insulin treatment restored the fertility of women with diabetes and was associated with a marked reduction in maternal mortality'.

The first true case of diabetes in pregnancy was published by Heinrich Gottleib Bennewitz of Berlin in 1824: following intrapartum fetal death, the woman delivered a 12-pound stillborn infant. According to Steven Gabbe: '[Life] expectancy improved dramatically for all diabetic patients with the discovery of insulin in 1921 by Frederick Banting and his collaborators, J.J.R. Macleod, James Collip and Charles Best. An eleven year old, Elsie Needham, became the first person to survive diabetic ketoacidosis. Gabbe quoted Banting's description in September 1922 of a patient with diabetes ... 'seventy-six pounds of the worst looking specimen of a wife I have ever seen ... she was a terrible looking specimen of humanity with eyes almost closed with edema, a pale and pasty skin, red hair that was so thin it showed her scalp ... her ankles were thicker than the calves of her legs and her body had sores where the skin was stretched thin over the bones. Above all she had the foulest disposition that I have ever known.' Banting treated the patient for her diabetes and she made a miraculous physical and emotional recovery and before long she was delivered of a healthy daughter.

Priscilla White of the Joslin Clinic developed the 'White classification of diabetes' based on her experience of diabetic women from the early 1930s. By the early 1940s the treatment and prospects for pregnant diabetics had improved somewhat but it was almost another half century before stable well-managed diabetic women could be assured of a (relatively) good outcome to their pregnancies. The Dublin physician, Ivo Drury summarized the difficulties of the early days of caring for pregnant diabetics in the poignantly entitled paper, 'They gave birth astride of a grave' (1989).

The thyroid gland and its disorders

The thyroid gland and its function in animals was the subject of numerous experiments from the late 1850s. The first approach was to remove the gland and observe the differences, if any, in animal behavior. George Murray (1891) then reported the first instance of injectable administration of thyroid gland extract in a hypothyroid subject. Kendall isolated thyroxin as the active principle of the thyroid gland in 1914 but it was found that the actual amount of thyroxin isolated per thyroid was so minute that it

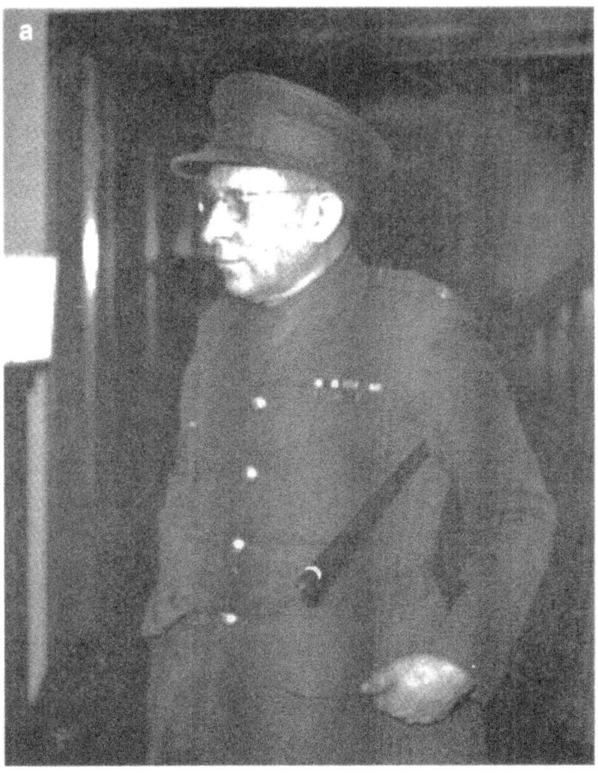

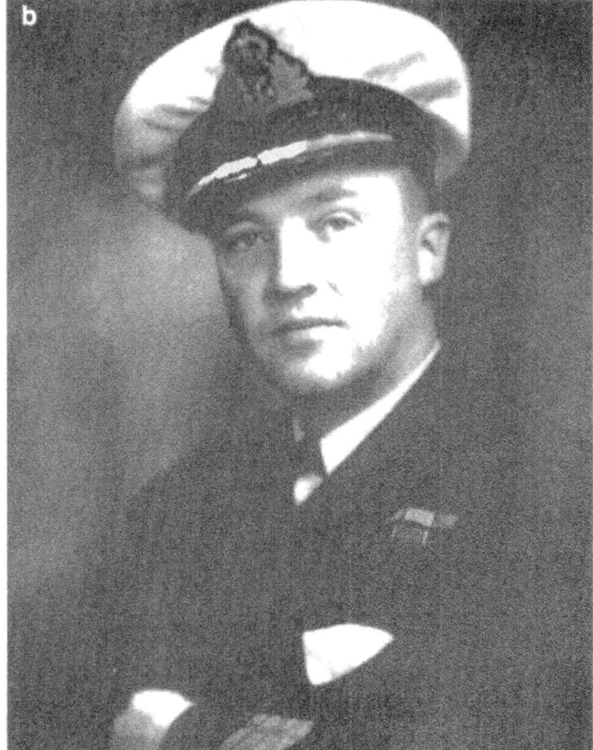

Figure 14 (a) Sir Frederick Grant Banting (b) Herbert Best

took three tons of pigs' thyroids to obtain 33 g of pure thyroxin (Kendall, 1929; Compeston and Pitt-Rivers, 1956). Harington and Barger established the formula and achieved the synthesis of thyroxin in 1927 (Medvei, 1993).

Research during the 1930s confirmed that removal of the thyroid gland from pregnant animals or the feeding of thyroid substance to pregnant rabbits induced histological changes in the thyroid glands of the fetuses. These experiments, together with the observation that thyroxin given to pregnant guinea pigs caused an increase in metabolism of the newborn offspring, demonstrating that the thyroid hormone crossed the placental barrier.

Thyroid function and pregnancy

Thyroid disease was said to affect approximately 1.5% of the female population, spanning all age groups. Niswander, Gordon and Berends (1972) estimated the prevalence of thyroid disease in pregnancy to be in the order of 0.7%, with spontaneous (or iatrogenic) hypothyroidism occurring four to five times more commonly than hyperthyroidism. As untreated thyroid disease is now rarely encountered in obstetric practice, the following observations by Howard Kelly and Alfred Beck provide an interesting background to the subject.

Howard Kelly described a condition known as adiposis dolorosa, otherwise known as Dercum's disease, that was characterized by the deposition of large masses of fat in various regions of the body, and was peculiar to women during the middle period of life. The thyroid gland showed a marked tendency towards atrophy and treatment with thyroid extract was found to bring about great improvement in patients with disease. He also reported that thyroid extract could be used for the treatment of menopause symptoms.

Alfred C. Beck, professor of obstetrics and gynecology at the Long Island College of Medicine, wrote a tract on 'Diseases of the ductless glands' in his textbook *Obstetrical Practice* in which he stated: 'Thyroid

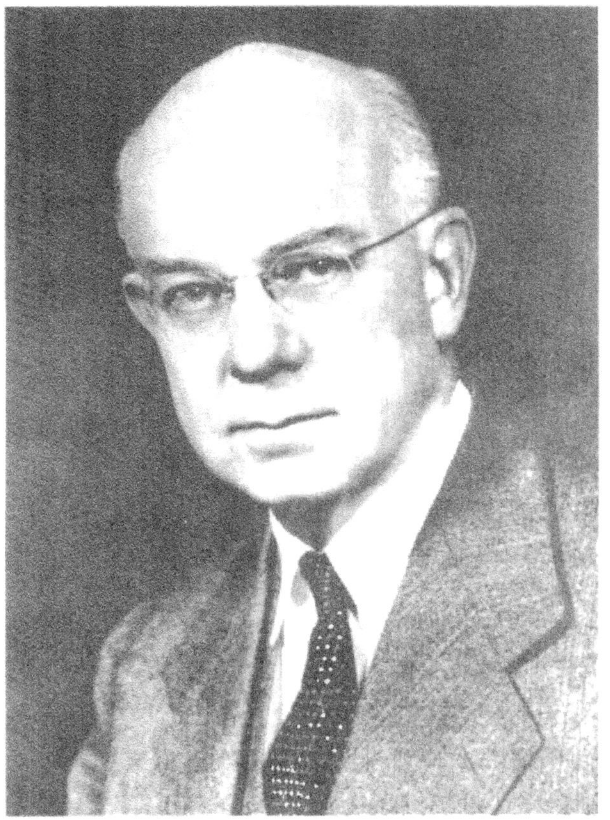

Figure 15 Edward Calvin Kendall (1886–1972)

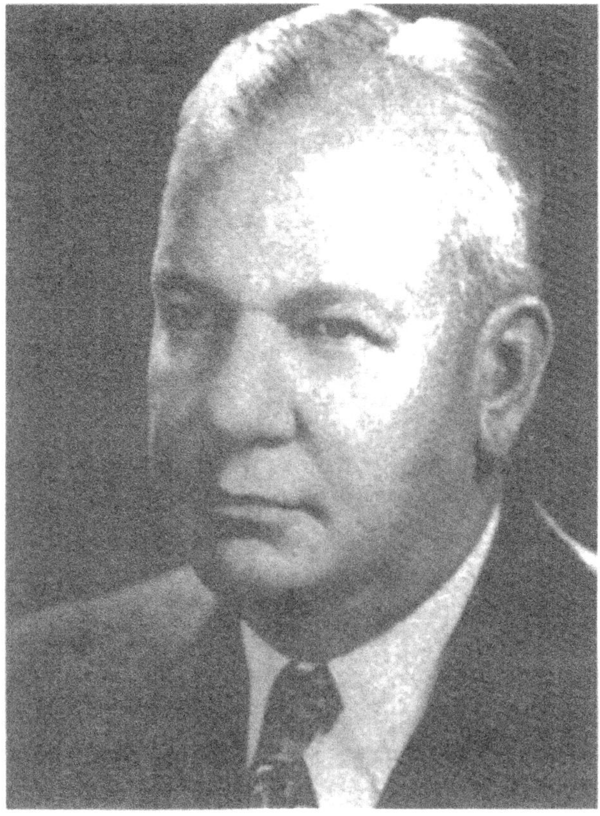

Figure 16 Alfred Beck

enlargement is demonstrable in the majority of pregnancies and disappears soon after delivery.' Colloid goiter was often seen as a complication of pregnancy in those regions where the disease was endemic. If the goiter was accompanied by marked hypothyroidism, Beck pointed out that 'spontaneous interruption of pregnancy may occur'. He continued: 'The children often have congenital goiter or are cretins, and the prophylactic use of iodine has been advocated for pregnant women living in goiter communities ... Women with exophthalmic goiter and toxic adenomas have a diminished fertility. When such patients do become pregnant the condition is usually aggravated and spontaneous abortion is not uncommon' (Beck, 1942). Iodine therapy and surgical treatment of the thyroid lessened the risk of complications. Therapeutic abortion was an option for those patients affected by the severe vomiting of thyrotoxicosis, a condition that was easily mistaken for hyperemesis gravidarum.

Hypothyroidism

A relationship between thyroid secretion and mammary gland function was noted in 1896 by Hertoghe, who reported a temporary stimulation of milk yield in a cow following administration of dried thyroid extract (Bowes, 1950). According to Beck (1942) it was demonstrated by J.C. Litzenberg and J.B. Carey in 1929 that some cases of habitual abortion were attributable to hypothyroidism and that the condition could be cured by the administration of thyroid extract. Thyroid extract was recommended for the treatment for amenorrhea in patients with obesity or if there were marked signs of hypothyroidism (Browne, 1950).

Hyperthyroidism

The incidence of hyperthyroidism in pregnant women was in the order of 0.2%. In the majority of patients, the thyrotoxicosis pre-dated pregnancy. In hyperthyroidism there is failure of ovulation and it was only with anti-thyroid therapy that affected women became fertile and eventually pregnant. Treatment of active thyrotoxicosis in pregnancy is imperative because the condition gives rise to higher incidences of toxemia, premature labor, and congestive heart failure. Perinatal mortality and morbidity were also significantly increased in the offspring of untreated patients. Antithyroid drugs for the treatment of hyperthyroidism in pregnancy were introduced by E.B. Astwood in 1951 (Sugrue and Drury, 1980) and carbimazole or methimazole have been the mainstay of treatment. Antithyroid drugs readily cross the placenta and in high doses can produce neonatal hypothyroidism and goiter.

Anticoagulants

Heparin

Heparin was discovered by a medical student, J. McLean of Johns Hopkins Medical School, in 1916. McLean was studying the clot-promoting activity of phosphatides, and was surprised to find that a liver preparation prolonged the clotting time. The name of the crude liver substance was derived from the Greek *hepar*, meaning liver, and 'in', a common ending for a chemical name (Laurence, 1973). Heparin was isolated by Howell in 1922, in whose laboratory McLean had been working (Jaques, 1978). It was found that heparin was present in many mammalian tissues. The lung is a rich source and commercial heparin is prepared from mammalian lung or liver.

Heparin was found to be an antithrombin, an antiprothrombin, and an antithromboplastin, and proved to be the most important, the safest, and the most certain of the anticoagulant drugs. A ready antidote existed in the form of a 1% solution of protamine sulfate. Unlike the dicumarol type of anticoagulants, the heparin molecule was too large to cross the placenta and was safe to use in pregnancy. The use of heparin *in vitro* to prevent blood from clotting led to its use to prevent venous thrombosis.

Heparin was first produced in a pure state in 1935 and large-scale studies were undertaken from 1938. Prophylactic pre-operative anticoagulant therapy was administered to patients undergoing gynecological surgery as early as the mid-1940s and it was demonstrated that the risk of venous thrombosis and/or pulmonary embolism was reduced. For those patients with established deep venous thrombosis or pulmonary embolism heparin treatment had a marked beneficial effect. It was suggested by Best in 1948 that low-dose heparin treatment might be a feasible form of therapy but it was not until the early 1970s that clinical trials led the way for this important development in the use of heparin in anticoagulant therapy (O'Reilly, 1985).

Dicumarol

The story of the discovery of coumarin was related by R.B. Hunter (1961) of the Department of Pharmacology and Therapeutics, Queen's College, Dundee, at a symposium on anticoagulant therapy held at the Royal Society of Medicine, London:

> 'On a Saturday afternoon in February, 1933, during a blizzard, a farmer in Wisconsin traveled over dangerous roads to visit the Agricultural Experimental Station, to try to get some help because his cattle were dying in great numbers. By mistake, he went into the biochemistry building which was Dr Link's department and dumped on the floor a dead calf covered with haematomas, a can of blood-stained milk and a bundle of sweet clover which was the only hay, because of the severe weather, that he had available to feed his cattle. This incident stimulated Link to consider this disease of cattle and try and find out what caused the bleeding'.

It transpired that the melilots (sweet clover) *Melilotus alba* and *Melilotus officinalis*, were introduced from Europe early in the twentieth century and planted on the plains of Dakota and Canada because they flourished on poor soil and were a substitute for corn in silage. Two decades later farmers in the region began to report a mysterious cattle disease characterized by hemorrhage, often copious, which, though sometimes spontaneous, more often followed trauma. In one case it was reported that 12 of 25 young bulls had died after castration – they had all bled to death.

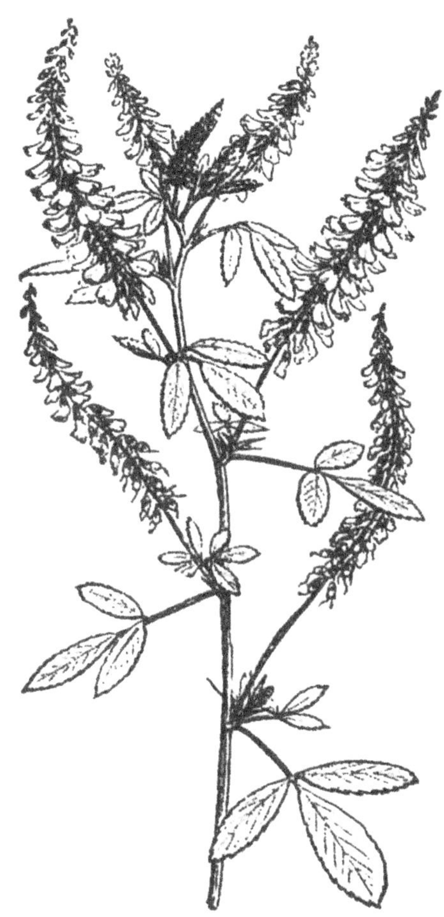

Figure 17 Melilotus

F.S. Schofield, a veterinary pathologist in Alberta, first described the disease and found that the abnormal bleeding only occurred in cattle which had eaten moldy sweet clover, while properly cured hay was harmless (Laurence, 1973). He discovered that the clotting time was prolonged and reported his observation to the *Journal of the American Veterinary Medical Association* in 1924. A number of years later L.M. Roderick, a veterinary surgeon in Dakota, showed that the alteration in the clotting time was due to a reduced crude prothrombin fraction in the blood. At the same time A.J. Quick introduced the one-stage prothrombin test that proved essential for further progress in unraveling the cause of the disease (Hollman, 1992).

K.P. Link of Wisconsin, where the disease was common, took up the search for the hemorrhagic agent in 1933. Six years later it was isolated in his laboratory by H.A. Campbell, at dawn, on 28 June 1939. The substance was shown to be a derivative of coumarin – the substance that gives new-mown hay its sweet smell – and was named bishydroxycoumarin, later to become the anticoagulant, dicumarol. Synthesis of dicumarol was first achieved on April Fools' Day 1940, and the synthetic and natural products were shown to be identical. Studies were soon carried out in Toronto and it was demonstrated that the new anticoagulant drug could prevent or dispel intravascular and extravascular clot formation in animals. The first clinical report on the use of dicumarol in humans was carried in *the Proceedings of the Mayo Clinic* in 1941.

Warfarin

Between 1946 and 1948 Dr Link and his laboratory staff reappraised the synthetic coumarin derivatives. They discovered an even better agent (known at first as No. 2) which had a uniform and potent anticoagulant action. Link, at that time suffering from tuberculosis, was researching rat poisons, and he proposed that No. 2 would be an ideal rodenticide. He renamed No. 2 'warfarin', the name being derived from the **W**isconsin **A**lumni **R**esearch **F**oundation and coum**arin**. Warfarin was found to be safer than dicumarol and was introduced into clinical practice in 1954. Parallel research demonstrated that vitamin K antagonized the anticoagulant effects of coumarin drugs and could be used as an antidote.

In obstetric practice drugs of the coumarin and the indanedione groups were found to cross the placenta and were associated with an 18% fetal mortality rate caused by fetal hemorrhage, either before or during labor. Fetal abnormality was also reported following the use of these drugs in early pregnancy. Bear in mind, however, that once puerperal sepsis had been conquered the commonest causes of maternal mortality were eclampsia and thrombo-embolic disease, and the anticoagulants have played a major role in the reduction of mortality and morbidity in women both in childbirth and gynecological procedures.

A SELECTION OF TWENTIETH CENTURY MATERIA MEDICA – DRUGS IN PREGNANCY

The risks associated with taking drugs have been recognized for millennia and the ancients banned the use of certain drugs in pregnant women, mainly based on the fact that some remedies were thought to induce miscarriage or premature labor. In the twentieth century society in general became acutely aware of the possible teratogenic effects of drugs and environmental toxins in the wake of the disasters following medication with agents such as stilbestrol and thalidomide. Despite this awareness, many women and their unborn are exposed to potential teratogens, and agencies such as the American College of Obstetricians and Gynecologists issue guidelines to professionals and the public alike. Governments have put stringent controls in place to protect the unborn, but the environment has been polluted as never before in history.

Eskes and associates (1985) advised in *Drug Therapy in Pregnancy* '[The] frequency of medication during pregnancy deserves continuous attention'. They went on to explain: 'This statement can be made because "obstetrics" can be blamed for at least two calamities: the thalidomide drama [Lenz, 1961] resulting in phocomelia, and the diethylstilbestrol (DES) story leading to adenosis and carcinoma of the vagina [Herbst *et al.*, 1971]. On the other hand, one must sometimes choose between Scylla and Charybdis because of maternal conditions such as hypertension, diabetes, renal transplantation, lupus erythematosus and others.' The recent papers, 'One Hundred Years of Pharmacovigilance' (Routledge, 1998) and 'Thalidomide – was the tragedy preventable?' (Dally, 1998), and the book *Adverse Effects of Herbal Drugs* (De Smet *et al.*, 1992) were among many publications that explored the issue of safety in prescribing for women and they make salutary reading.

Teratogens

The effect of a drug taken in pregnancy depends on its teratogenicity and on the timing of its administration. From the point of view of drug therapy, pregnancy may be divided into three intervals – conception to the 17th day, when exposure to harmful drugs will result either in abortion or intact survival; 18 to 55 days postconception, the period of organogenesis during which teratogens exert their worst effects; and after 56 days postconception, when drugs may affect fetal growth and/or function. The risk may be reduced by prescribing remedies that are known to be safe in pregnancy to all women of childbearing age. Preconception counseling of women on long-term treatment would be of benefit but up to 50% of all pregnancies are unplanned. The 'background rate' of congenital malformation in the general population has been determined as 1–3%, but the following drugs, chemicals and infections are all known teratogenic agents (ACOG Educational Bulletin, 1997) which could add to this figure.

Drugs and chemicals and their possible teratogenic effects

Alcohol

Growth restriction before and after birth, mental retardation, microcephaly, midfacial hypoplasia producing atypical facial appearance, renal and cardiac defects, various other major and minor malformations.

Androgens and testosterone derivatives (e.g. danazol)

Virilization of females, advanced genital development in males.

Angiotensin-converting enzyme inhibitors (e.g. enalapril, captopril)

Fetal renal tubular dysplasia, oligohydramnios, neonatal renal failure, lack of cranial ossification, intrauterine growth restriction.

Carbamazepine

Neural tube defects, minor craniofacial defects, fingernail hypoplasia, microcephaly, developmental delay, intrauterine growth restriction.

Cocaine

Bowel atresias, congenital malformations of the heart, limbs, face and genitourinary tract, microcephaly, intrauterine growth restriction, cerebral infarctions.

Coumarin derivatives (e.g. warfarin)

Nasal hypoplasia and stippled bone epiphyses (most common), also broad short hands with shortened phalanges, ophthalmic abnormalities, intrauterine growth restriction, developmental delay, anomalies of the neck and the central nervous system.

Diethylstilbestrol
Clear-cell adenocarcinoma of the vagina or cervix, vaginal adenosis, abnormalities of the cervix and uterus, abnormalities of the testes, possible infertility in males and females.

Folic acid antagonists (e.g. methotrexate and aminopterin)
Increased risk of spontaneous abortions, various anomalies.

Lead
Increased abortion rate, stillbirth.

Lithium
Congenital heart disease, in particular, Ebstein anomaly.

Organic mercury
Cerebral atrophy, microcephaly, mental retardation, spasticity, seizures, blindness.

Phenytoin
Intrauterine growth restriction, mental retardation, microcephaly, dysmorphic craniofacial features, cardiac defects, hypoplastic nails and distal phalanges.

Streptomycin and kanamycin
Hearing loss, eighth cranial nerve damage.

Tetracycline
Hypoplasia of tooth enamel, incorporation of tetracycline into bone and teeth, permanent yellow-brown discoloration of deciduous teeth.

Thalidomide
Bilateral limb deficiencies, anotia and microtia, cardiac and gastrointestinal anomalies.

Trimethadione and paramethadione
Cleft lip or cleft palate, cardiac defects, growth deficiency, microcephaly, mental retardation, characteristic facial appearance, ophthalmic abnormalities, limb, and genitourinary tract abnormalities.

Valproic acid
Neural tube defects (in particular, spina bifida), minor facial defects.

Vitamin A and derivatives (e.g. isotretinoin, etretinate, and retinoids)
Increased abortion rate, microtia, central nervous system defects, thymic agenesis, cardiovascular effects, craniofacial dysmorphism, microphthalmia, cleft lip and palate, mental retardation.

Infections and their potential teratogenic effects

Cytomegalovirus
Hydrocephaly, microcephaly, chorioretinitis, cerebral calcifications, symmetric intrauterine growth restriction, microphthalmos, brain damage, mental retardation, hearing loss.

Rubella
Microcephaly, mental retardation, cataracts, deafness, congenital heart disease (all organs may be affected).

Syphilis
Severe infection – fetal demise with hydrops; mild infection – detectable abnormalities of skin, teeth, and bones.

Toxoplasmosis
Possible effects on all systems but particularly chorioretinitis and central nervous system effects (microcephaly, hydrocephaly and cerebral calcifications), severity of manifestations depending on duration of disease.

Varicella
Possible effects on all organs, including skin scarring, chorioretinitis, cataracts, microcephaly, hypoplasia of the hands and feet, and muscle atrophy.

EPILOGUE

Sir Walter Langdon-Brown of Corpus Christi College, Cambridge delivered the Linacre Lecture for 1941 and his address was published in the same year. Entitled 'From Witchcraft to Chemotherapy', the lecture dealt with the history of herbal and other remedies. The society in which he lived, and the medicine and therapeutics of the age, seemed so advanced then that they could never be surpassed, but Langdon-Brown concluded: 'Let me end with a note of interrogation: the wisdom of one generation is often the foolishness of the next. What will coming generations think of ours?' At first, do no harm.

A SELECTION OF TWENTIETH CENTURY 'ALTERNATIVE MEDICATIONS'

(Extracted from *Squire's Companion to the British Pharmacopoeia*, 1908, and a selection of six modern books on Herbal Medicine).

Aconite root, agnus castus (chaste tree), agrimony, almond, aloes, amyl nitrite, angelica, anise (aniseed), astragalus, atropine sulfate.

Balm of Gilead, barberry, basil, bay laurel, belladonna, beth root, black hellebore, blue cohosh, borax, broom, bryony.

Calendula (marigold), cantharides, cardamom, castor oil plant, china root, Chinese angelica, chloral hydrate, codeine, common St John's wort, cumin.

Damiana, dandelion, datura seeds, deadly nightshade, dill, diluted hydrochloric acid, dittany, dong quai/du zhong (Chinese), dulse.

Echinacea, elder (elderberry), elecampane, ergot, eringo, ether, ethyl iodide, eucalyptus, evening primrose.

False unicorn root, fennel, fenugreek, ferrous sulfate, feverfew, flagyl, flax, flax seed, flexible collodion, fo-ti.

Galangal, gall, gentian, German chamomile, ginger, ginkgo (maidenhair tree), ginseng, golden seal, greater periwinkle, guaiacum resin, guelder rose.

Hawthorn, he shou wu (Chinese flowery knotweed), hemlock, henna, hibiscus flowers, huang bai, huang qi (milk vetch), giant hyssop, hydrangea, hydrastinine hydrochloride, hydrastis rhizome, hyoscyamus leaves.

Immune cleanser tea, Indian hemp, Indian (Egyptian) henbane, iodine, iodoform, ipecacuanha root, iron, ispaghula.

Jalap, Jamaica dogwood, joy tea, juniper.

Kale, kava kava, kefir, kelp, krameria root.

Lady's mantle, lady's slipper (valerian, American), lanolin, lapis lazuli, laudanum, lavender, lecithin, lesser periwinkle, life root, lime flowers, lovage.

Maidenhair, marigold, marijuana, marjoram, marshmallow, melilot, mercury, milkwort, motherwort, myrrh.

Nettle, nikkar nut, nitric acid, nutmeg.

Oak bark, onion, opium, orange, orris, osha root powder.

Paeony, parsley, peach, pellitory-of-the-wall, pennyroyal, phenyl salicylate, pipsissewa, plantain, poke root, primrose (evening), purslane.

Quaking aspen, queen's root.

Raspberry, reishi mushrooms, resin, rhubarb, rose, rue.

Saffron, sage, sassafras, savin, saw palmetto, scammony, sitz-bath, slippery elm, snakeroot, Solomon's seal, St John's wort.

Tamarind, tansy, *Taraxacum*, tea tree, terebene, thyme, tree of heaven (chun pi), turkey rhubarb root.

Umboshi plum paste, uva ursi.

Valerian, Venice treacle, vervain, vitamin E.

Water hyssop, white clay, white deadnettle, white peony (bai shao tao), white waterlily, white willow, wild lettuce, wild marjoram, witchhazel, wormwood.

Yam, yeast, yellow dock, yellow mercuric oxide ointment, yohimbene bark, yoni powder.

Zinc sulfate, zinc sulfocarbolate, zinc valerianate.

References

Abraham, G. E. (1983). Nutritional factors in the aetiology of the pre-menstrual tension syndromes. *J. Repr. Med.*, 28, 446–64

Albright, F., Bloomberg, E. and Smith, P. H. (1940). Post-menopausal osteoporosis. *Trans. Assoc. Am. Phys.*, 55, 298–305

Albright, F., Smith, P. H. and Richardson, A. M. (1941). Post-menopausal osteoporosis. Its clinical features. *JAMA*, 116, 2465–74

Allison, A. C. (1955). Danger of vitamin K to the newborn. *The Lancet*, 1, 669

ACOG (American College of Obstetricians and Gynecologists) (1997). Teratology. *Educational Bulletin*, No. 236. (Washington, DC: ACOG)

Anderson, E. Garrett (1907). Menopause. In *Green's Encyclopedia and Dictionary of Medicine and Surgery*, Vol. 6, pp. 332–5. (Edinburgh and London: William Green & Sons)

Avery, M. E. (1981). Corticosteroids: the case for their use. In *Pre-term Labour*, Elder, M. G. and Hendricks, C. H. (eds) Butterworth's *Int. Med. Revs. Obst. Gynecol.*, 1, pp. 176–86. (Boston and London: Butterworths)

Baskett, T. F. (1996). *On the Shoulders of Giants. Eponyms and Names in Obstetrics and Gynaecology*, Rubin, pp. 191–2. (London: RCOG Press)

Bates, C. P. (1971). Continence and incontinence. *Ann. R. Coll. Surgeon. Eng.*, **49**, 18–34

Bayer Pharma. Co. (1938). *Fifty Years of Bayer Remedies*, p. 27. (Leverkusen, Germany: Bayer)

Beck, A. C. (1942). *Obstetrical Practice*, pp. 78, 577–8, 578–84. (Baltimore: Williams & Wilkins Co.)

Berger, A. (1998). The rise and fall of Viagra. *BMJ*, **317**, 824

Bishop, P. M. F. (1950). Endocrine therapy. In Bowes, K. (ed.) *Modern Trends in Obstetrics and Gynaecology*, pp. 586–605. (London: Butterworth & Co.)

Blair-Bell, W. (1922). Endometrioma and endometriomyoma of the ovary. *J. Obstet. Gynaecol. Br. Emp.*, **29**, 443

Boolell, M., Gepi-Attee, S., Gingell, J. C. and Allen, M. J. (1996). Sildenafil, a novel effective oral therapy for male erectile dysfunction. *Br. J. Urol.*, **78**, 257–61

Bowes, K. (1950). *Modern Trends in Obstetrics and Gynaecology*, pp. 447–9, 521–33. (London: Butterworth & Co.)

Briggs, G. G., Freeman, R. K. and Yaffe, S. J. (1994). *Drugs in Pregnancy and Lactation*, 4th ed. (Baltimore: Williams and Wilkins)

Brindley, G. S. (1983). Cavernosal alpha-blockade: a new technique for investigating and treating erectile impotence. *Br. J. Psych.*, **143**, 332–7

Brindley, G. S. (1986). Pilot experiments on the actions of drugs injected into the human corpus cavernosum penis. *Br. J. Pharmacol.*, **87**, 495–500

Brown, J. R. (1964). A chronology of major events in obstetrics and gynecology. *J. Obstet. Gynaecol. Br. Common.*, **71**(2), 302–9

Browne, F. J. (1950). *Postgraduate Obstetrics and Gynaecology*, pp. 244–53. (London: Butterworth & Co.)

Brush, M. G. (1984). *Understanding Premenstrual Tension*, p. 11. (London: Pan)

Carter, B. (1962). Treatment of endometriosis. *J. Obstet. Gynaecol. Br. Common.*, **69**(5), 783–9

Centers for Disease Control (1992). Recommendations for the use of Folic Acid to Reduce the Number of Cases of Spina Bifida and other Neural Tube Defects. *Morbid Mortal Wkly. Rep.*, **41**(RR-14) 1: 7

Charatan, F. (1998). First pill for male impotence approved in US. *BMJ*, **316**, 1112

Cleaves, M. A. (1903). Radium: with a preliminary note on radium rays in the treatment of cancer. *Med. Rec.*, **64**, 601–10

Clinch, J. and Tindall, V. R. (1969). Effect of oestrogens and progestogens on liver function in the puerperium. *BMJ*, **1**, 602–5

Collip, J. B. (1923). The original method as used for the isolation of insulin in semipure form for the treatment of the first clinical cases. *J. Biol. Chem.*, **55**, 40

Compeston, N. and Pitt-Rivers, R. (1956). Thyroxine. *The Lancet*, **1**, 22–3

Cook, J. W., Dodds, E. C. and Hewett, C. L. (1933). A synthetic oestrus-exciting compound. (Letter to The Editor) *Nature*. (London), **131**, 56–7

Cooper, L. Z. (1968). Intrauterine infections. In Bergsma, D. (ed.) *Birth Defects Original Article Series*, Vol. IV(7), pp. 21–35. (New York: The National Foundation March of Dimes)

Crowley, P. (1995). Ante-natal corticosteroid therapy: a meta-analysis of the randomized trials, 1972–1994. *Am. J. Obstet. Gynecol.*, **173**, 322–35

Czeizel, A. E. and Dudas, I. (1992). Prevention of the first occurrence of neural-tube defects by peri-conceptional vitamin supplementation. *N. Eng. J. Med.*, **327**, 1832–5

Dally, A. (1998). Thalidomide – was the tragedy preventable? *The Lancet*, **351**, 1197–9

Dam, H., Dyggve, H., Hjalmar, M., Plum, P. (1952). The relation of vitamin K deficiency to haemorrhagic disease of the newborn. *Adv. Pediatr.*, **5**, 129–53

De Smet, P. A. G. M., Keller, K., Hansel, R., and Chandler, R. F. (1992). *Adverse Effects of Herbal Drugs*. (Berlin: Springer Verlag)

Dodds, E. C., Goldberg, L., Lawson, W., *et al.* (1938a). Oestrogenic activity of certain synthetic compounds. (Letter to The Editor) *Nature*. (London), **141**, 247–8

Dodds, E. C., Goldberg, L., Lawson, W., *et al.* (1938b). Oestrogenic activity of alkylated stilboestrols. (Letter to The Editor) *Nature*. (London), **142**, 34

Dodds, E. C., Goldberg, L., Lawson, W., *et al.* (1938c). Oestrogenic activity of esters of diethylstilboestrol. (Letter to The Editor) *Nature*. (London), **142**, 211–12

Dodds, E. C., Lawson, W. and Noble, R. L. (1938d). Biological effects of the synthetic oestrogenic substance 4: 4'-dihydroxy-alpha: beta-diethyl-stilbene. *The Lancet*, **1**, 1389–91

Draper, G. and McNinch, A. (1994). Vitamin K for neonates. The Controversy. *BMJ*, **308**, 867–8

Drury, M. I. (1989). They gave birth astride of a grave. *Diabet. Med.*, **6**, 291–8

Eardley, I., Morgan, R., Dinsmore, W., *et al.* (1996). Evaluation of the Efficacy of Sildenafil (Pfizer UK-92, 480), A new oral treatment for male erectile dysfunction (MED) in a double-blind, placebo-controlled study (Abstr.). *Eur. Urol.*, **30** (Suppl. 2), 355

Enhorning, G. and Robertson, B. (1972). Lung expansion in the premature rabbit fetus after tracheal deposition of surfactant. *Pediatrics*, **50**, 58–64

Eskes, T. A. A. B., Lijdam, W. S., Buys, M. J. R. M. and Van Rossum, J. M. (1985). Prospective study of the use of medication during pregnancy in the Netherlands. In Kab Eskes, T. and Finster, M. (eds) *Drug Therapy during Pregnancy*, pp. 1–8. (London: Butterworths)

Evans, W. C. (1996). *Trease and Evans Pharmacognosy*, pp. 448–9. (London: W. B. Saunders Co.)

Expert Advisory Group (1992). Folic Acid in the Prevention of Neural Tube Defects. (UK Department of Health)

Fido, M. and Fido, K. (1996). *The World's Worst Medical Mistakes*, pp. 14–27. (London: Seven Oaks Ltd.)

Flower, R. J., Moncada, S. and Vane, J. R. (1985). Drug Therapy of Inflammation. In Goodman Gilman, A., Goodman, L. S.,

Rall, T. W. and Murad, F. (eds) *Goodman and Gilman's The Pharmacological Basis of Therapeutics*, 7th ed., pp. 674–715. (New York: Macmillan Publishing Co.)

Fraser, J. R. (1925). Progress in gynecology in the last twenty years. *Surg. Gynecol. Obstet. Int. Abst. Surg.*, **40**, 452

Fuchs, A. R. and Wagner, G. (1963). Effect of alcohol on release of oxytocin. *Nature* (London), **198**, 93–5

Fuchs, F. and Stakemann, G. (1960). Treatment of threatened premature labor with large doses of progesterone. *Am. J. Obstet. Gynecol.*, **79**, 172–6

Fuchs, F. (1983). An Alphabet of Progress. Presidential Address to the New York Obstetrical Society. *Am. J. Obstet. Gynecol.*, **147**(3), 311–18

Gabbe, S. G. (1992). After Office Hours. A story of two miracles: the impact of the discovery of insulin on pregnancy in women with diabetes mellitus. *Obstet. Gynecol.*, **79**, 295–9

Gemzell, C. A., Diczfalusy, E., and Tillinger, K. J. (1958). Clinical effect of human pituitary follicle-stimulating hormone (FSH). *J. Clin. Endocrinol. Metab.*, **18**, 1333–48

Gingell, C., Jardin, A., Giuliano, F. A., *et al.* (1996). The efficacy of sildenafil. (Viagra), a new oral treatment for erectile dysfunction, demonstrated by four different methods in a double-blind placebo-controlled, multinational clinical trial (Abstr.). *Eur. Urol.*, **30**(Suppl. 2), 353

Golding, J., Greenwood, R., Birmingham, K., and Mott, M. (1992). Childhood cancer, intramuscular vitamin K. and pethidine given during labour. *BMJ*, **305**, 341–6

Golding, J., Paterson, M. and Kinlen, L. J. (1990). Factors associated with childhood cancer in a national cohort study. *Br. J. Cancer*, **62**, 304–8

Graham, J. (1984). *Evening Primrose Oil*, pp. 14–17. (London: Thorsons)

Greenblatt, R. B., Dmowski, W. P., Mahesh, V. B. and Scholer, H. F. L. (1971). Clinical studies with an anti-gonadotropin, danazol. *Fertil. Steril.*, **22**, 102–12

Greenblatt, R. B., Roy, S., Mahesh, V. B., *et al.* (1962). Induction of ovulation. *Am. J. Obstet. Gynecol.*, **84**, 900–9

Greenhill, J. P. (ed.) (1975). Progress in obstetrics and gynecology, 1921–75. In *The Year Book of Obstetrics and Gynecology*, pp. 9–15. (Chicago: Year Book Medical Publishers)

Greg, N. M. (1942). Congenital cataract following German measles in mothers. *Trans. Ophth. Soc. Austr.*, **3**, 35

Grieve, M. (1931). *A Modern Herbal*, p. 658. (London: Jonathan Cape)

Heiduschka, A. and Luft, K. (1919). The fat and oil in seeds of *Oenothera biennis* and one new linolenic acid. *Archiv der Pharmazie*, **257**, 33–69

Hellman, L. M. and Pritchard, J. A. (1971). Obstetrics in broad perspective. In *Williams' Obstetrics*, 14th ed. pp. 1–18 (London: Butterworths)

Herbst, A. L., Ulfelder, H. and Poskanzer, D. C. (1971). Adenocarcinoma of the vagina: association of maternal stilbesterol therapy with tumor appearance in young women. *N. Eng. J. Med.*, **284**, 878–81

Hertz, R. (1963). Folic acid antagonists: effects on the cell and the patient. clinical staff conference at NIH. *Ann. Intern. Med.*, **59**, 931–56

Hewitt, S. R. (1981). *Farewell – A personal review of 40 years*, Annual Report, Dept. Obstet. Gynaecol., Portiuncula Hospital. (Ballinasloe: Kelly's Printers)

Hibbard, B. M. (1964). The role of folic acid in pregnancy with particular reference to anaemia, abruption and abortion. *J. Obstet. Gynaecol. Br. Common.*, **71**(4), 529–739

Hibbard, E. D. and Smithells, R. W. (1965). Folic acid metabolism and human embryopathy. *The Lancet*, **1**, 1254

Hillman, R. S. (1985). Vitamin B12, folic acid, and the treatment of megaloblastic anaemias. In Goodman Gilman, A., Goodman, L. S., Rall, T. W. and Murad, F. (eds) *Goodman's and Gilman's The Pharmacological Basis of Therapeutics*, pp. 1323–37. (New York: MacMillan)

Hollman, A. (1992). *Plants in Cardiology*, pp. 8–9, 17. (London: British Medical Journal Publications)

Horrobin, D. F. (1983). The role of essential fatty acids and prostaglandins in the pre-menstrual syndrome. *J. Reprod. Med.*, **28**, 465–8

Hunter, R. B. (1961). Review of the action of oral anticoagulants on the blood coagulation mechanism. In G. W. Pickering (ed.) *Symposium on Anticoagulant Therapy*, pp. 2–13. (London: Harvey & Blythe)

Ingemarsson, I. (1984). Pharmacology of tocolytic agents. In Howie, P. W. and Patel, N. B. (eds) *The Small Baby. Clinics in Obstetrics and Gynaecology*, pp. 337–51. (London: W. B. Saunders & Co.)

Ishii, N., *et al.* (1986). Studies on male sexual impotence. Report 18. Therapeutic trial with prostaglandin E1 for organic impotence. *Nippon Hinyokika Gakkai Zasshi.*, **77**, 954–62

Jaques, L. B. (1978). Addendum: The discovery of heparin. *Seminars in Thrombosis and Haemostasis*, **4**, 350–3

Kelly, H. A. (1909). *Medical Gynaecology*, pp. 87–90, 89, 169–80, 231–2, 604–6. (London: Appleton & Co.)

Kendall, E. C. (1929). *Thyroxine*. (New York: Chem. Catalog. Co.)

Kistner, R. W. (1958). The treatment of endometriosis by inducing pseudo-pregnancy with ovarian hormones: A report of fifty-eight cases. *Fertil. Steril.*, **10**, 539–56

Knobil, E. (1980). The neuro-endocrine control of the menstrual cycle. *Recent Prog. Horm. Res.*, **36**, 53–88

Notice Board (1991). Congenital rubella – fifty years on. *The Lancet*, **337**, 668

Langworthy, O. R. (1936). A new approach to the diagnosis and treatment of disorders of micturition and diseases of the nervous system. *Int. Clin.*, **3**, 98

Lanier, A. P., Noller, K. L., Dekker, D. G., *et al.* (1973). Cancer and stilbesterol: a follow up of 1719 persons born 1943–1959 and exposed to estrogens *in utero*. *Mayo Clinic Procs.*, **48**, 793–9

Lauersen, N. H., Merkatz, I., Tejani, N., *et al.* (1977). Inhibition of premature labor: a multi-center comparison of ritodrine and ethanol. *Am. J. Obstet. Gynecol.*, **127**, 837–45

Laurence, B. (1955). Danger of vitamin K analogues to the newborn. *The Lancet*, **1**, 669

Laurence, D. R. (1973). *Clinical Pharmacology*, pp. 6.67–6.70, 23.1–23.15. (Edinburgh: Churchill Livingstone)

Laurence, K. M., James, N., Miller, M. H., Tennant, G. B. and Campbell, H. (1981). Double-blind randomised controlled trial of folate treatment before conception to prevent recurrence of neural tube defects. *BMJ*, **282**, 1509–11

Lechtenberg, R. and Ohl, D. A. (1994). *Sexual Dysfunction. Neurologic, Urologic and Gynecologic Aspects*, pp. 305–23. (Philadelphia: Lea & Febiger)

Lehman, J. (1944). Vitamin K as prophylaxis in 13,000 infants. *The Lancet*, **1**, 493–4

Lenz, W. (1961). Fragen aus der praxis. *Dtsche Med. Wochensch.*, **85**, 2555

Lewis, T. L. T. (1964). *Progress in Clinical Obstetrics and Gynaecology*, pp. 1–78, 383–99. (London: J. and A. Churchill Ltd.)

Liggins, G. C. and Howie, R. N. (1972). A Controlled trial of ante-partum glucocorticoid treatment for prevention of the respiratory distress syndrome in premature infants. *Pediatrics*, **50**, 515–25

Lunenfeld, B., Sulimovici, S., Rabau, E. and Eshko, A. (1962). L'indution de L'ovulation dans les amenorrhés hypophysaires par un traitement combaine de gonadotropines urinaires menopausiques et de gonadotropines chorionique. *C. R. Soc. Fr. Gynecol.*, **35**, 346–56

MacNaughton Jones, H. (1885). *Practical Manual of Diseases of Women and Uterine Therapeutics*, 2nd ed. (London: Bailliere, Tindall & Cox)

Mathews, F., Yudkin, P. and Neil, A. (1998). Folates in the peri-conceptional period: are women getting enough? *Br. J. Obstet. Gynaecol.*, **105**, 954–9

McBride, W. G. (1961). Thalidomide and congenital abnormalities. *The Lancet*, **2**, 1358

Medvei, V. C. (1993). *The History of Clinical Endocrinology*, pp. 232–5, 249–58. (London & New York: Parthenon Publishing)

Meldrum, D. R., Change, R. J., Lu, J., Vale, W. Rivier, J. and Judd, H. L. (1982). Medical oophorectomy using long acting GnRH agonist – a possible new approach to the treatment of endometriosis. *J. Clin. Endocrin. Metab.*, **54**, 1081–3

Meyer, T. C. and Angus, J. (1956). The effect of large doses of synkavit in the newborn. *Arch. Dis. Child.*, **31**, 212–15

Michal, V., Kramar, R. and Pospichal, J. (1977). Arterial epigastrico-cavernous anatomosis for the treatment of sexual impotence. *World J. Surg.*, **1**, 515–20

Millin, T. and Read, C. D. (1950). Gynaecological urology. In Bowes, K. (ed.) *Moderns Trends in Obstetrics and Gynaecology*, pp. 694–701. (London: Butterworth & Co.)

Mitchell, H. K., Snell, E. E. and Williams, R. J. (1941). The concentration of 'folic acid'. *J. Am. Chem. Soc.*, **63**, 2284

MRC Vitamin Study Research Group (1991). Prevention of neural tube defects: Results of the Medical Research Council Vitamin Study. *The Lancet*, **346**, 393–6

Mullner, M. (1998). Nobel Prize for Medicine awarded for work on nitric oxide. *BMJ*, **317**, 1031

Munro-Kerr, J. M., Johnstone, R. W. and Phillips, M. H. (1954). *Historical Review of British Obstetrics and Gynaecology. 1800–1950*, pp. 87–406. (Edinburgh & London: E. & S. Livingstone)

Murray, G. R. (1891). Note on the treatment of myxoedema by hypodermic injections of an extract of the thyroid gland of a sheep. *BMJ*, **2**, 796–7

Nilsson, L. and Rybo, G. (1971). Treatment of menorrhagia. *Am. J. Obstet. Gynecol.*, **110**, 713–20

Niswander, R. R., Gordon, M. and Berends, H. W. (1972). The women and their pregnancies. In *The collaborative perinatal study of the National Institute of Neurologic Disease and Stroke*, Vol. 1, pp. 246–9. (Philadelphia: W. B. Saunders)

Noller, K. L., Dekker, D. G., Lanier, A. P., *et al.* (1972). clear-cell adenocarcinoma of the cervix after maternal treatment with synthetic estrogens. *Mayo Clinic Proc.*, **47**, 629–30

O'Connor, D. G. (1987). Endometriosis. Singer, A. and Jordan, J. A. (eds) *Curr. Rev. Obstet. Gynaecol.*, **12**, 85–144. (Edinburgh: Churchill Livingstone)

O'Dowd, M. J. and Philipp, E. (1994). *The History of Obstetrics and Gynaecology*, pp. 21–40, 509–22, 531–92. (New York and London: Parthenon Publishing)

O'Reilly, R. A. (1985). Anti-coagulant, antithrombotic and thrombolytic drugs. In Goodman Gilman, A., Goodman, L. S., Rall, T. W. and Murad, F. (eds) *Goodman's and Gilman's The Pharmacological Basis of Therapeutics*, pp. 1338–59. (New York: MacMillan)

Padma-Nathan, H., Hellstrom, W. J., Kaiser, F. E., *et al.* (1997). Treatment of men with erectile dysfunction with trans-urethral alprostadil. medicated urethral system for erection (MUSE) study group. *N. Eng. J. Med.*, **336**, 1–7

Paulson, D. F. (1979). Oxybutynin chloride in the management of idiopathic detrusor instability. *South. Med. J.*, **72**, 374

Pittler, M. H. and Ernst, E. (1998). Trials have shown yohimbine is effective for erectile dysfunction. (Letter) *BMJ*, **317**, 478

Porter, R., Smith, W., Craft, I. L., Abdulwahid, N. and Jacobs, H. (1984). Induction of ovulation for *in vitro* fertilization using buserelin and gonadotropins. *The Lancet*, **2**, 1284–5

RCOG Guideline (1997). *Beta-agonists for the Care of Women in Pre-Term Labour.* (London: Royal College of Obstetricians and Gynaecologists)

Reid, K., Surridge, D. H. C., Morales, A., *et al.* (1987). Double-blind trial of yohimbine in the treatment of psychogenic impotence. *The Lancet*, **2**, 421–3

Ringer, S. (1888). *A Handbook of Therapeutics*, pp. 87–90, 604–6. (London: H. K. Lewis)

Rokitansky, C. von (1860). Ueber Uterusdrusen-Neubildung in Uterus und Ovarialsarcomen. *Zkk. Gesellsch. d. Aerzte zu Wien*, **37**, 577

Routledge, P. (1998). One Hundred Years of Pharmacovigilance. *The Lancet*, **351**, 1200–1

Royal College of Obstetricians and Gynaecologists (1996). Antenatal corticosteroids to prevent respiratory distress syndrome. *Guideline No. 7.* (London: RCOG)

Royal College of Obstetricians and Gynaecologists (July 1998). The management of recurrent miscarriage. *Guideline No. 17.* (London: RCOG)

Sampson, J. A. (1921). Perforating haemorrhagic (chocolate) cysts of the ovary. *Arch. Surg.*, 3, 245

Slattery, J. M. (1994). Why we need a clinical trial of vitamin K. *BMJ*, 308, 908–10

Smith, G. N. and Brien, J. F. (1998). Use of nitroglycerine for uterine relaxation. *CME Rev. Obstet. Gynaecol. Surv.*, 53(9), 559–65

Smithells, R. W. (1971). The prevention and prediction of congenital malformations. In MacDonald, R. R. (ed.) *Scientific Basis of Obstetrics and Gynaecology*, pp. 249–73. (London: Churchill Livingstone)

Smithells, R. W., Nevin, N. C., Seller, M. J., *et al.* (1983). Further experience of vitamin supplementation for prevention of neural tube defect recurrences. *The Lancet*, 1, 1027–31

Smithells, R. W., Sheppard, S., Schorah, C. J., *et al.* (1980). Possible prevention of neural-tube defects by peri-conceptional vitamin supplementation. *The Lancet*, 1, 339–40

Squire, P. W. (1909). *Squire's Companion to the British Pharmacopoeia*, 18th ed. (London: J. and A. Churchill)

Steer, C. M. and Petrie, R. H. (1977). A comparison of magnesium sulfate and alcohol for the prevention of premature labor. *Am. J. Obstet. Gynecol.*, 129, 1–4

Sugrue, D. and Drury, M. I. (1980). Hyperthyroidism complicating pregnancy: results of treatment by anti-thyroid drugs in 77 pregnancies. *Br. J. Obstet. Gynaecol.*, 87(11), 970–5

The American College of Obstetricians and Gynecologists (ACOG) (1994). *Committee Opinion*, pp. 176–86. (Washington: ACOG)

The Department of Health (1992). Folic acid in prevention of neural tube defects. *Reports from an Expert Advisory Panel.* (London: Department of Health)

Ulmsten, U., Andersson, K. E. and Wingerup, L. (1980). Treatment of premature labour with the calcium antagonist nifedipine. *Arch. Gynecol.*, 229, 1–5

Unger, W. (1917). Fats and oils in the seeds of *Oenothera biennis. Apotheker-Zeit.*, 32, 351–2

Virag, R. (1982). Intracavernosal injection of papaverine for erectile failure. (Letter). *The Lancet*, 2, 938

Virag, R., Fryman, D., Legman, M. and Virag, H. (1984). Intracavernous injection of papaverine as a diagnostic and therapeutic method in erectile failure. *Angiology*, 35, 79–87

Wesselius de Casparis, A., Thiery, M., Yo Le Sian, A., *et al.* (1971) Results of double-blind multi-center study with ritodrine in premature labour. *BMJ*, 2, 144–7

Westrom, L. and Bengtsson, L. P. (1970). Effect of tranexamic acid (AMCA) in menorrhagia with intra-uterine contraceptive devices. A double blind study. *J. Reprod. Med.*, 5, 154–61

Williams, J. W. (1903). *Obstetrics*, pp. 344–5. (Connecticut: Appleton and Lange)

Wilson, R. A. (1966). *Feminine Forever*, pp. 11–19. (Philadelphia & New York: M. Evans & Co. Ltd.)

Wootton, A. C. (1910). *Chronicles of Pharmacy*, p. 269. (London: MacMillan & Co.)

World Health Organization (1970). *World Health Outlines for Health.* (Geneva: WHO)

Zorgniotti, A. W. and Lefleur, R. S. (1985). Auto-injection of the corpus cavernosum with a vasoactive drug combination for vasculogenic impotence. *J. Urol.*, 133, 39–41

Section 4

Special Subjects

Anesthesia and analgesia and the curse of Eve

18

INTRODUCTION

Anesthesia was introduced to obstetrics by James Young Simpson, professor of midwifery at the University of Edinburgh, when he used ether to successfully conduct a pain-free delivery on 19 January 1847. However, Simpson's attention soon turned to chloroform which he first used in obstetrics on 8 November, of the same year. The use of anesthesia in obstetrics led to medical and moral controversies, with Simpson and his followers coming under the combined attack of the medical profession and the clergy. Simpson entered the fray in characteristically able fashion: using reasoned arguments, vehemence in debate and humanity. Simpson's opinions won through and the use of obstetric anesthesia became widespread.

In reviewing those early days of inhalation anesthesia, the historian Barbara Duncum of Oxford wrote 'by the middle of the year 1848 the practice of administering an anesthetic during labor was well established'. In reality, however, it was not until John Snow administered chloroform to Queen Victoria for the birth of Prince Leopold in April 1853 that anesthesia gained 'the seal of perfect propriety' in midwifery (Duncum, 1947 p. 177). The technique of 'Chloroform a la Reine' became fashionable and the relief of the pains of labor, the 'Curse of Eve', could at last be properly addressed.

SIR JAMES YOUNG SIMPSON

AND

CHLOROFORM

(1811—1870)

BY

H. LAING GORDON

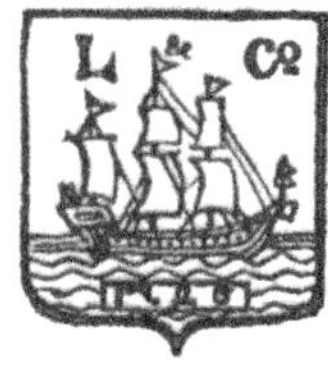

NEW YORK

T. FISHER UNWIN

91 & 93, FIFTH AVENUE

1897

Figure 1 Frontispiece from Laing Gordon's book on Simpson

Definition of anesthesia

Anesthesia is defined as a 'loss of feeling' and derives from the Greek term for 'insensibility' or 'lack of perception'. The word only came into general English usage in 1721, although Dioscorides c. 65 AD had used it in the modern sense when discussing the properties of mandragora. When William Morton discovered the anesthetic effects of ether, he called the substance 'letheon' which derived from the Greek for 'oblivion'. However, Oliver Wendell Holmes of Boston wrote to Morton on 21 November 1846 and suggested 'All I will do is to give you a hint or two as to names, or name, to be applied to the state produced, and to the agent. The state should, I think, be called anaesthesia ... the adjective will be anaesthetic' (Armstrong Davidson, 1970 p. 18). The suggested term was readily accepted by Morton and the medical profession and retained its original spelling until the early twentieth century when 'anaesthesia' became shortened to 'anesthesia' in America.

Pre-anesthetic analgesia

Although many analgesics substances were known, pain relief played a minor role in medicine, surgery and midwifery prior to the nineteenth century. The classical Greco-Roman belief regarded pain and suffering as a cosmic experience of gods and heroes, which seemed unrelated to ordinary mortals. In the Judeo-Christian belief, pain was seen as a means to salvation and was inflicted by a vengeful god as a punishment for sin (Adams, 1996 pp. 96–100).

Medicine and the long-held views on morality, as interpreted in the Bible, gradually became intertwined and so the use of analgesia was seen as being contrary, not only to religious, but also to medical belief. To recall how deeply embedded those beliefs were one only has to recall the tale of Eufame McAlyane who was executed in Scotland during the reign of James VI for attempting to relieve the pains of childbirth. It was alleged that Eufame had consulted and sought pain-relieving drugs from Annie Samson, who was thought to be a witch (Armstrong-Davidson, 1970 pp. 212–15).

The drugs which could have been used as analgesics were known since antiquity. 'The use of a soporific potions as a substitute for anesthesia', wrote Garrison (1924 p. 29) 'goes back to remote antiquity ... from the soothing Egyptian *nepenthe* to the *samme de shinta* of the Talmud, the *bhang* of the Arabian Nights, or the 'drowsy syrups' of Shakespeare's time, the soporific virtues of opium, Indian hemp (*Cannabis indica*), mandrake (*Atropa mandragora*), henbane (*Hyoscyamus*), dewtry (*Datura stramonium*), hemlock (*Conium maculatum*), and lettuce (*Lactuca sativa*), appear to have been well known to the Orientals and the Greeks; and in the thirteenth and fourteenth centuries, a mixture of some of these ingredients (*oleum de lateribus*) was formerly recommended for 'surgical anesthesia' by many of the medieval 'masters', including Theodoric in the

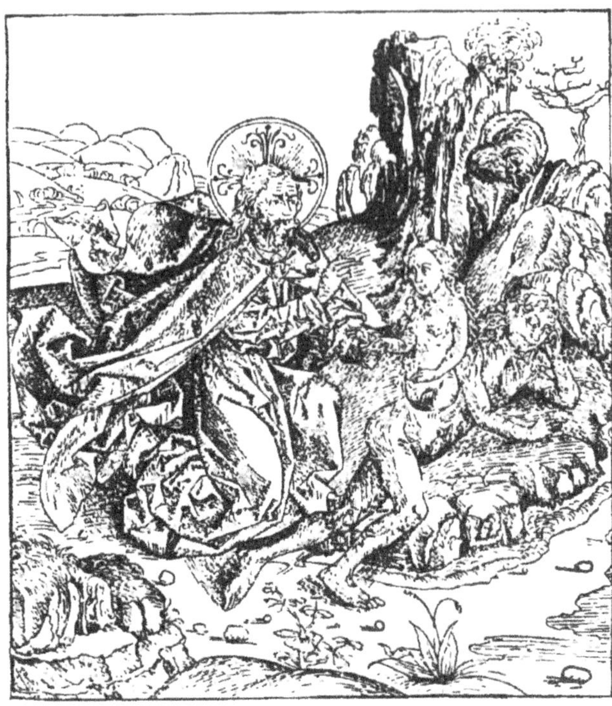

"And the Lord God caused a deep sleep to fall upon Adam, and he slept."

Figure 2 The Bible and anesthesia

form of a *spongia somnifera* or *confectio soporis* for inhalation'.

It is related in the Bible (Genesis 30: 14–16) that Rachel sought mandrake from Leah, but it is uncertain whether they were to ease the pangs of childbirth, or whether they were for use as aphrodisiacs or soporifics. The use of the soporific draught of Dioscorides (mandragora wine) and the soporific sponge of the Salernitans 'was unknown to Paré (1510–1590) and died out in the seventeenth century' but patients were frequently intoxicated with alcohol or opium to cause relaxation and to alleviate pain.

The traditional pharmacopoeias contained analgesic drugs which, with fungi, herbs, roots and alcohol, were available to midwives. Birth attendants sometimes used the ancient 'soporific sponges' containing a decoction of henbane, hemlock, mandragora and ground ivy, and which rendered women insensible or temporarily pain-free (Gelis, 1991 p. 153). Although Simpson (1848a pp. 209–51) was aware of the ancient anodynes and the use of opium he 'failed, however, in finding any trace whatever either of any practical attempts to abrogate or modify, by true anaesthetic means, the pains of labor'.

Opium, in the guise of tincture of laudanum (a term coined by Paracelsus in the sixteenth century) was being prescribed for some women in labor. Fielding Ould of Dublin, in *A Treatise of Midwifery, in Three Parts* of 1742, was one of the first obstetricians of relatively modern times to advocate its use. William Dewees of Pennsylvania, later called the 'father of American obstetrics', wrote in 1819 that opium was the favorite remedy of most accoucheurs, but he found that it weakened uterine contractions and he did not favor its use. His Doctoral thesis, 'The Means of Moderating or Relieving Pain during Parturition' was published in book form in 1808, demonstrating his lively interest in the subject (Findley, 1939 pp. 237, 215).

MIDWIFERY IN THE PRE-ANESTHETIC DAYS OF THE EARLY 1800s

To put midwifery problems of the early 1800s in perspective, I quote from John Burns, professor of surgery at the University of Glasgow, who wrote in those pre-anesthetic days (safe oxytocics were not yet available) that maternal mortality in labor occurred in one out of every 92 women, while one child in 18 was stillborn (Burns, 1820 pp. 423–4, 392–414). 'Tedious labor' (usually labor of more than 24 hours) was one of the main causes of maternal and perinatal mortality.

Delay in labor was most often encountered in primigravidae but also occurred in multigravidae, because of premature induction of labor, a treatment (introduced by Macauley of London in the 1700s) was advocated for women with a past history of difficult births and in those with deformed contracted pelves due to rickets, a disease common at that time. The treatments for 'tedious labor' were venesection, purgation and administration of opium, or manual dilatation of the cervix and lubrication of the birth canal with oil (Burns, 1820 pp. 392–414). Cesarean section was not an option as in the early 1800s, as it almost always resulted in maternal and fetal death.

Ringland (1870 p. 23) wrote that 'the forceps had fallen into disuse, and the perforator [used to 'decompress' the fetal head] and crotchet [a metal hook to extract the fetus] substituted' until forceps came back into fashion in the 1830s. And so, countless craniotomies and difficult forceps extractions were carried out on fully-conscious patients with resultant mental and physical injuries often followed by hemorrhage, sepsis and possibly death. Against this background, it is easy to understand that the introduction of anesthesia in labor had a major impact on the welfare of women, their unborn, their families and their attendants in labor.

Ether

Ether was independently discovered by both Paracelsus and by Valerius Cordus in the sixteenth century. William Morton of Boston demonstrated the anesthetic properties of ether on 16 October 1846 (Morton, 1846; 1847). During a trip to London, James Young Simpson met the surgeon Robert Liston who had performed a leg amputation on 21 December 1846, while the patient was anesthetized with ether. On his return, Simpson decided to extend the use of ether to midwifery. He pondered on the time interval over which ether could be given; what effects it might have on the mother and her uterus; and whether it would cause maternal hemorrhage or adverse effects on the welfare of the unborn. Despite his reservations, Simpson administered ether anesthesia to a midwifery patient, for the first time, on 19 January 1847, and reported the case in the March issue of the *Monthly Journal of Medical Science* (Simpson, 1847a p. 721), with an introduction paraphrased from Shakespeare:

> 'Not poppy, nor mandragora,
> Nor all the drowsy syrups of the world,
> Shall ever medicine thee to such sweet sleep'.

News of Simpson's momentous achievement spread quickly and soon afterwards the use of ether anesthesia in midwifery was reported in France by Fournier Deschamps, about 26 January, and by Paul Dubois of Paris (for a forceps delivery) on 13 February, 1847. In Germany, Professor Martin of Jena used anesthesia in midwifery on 24 February 1847. In the USA, the first

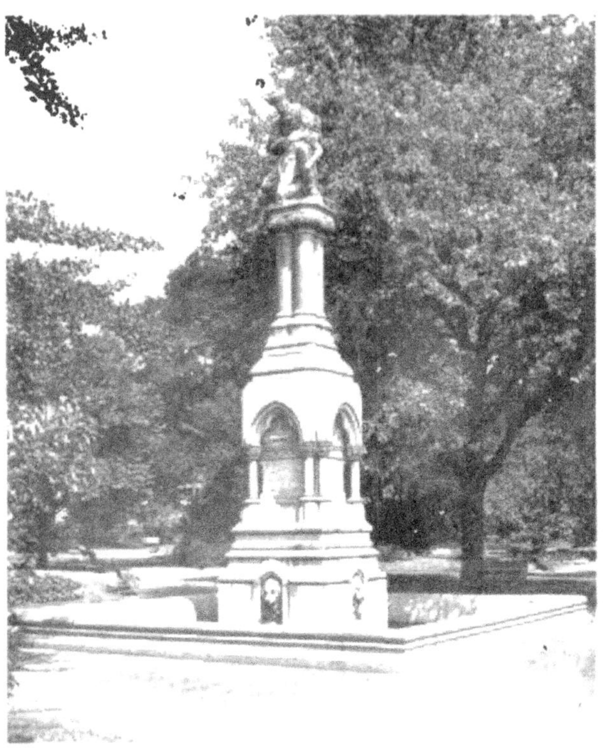

Figure 3 The Ether monument. From Raper, *Man Against Pain* (1945)

obstetrical anesthetic was undertaken by Dr Nathan C. Keep, a Boston dentist, on 7 April 1847. Walter Channing of Harvard followed, with anesthetic intervention for an instrumental delivery on 5 May of the same year, and went on to become the champion of anesthetic midwifery in America. His important *A Treatise on Etherization in Childbirth* was published in Boston in 1848. In Ireland, Alexander Tyler of Dublin used ether on a patient for instrumental delivery on 28 November 1847 (Simpson, 1848a pp. 209–51; Armstrong Davidson, 1970 p. 118). Paul Dubois of Paris concluded that the inhalation of ether could: suspend physiological labor pain; annul the pain of obstetric operations; did not adversely affect uterine contractions nor those of the abdominal muscles; diminished the resistance of the perineum; and did not appear to act unfavorably on the health of the infant (Simpson, 1848 pp. 209–51).

Despite his epoch-making advance, Simpson continued his quest for the 'ideal' obstetric anesthetic as ether was unpleasant to inhale and the lightly anesthetized patient was liable to vomit. Ether was also inflammable, not portable and was required in large quantities. Simpson wished to find a better anesthetic which would provide adequate analgesia without loss of consciousness. His attention turned to chloroform.

Chloroform

Chloroform was discovered independently and almost simultaneously by Samuel Guthrie of the USA ('Guthrie's sweet whisky') and also by Jonathan Pereira, Soubeiran in France and by Justus Leibig of Germany between 1831 and 1832. The chemical and physical properties of the substance, originally known as 'formyle chloride', were first correctly identified in 1834 by Jean-Baptise Dumas of France, who also introduced the name 'chloroform'. Jacob Bell used chloroform as an anesthetic in February 1847 and was followed by Pierre Flourens of France in March of the same year (Foy, 1889 pp. 34, 39).

Simpson had begun his search for an alternative to ether in the autumn of 1847 with the help of Thomas Keith and J. Matthews Duncan. They tested various chemicals but, on the suggestion of David Waldie, a Scots chemist working in Liverpool, they inhaled the vapors of chloroform on 4 November 1847. Simpson discovered that the substance was 'far stronger and better than ether' (Laing Gordon, 1897 p. 107). Four days later, Simpson used chloroform for the delivery of the wife of Dr Carstairs of Edinburgh and reported the event to the Medico-Chirurgical Society of Edinburgh on 10 November 1847 (Simpson, 1847c). News of the event spread rapidly and chloroform soon ousted ether from its preeminent position, while extending the employment of anesthesia in obstetrics.

Simpson found that, when compared to ether, chloroform was more rapid in its onset of action. It had a pleasant perfume and was agreeable to inhale. Much less was required and chloroform did not need a special inhaler. He advised that it should only be given during contractions and estimated that, on average, one ounce of chloroform per hour was necessary (Claye, 1939 p. 13). Looking to the future, Simpson was aware of the possible dangers of chloroform. 'Like many other agents, it may be powerful for evil as well as for good ... if exhibited in too

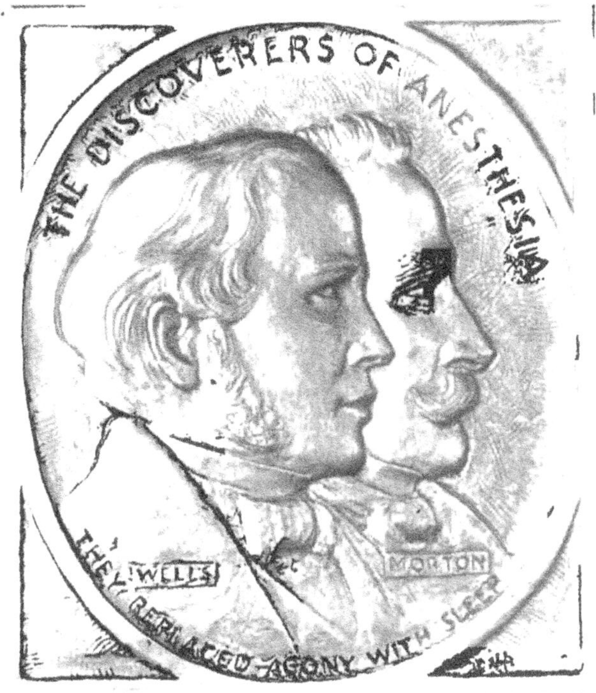
THE DISCOVERERS OF ANESTHESIA
WELLS
MORTON
THEY REPLACED AGONY WITH SLEEP

Figure 4 Medal depicting Wells and Morton

strong a dose ... it would doubtless produce serious consequences, and even death ... it is certainly far too powerful ... to be entrusted to ... unprofessional individuals' (Claye, 1939 p. 15). Hannah Greener, who died on 28 January 1848, was the first recorded mortality related to chloroform (Armstrong Davidson, 1970 p. 101).

The use of anesthesia in midwifery became widespread despite immediate concerns and later realization of toxicity of chloroform. At the Rotunda Hospital Dublin, Eliza Hughes was delivered by forceps while under the influence of chloroform on 18 February 1848 (Gardiner, 1995 pp. 180–5). Soon afterwards, John Denman (1849 pp. 107–42) reported a series of 50 cases from the same hospital. Such cases mirrored the experiences of many other accoucheurs in Europe and America.

In 1853 Queen Victoria sought the aid of John Snow, the first physician-anesthetist, and he administered chloroform to her during the birth of Prince Leopold, her eighth child, on 14 April of that year. Her Majesty's approval and praise of the procedure helped remove most of the remaining opposition to anesthesia in labor and chloroform gained widespread acceptance in obstetric practice. Soon after Simpson's death in 1870, Professor Gusserow of Berlin acknowledged that 'chloroform was the only anesthetic used over almost the entire world' (Claye, 1954 pp. 226–38).

Although ether was reintroduced in 1872, chloroform remained popular in hospital and domiciliary midwifery until the early 1960s. A common form of analgesia was two chloroform 'brisettes', crushed into a handkerchief and inhaled, for the delivery of the head. When chloroform was finally withdrawn the reasons cited were the risks of maternal mortality at induction or when emerging from anesthesia, and the long-term risk of liver failure.

CONTROVERSIES – MEDICAL AND MORAL

Medical

The introduction of anesthesia to surgery and obstetrics led to medical and moral controversies which captured the imagination of the general public. The French physiologist, François Magendie, held views similar to Pickford who claimed that 'pain during [surgical] operations is in the majority of cases even desirable; and its prevention or annihilation is, for the most part, hazardous to the patient' (Claye, 1939 p. 3). Simpson countered with the results of his investigations into the results of limb amputations (the commonest form of surgery at the time) performed without anesthesia in which 38% of patients died compared to an operative mortality 25% if amputation was performed under anesthesia. Simpson believed that the mortality and morbidity of surgery was reduced in anesthetized patients through the elimination of mental and physical shock.

The medical pundits pointed out that labor did not compare to surgical operations. They also claimed that anesthesia would increase the operative mortality in obstetrics and would be responsible for insanity, hemorrhage and convulsions in the mother and would promote idiocy in the neonate – if it were lucky enough to be born alive. It was argued that pain was a 'desirable, salutary and conservative manifestation of life force' (Miller, 1962 pp. 142–50).

In March of 1848, Charles Meigs wrote in the *Philadelphia Medical Examiner* that the pain of parturition was a 'physiological pain'. However, in his textbooks, *Females and their Diseases* and *Philadelphia Practice of Midwifery*, he wrote: 'there is no name for it but agony ... absolutely indescribable' (Simpson, 1848a pp. 215–16). During the height of the controversy, Meigs wrote a letter to Simpson stating that 'should I exhibit the remedy ... to prevent the physiological pain, and for no other motive, and if I should in consequence destroy only one of them, I should feel disposed to clothe me in sackcloth, and cast ashes on my head, for the rest of my days' (Montgomery, 1849 pp. 321–40).

Meanwhile, Ashwell (1848 vol. 1, pp. 291–2), an obstetrician at Guy's Hospital London, wrote that the use of anesthesia in obstetrics was an 'unnecessary interference with the providentially arranged process of healthy labor ... sooner or later, to be followed by injurious and fatal consequences', and he then also entered into the 'biblical' debate.

William Featherstone Montgomery, professor of midwifery to the King and Queen's College of Physicians in Ireland, famous for his *An Exposition of the Signs and Symptoms of Pregnancy* (1837), was drawn into the fray (Montgomery, 1849 pp. 321–40): 'I believe ... it would be no exaggeration to affirm, that the present age has witnessed no more remarkable event in medicine, than the application of anaesthetic agents'. But Montgomery then laid out his objections to the 'indiscriminate administration of anesthetic agents in midwifery'.

In the same year that Montgomery wrote his objections, Robert Shekelton of the Rotunda Hospital reported the use of chloroform in 56 cases on 4 January to the Dublin Obstetric Society and in the following year chloroform was used at the Rotunda for one in every 37 deliveries (O'Donel Browne, 1947 p. 269).

Merriman (1848) opposed the employment of anesthesia in natural labor as 'in savage nations ... child birth ... in almost every instance ... appears ... easily accomplished; the mother suffers little' and extolled the 'great superiority of allowing nature to conduct the whole process of the birth'. Simpson accused him of 'a deliberate act of omission' in refusing to administer analgesia to women in 'the agonies of labor'.

Simpson (1847a) made an impassioned plea for anesthesia in obstetrics and posed the question 'whether on any grounds, moral or medical, a professional man could deem himself justified in withholding [ether, for pain relief]'. He went on to quote Alfred Velpeau of France who described those 'piercing cries, that agitation so lively, those excessive efforts, those inexpressible agonies, and those pains apparently intolerable' which accompany the termination of natural parturition in the human mother.

On 1 December 1847 Simpson again addressed the Medico-Chirurgical Society of Edinburgh and prophesied that 'our patients will force it [obstetric anesthesia] upon the profession ... husbands will scarcely permit the sufferings of their wives ... women themselves will betimes rebel against enduring the usual tortures and miseries of childbirth, merely to subserve the caprice of their medical attendants' (Speert, 1957 pp. 744–9). Simpson also recalled the words of Galen, *dolor dolentibus inutilis est* (pain is useless to the pained) and further wrote that 'bodily pain ... is, with very few, if indeed any exceptions, morally and physically a mighty and unqualified evil' (Simpson, 1847b pp. 15, 145–312). 'Medical men may oppose for a time the superinduction of anesthesia, but they will oppose it in vain', wrote Simpson, 'for certainly our patients themselves will force the use of it upon the profession. The whole question is, even now, one merely of time' (Simpson, 1847d p. 13).

Notably absent from the debate was the voice of women, presumably because there were no female accoucheurs and the midwives of the time were either poorly educated or did not publish their comments. However, Wertz and Wertz (1989 p. 118) quoted one woman who wrote thus to the *Boston Medical and Surgical Journal* in 1866: 'One great reason for the aversion to child-bearing ... is the certain agony at the end ... If the blessed, benevolent suggestion of the use of chloroform could be adopted, the world would hear less of abortions'.

Moral

The moral pedants claimed that anesthesia in obstetrics was contrary to scriptural precept, as outlined in Genesis 3: 16: 'Unto the woman He said, I will greatly multiply thy sorrow and thy conception; in sorrow thou shalt bring forth children.' This Biblical passage became known as the 'Curse of Eve' although no sentence was cast on the woman and the scriptural passage does not contain the term 'curse'. One clerical opponent of anesthesia wrote: 'Chloroform is the decoy of Satan, apparently offering itself to bless women, but in the end it will poison society and rob God of the deep, earnest cries which arise in time of trouble for help' (Claye, 1954 pp. 226–38).

Simpson sought an interpretation of the original Hebrew, from which the seventeenth-century English version of the Bible was translated, and deduced that the word *etsebh* which the English scholars interpreted as 'sorrow' did not mean pain, rather it referred to 'muscular effort' (Simpson, 1847d p. 13). Not everyone agreed with his translation but many colleagues wrote pamphlets in support of his medical and moral views. Edward Murphy, professor of midwifery at University College London, and formerly assistant physician to the Dublin Lying-in Hospital, examined the crucial word 'sorrow' and wrote that, 'although man, who was 'cursed' and therefore destined to 'eat bread in 'sorrow' ... had managed 'to dine as comfortably as his means permitted, notwithstanding the curse' (Murphy, 1855 p. 3).

In his defense of anesthesia Simpson quoted Genesis 2: 21: 'and the Lord god caused a deep sleep to fall upon Adam; and he slept; and He took one of his ribs and closed up the flesh instead thereof'. Drawing a parallel with sleep and anesthesia, this passage proved to be a strong argument in Simpson's favor, although it was derided by Ashwell (1848 p. 291) who doubted that God used anesthesia during the creation of Eve, an event which occurred during the perfect Eden era, a time without suffering, prior to the 'fall from grace'.

The topic of pain relief in labor still generated much 'moral' discussion until recent times. Grantley Dick Read (1960 pp. 61–78) wrote that the classical scholars who translated the Bible during the reign of

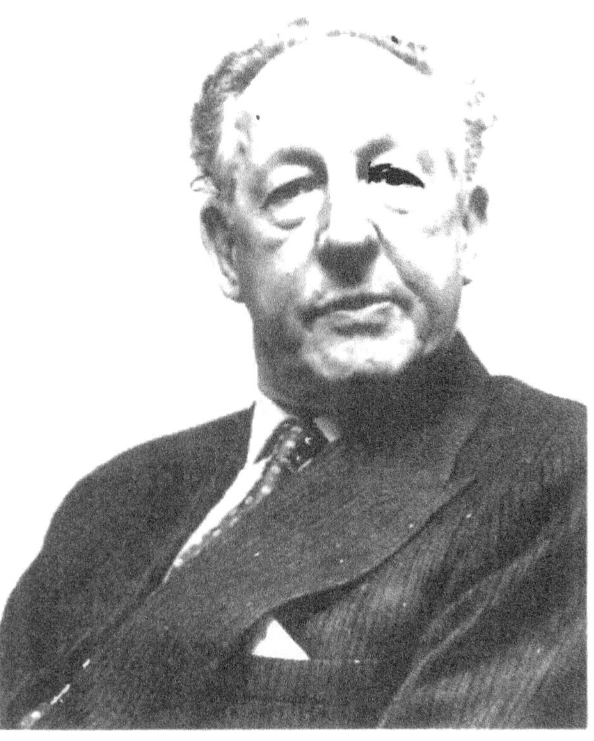

Figure 5 Grantley Dick Read (1890–1959)

James 1 (1604–1611) were heavily influenced by the inadequate obstetric care of their era and that the translations which referred to childbirth were in keeping with the accepted beliefs and experiences of the seventeenth century rather than biblical times. He also deduced that the original Hebrew referred to 'toil' rather than pain in labor and that while a woman's childbirth might always be strenuous 'it need not be painful'.

Jeffrey Boss (1962 pp. 508–13), in an article entitled 'The Character of Childbirth According to the Bible', investigated the so-called 'Curse of Eve' and provided a learned discussion on the topic. He considered the 31 biblical passages referring to parturition and pain and discussed the original roots of the Hebrew words (*etsebh* or *itsabhon*, *tsir*, *hebhel*, *tsarah*, *hul andke'ebh*) relating to childbirth. Boss concluded that 'the general picture ... is more akin ... to prophetic possession than to being physically hurt' while the wording of the 'so-called Curse of Eve is in favor of its referring to 'toil and trouble', and almost incompatible with there being any reference to physical pain'.

COMPARISON BETWEEN ANESTHESIA AND NO ANESTHESIA IN LABOR IN THE NINETEENTH CENTURY

Anesthesia was not subjected to clinical trials in the modern sense but the following results, culled from various clinical reports of the nineteenth century, are of interest.

Simpson (1848a pp. 209–51) reported on the favorable results of anesthesia from his own practice and from colleagues throughout Scotland, from Bristol, London, Dublin, Berlin and Vienna. He quoted the results of 7050 women in labor from the Dublin Lying-in Hospital when under the care of Collins in the preanesthetic era (1826–1833). The mortality rate for those mothers who delivered within two hours was 1 in every 320, but the death rate was 1 in every 11 women, when labor was prolonged beyond 20 hours. Maternal mortality in this group related to hemorrhage, sepsis and the shock of destructive operations or forceps births. Proponents of anesthesia in labor argued that delivery with well controlled analgesia could be effective in shortening labor (by allowing earlier manipulative intervention). This in turn would mean a more humane birth process and less blood loss and sepsis. An unpleasant exchange of views between Collins and Simpson was published in the *Provincial and Medical Surgical Journal* on 15 November 1848, and in four articles in the 'medical press'.

Joseph Clarke (1758–1834), in a personally-managed series over 44 years of practice in Dublin, reported 22 maternal deaths out of 3847 cases, of which only 8 were directly related to pregnancy – a maternal death rate of one per 447 cases (Collins, 1849 pp. 481–9).

Burns (1820 pp. 423–4) commented on the results of 'tedious labor' in primigravidae, and observed that, where labor was protracted for up to 50 hours, one mother in 13 died and, when labor exceeded 70 hours, 'one-eighth died, and nearly half of the children'. Where 'instruments were used, on account of tedious labor' almost half the mothers died.

Simpson (1848a pp. 209–51) wrote that 'the mortality accompanying labor is regulated principally by the previous length and degree of the patient's struggles' and he believed that proper analgesia would reduce such suffering and would allow easier intervention in protracted labor. This, for Montgomery (1849 pp. 321–40) raised the specter of the accoucheur 'with a bottle of chloroform in one pocket and a pair of forceps ... in another' who would 'play such fantastic tricks before heaven, as make the angels weep' (Montgomery, 1849 pp. 321–40).

Conclusions

Queen Victoria's decision to use chloroform during the birth of Prince Leopold on 7 April 1853, turned the tide of medical and lay opinion in favor of anesthesia. Later in the same year, John Snow was called to Lambeth Palace for the confinement of the daughter of the Archbishop of Canterbury – and he used chloroform to induce analgesia.

The use of anesthesia did not cause idiocy in newborn infants, as predicted, but it did lead to some maternal deaths, the causes of which were only effectively dealt with in the twentieth century. Thus those who opposed the concept of anesthesia for all laboring women, on the grounds of maternal safety, had a valid argument. While some mothers died, anesthesia was responsible for a large reduction in overall maternal and fetal mortality and morbidity. Selective use of safely administered anesthesia was what was required.

The development of safe cesarean section in the late nineteenth and early twentieth centuries was made possible because of the introduction of anesthesia to midwifery, allied with Listerism and also the technical surgical innovations of Porro in 1876, Max Sanger in 1882 and the contributions of those who followed. Gynecological surgery also became a reality.

A further success for chloroform was its use to control eclamptic fits which, when untreated, led to a maternal mortality rate of 20 to 60% (Browne, 1954 pp. 158–67). In January 1854, Lombe Atthill of the Rotunda Hospital published his personal observations on the *Use of Chloroform in labor and the Control of Convulsions* (O'Donel Browne, 1947 p. 240). Around the same time, Samuel Little Hardy introduced the 'chloroform douche' (Ringland, 1870 p. 32).

The rectal route was later favored for the sedatives employed in the control of eclampsia at the end of the nineteenth century.

OTHER INHALATION AGENTS

Ethylene, a gas first prepared by Becher in 1669, was reintroduced by Luckhardt and Carter of Chicago in 1923. It was widely used in obstetrics in America but was a highly explosive gas and was replaced by safer products. Cyclopropane, an expensive gas used in a completely closed-circuit apparatus, was also employed in obstetric analgesia. It was first prepared by the chemist Freund in 1882 and was introduced into clinical anesthesia in 1933. Trichlorethylene (Trilene), introduced in 1934, and methoxyflurane (Pentrane), first used in 1959, were both popular for a while.

Halothane (fluothane) was prepared and researched by Raventos (1956 p. 394) and was introduced to clinical practice by Johnstone (1956 pp. 392–410) of Manchester and by Bryce Smith and O'Brien of Oxford in the same year. Fluothane was widely evaluated and soon became the most popular obstetric anesthetic worldwide. It was more potent than chloroform or ether but was found to have uterine relaxing effects which could induce hemorrhage.

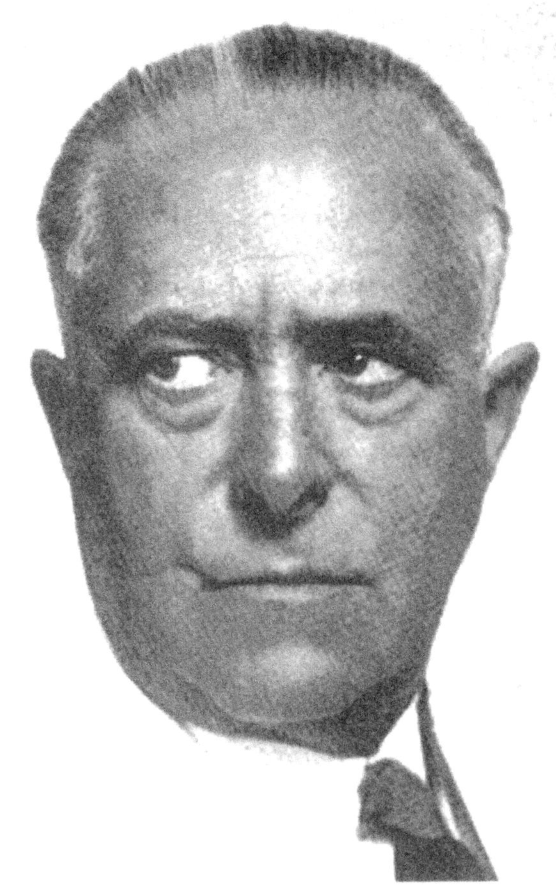

Figure 6 Carl Joseph Gauss (b. 1875). From Claye, *Evolution of Obstetric Analgesia* (1939)

TWILIGHT SLEEP

In his historical essay, *Twilight Sleep* (1939 p. 25–52), Andrew Claye recounted that 'von Steinbuchel (1902 pp. 1304–6) of Graz, stimulated by the work of Schneiderlein and Korff on scopolamine–morphine at Freiburg, tried out for the first time the effects of this combination of drugs in obstetric practice'. Morphine was used in a dose of 0.01 gm (approximately 1/7 grain) with scopolamine 0.0003/4 (1/216 to 1/162 grain), given hypodermically, two-hourly. Twilight sleep was the first improvement in pain relief in labor to follow chloroform.

At the instigation of Bernard Kroing, C.J. Gauss of Freiburg researched the technique of morphine-scopolamine narcosis and published his experiences of 500 cases (Gauss, 1906 pp. 579–631). It was Gauss who introduced the term 'twilight sleep' (*dammerschlaf*) which he defined as a state of 'light disturbance of consciousness in which the patient can perceive impressions but not apperceive them'.

The use of 'twilight sleep' spread extensively throughout Europe and America. W.H. Knipe read a paper on the subject to the New York Obstetrical Society (1914 p. 884) and there was further discussion at the New York Academy of Medicine in 1915. In England, the method was investigated by a Committee of the Section of Obstetrics and Gynaecology of the Royal Society of Medicine (1918 p. 1) and they found that it was possible to produce almost painless labor in rather less than half of the treated cases and considerable relief in all but 5% of the total. The chief risk was fetal asphyxia which related to the quantity of morphine used. Disadvantages included prolongation of labor and an increase in forceps deliveries. It was also apparent that treated patients required close monitoring throughout labor and that occasionally acute delirium occurred.

Various modifications of the technique were introduced. Other drugs were substituted for morphine: narcophen (morphine plus narcotine), pantopon (omnopon), barbiturates (pernocton, amytal and nembutal) and even strychnine, but the original regimen retained its popularity. Pituitary extract, recently available, was added to the regimen in an effort to reduce the incidence of forceps deliveries (Harrar and McPherson, 1914 p. 621). Finally, in the early 1920s 'twilight sleep' was combined with administration of acetylene during delivery. The Freiburg *dammerschlaf* retained its popularity until the 1940s.

Scopolamine

Scopolamine (and atropine) is a naturally occurring antimuscarinic alkaloid from the belladonna plant. Preparations of belladonna have been used in medications since antiquity and were known to be poisonous in higher dosage. Scopolamine (hyoscine) was isolated in 1871 and is mainly found in the shrub *Hyoscamus niger* (henbane). Linneaus named *Atropa belladona*, a species of belladonna, in memory of Atropos, the eldest of the three Fates who cuts the thread of life. *Atropa belladona* is also known as deadly nightshade and yields atropine, an alkaloid first isolated by Mein in 1831, synthesized by Willstatter in 1896 and later used as a premedication for anesthesia. Atropine is found in a variety of plants including *Datura stramonium*, variously known as jimson weed, thorn-apple and devil's apple.

Morphine

Morphine, together with codeine and papaverine, is among 20 distinct alkaloids derive from opium. Sertürner (1806 p. 47) isolated morphine from opium and named it after Morpheus, the Greek god of dreams. Opium is derived from the Greek word for 'juice', the drug being obtained from the juice of the poppy, *Papaver somniferum*. Morphine, introduced to midwifery in 1902, caused excessive fetal sedation which limited its use in labor. However, it proved to be

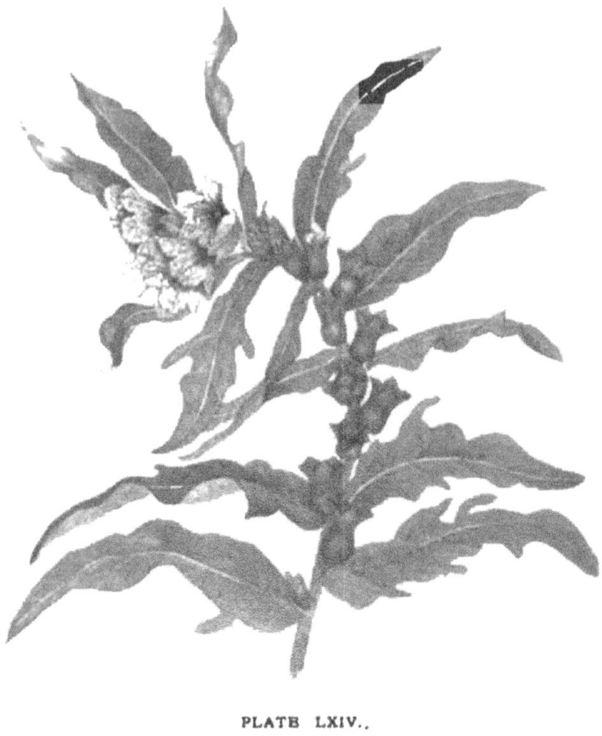

Figure 7 Henbane (*Hyoscyamus* sp.)

beneficial in post-delivery pain relief. Meconium, the first intestinal discharge of the neonate, is green–black in color and is named for its similarity to poppy juice (Greek ***mekonion***, diminutive of ***mekon***, poppy).

Gas in air and nitrous oxide

Gas and air, and later gas with oxygen, were the next great steps forward in obstetric analgesia. The method of administration, when perfected, could be used by laboring women in the presence of unsupervised midwives and thus constituted a major advance in the conquest of pain. This form of analgesia depended on the well known anesthetic gas, nitrous oxide, which also became much used in 'complete' general anesthesia.

Nitrous oxide was discovered by Joseph Priestley in 1772. Its analgesic properties were determined by Humphry Davy, during self-experimentation in 1800. Nitrous oxide was first used deliberately as an anesthetic by Horace Green in 1844. Andrews of Chicago combined nitrous oxide with oxygen in 1868, thus

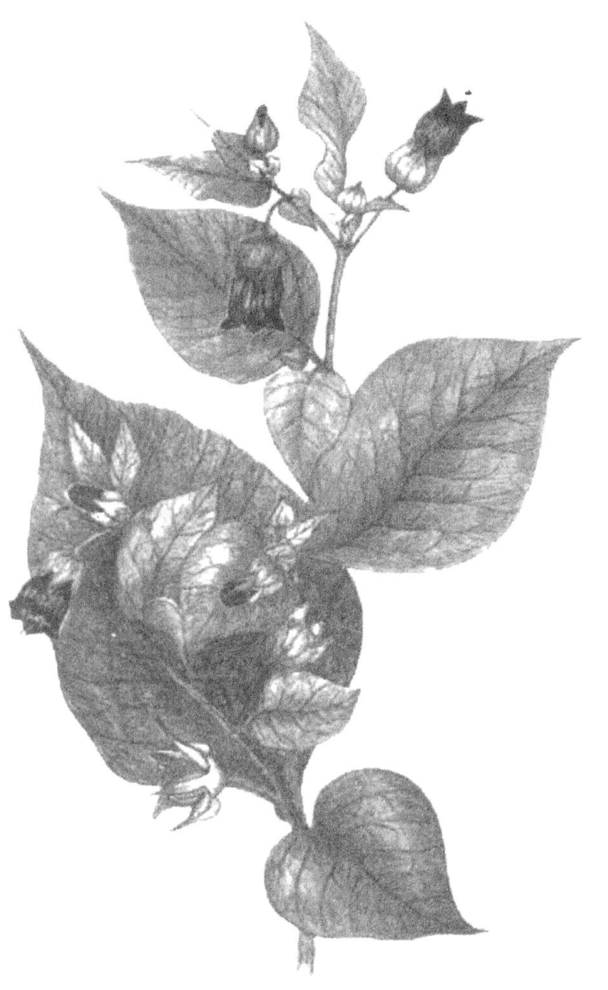

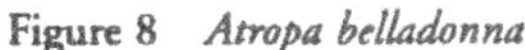

Figure 8 *Atropa belladonna*

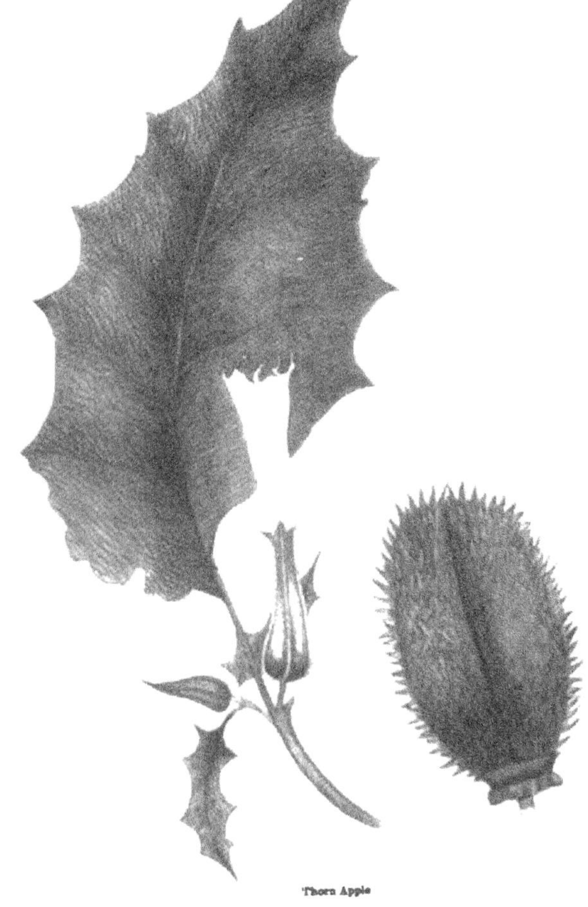

Figure 9 *Datura* sp.

enlarging its field of use enormously (Sykes, 1939 pp. 54–64).

Stanislav Klikovitch of St Petersburg, in 1881, was the first to use a combination of nitrous oxide and oxygen in obstetrics (Richards *et al.*, 1976 pp. 933–44). Self-administration of nitrous oxide in midwifery was reported by A.E. Guedel of California in 1911 (O'Dowd and Philipp, 1994 pp. 435–56). J. Clarence Webster (1915 pp. 812–13), and Frank W. Lynch (1915 p. 813) of Chicago used nitrous oxide analgesia in obstetrics and Lynch remarked that it was a safe substitute for the Freiburg method of 'twilight sleep'.

The next advance was introduced by R.J. Minnitt who, with Charles King of London, invented a nitrous oxide and air machine, an upgrade of McKeeson's intermittent flow apparatus (Minnitt, 1934 pp. 1313–18). (Grantley Dick Read introduced his concept of 'childbirth without fear' in the same year that Minnitt introduced the gas and air machine.) In 1936 the Royal College of Obstetricians recommended that midwives should be allowed to give gas and air and the Central Midwives Board agreed. A further improvement came when Tunstall of Aberdeen (1961 p. 964) introduced premixed nitrous oxide and oxygen in a single cylinder and this preparation replaced the older gas and air machines which were phased out about 1970.

A number of maternally activated inhalers were developed for various gases, including the Freedman

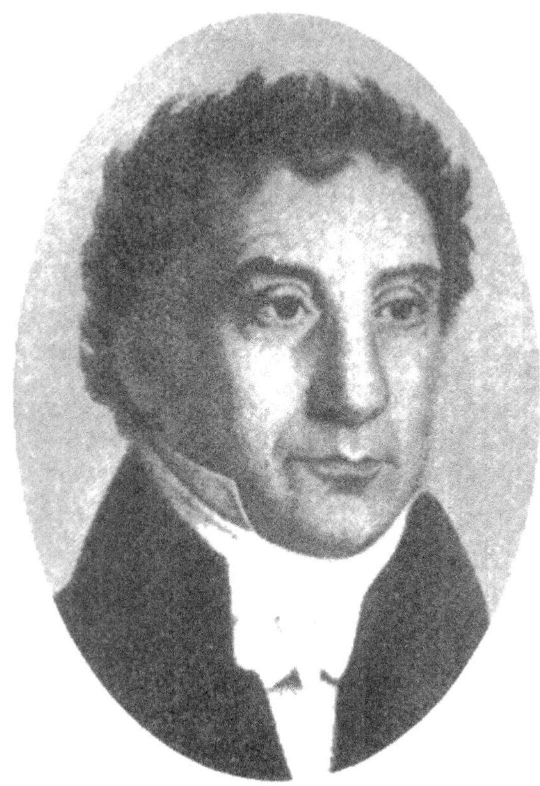

Figure 10 Adam Frederick William Sertürner (1783–1841). From Keys, *History of Surgical Anesthesia* (1945)

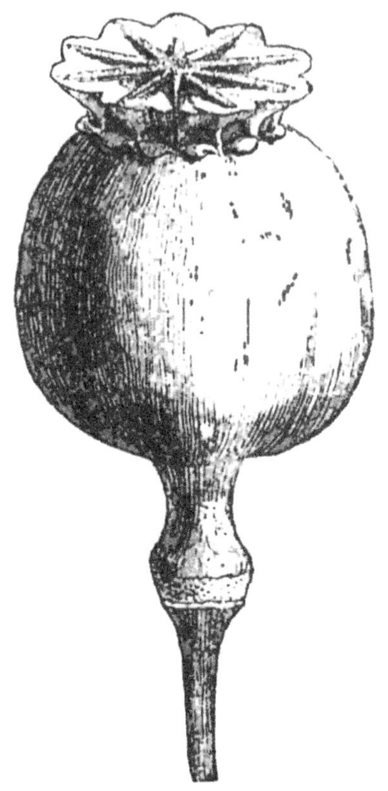

Figure 11 Opium poppy seed capsule

inhaler of 1943 and the Emotril and Tecota mark six machines of 1955. However, the Entonox apparatus (50% nitrous oxide and 50% oxygen) provides the only inhalational agent available for self administered analgesia, since approval for the other methods was withdrawn.

SEDATIVES

Sedatives were introduced to lessen pain, reduce apprehension and to abolish the memory of labor. They could, however, inhibit uterine action and depress respiration in the newborn. Sedatives were helpful in the early stages of labor, often allowing the patient to sleep between contractions.

Chloral hydrate

A great favorite for many years was chloral hydrate, a hypnotic which was introduced by Liebrich of Berlin in 1869. Chloral hydrate was reputed to have a relaxing influence on the rigid cervix. The drug was often combined with tincture of opium and formed the basis of what in many maternity hospitals was euphemistically termed 'mother's mixture'. It was also sometimes combined with potassium bromide, the latter being the first synthetic sedative introduced to medical practice (1853). The tablet form of chloral (dichloral phenazonum) was known as 'welldorm'.

Opium, morphine and scopolamine

Opium and morphine were used as sedatives but great caution was necessary as the newborn was likely to be oversedated and prolonged neonatal apnea was common. Hyoscine (scopolamine) was used alone to good effect or in combination with morphia to induce 'twilight sleep'.

Barbiturates

This group of drugs was based on barbituric acid, described in 1882 by Conrad and Guthzeit. Emil Fischer and von Mehring introduced barbitone (barbital) in 1903. Phenobarbitone was introduced in 1912. The barbiturates proved very successful and over 50 types were introduced commercially. Three groups were described: ultra-short acting (e.g. thiopentone, later famed for its use as an agent to induce anesthesia), medium acting (e.g. sodium amytal), and long-acting (including barbitone and phenobarbitone). Barbiturates were dominant in the sedative market until the introduction of the benzodiazepines in 1961.

Nembutal (pentobarbitone) was the most-used barbiturate and in the 1930s many investigators, including Irving, Berman and Nelson (1934 p. 1) of the Boston Lying-in Hospital, reported favorably on its use in their observations of 860 patients. Overall, it was found that complete amnesia was obtained in 86% of mothers and in the remainder only isolated incidents were remembered. However, 37% of neonates were noticeably sedated at birth. Nembutal was used in combination with other drugs and the best results were obtained when it was used with hyoscine.

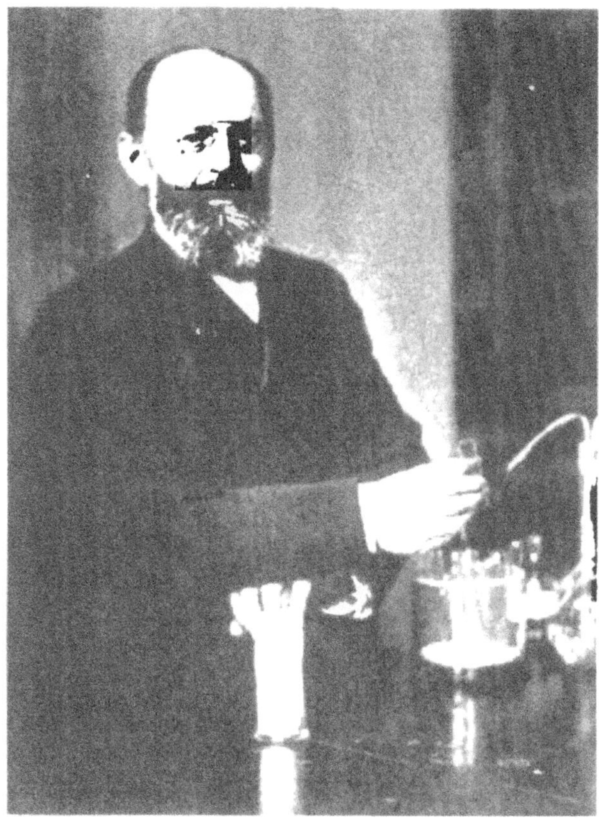

Figure 12 Emil Hermann Fischer (1852–1919). From Keys, *History of Surgical Anesthesia* (1945)

Phenothiazines

The phenothiazine derivatives were synthesized during the years 1945–1951 and included chlorpromazine (largactil) and promethazine (phenergan) which promoted sedation while also relieving nausea and vomiting. A third member of the group, promazine (sparine), also had analgesia potentiating effects and was employed extensively in labor. The phenothiazines were used in anesthesia by Laborit and Huguenard of France in 1951 and they coined the term 'lytic cocktail' for the mixture containing pethidine, chlorpromazine and promethazine. The lytic cocktail became one of the drug treatments for eclampsia.

Rectal sedatives

Pirogoff of St Petersburg in Russia advocated the use of ether vapor per rectum in 1847, and Samuel Hardy of Dublin invented the 'chloroform douche' soon afterwards (Ringland, 1870 p. 32). A number of other drugs were administered by rectal injection to produce a state somewhat similar to basal narcosis. While the drugs were all well absorbed per rectum they had the disadvantage that patients often remained stuporous for many hours after delivery.

Ether–oil

Gwathmey's ether–oil mixture, introduced in 1913, was widely employed in America but failed to maintain its reputation and was little used after the mid-1940s (Gwathmey, 1935 p. 2044).

Paraldehyde

Discovered by Wiedenbusch in 1829, paraldehyde was introduced into medicine by Cervello in 1882 and was administered rectally in oil by Rowbotham in 1928 (Lee and Atkinson, 1968 pp. 109–110) but

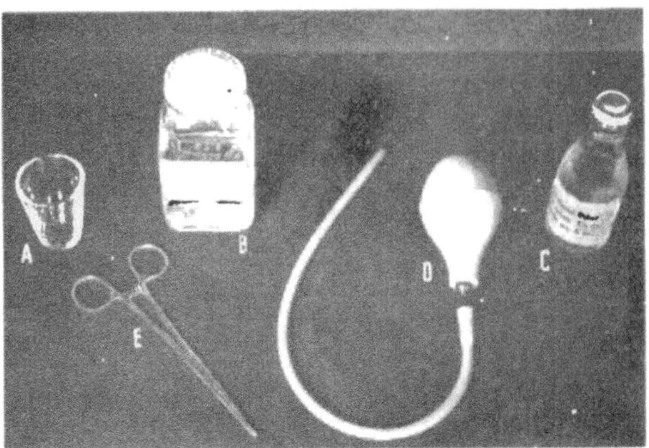

Figure 13 Rectal sedatives. From Lull and Hingson, *Control of Pain in Childbirth* (1945)

experience with the drug in obstetric analgesia was not encouraging.

Avertin (bromethol)

Synthesized by Willstaeter and Duisberg in 1923, avertin was popular, for a time as a sedative in early labor. It was later found to be of value in the treatment of eclampsia.

Pethidine/meperidine/demerol

Pethidine, a synthetic analgesic drug, was introduced by Eisleb and Schaumann of Germany in 1939. Originally marketed under the trade name of dolantin, it became known as pethidine in England and as demerol or meperidine in America. The drug was first used in labor by Benthin in 1940 (Lee and Atkinson, 1968 p. 621).

Encouraging reports by Gilbert and Dixon (1943 p. 320) and others soon appeared in the American literature and in England Cripps *et al.* (1944 p. 498) and Barnes (1947 p. 437) published similar results. The maternal and fetal respiratory depressant side-effects of pethidine could be counteracted by levallorphan tartrate (Lorphan), a drug synthesized by Schneider and Hellerbach in 1950. Levallorphan 1.25 mg was combined with pethidine 100 mg and marketed as pethilorphan. Although popular for a while, pethilorphan had reduced analgesic potency and could actually increase respiratory depression.

Pethidine was combined with hyoscine to induce twilight sleep and, with a range of other drugs, to increase its analgesic efficacy (e.g. with sparine), or to reduce its potential to cause vomiting. The drug could be administered orally, by intramuscular injection, or intravenously. Midwives were allowed to use pethidine without direct supervision. It soon became the most popularly prescribed analgesic in midwifery and is still a market leader. Pethidine, and morphia, were important analgesics for self-administration post-operatively in what became known as 'patient controlled analgesia'.

Ataralgesia

Atarexic (Greek *ataraxia*, peace of mind) drugs were combined with pethidine by Hayward-Butt (1957 p. 972) and he coined the term 'ataralgesia'. He used pecazine (pectal), a phenothiazine derivative, with the intention of combining very effective pain relief while retaining normal physical and mental functions. This appeared to be an ideal situation, especially for obstetric cases, and was in vogue for about 20 years. Promazine (sparine) was another much used ataractic drug. Ataralgesia was overtaken by conduction analgesia and also by the increasing safety of general anesthesia.

Pentazocine

Known as fortral or talwin, pentazocine was first described in 1959. Filler and Filler (1966 p. 224) reported that 45 mg of the drug given intravenously during labor produced an acceptable degree of analgesia and did not affect the fetus to the same degree as pethidine. Despite its merits, pentazocine did not become popular in obstetrics.

LOCAL AND CONDUCTION ANALGESIA

Cocaine, an alkaloid in the leaves of *Erythroxylon coca*, a shrub from the Andes mountains of Bolivia and Peru, had been used for its narcotic effects by the local inhabitants for many centuries. However, it was not until 1860 that Albert Niemann purified and named the drug. One Moreno y Maiz, surgeon in chief to the Peruvian army, discovered its local anesthetic effect some eight years later. The clinical use of this new alkaloid was investigated by Karl Köller in 1884 at the suggestion of Sigmund Freud (O'Dowd and Philipp, 1994 p. 439). A synthetic substitute, procaine, was introduced in 1905 by Einhorn and colleagues.

Stiassny introduced local anesthesia to obstetric practice in 1910 when he described the application of cocaine to the vulva to relieve labor pains (Claye, 1954 p. 237). George Gellhorn (1927 p. 105) of St Louis, Missouri used local anesthesia in an effort to allay pelvic pain of the second stage of labor and also applied it during perineal repair.

The introduction of local anesthetic agents had a major impact on analgesia in midwifery. Not only was perineal infiltration possible but spinal analgesia (Kreis, 1900 p. 724); pudendal nerve block (Muller, 1908); caudal analgesia (Stoekel, 1909 p. 1); paracervical nerve block (Gellert, 1926 p. 143), and lumbar extradural analgesia (Graffagnino and Seyler 1938 p. 597) all became a reality in obstetrics.

Epidural analgesia

In North America, regional analgesia was popularized by Cleland, a Canadian obstetrician, who reported the relief of labor pain by lower thoracic paravertebral injections (Cleland, 1933 p. 51). During the Second World War, Hingson and Edwards of New York developed a technique of continuous caudal analgesia and the method became popular throughout America (Hingson and Edwards, 1942 p. 301). In the same year, Manalan (1942 p. 564) developed the concept used by Eugen Aburel of Rumania of inserting a silk ureteric catheter via a needle into the caudal space. Flowers *et al.* (1949 p. 181) adapted the technique and passed a ureteric catheter into the lumbar epidural space. Tuohy (1945 p. 834) extended the technique and invented a special needle for easier passage of a catheter. Because of the dangers of general anesthesia and the sedative effects of analgesic drugs on the neonate, it appeared that conduction analgesia, which was relatively free of major side effects, would soon become the pain relief of choice in labor and for instrumental and cesarean section deliveries. However, many technical advances were necessary along the way to overcome some of the negative aspects of epidural blockade.

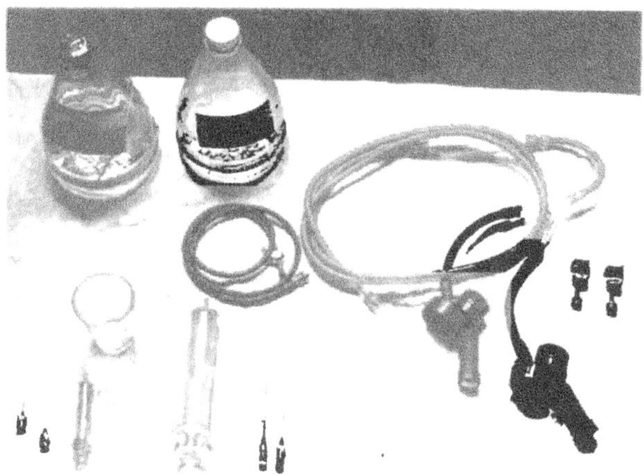

Figure 14 Caudal blocks. From Lull and Hingson, *Control of Pain in Childbirth* (1945)

The headache which followed inadvertent dural puncture was a disagreeable and disabling event which occurred in at least 0.5% of epidural patients. A partial solution was offered by Rice and Dobbs (1950 p. 17) who first described epidural injection of saline to combat the problem. The technique was enhanced by Gormley (1960 p. 565) who injected autologous non-anticoagulated blood by epidural injection to seal the rent in the dura and thus stop leakage of cerebrospinal fluid which led to the low tension dural tap headache. Improvements in epidural needles and catheters also helped.

The introduction of bupivacaine, a long-acting local anesthetic (Teluvio, 1963 p. 513) and its later enhancement by the addition of the opioids, fentanyl and morphine (Justins *et al.*, 1982 p. 409), were important milestones in the search for the perfect epidural anesthetic. The introduction of 'ambulatory epidurals' helped to increase patient satisfaction and more mothers experienced normal births because they retained the sensation of perineal pressure during the second stage of labor. Continuous infusion pumps also helped to increase the analgesic efficiency of 'standard epidurals'.

Spinal analgesia

The New York neurologist J. Leonard Corning (1855–1923) first induced spinal analgesia when he

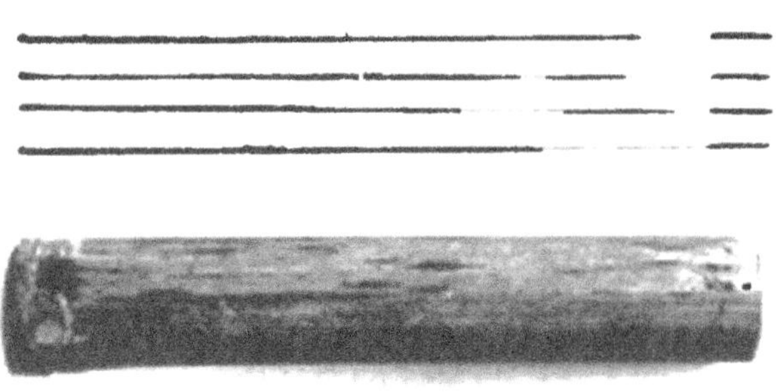

Figure 15 Curare darts and quiver

accidentally pierced the dura and injected cocaine close to the spinal cord of a dog. He later repeated the experiment deliberately and thus discovered the efficacy of what he termed 'spinal anesthesia'. He later wrote in an article in the *New York Medical Journal*: 'Be the destiny of this observation what it may ... it has seemed to me on the whole, worth recording' (Lee and Atkinson, 1968 p. 380). Kreis of Germany first used spinal analgesia for an operative vaginal delivery in 1901, and Pitkin of America popularized its use and introduced the hyperbaric technique in 1928. Contamination of analgesic solutions by phenol led to cases of paraplegia in a small number of patients. As a result, spinal analgesia fell out of favor for many years in England, although still used extensively in obstetrics in America. Despite the initial setback, the technique was found to have a good safety record and became the anesthetic of choice for pain relief during cesarean sections.

Muscle relaxants

Harold Griffith and Enid Johnson of Montreal, on the advice of Lewis Wright, introduced curare as a muscle relaxant in anesthesia, a significant advance which allowed safer anesthesia (Griffith and Johnson, 1942 pp. 418–20). Curare, an arrow poison extracted from various plants including *Strychnos toxifera*, was first described in the Western world in 1516 by the Italian, Peter Martyr of d'Anghera, after his observation of its use by native Amerindians (see Hughes, 1989 pp. 257–67 for a good account).

ANESTHESIA AND MATERNAL MORTALITY

Although anesthesia was responsible for saving many lives, it was also a direct cause of maternal mortality. In the early days, anesthesia was administered by clinicians or junior members of staff who had little or no experience of the technique and many mothers were subjected to its effects late in labor or after significant blood loss and during the course of eclampsia or other significant maternal complications. Many were anesthetized soon after the ingestion of food. In pre-curare days induction of general anesthesia was much more hazardous, particularly with obstetric patients.

As late as the 1960s about 4% of maternal deaths were due to the complications of anesthesia. Inhalation of vomit was the major cause in almost half of these cases, and usually occurred in the interval between induction of anesthesia and intubation of the trachea. Mendelson (1946 pp. 191–204) wrote about the often fatal results of acid inhalation. This led to the use of apomorphine to induce vomiting or to emptying of stomach contents by nasogastric tube. Antacids, histamine type 2 receptor antagonistic drugs, which increased gastric motility and sodium bicarbonate or citrate were all used. Sellick (1961 pp. 404–6) introduced cricoid pressure with compression of the esophagus and his maneuver was widely adopted. Modifications in premedication and induction agents; introduction of safer depolarizing and anesthetic agents; combined with better training for obstetric and anesthetic staff; the gradual displacement of general anesthesia by epidurals and later by spinal analgesia for cesarean section delivery; and a general improvement in patient's health had a major impact on the reduction of maternal mortality due to anesthesia.

BIOGRAPHIES

James Young Simpson (1811–1870)

On the 7th of June 1811, the local doctor attended during the birth of James Young Simpson and made the following entry in his case-notes: '275, June 7th, Simpson, David, Baker, Bathgate, Wife Mary Jarvis, *aet.* 40, Lab. nat. easy rapid 8th child. Natus 8 o'clock. *Uti veniebam natus.* Paid 10s. 6d.' (Miller, 1962 pp. 142–50). Simpson was born in West Lothian, near

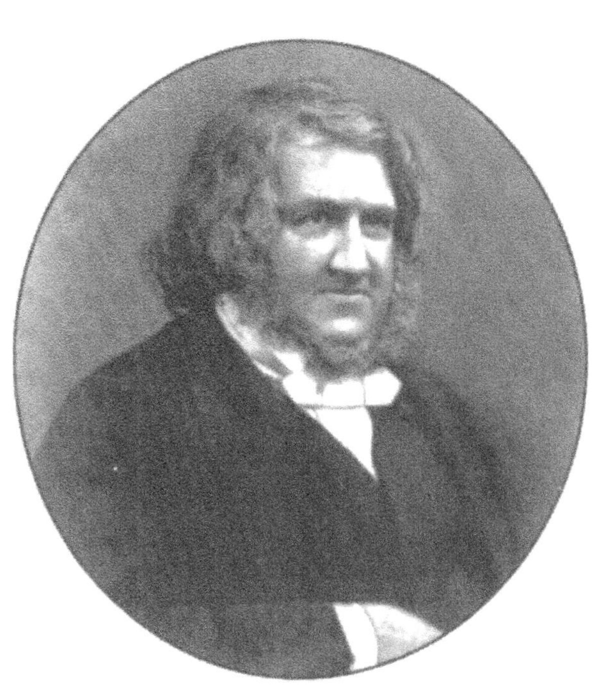

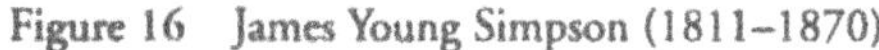

Figure 16 James Young Simpson (1811–1870)

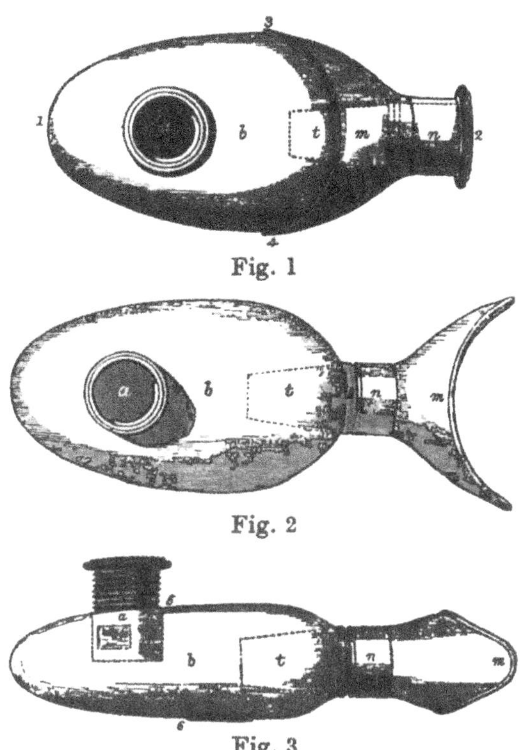

Figure 17 Simpson's ether apparatus. From Claye, *Evolution of Obstetric Analgesia* (1939)

Edinburgh, in 'straitened rather than easy or comfortable' circumstances but, due to the ambition and financial contributions of family members, he was sent to college in Edinburgh at the age of 14. Simpson enrolled as a student in the Arts Faculty but two years later moved to the Faculty of Medicine and qualified as a Member of the Royal College of Surgeons when he was still only 18 years old.

Later, on completion of his doctorate in medicine, he worked as an assistant to the pathologist, Professor Thomson, who suggested that Simpson should consider a career in obstetrics. Simpson attended the midwifery classes of the renowned Professor Hamilton and soon read his first important paper: 'Diseases of the placenta' to the Royal Medical Society in 1832. Three years later, after a short tour of hospitals in London and France, he returned to Edinburgh and commenced private practice. In 1839, at the age of 28, he was elected to the chair of midwifery, recently vacated by Hamilton. The election was fiercely contested, with Simpson winning by one vote over his rival, Evory Kennedy of Dublin (Hale-White, 1935 pp. 143–58).

Although Simpson was an eminent teacher, researcher and innovator with protean medical and non-medical interests, he is chiefly remembered for his introduction of anesthesia to midwifery. Simpson was motivated by a desire to alleviate the pains of laboring women and was spurred on by the memory of a mastectomy he witnessed during his student (pre-anesthetic) days. William Morton's demonstration of the anesthetic properties of ether on 16 October 1846, prompted Simpson to research its effects in midwifery and three months later on 19 January 1847, he became the first ever to administer a general anesthetic in obstetrics. The ensuing controversy had few equals in the annals of medicine (Simpson, 1856 p. 463). Undaunted, Simpson continued his research and tested the anesthetic properties of chloroform on

4 November 1847. In a landmark event he introduced the anesthetic to obstetric practice four days later.

In 1847, at the age of 36, Simpson was appointed physician to the Queen in Scotland and, by chance, the letter notifying him of this honor arrived 'at the very hour when he was administering the first anesthetic ever given to a woman in labor' (Moir, 1964 pp. 171–9). Simpson became a legendary figure and his home at 52 Queen Street, Edinburgh, became a center of medical and social activity. His residence and the local hotels were filled with his patients, and with famous visitors from all over the world who had come to seek his help and advice. In 1866 Simpson was created a Baronet, the inscription on his coat of arms reading *Victo Dolore* (pain conquered). A local wit suggested that Simpson's coat-of-arms should show 'a wee naked bairn' with the legend 'Does your mither know you're oot?' (Graham, 1951 p. 488).

The main cause of maternal mortality during Simpson's time was puerperal sepsis. To reduce the risk of sepsis he advocated Semmelweis' doctrine of hand disinfection before treating obstetric cases. Simpson was also aware of the changes being wrought by his contemporary, Lister, in the field of antisepsis. When Simpson became professor in Edinburgh in 1839 the maternal mortality rate was 1%. The rate dropped steadily during his professional career to a figure which remained constant until the introduction of chemical and antibiotic therapy 79 years later (Miller, 1962 pp. 142–50).

Simpson is remembered eponymously for his obstetric forceps which he first demonstrated in 1848 (Simpson, 1848b p. 193; Speert, 1957 pp. 744–9) and he also experimented with an 'air tractor', an early form of vacuum extractor (Duns, 1873 p. 288). He invented a cranioclast, a uterine sound and a sponge tent for dilating the cervix. He was one of the first to advise the importance of bimanual pelvic examination in gynecology (Simpson, 1850 p. 3).

Simpson wrote articles on archeology and he became an ardent antiquarian. He also wrote papers on hospital design, mesmerism, homeopathy and acupressure. In time he became engrossed in literature, in medical reforms and in politics and served as president of the Edinburgh Obstetrical Society from 1841 to 1858.

James Young Simpson developed coronary heart disease and died on 6 May, 1870, at the age of 59. It was proposed that this great man of medical history would be buried in Westminster Abbey but his wife declined that national honor for him and he was interred in Warriston Cemetery in Edinburgh, along with five of his children who had predeceased him. Asleep, in the arms of Morpheus, the god of dreams. A bust of Simpson, erected in Westminster Abbey, carries the inscription:

> 'To whose Genius and Benevolence
> The world owes the blessings derived
> From the use of Chloroform for
> The relief of suffering.
> Laus Deo.'
>
> Laing Gordon (1897 p. 219)

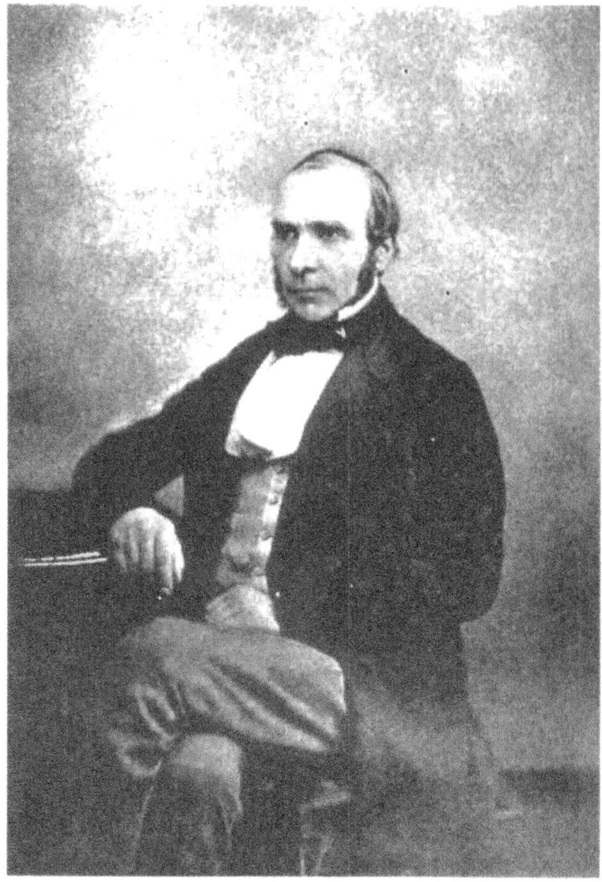

Figure 18 John Snow (1813–1858). From Keys *History of Surgical Anesthesia* (1945)

John Snow (1813–1858)

John Snow of York, a London graduate of 1844, famed for his work on cholera, is best remembered for his administration of chloroform to Queen Victoria for the births of Prince Albert in 1853 and Princess Beatrice in 1857. On both occasions, Snow was called upon by Sir James Clark, the Queen's physician, and in both cases the obstetrician was Charles Locock. In his diary Snow wrote that 'The chloroform was inhaled [by the Queen] for 53 minutes with each pain … [without] removing consciousness' (Atkinson, 1970 pp. 197–9) so, while this is one of the most famous anesthetics in history, it was only analgesia in reality. The Queen was later quoted as saying, 'Dr Snow gave the blessed chloroform and the effect was soothing, quieting and delightful beyond measure' (Secher, 1990 pp. 242–6)

Snow is regarded as the first physician–anesthetist and he researched and wrote extensively on 'Narcotism by the Inhalation of Vapours'. For an extensive bibliography see Ellis (1991 pp. 23–26). David Shephard (1995) also penned a biography of this remarkable Victorian physician and medical scientist.

Stanislav Klikovitch (1853–1910)

The pioneer of nitrous oxide and oxygen analgesia, Stanislav Klikovitch, was born of Polish parents on 31 August 1853 in Vilno, a province of Russian-occupied Poland. He graduated *cum eximia laude* as a physician and surgeon from St Petersburg University in 1876. Shortly afterwards he began his studies on nitrous oxide, for which he gained his MD in 1881. Nitrous oxide was a well known anesthetic agent at the time of Klikovitch's research but it was he who introduced the concept of mixing the gas with oxygen to provide analgesia without loss of consciousness or risk of hypoxia.

Following animal experimentation and clinical research using nitrous oxide and oxygen for asthmatic patients, Klikovitch, then house surgeon to Professor Botkin at the clinic for Internal Diseases, studied the effects of the gas mixture on 25 women in labor in the maternity clinic of Professor Slavyansey. Klikovitch concluded that the method was safe; it had analgesic action in all stages of labor; consciousness was not lost; there was absence of vomiting; the anesthesia did not have a cumulative effect; and the presence of a physician to administer the anesthetic was not necessary.

Klikovitch's promising academic career was interrupted by the unsettled political climate of the time and he worked as a military doctor in a number of European countries over the next 25 years. Evacuated to Kazan following the Revolution of 1905, he died as the result of a stroke on 2 February 1910, aged 56 years (Richards, Parbrook and Wilson, 1976 pp. 933–40).

EPILOGUE

Many great men and women devoted their lives to the study and treatment of pain in labor. Foremost among them was James Young Simpson, a robust dynamic individual who became embroiled in controversy, a situation to which he was not adverse, and which prompted the following comment in one of his obituary notices: 'It was a Scotch dog of whom it is mentioned that he was moody and unhappy because "he could not get eneugh o'fechting"' (Moir, 1964 pp. 171–9).

> 'If the object of the medical practitioner is really two-fold, as it has always, until of late, been declared to be, "the alleviation of human suffering and the preservation of human life", then it is our duty, as well as our privilege, to use all legitimate means to mitigate and remove the physical sufferings of the mother during parturition.'
>
> J.Y. Simpson.

References

Adams, A. K. (1996). The belated arrival, from Davy (1800) to Morton (1846). *J. R. Soc. Med.*, 89, 96–100

Armstrong Davidson, M. H. (1970). *The Evolution of Anesthesia*, pp. 18, 101, 118, 212–15. (Altringham, UK: John Sherratt and Son Ltd.)

Ashwell, S. (1848). Observations on the use of chloroform in natural labour. *Lancet*, 1, 291–2

Atkinson, R. S. (1970). The Lost Diaries of John Snow. *Proceedings of the 4th World Congress of Anesthesia*, pp. 197–9. (Rotterdam: Excerpta Medica)

Barnes, J. (1947). Pethidine in labour: Results in 500 cases. *BMJ*, 1, 437–42

Boss, J. (1962). The Character of Childbirth According to the Bible. *J. Obstet. Gynaecol. Br. Common.*, 19(3), 508–13

Browne, F. J. (1954). Toxaemias of Pregnancy. In Munro Kerr, J., Johnstone, R. W. and Phillips, M. H. (eds) *Historical Review of British Obstetrics and Gynaecology*, pp. 158–67. (London: Livingstone)

Burns, J. (1820). *The Principles of Midwifery, including the Diseases of Women and Children*, 5th ed. pp. 392–414, 423–4. (London: Longmans)

Claye, A. M. (1939). *The Evolution of Obstetric Analgesia*, pp. 13, 15, 3.25–52. (London: Oxford University Press)

Claye, A. M. (1954). Obstetric Anesthesia and Analgesia. In Munro Kerr, J., Johnstone, R. W. and Phillips, M. H. (eds) *Historical Review of British Obstetrics and Gynaecology*, pp. 226–38. (London: Livingstone)

Cleland, J. P. (1933). Paravertebral Anesthesia in Obstetrics, experimental and Clinical basis. *Surg. Gynecol. Obstet.*, 57, 51–4

Collins, R. (1849). A short sketch of the life and writings of the late Joseph Clarke. *Dublin Quart. J. Med. Sci.*, 14, 481–9

Committee of the Section of Obstetrics and Gynaecology of the Royal Society of Medicine (1918). Report on Scopolamine–Morphine Analgesia in Labour. *Proc. R. Soc. Med. Obstet. Gynaecol. Sec*, pp. 1–44

Cripps, J. A. R., Hall, B. and Haultain, W. F. T. (1944). Analgesia in labour. *BMJ*, 2, 498–500

Denman, J. (1849). A Report on the Use of Chloroform in Fifty-Six Cases of Labour at the Rotunda Lying-in Hospital. *Dublin J Med. Sci.*, 8, 107–42

Duncum, B. M. (1947). *The Development of Inhalation Anesthesia*, p. 177. (London: Oxford University Press)

Duns, J. (1873). *A Memoir of Sir James Young Simpson*, pp. 288–9. (Edinburgh: Edmonston and Douglas)

Ellis, R. H. (1991). *On Narcotism by the Inhalation of Vapours by John Snow, 1848–1851.* A facsimile edition, pp. 23–26. (London: Royal Society of Medicine)

Filler, W. W. and Filler, N. W. (1966). Effect of a potent non-narcotic analgesic agent (Pentazocine) on uterine contractility and fetal heart rate. *Obstet. Gynecol.*, 29, 224–32

Findley, P. (1939). *Priests of Lucina: the Story of Obstetrics*, pp. 215, 237. (Boston: Little, Brown and Co.)

Flowers, C. E., Hellman, L. M. and Hingson, R. A. (1949). Continuous peridural anesthesia for labor, delivery and caesarean section. *Anesth. Analg.*, 28, 181–9

Foy, G. (1889). *Anaesthetics, Ancient and Modern*, pp. 34, 39. (London: Balliere, Tindall and Cox)

Gardiner, J. (1995). Anesthesia and Analgesia at the Rotunda. In A. Browne (ed.) *Masters, Midwives and Ladies-in Waiting: The Rotunda Hospital 1745–1995*, pp. 180–5. (Dublin: A. and A. Farmer)

Garrison, F. H. (1924). *An Introduction to the History of Medicine*, pp. 29–30. (Philadelphia and London: W. B. Saunders Co.)

Gauss, C. J. (1906). Geburten im kunstlichen Dammerschlaf. *Archiv. f. Gyn.*, 78, 579–631

Gelis, J. (1991). *History of Childbirth*, Translated by Rosemary Morris. p. 153. (Cambridge: Polity Press)

Gellert, P. (1926). Aufhebung der Wehenschmerzen und Wehenuberdruck. *Monatsschrift fur Wchnschr. Geburts. Gynakol. Berlin.*, 73, 143–61

Gellhorn, G. (1927). Local Anesthesia in Gynecology and Obstetrics. *Surg. Gynec. Obst.*, 45, 105–9

Gilbert, G. and Dixon, A. B. (1943). Observations on demerol as an obstetric analgesic. *Am. J. Obstet. Gynecol.*, 45, 320–6

Gormley, J. B. (1960). Treatment of Postspinal Headache. *Anesthesiology*, 21, 565–6

Graffagnino, P. and Seyler, L. W. (1938). Epidural anesthesia in obstetrics. *Am J. Obstet. Gynecol.*, 35, 597–602

Graham, H. (1951). *Eternal Eve. The History of Gynecology and Obstetrics*, p. 488. (New York: Doubleday and Co.)

Griffith, H. R. and Johnson, G. E. (1942). The use of curare in general anesthesia. *Anesthesiology*, 3, 418–20

Gwathmey, J. T. and McCormack, C. O. (1935). Ether-oil rectal analgesia in obstetrics. *JAMA*, 105, 2044–7

Hale-White, Sir W. (1935). Sir James Young Simpson. In *Great Doctors of the 19th Century*, pp. 143–58. (London: Edward Arnold & Co.)

Harrar, J. A. and McPherson, R. (1914). Scopolamine–narcophin seminarcosis in labor. *Am. J. Obstet. Gynecol.*, 70, 621–30

Hayward-Butt, J. T. (1957). Operations without anesthesia. *Lancet*, 2, 972–4

Hingson, R. A. and Edwards, W. B. (1942). Continuous caudal anesthesia during labor and delivery. *Anesth. Analg.*, 21, 301–11

Hughes, R. (1989). Development of skeletal muscle relaxants from the curare arrow poisons. In Atkinson, R. S. and Boulton, T. B. (eds) *The History of Anaesthesia*, pp. 257–67. (London and New York: RSM and Parthenon Publishing)

Irving, F. C., Berman, S. and Nelson, H. B. (1934). The barbiturate and other hypnotics in labor. *Surg. Gynecol. Obstet.*, 58(1), 1–11

Johnstone, M. (1956). The human cardiovascular response to flouthane anesthesia. *Br. J. Anaesth.*, 28, 392–410

Justins, D. M., Francis, D., Houlton, P. G. and Reynolds, F. (1982). A controlled trial of extradural Fentanyl in labour. *Br. J. Anaesth.*, 54, 409–14

Knipe, W. H. (1914). The Freiburg method of dammerschlaf or twilight sleep. *Am. J. Obstet. Gynecol.*, 70, 884–909

Kreis, O. (1900). Uber Medullarnarkose bei Gebarenden. *Zentbl. gynakol.*, 28, 724–9

Laing Gordon, H. (1897). *Sir James Young Simpson and Chloroform (1811–1870)*, pp. 107, 219, 291. (London: T. Fisher Unwin)

Lee, J. A. and Atkinson, R. S. (1968). *A Synopsis of Anesthesia*, 6th ed. pp. 109–10, 380, 621. (Bristol: John Wright & Sons Ltd.)

Lynch, F. W. (1915). Nitrous oxide gas analgesia in obstetrics. *JAMA*, 10, LXIV, 813

Manalan, S. A. (1942). Caudal block anesthesia in obstetrics. *J. Indiana Med. Assoc.*, 35, 564–5

Minnitt, R. J. (1934). Self administered analgesia for the midwifery of general practice. *Proc. Soc. Med.*, 27, 1313–18

Mendelson, C. L. (1946). Aspiration of stomach contents into lungs during obstetric anesthesia. *Am. J. Obstet. Gynecol.*, 52, 191–204

Merriman, S. W. J. (1848). *Arguments against the Indiscriminate Employment of Anaesthetic Agents in Midwifery.* (London: John Churchill)

Miller, M. (1962). Sir James Young Simpson. *J. Obstet. Gynaecol. Br. Common.*, 69, 142–50

Moir, J. C. (1964). Sir J. Y. Simpson – His Impact and Influence. *J. Obstet. Gynaecol. Br. Common.*, 71, 171–9

Montgomery, W. F. (1849). Objections to the indiscriminate administration of anaesthetic agents in midwifery. *Dublin Quart. J. Med. Sci.*, 15, 321–40

Morton, W. G. (1847). *Remarks on the Proper Mode of Administering Sulfuric Ether by Inhalation.* (Boston: Dutton and Wentworth)

Morton, T. G. (1846). *Circular. Morton's Letheon.* (Boston: Dutton and Wentworth)

Murphy, E. W. (1855). *Chloroform in Childbirth*, pp. 3, 177. (quoted by Duncum, 1947)

O'Dowd, M. J. and Philipp, E. E. (1994). *The History of Obstetrics and Gynaecology*, pp. 435–56. (New York and London: Parthenon Publishing)

Ould, F. (1742). *A Treatise of Midwifery, in Three Parts.* (Dublin: O. Nelson and C. Connor)

O'Donel Browne, T. D. (1947). *The Rotunda Hospital 1745–1945*, pp. 240, 269. (Edinburgh: Livingstone)

Priestley, W. O. and H. R. Storer (eds) (1855). *The Obstetric Memoirs and Contributions of James Young Simpson*, Vol. 2, p. 463. (Philadelphia: Lippincott)

Raventos, J. (1956). The action of Fluothane – a new volatile Anaesthetic. *Br. J. Pharmacol. Chemother.*, 11, 394–410

Read, G. D. (1960). *Childbirth Without Fear. the Principle's and Practice of Natural Childbirth*, 4th ed. pp. 61–78. (London: Heinemann Ltd.)

Rice, G. G. and Dobbs, C. H. (1950). The use of Peridural and Subarachnoid Injections of Saline solution in the Treatment of severe postspinal headache. *Anesthesiology*, 11, 17–23

Richards, W., Parbrook, G. D. and Wilson, J. D. (1976). Stanislav Klikovitch (1853–1910), Pioneer of nitrous oxide and oxygen analgesia. *Anesthesia*, 31, 933–44

Ringland, J. (1870). *Annals of Midwifery in Ireland*, pp. 23, 24, 32. (Dublin: John Falconer)

Secher, O. (1990). Chloroform to a Royal Family. In Atkinson, R. S. and Boulton, T. B. (eds) *The History of Anaesthesia*, pp. 242–6. (London: Royal Society of Medicine and Parthenon Publishing)

Sellick, B. A. (1961). Cricoid pressure to control regurgitation of stomach contents during induction of anesthesia. *The Lancet*, 2, 404–6

Sertürner, F. W. (1806). Darstellung der reinen Mohnsaure (Opiumsaure) nebst einer chemischen untersuchung des opiums. *J. Pharm. f. Aerzte Apothexer.*, 14, 47–93

Shephard, D. A. (1995). *John Snow. Anaesthetist to a Queen and Epidemiologist to a Nation. A Biography.* (Cornwall, Canada: New Point Publishing)

Simpson, J. Y. (1847a). Notes on the Employment of the Inhalation of Sulphuric Ether in the Practice of Midwifery. *Month. J. Med. Sci.*, 1X, 639–40, 721–8, 794–5

Simpson, J. Y. (1847b). Etherization in Surgery. Part 1. *Month. J. Med. Sci.*, 15, 145–66

Simpson, J. Y. (1847c). *Account of a New Anaesthetic Agent, as a Substitute for Sulphuric Ether in Surgery and Midwifery.* (Edinburgh: Sutherland and Knox)

Simpson, J. Y. (1847d). *Answer to the Religious Objections advanced against the Employment of Anaesthetic Agents in Midwifery and Surgery*, p. 13. (Edinburgh: Sutherland and Knox)

Simpson, J. Y. (1847e). *Remarks on the Superinduction of Anesthesia in Natural and Morbid Parturition*, p. 13. (Edinburgh Sutherland and Knox)

Simpson, J. Y. (1848a). Report on the Early History and Progress of Anaesthetic Midwifery. *Month. J. Med. Sci.*, xciv, 209–51

Simpson, J. Y. (1848b). On the Mode of Application of the Long Forceps. *Month. J. Med. Sci.*, 26, 193–6

Simpson, J. Y. (1850). On the Detection and Treatment of Intra-Uterine Polypi. *Month. J. Med. Sci.*, 10, 3–21

Speert, H. (1957). Obstetrical–gynaecological eponyms: James Young Simpson and his obstetric forceps. *J. Obstet. Gynaecol. Br. Emp.*, 64, 744–9

Steinbuchel, V. (1902). Vorlaufige Mitthrilung uber die Anwendung Skopalomin-Morphium-Injektionen in der Geburtshulfe. *Zentralbl. f. Gyn.*, xxvi, 1304–6

Stoekel, von W. (1909). Uber Sakrale Anasthesie. *Zentbl. f. Gyn.*, 33, 1–15

Sykes, W. S. (1939). More inhalation Anaesthetics. In Claye, A. M. (ed.) *The Evolution of Obstetric Analgesia*, pp. 54–64. (London: Oxford University Press)

Teluvio, L. (1963). A new long-acting local anaesthetic solution for pain relief after thoracotomy. *Ann. Chir. et Gynec. Fenniae*, 52, 513–20

Tunstall, M. E. (1961). The use of a fixed nitrous oxide and oxygen mixture from one cylinder. *The Lancet*, 2, 964

Tuohy, E. B. (1945). Continuous spinal Aanesthesia: A new method of utilising a ureteral catheter. *Surg. Clin. N. Am.*, 25, 834–40

Webster, J. C. (1915). Nitrous oxide gas analgesia in obstetrics. *JAMA*, 64(10), 812–13

Wertz, R. E. and Wertz, D. C. (1989). *Lying-In: A History of Childbirth in America*, p. 118. (New Haven and London: Yale University Press)

19

Antiseptics, antibiotics and chemotherapy

INTRODUCTION

One of the main causes of mortality in women from earliest days was infection. Whether it occurred in the guise of childbed fever, the great pockes or consumption it mattered not, as treatments prior to the nineteenth century were largely ineffective. The introduction of antiseptics, chemotherapy, antibiotics and antiviral agents led to an unbelievable reduction in mortality and morbidity.

There was an awareness of infection from earliest times and treatment was offered with substances such as the antiseptic remedies of frankincense and myrrh, but they were insufficient in severe cases. The ancient Egyptians attributed the septic process to worms. Similar concepts evolved in different societies but it was not until the nineteenth century that the etiology of infection was elucidated. Once the cause was understood, intensive efforts were set in motion to find agents to combat infection and so antiseptics, chemotherapy, antibiotics and antivirals were discovered in turn and soon joined the materia medica of women. The agents treated puerperal sepsis, tuberculosis and the venereal diseases.

Alexander Fleming discovered penicillin in 1928 in a mold that contaminated a petri dish in his laboratory. The mold belonged to the genus *Penicillium* – later identified as *Penicillium notatum*, a species of fungus that was first isolated from the decaying leaves of the blue labiate *Hyssopus officinalis*, by the Swedish scientist Westling. Hyssop is an ancient herb, mentioned several times in the Old Testament for purification, although the Biblical references may possibly be to *Origanum aegypticum* or to *Origanum syriacum*, rather than to *Hyssopus officinalis*. Penicillin therapy was pioneered by Howard Florey and Boris Chain. It was found to be a much superior drug to Prontosil which it replaced in 1940.

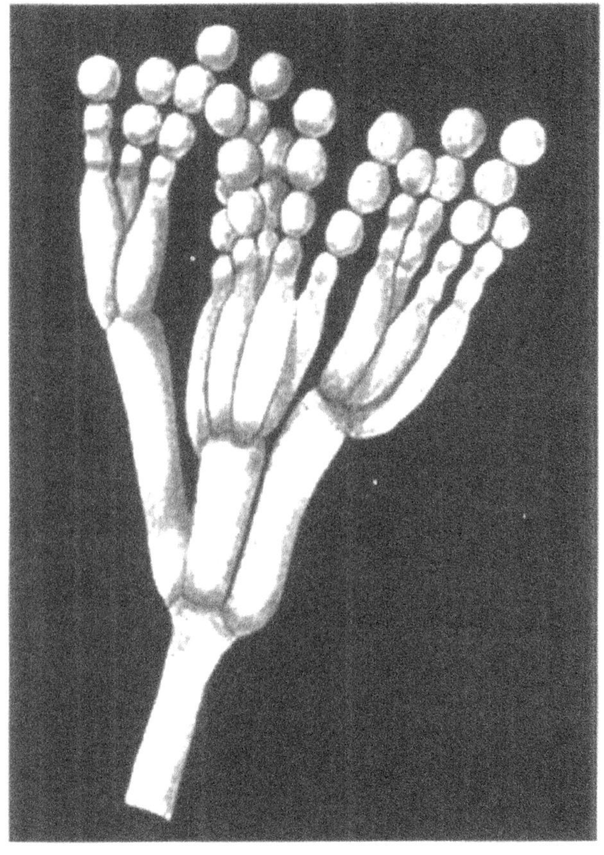

Figure 1 Penicillium mold. From Fleming, *Penicillin, its Practical Application* (1946)

CHILDBED OR PUERPERAL FEVER

In an essay on *Puerperal priority*, Gerald Weissmann (1997) of New York wrote 'at the dawn of the twentieth century 2000 women were lost each year in England and Wales from puerperal fever ... In 1966 only 3 of every 100 000 women in the industrialized world died of puerperal sepsis'. However, in less well-developed countries, due to lack of antiseptics,

OXFORD MEDICAL PUBLICATIONS

ANTIBIOTICS

A SURVEY OF PENICILLIN, STREPTOMYCIN, AND OTHER ANTIMICROBIAL SUBSTANCES FROM FUNGI, ACTINOMYCETES, BACTERIA, AND PLANTS

BY

H. W. FLOREY, M.A., M.D., Ph.D., F.R.S.
E. CHAIN, M.A., Ph.D., F.R.S.
N. G. HEATLEY, M.A., Ph.D.
M. A. JENNINGS, M.A., B.M.
A. G. SANDERS, M.A., M.B., D.Phil.
E. P. ABRAHAM, M.A., D.Phil.
M. E. FLOREY, M.B., B.S.

VOLUME I

GEOFFREY CUMBERLEGE
OXFORD UNIVERSITY PRESS
LONDON NEW YORK TORONTO
1949

Figure 2 Frontispiece from Florey's book on antibiotics

chemotherapy, antibiotics, antiviral agents, suitable sanitation and social structure, the rate was a 100 times higher.

Childbed fever, described from earliest times, usually occurred soon after the birth and few women survived. In the seventeenth century Thomas Willis introduced the phrase 'puerperarum febris' and the term 'puerperal fever' was finally popularized in 1716 by Edward Strother and replaced the previously used descriptive terms 'childbed fever' and 'lying-in fever'

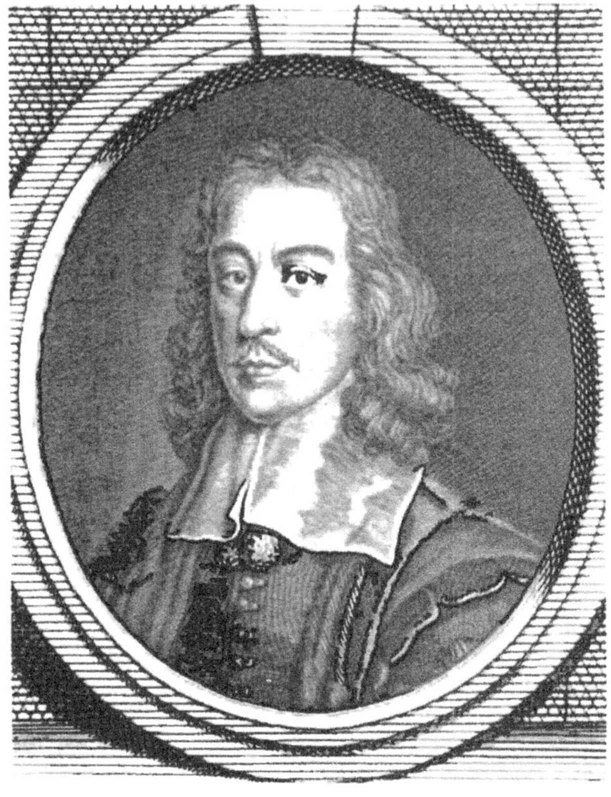

Figure 3 Thomas Willis (1621–1675)

over the next two centuries. The first treatment to adequately restrain the ravages of puerperal fever and other infections was Prontosil rubrum. Introduced to clinical practice in 1935 by Gerhard Domagk, Prontosil was first successfully used by Leonard Colebrook and Maeve Kenny in 1936. The maternal mortality figures plummeted in unprecedented fashion.

The Hippocratic Corpus

Hippocrates of Cos was born c. 460 BC and became the most famous of all the Greek physicians. He and his followers were responsible for a body of medical writings known as the *Hippocratic Corpus*. The collection consisted of about 60 treatises most of which were written between 430 and 330 BC.

Descriptions of puerperal or childbed fever are contained in the *Hippocratic Corpus*. Five cases followed childbirth and two developed after miscarriage.

Pessary treatment was noted in two cases for relief of genital pain. None of the women were named but two were identified by their husband's name and one by a household name. Only one of the seven women survived. The case studies were written in great detail and were contained in the portion of the *Hippocratic Corpus* known as the 'Epidemics'.

Soranus of Ephesus second century AD

This great gynecologist of antiquity had an intimate working knowledge of puerperal fever and realized that the condition frequently had its base in the uterus, although he was also aware of the toxic effects of breast abscess. He recognized that 'there are many conditions which precede the inflammation of the uterus, but the more frequent are cold, likewise pain, miscarriage, and a badly managed delivery, none of which make any difference in the treatment ... Inflammation [phlegmone] derives its name from inflame [phlegein], and not, as Democritus said, from phlegm [phlegma] being its cause'. Soranus mentioned the symptoms and signs of puerperal fever in great detail and offered various treatments. His materia medica included relaxing or warm olive oil, relaxing clysters, cupping, fomentations, leeches, poultices, scarification and wine. When fever and pain developed he prescribed the juice of nightshade (Temkin, 1956). Nightshade (*Atropa* sp.) is the narcotic herb from which atropine was obtained.

The Middle Ages and after

Inflammation of the uterus was recognized as a problem throughout the Middle Ages and juice of black nightshade continued to be an important treatment. Also availed of were herbal medications with linseed or fenugreek, medicated plasters, venesection and various other remedies (Rowland, 1981). The cause of puerperal fever was not understood but the prevailing notion was that it was due to lochial retention. Thomas Raynold (1545) in *The Byrth of Mankynde* was of the opinion that 'yfy woman haue the ague [fever] after her labor, for that cometh of lyke cause by retention of the flowres'.

François Mauriceau (1686) in his *The Diseases of Women with Child* wrote that 'Very often the stopping of the lochia, (of which we have lately discoursed, and especially at the beginning of Child-bed) doth cause an Inflammation to the Womb, which is a very dangerous Disease, and the death of most of the Women to whom it happens'. Mauriceau gave a graphic description of the symptoms and signs and related that 'If she do not die of it, an Abscess will be made there ... which will make her lead a miserable life the rest of her days'. His approach was to use a cooling diet, herbal medications, venesection and detersive (cleansing) injections to carry off the corrupt matter and retained lochia.

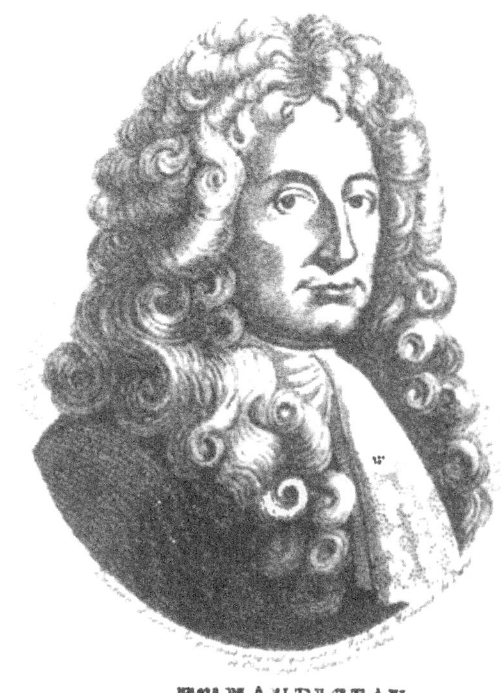

Figure 4 François Mauriceau (1637–1709). From Findley, *Priests of Lucina* (1939)

The eighteenth century

John Burton (1751) and John Leake (1772) were among the first to recognize that puerperal fever was a contagious disorder (Burton was satirized by the writer Laurence Stern as Dr Slop in his book *Tristram Shandy*).

Charles White, surgeon and man-midwife of Manchester, England, developed the hypothesis that the uterus became inflamed because putrid matter was conveyed by the examining practitioner through the birth canal to the site of placental separation (Cutter and Veits, 1964). He was the first to advocate the necessity of absolute cleanliness in the lying-in chamber. In chapter six of his *A Treatise on the Management of Pregnant and Lying-in Women* (1773), White wrote about the prevention of puerperal fever and advocated the isolation of infected patients, and the importance of adequate ventilation. He advised that the patient should sit upright to encourage free flow of the lochia and he designed a special bed and chair for the patient to recline on. The lying-in chamber was to be kept scrupulously clean. The bedding and curtains were washed and the floor and woodwork cleansed with vinegar, after which the room was stoved with brimstone.

The Scottish obstetrician, Alexander Gordon, dedicated his *A Treatise on the Epidemic Puerperal Fever of Aberdeen* (1795) to his friend and teacher, Thomas Denman. Gordon had closely observed the Aberdeen epidemic of puerperal fever of 1793 and was aware that women who fell prey to the disease had been visited or delivered by practitioners who had previously attended patients affected with the disease.

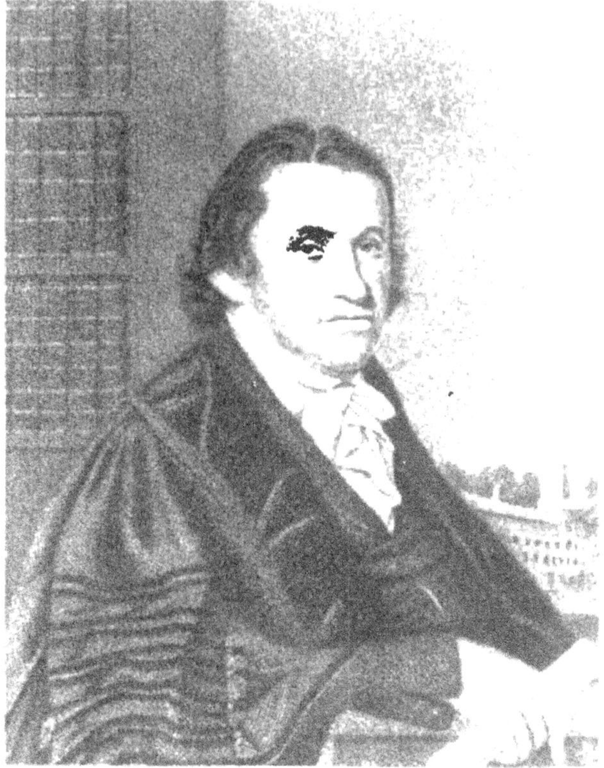

Figure 5 Samuel Bard (1742–1821). From Findley, *Priests of Lucina* (1939)

The nineteenth century

In the early part of the nineteenth century a number of obstetric authors wrote on the contagious nature of puerperal fever. At that time there was no demonstrable 'germ theory' so their explanations were entirely non-specific. Many notable obstetricians were offended by the notion that they could be responsible for spreading the disease and came out in strong opposition against the theory of contagion. Despite the furore that developed the pro-contagionists introduced effective practical programs to reduce the incidence of puerperal fever.

Thomas Denman (1801) in his *An Introduction to the Practice of Midwifery* wrote of puerperal fever and its contagious nature 'and being now fully proved ... and often have been conveyed by midwives or nurses, from one patient to another'. He also stated that the word 'erysipelas' was probably given by the ancients to this disease, without any intention to denote a specific kind of inflammation. It was later proven that erysipelas or 'red-skin disease' (an acute febrile contagious disease) was due to infection with the hemolytic streptococcus, the bacterial source of most cases of puerperal sepsis. Thomas Denman was the first licentiate in midwifery of the College of Physicians. He was appointed in 1769 as physician midwife to the Middlesex Hospital.

Samuel Bard of New York, wrote the first American textbook of obstetrics, *A Compendium of the Theory and Practice of Midwifery* (1807). In it Bard gave a detailed account of childbed fever 'The puerperal fever begins with cold chills, succeeded by great heat, and accompanied by its characteristic symptom, a remarkable soreness of the belly ... This soreness is generally confined, at first, to the parts over the womb, just below the navel; at other times, it extends more generally over the abdomen, and sometimes affects the bladder, so as to occasion a frequent and painful discharge of the urine; and the rectum, bringing on a frequent and painful urging to stool. ... The soreness and pain increase, the belly swells, the secretion of the milk, and the natural discharges are checked or suppressed, and the patient dies of a sudden mortification, or the disease runs rapidly into a putrid state'.

Samuel Bard advised 'putting a end to the chill as soon as possible' with cold drinks. His materia medica for the disease included antimony (a powerful diaphoretic), ipecacuanha to induce daily vomiting, laudanum (morphine), Peruvian bark (contains quinine, an analgesic and antipyretic), and a number of other medications, some of which were to induce purgation, and finally, venesection. 'For a more particular description of this disease, than is consistent with my design, I must refer my reader to the admirable writings of Mr White of Manchester, and Dr Denman.'

Robert Collins (1841), Master at the Dublin Lying-in Hospital (later called the Rotunda) was faced with an epidemic outbreak of puerperal fever in 1829. The trend towards delivery in hospital, introduced as a safety measure for poor and underprivileged women, exposed them to cross-infection and thus a higher degree of puerperal sepsis. Collins was aware that 'when met within lying-in hospitals, [it] is singularly alarming, proving fatal to a vast majority of those attacked under every mode of treatment as yet recommended'. Meanwhile, within private practice in higher class Dublin the disease was scarcely known.

Collins introduced an intensive cleansing and purification plan for the hospital. Each room was treated with chlorine gas. Chloride of lime was painted on the floors and woodwork and 48 hours later the rooms were washed with fresh lime and thoroughly ventilated. All blankets and linen were cleansed and then cooked in a stove at 120 to 130 °F. New patients to a room were greeted with blankets, quilts and linen that had been hung in chlorine gas. Through his intensive antiseptic endeavors he was able to write that 'for the four remaining years of my Mastership we did not lose a single patient from this disease'. Collins' materia medica included calomel (mercurous chloride, antiseptic, diuretic, and purgative), ipecacuanha (diaphoretic and emetic) and opium accompanied by warm bathing and leeching.

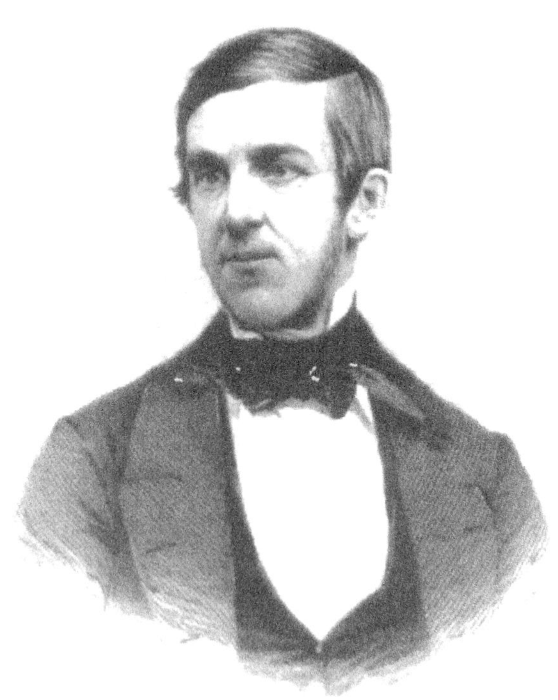

Figure 6 Oliver Wendell Holmes (1809–1894)

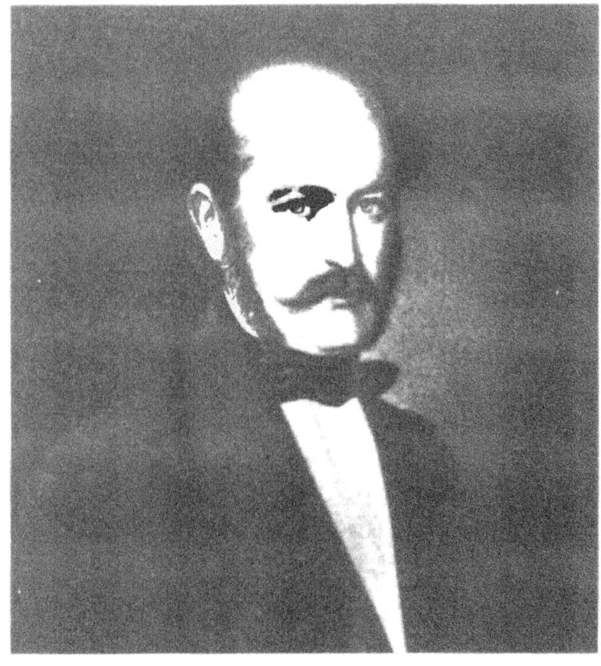

Figure 7 Ignaz Phillipp Semmelweiss (1818–1865). From Findley, *Priests of Lucina* (1939)

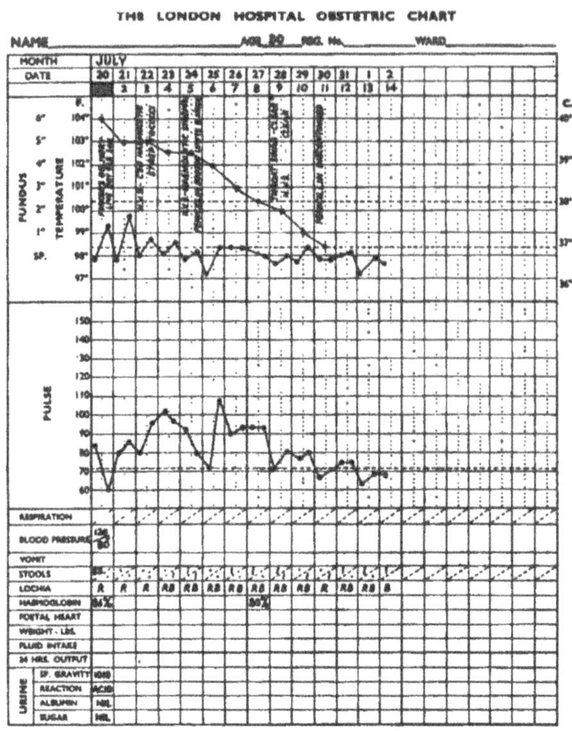

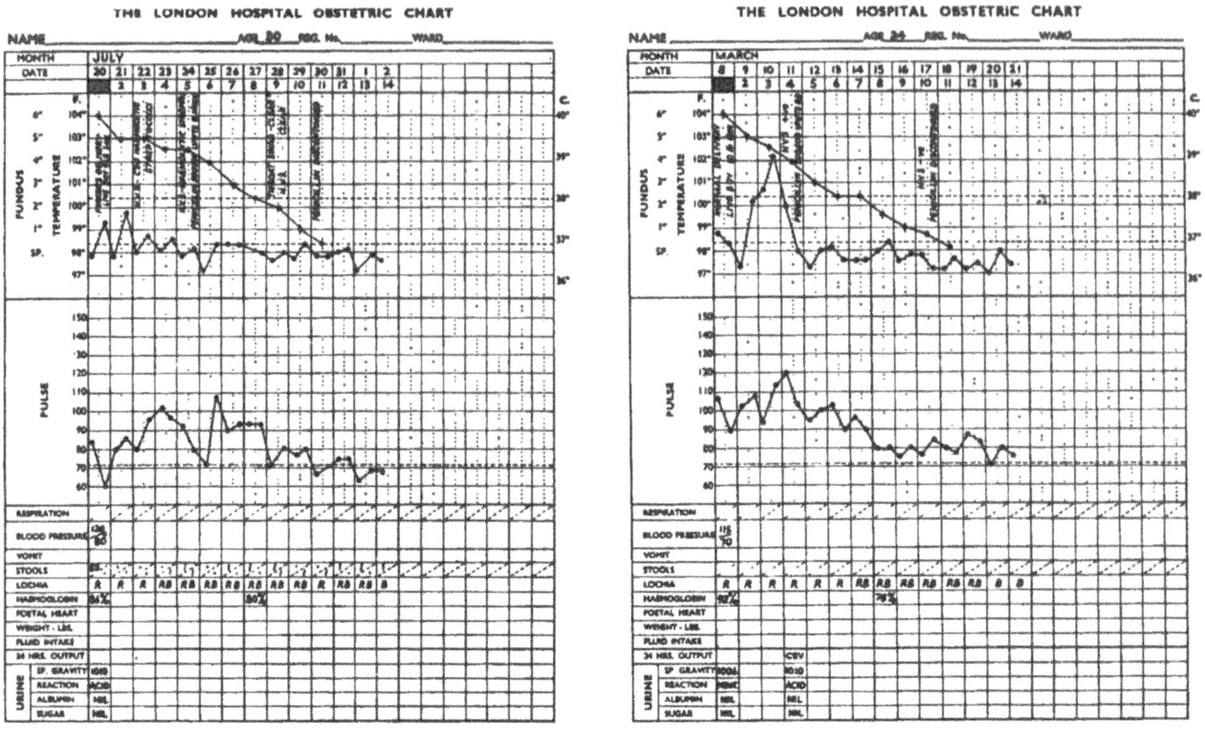

Fig. 291. Chart of a Case of Slight Uterine Infection following forceps delivery. The fever subsided spontaneously before penicillin was begun. High vaginal swabs and catheter specimens of urine taken on the second and fourth days of the puerperium all cultured profuse growths of hæmolytic streptococci. After four days penicillin therapy further specimens were sterile. The mild clinical character of the infection might have led to spread of the infection to other parturient women if room isolation had not been instituted from the outset.

Fig. 292. Chart of an Initially Severe Case of Uterine Infection following normal spontaneous delivery. A high vaginal swab on the third day of the puerperium yielded a profuse growth of hæmolytic streptococci on culture. The fever subsided within twenty-four hours of the institution of penicillin therapy. A further high vaginal swab on the ninth day of the puerperium was sterile on culture.

Figure 8 London Hospital charts. From Brews, *Eden & Holland's Manual of Obstetrics* (1957)

In America, Oliver Wendell Holmes (1843) wrote to the readers of the *New England Quarterly Journal of Medicine* in forceful terms: 'In collecting, and forcing and adding to the evidence accumulated on this most serious subject, I would not be understood to imply that there exists a doubt in the mind of any well-informed member of the medical profession as to the fact that puerperal fever is sometimes communicated from one person to another, both directly and indirectly'. Unfortunately, his views on the contagiousness of puerperal fever were nullified in large measure by opposition from the Philadelphia professors of midwifery, Charles D. Meigs of the Jefferson Medical School and Hugh Lennox Hodge of the University of Pennsylvania, who did not agree with his claims.

In Europe, Ignaz Philipp Semmelweis (1847/48, 1849, 1861; The 1847/48/49 papers were written for Semmelweis by his friend, Ferdinand von Hebra, editor of the magazine) a Hungarian working in Vienna, investigated puerperal sepsis and developed five doctrines, the most important of which (his Lehre 1) was that puerperal fever could be transmitted by 'cadaveric particles' adhering to students or physicians hands and carried from the autopsy room to pregnant women in the labor room or lying-in ward (the other four doctrines incorporated previous and current views on the topic). As Semmelweis concluded that the doctors and students of Vienna's first obstetrical clinic were 'carriers of decomposed matter … [on] the examining finger' he instituted a program of hand-washing with chlorinated lime between autopsy work and examining of patients to reduce the spread of infection. Soon afterwards, a 10% decline of mortality from puerperal sepsis was noted. By a cruel twist of fate, Semmelweis contracted an infection of his right hand and died from the same form of sepsis that he had sought so hard to eradicate in women.

Joseph Lister's use of antisepsis in surgery began in 1865, some four years after Semmelweis published his treatise on puerperal fever. In the year of Semmelweis' untimely death, J.L. Bischoff of Basel applied the Listerian principles to midwifery. Carbolic washing of hands, and carbolic-acid impregnated dressings and pads were employed, and although not defeated, the incidence of puerperal sepsis was reduced. In 1874 the famed Viennese surgeon Theodor Billroth identified a bacteria, soon to be called *Streptococcus* (Greek, *strepto*, twisted; *kokkus*, berry) in a sample of pus. Then Louis Pasteur (1879) of France discovered that the *Streptococcus* was the cause of puerperal sepsis. Beginning in 1918, Rebecca Lancefield of the Rockefeller Institute in New York developed the method of distinguishing between different varieties of hemolytic streptococci (Hare, 1970) and her system was combined with that of Griffith in the 1930s. The management of puerperal fever continued to be primarily by prevention, and no effective treatment was available until the introduction of Prontosil in 1935 by Gerhard Dogmak and its clinical use by Leonard Colebrook and Maeve Kenny of London in 1936.

TUBERCULOSIS

The term 'tuberculosis' was introduced by J.L. Schoenlein, professor of medicine at Zurich, in 1839. The disease takes its name from the Latin *tuberculum*, diminutive of tuber, a little swelling or nodule, being based on the pathological appearance of the circumscribed tuberculous lesion. In the ancient world the Greeks knew the disease as 'phthisis' i.e. to waste away. Later, during the Middle Ages, tuberculous infection of the lymph nodes in the neck was termed 'scrofula', the Latin word for brood sow, as it was thought that the animals were prone to carry the disease. An alternative name was the 'Kings Evil', and the condition was supposed to be healed by the touch of a monarch. In the sixteenth century the Parisian physician Jean Fernel carried out postmortem studies on 'consumption' and identified the disease with the chest cavity.

Epidemics of pulmonary tuberculosis swept through Europe from the sixteenth through the twentieth centuries. In the 1800s it was estimated that about 20% of all deaths from disease were due to tuberculosis. Robert Koch (1882) discovered the bacterial agent responsible for the disease to be *Mycobacterium tuberculosis*. No treatment was available for the disease but from the mid-nineteenth century a 'sanitarium movement' advocated rest, sunshine and good nutrition. This form of remedy was popular until the time of the Second World War. Surgical treatment, by inducing lung collapse, became popular in the 1920s and was extensively used for over 30 years.

The various forms of tuberculosis took their names from the gross appearance of the lesions that the disease was associated with, e.g. miliary, ulcerative, papillary or interstitial forms. Apart from the lung-fields, tuberculosis affected other tissues and of course the genital tract. Tuberculosis of the fallopian tubes accounted for 90% of all lesions of the female reproductive system. The endometrium was also affected, usually on a cyclical basis by spread from the oviducts, and evidence of the disease was found in up to 6% of endometrial biopsies obtained from women complaining of sterility.

Leon Charles Calmette with C. Guerin and B. Weill-Halle produced a vaccine (BCG: Bacille Calmette–Guerin) in 1906 that was introduced as a prophylactic against tuberculosis in children in 1921 (Calmette *et al.*, 1924, 1927). The vaccine became widely available after 1928. Chemotherapy, in the form of streptomycin, was introduced by Selman Abraham Waksman of Rutgers University (Schatz, Bugie and Waksman, 1944). Para-aminosalicylic acid (PAS) was developed between 1946 and 1948 by Jorgen Lehmann of Sweden. Isoniazid was isolated in Germany in 1950 and in the following year in America.

The mortality caused by puerperal sepsis in the 'developed' world was virtually eliminated by Prontosil and penicillin, and pulmonary tuberculosis became the most frequent cause of death among women of childbearing age in the 1940s. As a result of strict preventive measures, and effective chemotherapy, the incidence of tuberculosis was drastically reduced over the next 40 years. The advent of the acquired immune deficiency syndrome (AIDS) led to increased rates of tuberculosis in immuno-compromised patients. The tuberculosis story was the subject of a recent book by Frank Ryan (1992).

VENEREAL DISEASE AND ITS TREATMENT

The word venereal is derived from the Latin, *venerus*–Venus, Veneris, the goddess of love; connected with the Latin *venerari*, to worship. Venereal, or sexually transmitted diseases have been recorded for thousands of years. The most common forms were gonorrhea and syphilis.

Syphilis

The history of syphilis dates from about 1493. It was variously known as the 'French pockes; the 'Portuguese sickness'; the 'Great pockes' – because its consequences were significantly worse than smallpox – and eventually became known as 'the pox'. The name syphilis derives from a poem written in 1530 by an Italian physician, Girolama Fracastoro, of Verona. Millions of people died from epidemics of syphilis over the centuries. In the twentieth century syphilis was a major killer worldwide until the 1950s.

Mercury

In 1496 Georgio Sommariva, a Veronese physician, used mercury to treat syphilis. It was later stated that 'a night with Venus meant a lifetime with Mercury'. Mercury could be taken as an oral preparation, administered by fumigation, or rubbed into the skin. It was effective but poisonous and caused symptoms as bad as the disease. Its effects were known as 'salivation' or the 'salivary cure' and the heavy flow of saliva induced by the mercury was thought to wash out the syphilitic poison.

Guajacum

This exotic treatment was introduced from the West Indies in 1508. For many years it was thought to treat syphilis and, as it had no major side effects, it became very popular (see Chapter 26).

Iodides

Iodine was discovered in 1811 by the French chemist, Bernard Courtois, although the seaweed and burned sponge from which it came had been used medicinally for many years. Iodides began to be used in the treatment of syphilitic ulcers in the early nineteenth century. Iodides retained their popularity well into the twentieth century.

Organic arsenicals

Ehrlich and Hata (1910) introduced the organic arsenicals for the treatment of syphilis and spectacular results were obtained from the use of '606' (Salvarsan). Initially, arsphenamine was used as a single dose treatment but relapses occurred. Eventually it was proposed that treatment should continue for at least a year. Arsphenamine and the organic arsenicals were successfully used until 1943.

Bismuth

Two Paris physicians, Sazerac and Levaditi, injected sodium and potassium bismuth tartrate into syphilitic rabbits. They showed that a good response was obtained in both early and late syphilitic infection. Bismuth became such an important part of the materia medica that it replaced mercury. At one stage there was a choice of over a hundred different preparations of bismuth. For many years syphilis was treated with combinations of arsenicals, bismuth and mercury. Treatment with penicillin began in 1943.

Gonorrhea

Galen (c. AD 130–200) was the first to use the term 'gonorrhea' and is said to have used theriac for inflammation. The disease was described by Aetius in the sixth century AD and he detailed the treatment of pelvic abscess. In France the disease was known as 'La chaude pisse' (hot piss) and the word 'clap' dates back to the late fourteenth century. Gonorrhea was the dominant venereal disease in Europe until the syphilis epidemic began. Although not as destructive as syphilis, gonorrhea had a major impact on women's reproductive health. The relationship between gonorrhea and pelvic sepsis was first demonstrated in the nineteenth century and the Breslau bacteriologist, Albert Neisser (1879) discovered the causal organism.

Herbal remedies for gonorrhea

Dandelion, flax, jujube, lettuce, liverwort, maiden hair, marshmallow, melon, poppy, purslane, strawberries, violets, waterlilies,

Mercury was found not to be helpful. In the male, urethral lavage and passage of medicated urethral sounds were used to relieve the accompanying urethral strictures. In the female, vaginal irrigation of acriflavine, astringents, lime water, mercurochrome and potassium permanganate were prescribed. Vaccine therapy was introduced at the time of the First World War and was particularly used in women. No effective cure for gonorrhea was found until 1937 when the sulfonamides were introduced. Sulfonamide resistance soon occurred but penicillin, to which the organism was sensitive, became available in 1943.

Genital warts

Treatment consisted of surgical removal or cautery until the introduction of podophyllin by the US Army doctor, I.W. Caplan (1942).

Chlamydia trachomatis

Sulfonamides had a 50% success rate in eradicating *Chlamydia trachomatis*, but penicillin was ineffective. In the early 1950s the treatment of choice became the tetracyclines, and the preferred first line treatment was doxycycline.

Herpes simplex

Acyclovir, a nucleoside analogue, was introduced in the early 1980s. For patients who had more than six recurrences per year, continuous suppression using acyclovir 400 mg twice daily was successful in preventing most. Two new nucleoside analogue pro-drugs, valacyclovir and famcyclovir came into use in the late 1990s. During pregnancy, azithromycin or erythromycin were used.

Bacterial vaginosis
Metroidazole or clindamycin.

Trichomoniasis
Metronidazole.

Group B Streptococcus
Penicillin VK.

ACQUIRED IMMUNE DEFICIENCY SYNDROME (AIDS)

Acquired immune deficiency syndrome was first recognized in Los Angeles and New York in 1981, although the causative human immuno-deficiency virus (HIV) had first appeared in the USA and Western Europe in 1978, and in Central Africa about 1972. By 1997 it was estimated that there were at least 23 million people with HIV infection while a further 8500 men, women and children were infected daily. Other statistical projections indicated that by the year 2000, five million children would be infected and five to ten million would have been orphaned as a result of maternal AIDS (WHO, 1995; Chin and Mann, 1997). The prevalence of HIV infection of women in the childbearing years varied from 0.1% in the United Kingdom, Canada and Australia to more than 30% in the more severely affected African nations.

Treatment

Everett Koop (1986), Surgeon General of the US Public Health Service, produced a report on acquired immune deficiency syndrome in which he estimated that 270 000 cases of AIDS would have occurred by 1991, of which over 50% would have died. The cost to medical and other supportive services would lie somewhere between eight and 16 billion dollars. Everett Koop held out no promise of treatment and wrote that information and education were the only weapons in the ongoing struggle against the disease.

In the following year, the antiviral drug Zidovudine, a thymidine derivative, was licensed for use but single-agent treatment was of limited success. From 1996 combination therapy of Zidovudine with Lamivudine was successfully used for most parenteral exposures (Easterbrook, 1997). Protease enzyme inhibitors were released in the same year. As of February 1997, 18 anti-retroviral drugs were available (thus 856 possible triple permutations) that could suppress the HIV virus almost completely, when used in combination therapy (Dillner, 1997). The drugs were of three main types.

Anti-retroviral therapy

Nucleoside reverse transcriptase inhibitors (NRTI)
Didanosine, lamivudine, stavudine, zalcitabine, zidovudine

Non-nucleoside reverse transcriptase inhibitors (NNRTI)
Delaviridine, mevirapine

Protease inhibitors
Indinavir, ritonavir, saquinavir.

Prophylaxis

Anti-retroviral therapy has been widely used since the early 1990s after incidents of occupational exposure to HIV. Medication with Zidovudine, 1g per day for three to four weeks, reduced the odds of seroconversion by almost 80% (Case–control Study of HIV Seroconversion, 1995).

Vaccine therapy

One method to prevent the disease would be the application of an AIDS vaccine. A live attenuated vaccine based on a strain of Simian immunodeficiency virus had long been considered the best hope. However, it was discovered in 1995 that the weakened virus eventually triggered the Simian version of AIDS when given to baby monkeys (Gottlieb, 1998).

Pregnancy and HIV infection

The American College of Obstetricians and Gynecologists (1997) stated that 'By mid-1995, more than half a million persons in the United States had been reported as having acquired immunodeficiency syndrome (AIDS), of whom approximately 14% were women … In 1994 HIV infection was the third leading cause of death among women 25–44 years old and the fifth leading cause of death in girls 1–4 years old. The prevalence of HIV infection in women giving birth in the United States in 1993 was about 1.6 per thousand'.

Perinatal or vertical transmission of HIV

The problem of perinatal transmission was first reported in 1982 (Buehler *et al.*, 1989) and it was discovered that the rate was about 25%. Approximately 6000 women of childbearing age, mostly living in the developing world, acquired HIV infection every day. As approximately 98% of HIV infected children had acquired HIV from the mother during pregnancy, at delivery, or through breast feeding, prevention of the 25% mother-to-child transmission (MTCT) became a major health priority. The presence of the virus in blood and mucus of the vagina increased the risk of HIV transmission during the passage of the fetus through the birth canal. Mother-to-child transmission at the time of birth was the primary route of HIV infection among infants and young children and it was estimated that 1000 babies a day became infected with HIV. According to the ACOG (1997) report, 'Mother-to-child transmission of HIV can occur during pregnancy or through breast feeding. Infection can occur as early as the eighth week of gestation, although perhaps 50% or more of perinatal infections occur during labor and delivery … rupture of membranes has been linked to increased rates of mother to child transmission of HIV'.

Prevention of perinatal transmission of HIV

Vitamin A

A role for vitamin A in HIV transmission has been suggested by the results of a study showing that vitamin A deficiency was associated with increased transmission (Semba *et al.*, 1994).

Chlorhexidine

It was found that chlorhexidine disinfection of the vagina was associated with a reduction from almost 40% of MTCT to 25% in women with premature rupture of the membranes (Taha *et al.*, 1997).

Zidovudine

An intensive regiment of Zidovudine prenatally, intrapartum and postnatally significantly reduced mother-to-child transmission (Connor *et al.*, 1994). In the Bangkok Perinatal HIV Study, oral Zidovudine, given during late pregnancy and labor to non-breast feeding women reduced the rate of mother-to-child transmission of HIV by 51% (CDCP, 1998). Breast feeding is responsible for around one-third of cases of maternal transmission. Cost of prophylaxis was a major problem for some Third World countries (Sidley, 1998).

The history of venerealogy was related by J.D. Oriel in his *The Scars of Venus* (1994); by Claude Quetel in his *History of Syphilis* (1990); by Virginia Berridge and Philip Stronge in their *AIDS, and Contemporary History* (1993); and there is an overview in the *History of Obstetrics and Gynaecology* by Michael O'Dowd and Elliot Philip (1994).

ANTISEPSIS

The word antisepsis is derived from the Greek, 'against putrefaction'. An antiseptic came to mean a substance that would inhibit the growth of microorganisms without necessarily destroying them. According to Roderick McGrew (1985) 'the word antiseptic was first used in an English pamphlet entitled *An Hypothetical Notion of the Plague and Some Out of the Way Thoughts About It*, published in 1721 by a Mr Place'.

Over the centuries, our predecessors discovered through trial and error, that certain agents could treat inflammation. Since the days of ancient Egypt, balsams, gums, resins and spices were used to treat wounds and inflamed areas after childbirth, and to arrest decomposition. Benzoin, frankincense, myrrh, styrax and turpentine were popularly used as were vinegar and wine and it is now appreciated that most, if not all of these agents, have antiseptic properties. Carbolic acid (from coal tar) and iodine (from seaweed) were both introduced in the nineteenth century and had a major impact on the control of obstetrical and surgical infections. Once the contagious nature of infection was proved in the late nineteenth century, strict antiseptic methods were adhered to. Hand-washing prior to surgery and obstetrical examinations was soon followed by the use of rubber gloves and the wearing of masks and suitable gowns for the operators. Helmuth Bottcher (1963) in his book entitled *Miracle Drugs, A History of Antibiotics* related the story of antiseptics through the ages.

Some antiseptics in the early twentieth century

Alcohol, boric acid, bromine, carbolic acid, charcoal, chlorinated soda, chlorine, chloride of lime, corrosive sublimate, creosote, ferric chloride, iodine, mercury, nitric acid, phenol, silver citrate, sodium chloride, sugar, tannic acid, vinegar, zinc chloride and zinc cyanide.

Carbolic acid

The antiseptic properties of carbolic acid (phenol, obtained from the distillation of coal tar) were discovered by François Jules Lemaire (1860). Five years later carbolic acid came to the attention of Joseph Lister (later Baron Lister) who became professor of surgery at Glasgow in 1861. Lister was also aware of the work of the French chemist, Louis Pasteur, who at that time was researching the cause of fermentation in beer, milk and wine. Pasteur found that microorganisms caused the fermentation, and went on to prove that they were also responsible for infection and putrefaction.

Lister had observed that half of all surgical cases treated by amputation died from infection. He developed a theory that organisms borne in the air caused putrefaction in the wound that, in turn, led to severe illness and sometimes to death. Lister covered wounds with a dressing that contained the recently discovered carbolic acid and found that infection could be prevented. In 1867 Lister devised an 'antiseptic curtain' of carbolic acid spray for use during operating that also helped to reduce the rates of surgical infection. Despite his success, his contemporaries were highly critical and his methods were not accepted until it was shown in 1874 that pus contained 'germs'.

Iodine

This popular antiseptic was discovered by Bernard Courtois of France in 1811. It was used in the treatment of wounds and as a finger dip for surgeons. Iodoform was discovered by George Simon Serullas (1822).

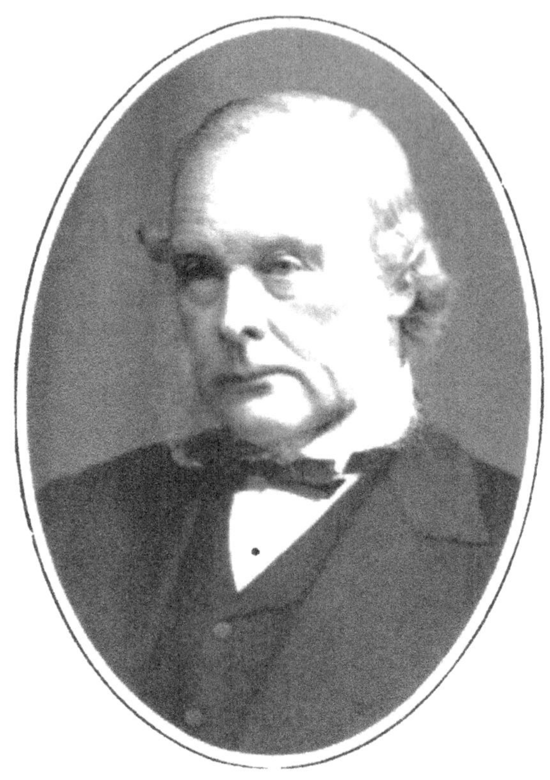

Figure 9 Lord Joseph Lister (1827–1912)

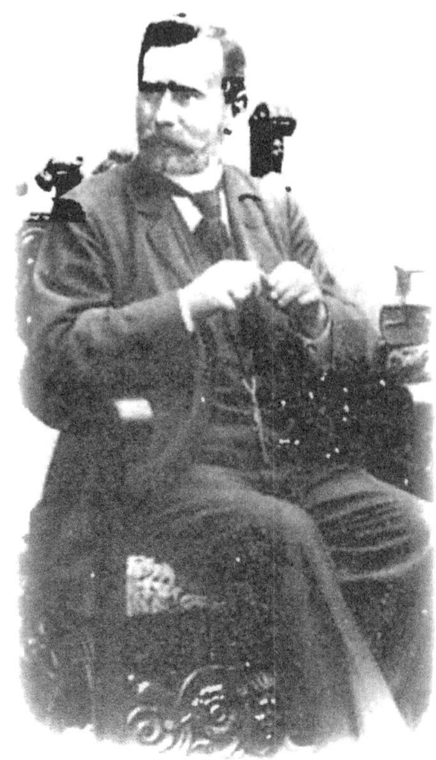

Figure 10 Paul Ehrlich (1854–1915)

Sixty years later Albert von Mosteig-Moorhof (1882) introduced the idea of impregnating surgical dressings with iodoform (See also Chapter 16).

CHEMOTHERAPY

The term 'chemotherapy' was introduced by Paul Ehrlich. In its strictest sense, chemotherapy is the treatment or prevention of disease by chemical disinfection or inhibition of the pathogenic agencies but without serious toxic effects on the patient. Although chemotherapy is currently associated with cancer treatment, the term also related to combined therapy for pulmonary tuberculosis and the use of agents to limit or destroy the multiplication of many disease causing bacteria.

Salvarsan

In the century that the general theory of infective disease evolved, the eminent bacteriologist Robert Koch discovered that mercuric chloride was superior to carbolic acid in disinfection (Koch, 1881). He called attention to variations in the bactericidal effect of different disinfectants and raised the question as to why antiseptics that destroyed bacteria in laboratory conditions failed to do so in the living organism. Koch's queries led Paul Ehrlich of Frankfurt to study various chemicals that could be bound to bacteria, and destroy them, but that would have no toxic effect on the host. Ehrlich experimented with dyes and successfully treated malaria with methylene blue. He then began the long search for chemicals that would be effective against syphilis. After many experiments Ehrlich and his collaborator, Sahachiro Hata, discovered that the 606th preparation they tried proved successful against syphilis. The arsenical compound was marketed as Salvarsan in 1910 (Ehrlich and Hata, 1910) and it became the first specific treatment of worth for syphilis. The side effects of treatment were formidable but fortunately the era of arsenotherapy in the treatment of syphilis was short-lived.

Prontosil rubrum

Prior to 1935 the only compounds available for chemotherapy were antimony, arsenicals, emetine, quinine and quinicrine but research continued in search of the ultimate compound. Gerhard Domagk, research director for the German Bayer Company, experimented with the metal-based compounds antimony, arsenic, gold and tin in an effort to discover a compound similar to, or better than, Salvarsan. The Bayer Company produced azo-dyes and Domagk turned his attention to them. During his investigation of a new dye compound he identified that it had antibacterial effects. After further refinement the new drug was introduced by Domagk (1935) and traded under the name, Prontosil rubrum. The drug had a marked antibacterial effect on streptococci.

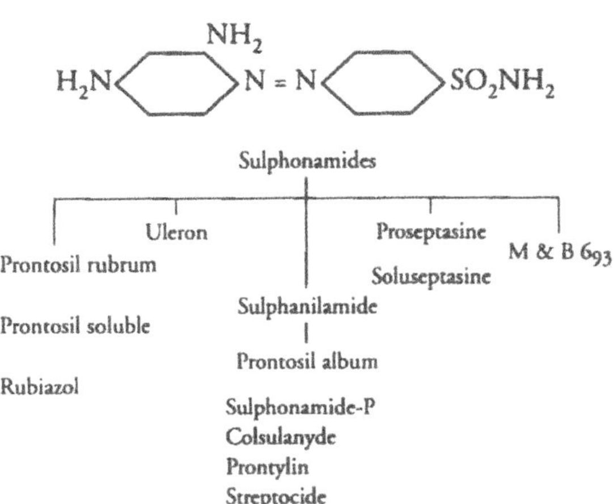

Figure 11 Prontosil rubrum. From Rolleston and Moncrieff, *Essentials of Modern Chemotherapy* (1941)

Colebrook, Kenny, prontosil and puerperal sepsis

Leonard Colebrook, of the Medical Research Council, and Maeve Kenny (1936), resident medical officer at Queen Charlotte's Hospital, London, wrote of their experience with Prontosil in the treatment of puerperal infections and experimental infections in mice. They detailed the case histories of 38 women with puerperal sepsis who were admitted to the isolation unit at Queen Charlotte's. The patients were given oral, intravenous or intramuscular Prontosil. The maternal mortality in the Prontosil-treated group was 8% compared to 26.3% mortality in 38 cases admitted immediately prior to the use of the drug. They found that Prontosil was well tolerated and that it retarded, though did not suppress, the growth of *Streptococcus*.

When Prontosil became generally available and prescribed for women with puerperal sepsis, the mortality figures for the disease plummeted. The cure for the commonest killer of women in childbirth was at hand.

During their study of Prontosil, Colebrook and Kenny found that during therapy the patients' skin had acquired 'a slightly red or terra-cotta tinge in several of the cases who received large doses of the drug. The urine is always deeply tinged by the dye during the treatment'. The vivid color was caused by the non-active dye component of the Prontosil. It was soon discovered that sulfanilamide was the clinically active portion and that drug went on to replace Prontosil as the treatment of choice in puerperal sepsis. The discovery that sulfanilamide had antibacterial effects led to experimentation with other sulfas and soon sulfathiazole and sulfadiazine were introduced.

Leonard Colebrook was also responsible for the introduction of chloroxylenol, a chemical related to carbolic acid, as suitable antiseptic to kill streptococci on the bare hands. The antiseptic became known as Dettol (Hare, 1970).

ANTIBIOTICS

An antibiotic is defined as a soluble substance derived from a mold or bacterium that inhibits the growth of other microorganisms (Hensyl, 1990). In 1887 Pasteur and Joubert observed that the growth of certain airborne organisms inhibited the growth of the anthrax bacillus and suggested that this fact might be of importance in therapeutics. It was also noticed that an attack of erysipelas had beneficial therapeutic effects in patients with chronic syphilis. Being aware of those facts, Rudolf Emmerich injected streptococci from an erysipelas patient into rabbits who were infected with anthrax. The inoculation countered the anthrax infection in over half of the rabbits. Similar experiments were carried out by a number of other investigators and in 1899 Emmerich and Loew extracted pyocyanase from cultures of *Pseudomonas*.

Pyocyanase was destructive against anthrax, diphtheria, typhoid, and plague (Newman Dorland, 1932).

Paul Vuillemin coined the word 'antibiosis' in 1889 to describe the natural condition whereby one microbe destroyed another to preserve its own existence. He called the active agent the 'antibiote'. Selman Waksman introduced the English word 'antibiotic' in 1945 and he suggested that the term be applied to describe a chemical substance of microbial origin that possesses 'antibiotic' powers. Penicillin was the first of the modern antibiotics to be discovered and derived its name from molds of the genus Penicillium. Newman Dorland (1932) described Penicillium as a genus of molds which develop fruiting organs resembling a broom, or the bones of the hand and fingers. Thus the Latin, *Penicillium*, brush, gave penicillin its name.

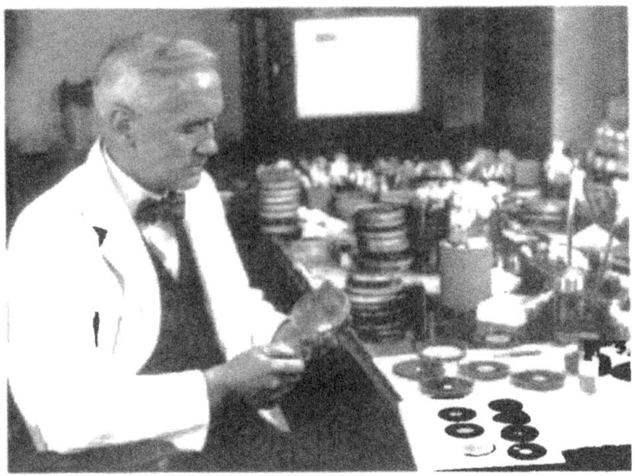

Figure 12 Sir Alexander Fleming (1881–1955). From Goldsmith, *The Road to Penicillin* (1946)

The discovery of penicillin

In a paper on his discovery of penicillin, Alexander Fleming (1944) of the Inoculation Department, St Mary's Hospital, London, wrote that he had been deeply interested during the whole of his career in the destruction of bacteria by leukocytes. During the First World War he had spent much time investigating problems in connection with septic wounds. He described how in 1922 he had isolated lysozyme a powerful antibacterial agent that occurred naturally in human tissues and secretions.

Fleming (1929) recounted that in September 1928 'while working with *Staphylococcus* variants a number of culture plates were set aside ... around a large colony of a contaminating mold the *Staphylococcus* colonies became transparent and were obviously undergoing lysis ... the antibacterial substance produced by the mold was a remarkable one and demanded further investigation'. Fleming related that the mold belonged to the genus Penicillium – later identified as *Penicillium notatum*, a species of fungus that was first isolated from the decaying leaves of the blue labiate hyssop, by the Swedish scientist Westling.

Fleming wrote that the active agent was readily obtained and the name 'penicillin' had been given to filtrates of broth cultures of the mold. The diphtheria bacillus, gonococcus, meningococcus, pneumococci, staphylococci and streptococci were very sensitive to the effects of penicillin. As it was found to be nontoxic to animals in large doses, and did not interfere with leukocyte function, Fleming suggested that it would be an effective antiseptic for application to or injection into areas infected with penicillin-sensitive microbes.

The further development of penicillin

J. David Oriel (1994) wrote that the first clinical observation of the antibacterial action of Penicillium was made by the surgeon, Joseph Lister, in the 1870s when he used fungal culture extracts to treat localized infections. Wainright and Swan (1986) related that, in 1930, Cecil George Paine, a bacteriologist in Sheffield, England, used a crude preparation of *Penicillium notatum* to treat gonococcal ophthalmia neonatorum in two infants. However, it was not until 1938 that a team of young scientists at the Sir William Dunn School of Pathology, Oxford, led by the pathologist Howard W. Florey of Adelaide, and the biochemist Ernst B. Chain, a German émigré, began a long-term research project on microbial antagonists. In a paper entitled 'Penicillin as a chemotherapeutic agent', Chain, Florey, *et al.* (1940) explained how they had derived a brown powder, freely soluble in water from Penicillium culture. Although not yet a pure substance, they concluded that penicillin was active *in vivo* against streptococci and staphylococci.

In the following year Abraham, Florey and associates followed up their original article with further observations on penicillin in which they compared the superior antibacterial activity of penicillin to the sulfonamides. They included their method of small-scale production in the paper. To increase the supply of Penicillium mold, Florey and his team debated whether they should use metal dishes instead of their small glass laboratory appliances. Unfortunately, the Penicillium did not survive contact with the metal but it was soon discovered that the mold grew very well in enamel-covered bedpans.

The first human experimentation with penicillin occurred on 27 January 1941 when an asymptotic woman was injected with 100 mg of the preparation. Disappointingly, she developed a rigor and felt unwell. The rigor was due to a pyrogen contaminant that was later separated out by chromatography. The first treatment with penicillin, some of which had been recovered from the urine of research subjects, began on 1 February 1941 for a policeman with an advanced staphylococcal infection, complicated by an overgrowth of streptococcus. He responded well and the infection began to settle. The meager supplies of penicillin were soon used up, so the infection relapsed and the policeman died. It was later related that an Oxford professor referred to penicillin as a remarkable substance, grown in bedpans and purified by passage through the Oxford police force.

Florey and his colleagues sought the aid of the British Government and pharmaceutical industry to research methods of producing large quantities of pure penicillin. However, due to the financial crisis of the on-going Second World War, little interest was shown. In 1941 Florey and Norman C.H. Heatly visited the United States to develop methods for producing penicillin in quantity. The US Department of Agriculture referred them to their Northern Region Research Laboratory in Peoria, Illinois. It was found that by adding corn-steep liquor, a by-product of corn starch manufacture, the penicillin yield could be increased ten fold. Also, more productive strains of Fleming's Penicillium were discovered and Penicillium mold was grown in deep tanks rather than on the surfaces of media in shallow dishes. The three pharmaceutical companies, Merck & Co., E.R. Squibb & Sons and the Charles P. Pfizer Company, cooperated in developing penicillin. By early 1943 sufficient penicillin was produced to treat about 100 cases, but by 1944 production had escalated to three hundred billion units of penicillin per month. In June 1944, when the allies invaded Europe, there were sufficient stocks of penicillin to treat all severe American and British casualties and in the following year penicillin was released for use in the civilian market.

Meanwhile, in 1943, John F. Mahoney of the US Public Health Service was provided with some penicillin by the Oxford investigators. Mahoney and his colleagues, Arnold and Harris, (1943) demonstrated the effectiveness of penicillin in the treatment of syphilitic rabbits and then reported their treatment of four patients with primary syphilis. The treponemes which cause the disease disappeared from the syphilitic skin sores within a few hours, and serological tests for syphilis rapidly became negative. In the same year, barely a quarter of all patients with gonorrhea were being effectively cured by sulfonamides. Penicillin was introduced as treatment for gonococcal urethritis and soon proved to be the most effective drug for gonorrhea ever tried (leading article, *Lancet*, 1944). As a further demonstration of its efficacy in syphilis, Goodwin and Moore (1946) treated 57 pregnant luetic women with penicillin and their infants were born without the stigmata of syphilis. A two-volume publication, *Antibiotics. A Survey of Penicillin, Streptomycin and other anti-microbial substances from Fungi, Actinomycetes, Bacteria and Plants*, produced by Howard Florey and associates (1949) is the definitive source for the vast amount of early data on anti-microbials.

Antibiotic resistance

The first cases of penicillin resistance in staphylococci were noted in early 1942 and soon thereafter for streptococci and gonococci. The responsible agent was penicillinase (beta lactamase), an enzyme obtained in 1939 from a strain of *Bacillus cereus*; formerly used in the treatment of slowly developing or delayed penicillin reactions. The search then began for new and better penicillins and other non-Penicillium derived antibiotics that would be penicillinase resistant. Interestingly enough, the problem of resistance is not new. Antibiotic-resistant bacteria were isolated from deep within Canadian glacial ice estimated to be 2000 years old (Dancer, Shears and Platt, 1997).

Bacterial resistance to antibiotics became a major problem in the mid- and late twentieth century, amidst calls for their prudent use, Robin Fox, editor of the *Journal of the Royal Society of Medicine*, in a leading article entitled 'The post-antibiotic era beckons' (1996), wrote of a new breed of antimicrobials, the magainins. Discovered in 1987 in the skin secretions of frogs and toads, the magainins are peptides with activity against a wide range of bacteria and fungi. Fox theorized that this new class of agents could save us from the threatened post-antibiotic era but added a note of caution, 'If history repeats itself, the magainins will be sold as widely as possible; they will be misused; and resistant organisms will emerge. Frogs will wish they had kept their secret'.

A SELECTION OF ANTIMICROBIAL AGENTS

Sulfonamides

The term 'sulfonamide' is derived from para-amino-benzo-sulfonamide (sulfanilamide). Prontosil was patented by Klarer and Mietzsch in 1932. Domagk (1935) discovered its chemotherapeutic value. Leonard Colbrooke and Maeve Kenny (1936) reported the successful treatment of puerperal sepsis by Prontosil.

Penicillin

In 1928 Alexander Fleming (1929) isolated penicillin from the mold, *Penicillium notatum*, a fungus known to inhabit decaying hyssop leaves. Howard Florey, Ernst Chain and associates developed penicillin as a drug from 1938 and it was introduced to medicine in 1940. Subsequently, various forms of penicillin were developed including benzylpenicillin and phenoxymethyl (penicillin V). The semisynthetic penicillins were obtained by enzymatic removal of a penicillin side chain followed by re-esterification with other acids. This group included cloxacillin, dicloxacillin, floxacillin, methicillin, nafcillin and oxacillin. Another group, the aminopenicillins, included ampicillin and amoxycillin.

Cephalosporins

Guiseppe Brotzu, of the University of Caligari, hypothesized in the mid-1940s that the apparent periodic clearance of microorganisms from the vicinity of a sewage outlet at Caligari was due to the inhibitory effects of substances produced by the fungus *Cephalosporium acremonium chrysogenum*. The substance was identified as cephalosporin C by researchers in Oxford. And so the family of cephalosporins was born. Modified cephalosporins included cephalexin, cephradine, cefaclor, cefadroxil, and others.

Aminoglycosides

The aminoglycosides were all derived from soil organisms. Selman A. Waksman, Albert Schatz and Betty Bugie investigated the Streptomycetes, close relatives of the Actinomycetes. They isolated streptomycin from a strain of *S. griseus* mold obtained from a chicken run. In 1949 Waksman and Lechevalier isolated neomycin from *S. fridiae*. Umezawa and associates, in Japan, discovered kanamycin in samples of *S. kanamyceticus* in 1957. Gentamycin was isolated from *Micromonospora purpurea* (Actinomycete) and described in 1963.

Tetracyclines

The tetracycline antibiotics were developed from systematic screening of soil samples collected from many parts of the world. The sources were *Streptomyces* species, *S. aureofaciens* and *S. rimosus*. The first of the group introduced to clinical practice was chlortetracycline in 1948. Then in 1950 came oxytetracycline and tetracycline in 1952.

Chloramphenicol

This toxic antibiotic, reserved for life-threatening infections, was obtained by Burkholder in 1947 from soil samples collected in Venezuela that contained the Actinomycete, *Streptomyces venezuelae*, but is now obtained by artificial synthesis.

Macrolides

An alternative therapy was found for penicillin-sensitive patients in erythromycin. In 1952 McGuire and associates isolated the antibiotic from *Streptomyces erythreus*, obtained from a soil sample collected in the Philippines. This group also contains the anti-fungal, nystatin.

Peptides

Principally obtained from the *Bacillus* species this group includes bacitracin. The antibiotic was isolated from *B. subtilis* and *B. licheniformis* found in the damaged tissue and street dirt removed from the compound fracture of a young girl named Tracey, in 1943. The name bacitracin comes from 'Bac' and 'Tracey'. Another of this group of antibiotics is polymyxin B and named after *B. polymyxa*, discovered in 1947, in a soil sample obtained from Fukushima Prefecture, Japan.

Antifungal agents

Amphotericin B was found in 1956 by Vandeputte and colleagues in a soil sample that contained the Actinomycete, *Streptomyces nodosus*.

Nystatin was named in 1954 by Dutcher when he obtained the antifungal agent from *Streptomyces noursei* contained in a soil sample in New York State (Ny stat in).

Griseofulvin was discovered by Raistrick and his colleagues in 1939 in an isolate of *Penicillium griseofulvum*. Griseofulvin was first used to treat fungal disease in plants and it was not until 1958 that it was employed in the treatment of animal and human mycoses.

Clotrimazol and the newer antifungal agents are synthetic.

Cytotoxic antibiotics

Actinomycin D and other cytotoxic antibiotics were obtained from various *Streptomyces* species by Waksman and Woodruff in 1940.

Non-microbial sources of antibacterials

Lichens
These have antifungal and bacteriostatic properties related to the osmic and vulpinic acid content.

Monocotyledons
The antibiotic action of garlic is related to its sulfur-containing amino acid, alliine.

Dicotyledons
A number of genera in this plant group contain antibiotics including hops, which contains the ketones, lupulene and humulene.

Marine organisms
Many marine organisms, including the fungus *Cephalosporium acremonium* and *Streptomyces tenjimariensis* SS-939 (and others) have proven antimicrobial activity. Marine organisms are also known to contain antiviral, antitumor, anticoagulant, antiparasitic and anti-inflammatory compounds. They are also the original source of prostaglandins (from the soft coral *Plexaura homolalla*). Seaweeds contain iodine and vitamins and sterilized stipes of *Laminaria digitata* (known as laminaria tents) has been used to dilate the uterine cervix in abortion, in induction of labor and for treatment of primary dysmenorrhea.

Metronidazole

This antimicrobial was discovered as azomycin (2-nitroimidazole) in 1955 by Nakumara, and synthesized in 1959. Metronidazole (Flagyl) was found to have high activity against *Trichomonas vaginalis*, *Entaemeba histolytica* and other microorganisms.

BIOGRAPHIES

Gerhard Domagk (1895–1964)

An extract from an obituary notice for Gerhard Domagk read as follows: 'He became a notable figure in the world of medical science by his reporting (1935) an experiment which made a landmark in the control of bacterial infections. He showed that mice, which usually died within a day or two of an intraperitoneal injection of a culture of streptococci, could survive in good health if they were given a single dose of a single red dye. That at once raised the question would the same drug be effective against the common infections of human beings by similar streptococci?' (Colebrook, 1964).

Domagk was born in the province of Brandenburg, and studied at Kiel University, shortly before the First World War. He was wounded in 1915 and transferred from his Grenadier Regiment to the Medical Corps. Domagk returned to Kiel after the war and graduated in medicine in 1921. He worked at the Pathology Department of the University of Greifswald and then joined the staff of I.G. Farbenindustrie (Bayer dye works) at Wuppertal–Elberfeld where he was appointed Director of Research in 1927, at the age of 32. He carried out research in experimental pathology and bacteriology and continued in the post for the following 37 years.

Domagk's company decided to investigate chemical agents to see which could be used against the most common fatal bacterial infections. Domagk investigated a red azo-dye combined with a sulfonamide radical that had been synthesized by Fritz Mietsch and Joseph Klarer in his own company some years previously, and known as prontosil rubrum. Domagk and his team discovered that prontosil rubrum effectively treated mice which were infected with streptococci. It was already known that streptococci were the cause of puerperal and acute rheumatic fevers, septicemia, cellulitis, erysipelas and inflammatory conditions of the respiratory tract and ear. Clinical testing in humans soon revealed that meningococcal, gonococcal and hemolytic streptococcal infections could all be treated with prontosil.

Domagk completed a survey of the various sulfonamide derivatives and in later life became interested in chemicals and the treatment of cancer. Domagk married Gertrude Strube in 1925. One of their four children was cured of a very severe streptococcal infection by prontosil during the early days of Domagk's research. Domagk was awarded the Nobel Prize for Physiology or Medicine in 1939 in recognition of his pioneering work and was the recipient of many other honors. His colleagues at the Bayer Foundation wrote that 'Domagk devoted himself to the goal of pure medicine to help mankind in disease'. His bibliography ran to seven pages of publications and was included in the obituary penned by Leonard Colebrook.

Sir Alexander Fleming (1881–1955)

Alexander Fleming, born on 6 August 1881, was the youngest of the eight children of an Ayrshire farmer, Hugh Fleming, and his second wife Grace (née Morton). He was educated at the village school in Darvel and for a further two years at Kilmarnock Academy.

Fleming graduated MB in 1908 from London University and a year later took the FRCS. Although he graduated as a surgeon he was invited by Sir Almroth Wright, professor of pathology at St Mary's, to join the Inoculation Department research laboratory. Fleming and Leonard Colebrook (1911) were the first to report on the use of Ehrlich's newly discovered Salvarsan (606) for the treatment of syphilis in Great Britain. During the First World War Fleming served in the Royal Army Medical Corps and worked with Almroth Wright and his team at a laboratory at Boulogne, where Fleming conducted experiments on antiseptics in the treatment of war wounds.

When the War ended, Fleming returned to St Mary's. Towards the end of 1921 he discovered the substance lysozyme, that was present in tissues and was capable of dissolving certain bacteria, an event that intensified his interest in antisepsis and antibiotics. In 1922 he was appointed professor of bacteriology in the University of London, the post being tenable at St Mary's. In 1928 he discovered the antibacterial effects of penicillin. In his 1944 paper on the discovery of penicillin he paid tribute to Florey and Chain: 'its use for practical therapeutic purposes remained in abeyance until the Oxford workers started their investigations'.

During his long career at St Mary's he made many notable contributions to medical progress and was a co-recipient, with Florey and Chain, of the Nobel Prize for Physiology or Medicine in 1945. Fleming was knighted in 1944 and was the first foreign citizen to receive the United States Medal of Merit (Allison, 1956; Colebrook, 1956; Cruickshank, 1956; Dale, 1955).

POSTSCRIPT

The mold used by Sir Alexander Fleming to develop penicillin went under the hammer in Christie's auction house in London in 1998 and was purchased by an American for £8050. The mold plate is engraved on its underside with the inscription 'the mold that makes Penicillin, Alexander Fleming, 1954' and was written a year before Fleming's death.

References

Allison, V. D. (1956). Obituary Notice. Sir Alexander Fleming. *J. General Microbiol.*, **14**, 1–13

American College of Obstetricians and Gynecologists (1997). Human immuno-deficiency virus infections in pregnancy. *Int. J. Obstet. Gynecol.*, 57, 73–80

Bard, S. (1807). *A Compendium of the Theory and Practice of Midwifery*, pp. 192–9. (New York: Collins and Perkins)

Berridge, V. and Strong, P. (1993). *AIDS: A Contemporary History*. (Cambridge: Cambridge University Press)

Bottcher, H. M. (1963). *Miracle Drugs. A History of Antibiotics*, p. 69. (London: Heinemann)

Buehler, J. W., Berkelman, R. L. and Curran, J. W. (1989). Reporting of AIDS; tracking HIV morbidity and mortality. *JAMA*, **262**, 2896–7

Burton, J. (1751). *An Essay Toward a Complete New System of Midwifery, Theoretical and Practical*. (London: J. Hodges)

Calmette, L. C. A., Guerin, C. and Weill-Halle, B. (1924). Essai D'immunisation contre l'infection tuberculeuse. *Bull. Acad. Med.*, (Paris) 3 Ser., 91, 787–96

Calmette, L. C. A., Guerin, C., Negre, L. and Boquet, A. (1927). Sur la Vaccination Preventive des Enfants Nouveau-Nes Contre la Tuberculose par le BCG. *Ann. Inst. Pasteur*, 41, 201–32

Case–Control Study of HIV zero conversion in health-care workers after percutaneous exposure to HIV-infected blood. France, United Kingdom and United States. January 1988–August 1994. (1995). *MMWR*, 44, 929–33

Centers for Disease Control and Prevention (1998). Administration of zidovudine during late pregnancy and delivery to prevent perinatal HIV transmission – Thailand 1996–1998. *MMWR*, 47, 151–4

Chadwick, J. and Mann, W. N. (1983). *Hippocratic Writings*. Translation, pp. 104, 105, 119, 120, 128, 137. (London: Penguin Books)

Chain, E., Florey, H. W., Gardner, A. D., Heatley, N. G., Jennings, M. A., Orr-Ewing, J. and Sanders, A. G. (1940). Penicillin as a chemotherapeutic agent. *The Lancet*, August 24, 226–8

Chin, J. and Mann, J. M. (1997). Global Surveillance and Forecasting of AIDS. *Bull. WHO*, **336**, 1–7

Colebrook, L. and Kenny, M. (1936). Treatment of human puerperal infections, and of experimental infections in mice, with prontosil. *The Lancet*, **1**, 1279–86

Colebrook, L. (1956). Alexander Fleming, 1881–1955. *Biogr. Mem. Fellows R. Soc.*, **2**, 117–27

Colebrook, L. (1964). Gerhard Domagk, 1895–1964. *Biogr. Mem. Fellows R. Soc.*, **10**, 39–50

Collins, R. (1841). *A Practical Treatise on Midwifery*, Containing the result of 16 654 births, occurring in the Dublin Lying-in Hospital during a period of seven years commencing November, 1826. pp. 228–74. (Boston: William D. Ticknor)

Connor, E. M., Sperling, R. S., Gelber, R., Kiselev, P., Scott, G., *et al.* (1994). Pediatric AIDS clinical trail group protocol 076 study group. Reduction of maternal-infant transmission of human immuno-deficiency virus type 1 with zidovudine treatment. *N. Eng. J. Med.*, **331**, 1173–80

Cruickshank, R. (1956). Obituary Notice. Sir Alexander Fleming. *J. Pathol. Bacteriol.*, 72, 697–708

Dale, H. H. (1955). Obituary. Sir Alexander Fleming. *BMJ*, **1**, 732–5, 795

Dancer, S. J., Shears, P. and Platt, D. J. (1997). Isolation and characterization of coliforms from glacial ice and water in Canada's High Arctic. *J. Appl. Bacteriol.*, 82, 597–609

Denman, T. (1801). *An Introduction to the Practice of Midwifery*, Vol. 2, pp. 444, 493. (London: J. Johnson)

Dillner, L. (1997). HIV may be eliminated from reservoirs of infection in the Body. *BMJ*, **314**, 1436

Domagk, G. (1935). Ein beitrag zur Chemotherapie der Bakterillen infektionen. *Dtsch. Med. Wochsch.*, **61**, 250–3

Easterbrook, P. and Ippolito, G. (1997). Prophylaxis after occupational exposure to HIV. *BMJ*, **315**, 557–8

Ehrlich, P. and Hata, S. (1910). *Die experimentelle Chemotherapie der Spirillosen (Syphilis, Ruckfallfieber, Huhnerspirillose, Frambosie)* (Berlin: J. Springer)

Fleming, A. and Colebrook, L. (1911). On the use of Salvarsan in the treatment of syphilis. *The Lancet*, **1**, 1631

Fleming, A. (1929). On the anti-bacterial action of cultures of a *Penicillium*, with special reference to their use in the isolation of *B. influenzae*. *B. J. Exp. Pathol.*, X(4), 226–37

Fleming, A. (1944). The Discovery of Penicillin. *Br. Med. Bull.*, **2**, 4–5

Florey, H. W., Chain, E., Heatley, N. G., Jennings, M. A., Sanders, A. G., Abraham, E. P. and Florey, M. E. (1949). *Antibiotics*. Two Volumes. (London: New York, Toronto: Geoffrey Cumberlege, Oxford University Press)

Fox, R. (1996). The Post-Antibiotic Era Beckons. *J. R. Soc. Med.*, **89**, 602–3

Goodwin, M. S. and Moore, J. E. (1946). Penicillin in prevention of pre-natal syphilis. *JAMA*, **130**, 688–94

Gordon, A. (1795). *A Treatise on the Epidemic Puerperal Fever of Aberdeen*. (London: G. G. & J. Robinson)

Gottlieb, S. (1998). Where now for AIDS Vaccines? *BMJ*, **317**, 163

Hare, R. (1970). *The Birth of Penicillin and the Disarming of Microbes*, p.132. (London: Allen & Unwin Ltd.)

Hensyl, W. R. (ed.) (1990). *Stedman's Medical Dictionary* 25th ed. p. 93. (Baltimore: Williams and Wilkins)

Holmes, O. W. (1843). The Contagiousness of Puerperal Fever. *N. Eng. Quart. J. Med. Surg.*, **1**, 503–30

Kaplan, I. W. (1942). *Condylomata acuminata. New Orleans Med. Surg. J.*, **94**, 388–90

Koch, R. (1881). Ueber Desinfection. *Mitt. K. Gesundheitsamte*, **1**, 234–82

Koch, R. (1882). Die aetiologie der Tuberkulose. *Berl. Klin. Wochschr.*, **19**, 221–30

Koop, C. E. (1986). The Surgeon General's Report on the Acquired Immune Deficiency Syndrome. *JAMA*, **256**(20), 2784–9

Leading Article (1944). Penicillin in gonorrhoea. *The Lancet*, **1**, 345–6

Leake, J. (1772). *Practical Observations on the Child-bed Fever*. (London: J. W. Walter)

Lemaire, F. J. (1860). *Du Coaltar Saponine, Desinfectant Energique*. (Paris: Germer-Bailliere)

Mahoney, J. F., Arnold, R. C. and Harris A. D. (1943). Penicillin treatment of early syphilis – a preliminary report. *Am. J. Public Health*, **33**, 1387–91

Mauriceau, F. (1686). *The Diseases of Women with Child*, pp. 334–7. Translated by Hugh Chamberlen. (London: John Darby)

Mosteig-Moorhof, A. Von (1882). Der Jodoform-Verband. *Samml. Klin. Vortr., Leipzig*, **211**. (Chir., 68), 1811–4

McGrew, R. E. (1985). *Encyclopedia of Medical History*, pp. 246–50. (London: Macmillan Press)

Neisser, A. (1879). Ueber eine der Gonorrhea eigentumliche Micrococcusform. *Centralbl. F. D. Med. Wissensch.*, **17**, 497–500

Newman Dorland, W. A. (1932). *The American Illustrated Medical Dictionary*, pp. 953, 1062. (Philadelphia and London: W. B. Saunders Co.)

O'Dowd, M. J. and Philipp, E. (1994). *The History of Obstetrics and Gynaecology*, pp. 219–47. (New York and London: Parthenon Publishing)

Oriel, J. D. (1994). *The Scars of Venus*. (London: Springer-Verlag)

Pasteur, L. (1879). Septicemie Puerperale. *Bull. Acad. Med.*, (*Paris*) 2 Ser., **8**, 505–8

Quetel, C. (1990). *History of Syphilis*. (Cambridge: Polity Press)

Raynold, T. (1545). *The Byrth of Mankynde*, Folio 77. (London: Tho. Ray)

Rowland, B. (1981). *Medieval Woman's Guide to Health*, pp. 115–19. (London: Croom Helm)

Ryan, F. (1992). *Tuberculosis: The Greatest Story Never Told*. (Worcestershire, UK: Swift Publishers)

Schatz, A., Bugie, E. and Waksman, S. A. (1944). Streptomycin, a Substance exhibiting antibiotic activity against gram-positive and gram-negative bacteria. *Proc. Soc. Exp. Biol.*, (*N.Y.*), **55**, 66–9

Semba, R. D., Miotti, P. G., Chiphangwi, J. D., *et al.* (1994). Maternal vitamin A deficiency and mother to child transmission of HIV-1. *The Lancet*, **343**, 1593–7

Semmelweis, I. P. (1861). *Die Aetiologie, der Begriff und de Prophylaxis des Kindbettfiebres*, pp. 554–61. (Leipzig: C. A. Hartleben)

Semmelweis, I. P. (1847/48). Hochst wichtige erfahrungen uber die aetiologie der in Gebaranstalten Epidemischen Puerperal Feber. *Z. K. K. Ges. Aerzte Wien*, **4**(2), 242–4

Semmelweis, I. P. (1849). Hochst wichtige erfahrungen uber die aetiologie der in Gebaranstalten Epidemischen Puerperal Feber. *Z. K. K. Ges. Aerzte Wien*, **5**, 64–5

Serullas, G. S. (1822). Memoire sur l'iodure de potassium, l'acide hydriodique et sur un compose nouveau de carbone, d'iode et d'hydrogene. *Ann. Chim. Phys.*, **2**, Ser., **20**, 163–8

Sidley, P. (1998). South African AIDS plan criticized. *BMJ*, **317**, 1032

Taha, T. E., Biggar, R. J., Broadhead, R. L., *et al.* (1997). Effect of cleansing the birth canal with antiseptic solution on maternal and newborn morbidity and mortality in Malawi: clinical trial. *BMJ*, **315**, 216–20

Temkin, O. (1956). *Soranus Gynecology*, pp. 143–8. (Baltimore & London: The Johns Hopkins University Press)

Wainright, M. and Swan, H. T. (1986). C. G. Paine and the earliest surviving clinical records of penicillin therapy. *Medical History*, **30**, 42–56

Weissmann, G. (1997). Puerperal Priority. *The Lancet*, **349**, 122–5

White, C. (1773). *A Treatise on the Management of Pregnant and Lying-in Women*. (London: E. & C. Dilly)

World Health Organization AIDS – Global Week. (1995). *Weekly Epidemiol. Rec.*, **70**, 353–5

Blood transfusion and rhesus disease

20

INTRODUCTION

It is a truism that blood transfusion had a major impact on the materia medica of women in the twentieth century, sufficient to promote the life-supporting red liquid to the ranks of an ambrosia for mere mortals. The medical historian Harvey Graham (a pseudonym for an eminent British surgeon and medical writer) declared that 'Blood transfusion may be said to have solved the problems of haemorrhage. Its effects have been most dramatic in cases of post-partum haemorrhage'. Blood transfusion 'also proved its worth in cases of placenta praevia ... [and] whenever caesarean section is performed' (Graham, 1950). Transfusion was a life-saver in many cases of maternal hemorrhage and of course many infants affected by congenital hemolytic anemia were rescued by exchange blood transfusion. In the 'developed' world the availability of antibiotics and blood replacement therapy reduced maternal mortality rates from almost 800 per 100 000 births in the 1920s to less than 20 per 100 000 in the late 1980s.

In the early nineteenth century Paul Scheel (1773–1811) wrote a history of the achievements in the field of intravenous injections and transfusions since the seventeenth century. His two-volume work entitled *Die Transfusion des Blutes und Einsprutzung der Arzneyen in die Adern* (Copenhagen: F. Brummer) 1802–1803 was improved by the addition of a third volume in 1828 by J.F. Dieffenbach. The details of the 'History of Blood Transfusion' from antiquity until the early 1940s were related by Nobel Suydam Maluf (1954) in the *Journal of the History of Medicine.*

The history of congenital hemolytic (rhesus disease) has played itself out almost entirely in this century and John T. Queenan (1971) of New York wrote that 'in the short span of three decades, we have witnessed discovery of the Rh antigens; systematic detection of Rh immunization; exchange transfusions; preterm delivery; amniotic fluid analysis; intrauterine transfusion; and, finally, prevention of Rh immunization'. In the United Kingdom it was estimated that deaths attributed to rhesus immunization had fallen from a figure of 46 per 1000 births before 1969 to 1.6 per 1000 in 1990 due to the introduction of RhoGam (anti-D) (Mollison *et al.*, 1997).

MYTHOLOGY

According to Harvey Graham (1950) 'The idea of blood transfusion was an old one, as old as Medea who, according to an ancient myth, was able to renew youth by transfusion'. In ancient Rome, Ovidius, the Roman poet, related that Princess Medea rejuvenated the aged Prince Aeson by slitting his throat, exsanguinating him, and then filling his ancient veins with rich elixir of witches' brew. That story may have led on to the vampiric custom of drinking the blood of fallen gladiators, or that obtained from slitting the veins of youths, as rejuvenating potions. In the centuries that followed the fall of Rome there were many instances of blood being given as an oral medication. Many gods of Europe, Asia and parts of Africa sucked or drank blood and the European myth of vampirism may have had its origin in the legend of Gilgamesh of ancient Babylonia. In pre-Columbian Mexico the vampires were women who died in childbirth. The red-headed Dublin writer Abraham Stoker (1847–1912) created the ultimate European bloodsucker, Dracula.

A medical episode from the *Tain Bo Cuailnge* (The Cattle Raid of Cooley), an epic Irish Iron Age tale, tells the story of the warrior Cethern, a friend of the hero of the Tain, Cuchulainn by name. During a cattle raid Cethern was set upon by two great warriors and, being badly wounded, he turned for advice to the healer Fingin. Cethern was given the choice to either treat his sickness for a whole year and live out his normal life span, or to get enough strength quickly in three days and three nights to fit him to fight his enemies. The healer went to Cuchulainn with a request for bone marrow. Cuchulainn took what cattle he could round up and made a mash of marrow out of their bones. Cethern was steeped in the mixture for three days and nights. The marrow found its way through the many lacerations in his skin and, following his successful 'transfusion', he made a marvelous recovery, re-engaged in battle and wrought havoc among his enemies until he eventually succumbed (Kinsella, 1970).

THE EARLY DAYS

Andreas Libavius (1546–1616)

According to Nobel Maluf (1954) of the Columbia Presbyterian Hospital, New York, the first description of transfusion was that of Andreas Libavius of Halle in Saxony, a chemist/physician and Director of the College at Coburg. In 1615 he described the passage of arterial blood from a youth into the artery of an aged man via silver tubes, as a rejuvenating technique. The technique was copied by a number of European physicians.

William Harvey (1578–1657)

William Harvey conducted crucial experiments on animals that established the existence of the pulmonary and general circulations in 1616. His findings were outlined in his *Exercitatio Anatomica de Motu Cordis et Sanguinis* (1628). It is generally held that the discovery of the circulation of the blood was the greatest physiological event of all time. William Harvey studied at Cambridge and completed his medical education at Padua, the leading European school of medicine. In 1602, he returned to England and began medical practice in London. Sixteen years later he was appointed Physician Extraordinary to James I and later to Charles I. Harvey was a skilled anatomist and embryologist and in his *De Generatione Animalium* (1651) he formulated the first fundamentally new theory of generation since antiquity. Harvey's work on the circulation led to the first attempted blood transfusion some 50 years later.

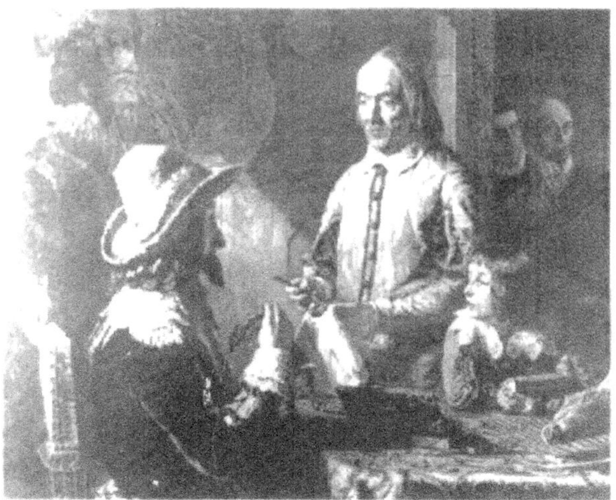

Figure 1 William Harvey (1578–1657)

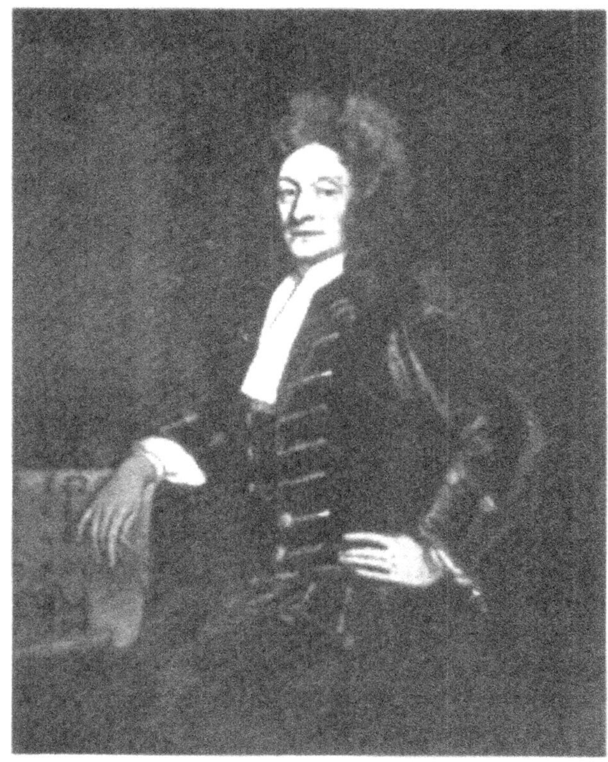

Figure 2 Sir Christopher Wren (1632–1723). From Keys, *History of Surgical Anesthesia* (1945)

Sir Christopher Wren (1632–1723)

Another influential scientist of the time was Sir Christopher Wren. He was one of the first to document intravenous therapy when he injected ale and wine into a hunting dog until it became extremely drunk. Wren was a renowned English architect, mathematician and scientist who redesigned many of the great churches of London after the Great Fire of 1666, the most famous of which was St Paul's Cathedral, completed in 1710. Wren was educated at Oxford University and became Professor of Astronomy at Gresham College, London.

Jean Denis (d. 1704)

Jean Baptiste Denis of Montpellier, philosopher and mathematician, and physician to Louis XIV, succeeded in making the first successful blood transfusion in a human. This was on the 15 of June 1667, in a 15-year-old boy who was in a shocked condition as a result of repeated purgings and more than 20 venesections administered by his physicians. Denis transfused 9 ounces of lamb's blood, from the carotid artery. The youngster improved and there were no long-lasting effects (Denis, 1667).

In 1667 Denis transfused a male house-servant, Antoine Mauroy, with calf's blood in an attempt to dampen the newly-wed's extramarital affairs. The calf was chosen as the animal was so docile and it was hoped that the calf's spirit would pass over in its transfused blood. As luck would have it, all went well with the procedure, and so, for good measure, it was repeated on a second occasion. However, Mauroy developed chest pain and passed dark bloody urine – the first reported blood transfusion reaction. Despite the novel treatments, the man continued his wayward romps and his agitated wife insisted upon another blood transfusion. The man died on the following night and Jean Denis was tried for manslaughter, but exonerated. Blood transfusion fell into disrepute and some years later the French Parliament prohibited the technique, until the nineteenth century.

Johann Sigmund Elsholtz (1623–1688)

Jean Denis' German contemporary, Johann Sigmund Elsholtz, conducted similar transfusion experiments and his book, *Clysmatica Nova, Oder Newe Clystier-Kunst* (1665), dealt with intravenous infusion of medications and also blood transfusion, although it is uncertain if he actually conducted blood transfusions himself. The book contained the first illustration of an intravenous injection into a man, using a syringe. Elsholtz, who was physician to the Baron of Brandenburg, suggested that blood transfusions exchanged between husband and wife might settle marital discord (Maluf, 1954).

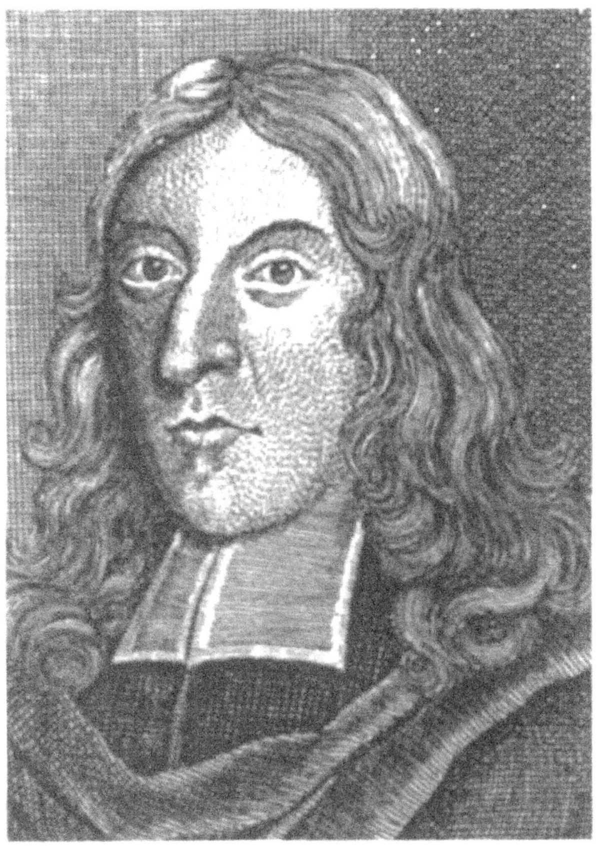

Figure 3 Richard Lower (1631–1691)

Richard Lower (1631–1691)

Although he attempted his first animal blood transfusion in February 1665, Richard Lower did not describe it until the following year, in the *Philosophical Transactions* (1665–66). Some five months after Jean Denis first transfused blood into a human, Lower and Edmund King, on 23 November 1667 transfused sheeps' blood into a Bachelor of Theology from Cambridge whose brain was considered 'a little too warm'. The proximal portion of a sheep's carotid was canulated with a silver tube; a similar tube was inserted into the man's vein; both silver tubes were connected by quills. After the operation the man found himself quite well (Lower, 1667). This was the first transfusion of blood performed in a human in England (Maluf, 1954). The event was witnessed by the English diarist Samuel Pepys (Pepys, 1972).

Lower recorded direct blood transfusion in animals in his *Tractatus de Corde* (1669). He detailed the first exchange transfusion of blood between two dogs. In his experiments Lower also used sheep's blood for transfusion, 8 to 16 ounces at a time. Most of his blood transfusions were homologous, that is, between animals of the same species.

James Blundell (1790–1877)

Interest in the therapeutic aspects of blood transfusion was aroused again in the eighteenth century. The London-based obstetrician, James Blundell, observed at first hand the disastrous consequences of obstetric hemorrhage. Moved by the plight of women who developed hypovolemic shock and died from postpartum hemorrhage, Blundell (1818) set about experimenting with transfusion techniques in dogs and soon published his first paper on the topic. In the early days of his experimentation he championed the notion of indirect transfusion. Blood was removed from the femoral artery of the donor dog with a specially constructed 2-ounce syringe and then injected into the femoral vein of another dog.

Blundell (1819) carried out the first transfusion of human blood at the beginning of the nineteenth century. Twelve to 14 ounces of blood from several donors were passed via a funnel and syringe, but the male recipient died 56 hours later. Blundell (1828) made the first human-to-human transfusion in which the patient did not die and reported this momentous achievement to the *Lancet*. His patient was a woman suffering from hemorrhage during childbirth, and he secured a surprisingly favorable result. He subsequently described about 10 cases over the following decade (Blundell, 1828–29).

Blundell suggested blood transfusion only for hemorrhage which endangered life and he was one of the first to proclaim that that blood could not be shared between animals and humans. He taught that blood transfusion would prevent death from hemorrhage; that only human blood should be transfused; and that venous blood was as satisfactory as arterial

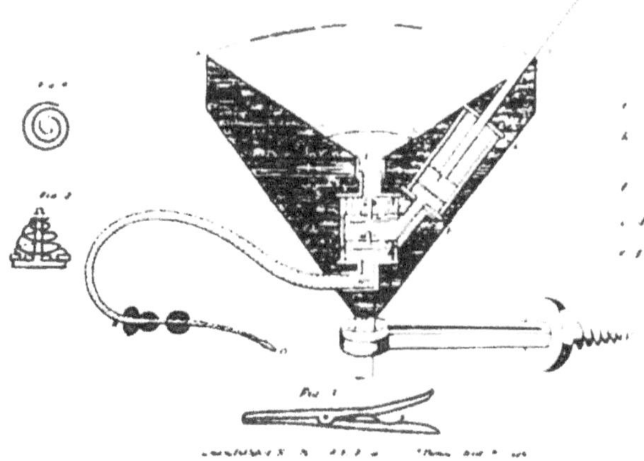

Figure 4 James Blundell's impellor

blood. Blundell's defended his stance on blood transfusion in a realistic fashion: 'the more the discussion, the more objection and defense it has to undergo, the better. If it be grounded in error let it perish; if in just principles, it must survive' (1834). Despite his innovative work on the subject Blundell's successors at Guy's Hospital rarely carried out blood transfusions. They, and many of their colleagues, resorted to the less risky procedure of saline infusion in the bleeding patient (Munro Kerr, 1954).

Blundell (1827) was one of the first to advise hysterectomy at the time of cesarean section in an effort to diminish the mortality associated with the operation. He also first recommended the lateral division of the fallopian tubes as a method of contraception to prevent the hazards of dystocia in women with contracted pelves (Blundell, 1834). He (1839) believed that puerperal fever was passed on by 'Gossiping friends, wet nurses, monthly nurses, the practitioner himself, these are the channels by which, as I suspect, the infection is principally conveyed', and he was also a pioneer of ovariotomy in animals.

BLOOD PRESSURE

Stephen Hales (1677–1761), an English clergyman, conducted seminal work on the elucidation of the principles of blood pressure. Using brass pipes and glass tubes inserted in the left crural artery, he found that the blood rose to 8 feet and 3 inches above the level of the left ventricle of the heart, and that the blood rose and fell between 2 and 4 inches with each heart beat. In 1828, Jean Leonard Marie Poiseuille of Paris improved upon Hale's method by substituting a mercury manometer. It later became apparent that the measurement of blood pressure was a valuable test in the diagnosis and monitoring of treatment in cardiovascular shock related to blood loss.

ANTICOAGULANTS

A major problem with blood transfusion was the normal process of coagulation. The English obstetrician John Braxton Hicks (1823–1897) found he could counteract the coagulation process by mixing blood with a solution of phosphate of soda. No side effects occurred in animals transfused with blood and phosphate of soda, so Hicks then tried anticoagulated blood in three women with obstetrical hemorrhage. The patients rallied temporarily but all eventually died from shock (Hicks, 1868, 1869). Hicks (1872) is better known for the eponymous Braxton Hicks (uterine) contractions that may be noted by women throughout pregnancy.

In the early 1900s it was discovered that whipping or twirling of blood resulted in deposition of fibrin on the churning instrument and that blood clotting could be prevented. The incoagulable defibriniated blood was capable of resuscitating animals or humans in shock due to hemorrhage but it became general opinion that whole blood would be a better treatment. Arthur Ronald Kimpton and James Howard Brown (1913) reported a novel approach to the problem of apparatus-induced coagulation when they used instruments lined with paraffin wax to prevent blood clotting during transfusion.

In the following year Albert Hustin (1914) of Belgium reported the use of sodium citrate and glucose to prevent coagulation of blood in an anemic 20-year-old who had suffered a bowel hemorrhage. Shortly afterwards, Luis Agote (1915) of Buenos Aires was one of a number of clinicians to popularize the transfusion of citrated blood and soon Braxton Hicks' phosphate of soda became obsolete. The advent of citrated blood popularized both direct and indirect blood transfusion and also meant that blood could be stored in a cold bank. Significant experience of citrated blood transfusion only began following 2 April 1917 when the USA joined the Allies in the First World War. In 1922 it was shown that citrated human blood could be kept in good condition in an ice box for a period of up to 4 weeks.

During the 1920s and 1930s, blood transfusions were followed by febrile and 'chill' reactions in 20% of cases. Febrile reactions were attributed to the inherent nature of the process of blood transfusion and the possible toxicity of citrate. Richard Lewisohn and N. Rosenthal (1933) of New York were aware that febrile reactions also followed the transfusion of plain dextrose. When the transfusion apparatus was properly cleansed and sterilized, and triple-distilled water used to dissolve the citrate, the incidence of chills and fevers fell to 1%.

Transfusions of human cadaver blood were attempted in Russia in the 1930s but did not prove practicable. Howkins and Brewer (1939), of London and Cambridge, respectively, experimented with transfusion of placental blood. They found that the average placenta could yield about 50 ml of blood, but contamination was present in a quarter of cases so transfusion of the product was not safe.

The first blood bank in the United States was set up at the Mayo Clinic, Rochester, in 1935 (Maluf, 1954). Soon afterwards, Bernard Fantus (1937) described the establishment of a Blood Bank at the Cook County Hospital. Around the same time, blood banks were set up in Europe and Russia. During the Spanish Civil War (1937–1939) blood was stored in large refrigerators and during that conflict transfusion of stored blood had a remarkable impact in the reduction of deaths from hemorrhage. Blood transfusion became widely available towards the end of the Second World War.

METHODS OF TRANSFUSION

In the early days, the transfusionist withdrew blood from a donor via a syringe and injected it into the recipient's vein. As the technique advanced it became a very complicated affair. The median basilic veins were dissected in both recipient and donor. An anastomoses was formed between both and blood flow was halted when it was estimated that sufficient blood had gone to the recipient. A Leipzig internist, Hugh Wilhelm von Ziemssen (1892), introduced hollow metal needles for collection of blood from donor veins. He then transfused the blood by subcutaneous injection but later resorted to intravenous injection of

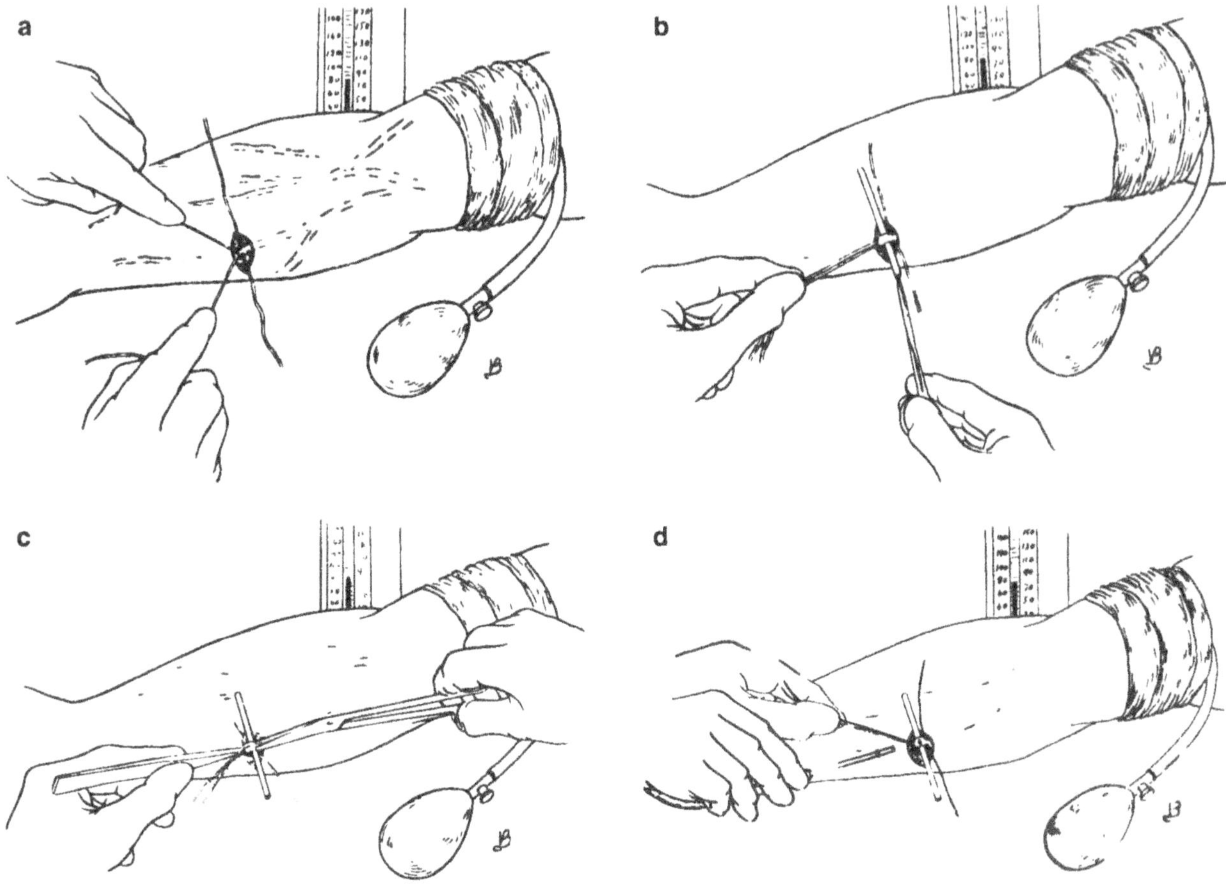

Figure 5 Methods of blood transfusion. From Bonney, *A Textbook of Gynaecological Surgery* (1947)

blood through the same hollow needles. His technique was not copied until well into the twentieth century.

In the meantime, transfusion became an experimental procedure requiring a high degree of surgical skill. Innovators in the field were the Americans, Alexis Carrel (1873–1944) and George Crile (1864–1943). They connected the donor's arterial system directly to the recipient's venous system. The technique of vascular anastomosis was accomplished by the use of guide sutures and intima-to-intima apposition of artery and vein to reduce the problem of blood clotting during transfusion (Carrel, 1907). Groups of skilled transfusionists who performed direct transfusions abounded in the larger cities until the advent of blood banking and the re-introduction of the needle cannula by E. Lindeman (1913), an internist at the Bellevue Hospital.

The importance of blood loss and its relationship to shock was investigated by Crile before the First World War. At that time, hypovolemic shock was treated with cardiotonics and infusions of saline or glucose solutions. During the First World War it was found that infusions of gum acacia were preferable. The Swedish researchers Anders Gronwall and Bjorn Ingleman (1944) introduced dextran as a plasma substitute.

BLOOD GROUPS

It was known from the seventeenth century that incompatible blood transfusions caused disastrous reactions, including kidney damage and death, but it was not until the twentieth century that sufficient progress was made in the understanding of immunology to explain what the actual problem was. An answer was in sight when in 1875 the German physiologist Leonard Landois demonstrated that the black urine that was passed following transfusion of blood from a different species was due to breakdown of the

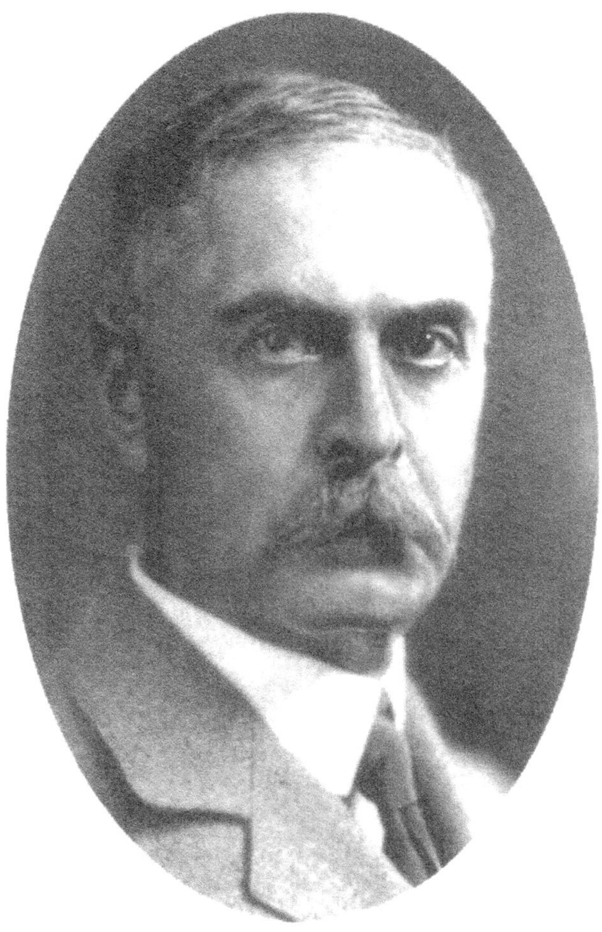

Figure 6 Carl Landsteiner (1868–1943)

incompatible red blood cells and their subsequent elimination through the renal tract (O'Dowd and Philipp, 1994).

What happened in the different animal species also occurred with humans and a person's blood could not always be given to another human with safety. The reason for that incompatibility was finally explained by Carl Landsteiner (1900) of the Institute of Pathological Anatomy at the University of Vienna. He and his coworkers demonstrated that mixing red cells of one person with the serum taken from another sometimes resulted in agglutination, that is, a clumping together of the red cells and later called isoagglutination. They discovered, in a study of 22 adults, that human blood contained naturally occurring antibodies which reacted with antigens of other humans (Landsteiner, 1901). Those red cell antigens were named A and B and due to Landsteiner's experiments the classical A B O blood group system was formulated. The original ABO classification divided the human race into four groups, A, B, AB and O. Group O had neither A nor B antigens on their red cells, and could donate blood with safety to persons of all groups and became known as universal donors. Group AB individuals had neither anti-A nor anti-B in their serum and could receive blood of any group with safety and were known as universal recipients.

In 1908, Ottenberg of the Laboratory of Biological Chemistry at Columbia University, began to test the blood of both potential donor and recipient before each transfusion, and in his paper in the *Journal of Experimental Medicine* (1911) he endorsed the use of preliminary agglutination tests before blood transfusions. In the same year he coined the term 'universal donor'.

In 1927 other human blood systems were found and given the names M, N and P. By 1928 Landsteiner had discovered that instead of the four groups he initially proposed there were at least 36 varieties. Landsteiner's discovery of the existence of definite blood groups opened the way for safety in blood transfusion, as proper crossmatching eliminated the problem of blood group reactions, and so transfusion was safe between persons of the same blood group. In recognition of his research on blood groups and immunology Landsteiner, originally from Vienna but domiciled in the USA, received the Nobel Prize for Physiology or Medicine in 1930. As time went by, further progress was made and other important blood groups were discovered, including the Lutheran system of 1945; the Kell and Lewis of 1946; Duffy of 1950 and the Kidd system of 1951 (Lawler and Lawler, 1957).

BLOOD TRANSFUSION IN OBSTETRICS

In olden days writers referred to binding of the limbs with bandages and this became known as 'autotransfusion' (Munro Kerr, 1954), while the practice of umbilical cord milking was used for resuscitation of the newborn. The first real obstetric interventions came with the research of James Blundell and John Braxton Hicks in the early nineteenth century. Many other obstetricians were also interested in the potential applications of blood transfusions. Walter Channing (1848) of Boston, famed for his work on anesthesia and analgesia in pregnancy, gave an early description of hemolytic anemia in pregnancy and suggested the possibility that blood transfusion could be helpful.

In 1877 Lombe Atthill of the Rotunda Hospital, Dublin, recommended blood transfusion in the treatment of postpartum hemorrhage (O'Donel Browne, 1947) at a time when that particular complication was dreaded by mothers and obstetricians alike. At the dawn of the twentieth century, John Whitridge Williams (1903), professor of obstetrics at Johns Hopkins, wrote in his tract on postpartum hemorrhage that elevation of the foot of the bed and the application of hot bottles or bricks to the extremities will be all that is needed. 'In more severe cases, the administration of one-thirtieth grain of strychnine hypodermically, is attended by excellent results, supplemented by hypodermic injections of whisky or ether. Hot rectal enemata of equal parts of black coffee and salt solution are also valuable'.

'When the patient is profoundly shocked, a sterile normal salt solution in large quantities – 500 cc being injected under each breast – will prove the best restorative. When the condition is very serious and a suitable cannula is available, even more striking results may be obtained by administering it intravenously.' Perchloride of iron, or glycerin, or ice cold or very hot water were applied as intrauterine styptic douches in cases of postpartum hemorrhage in an effort to control the blood loss, but blood transfusions were not available for volume replacement. The douches and the instrumentation involved often led to sepsis and death.

Blood transfusion was not only of major benefit in cases of postpartum hemorrhage but also in those instances of ruptured ectopic pregnancy. The Charity Hospital of Louisiana, New Orleans, surveyed 1000 cases of ectopic pregnancy that were treated from 1906 to 1946. It was discovered that the maternal mortality fell from almost 13% to just about 3% due to the use of blood transfusion. W.A. Scott reviewed almost 13 000 deliveries from the Toronto General Hospital between 1931 and 1943. Of nine women who had lost more than a liter of blood and who showed all the signs of severe shock, six died. Thanks to prompt transfusion there were no deaths in 190 women who had lost up to a liter of blood (Graham, 1950).

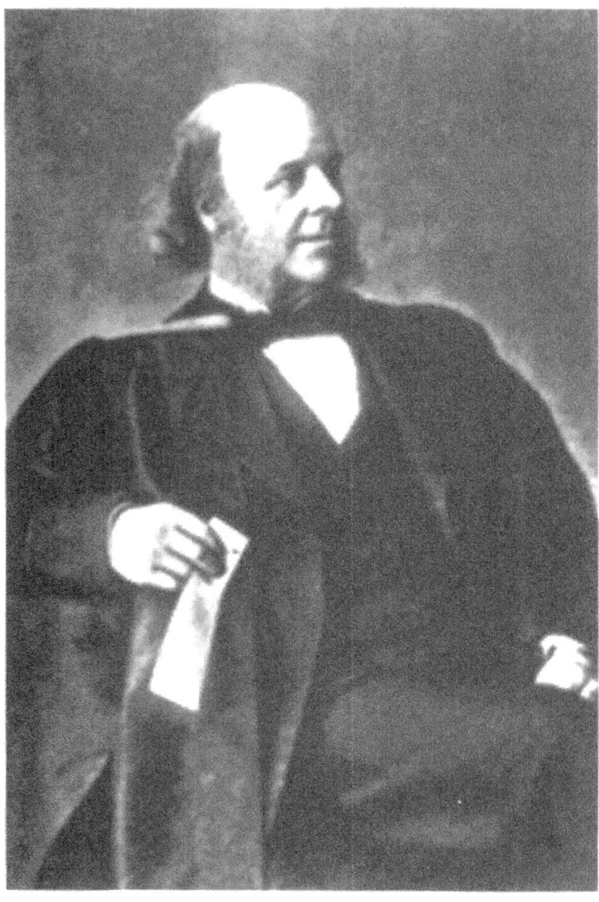

Figure 7 John Braxton Hicks (1825–1897)

Harmful effects of blood transfusion

Severe illness or death, related to incompatibility, were the main side effects of blood transfusion in the early days of the technique. Febrile reactions were related to improper sterilizing techniques. Many patients were under- or over-transfused. Unexpected non-fatal immune reactions also occurred and, until the rhesus factor was discovered, many rhesus-negative mothers were adversely affected by transfusion of ABO compatible, but rhesus-positive blood. In recent times the focus dwelt on the transmission of viral infections via blood products.

So, although blood and blood products such as red cells, platelets, fresh frozen plasma and anti-D (Rho-gam) have saved countless lives and averted untold morbidity, those same products also had the potential to cause harm. It is estimated, in the United States for instance, that about 4% of patients who received a blood transfusion were infected with hepatitis C virus (that may lead to hepatic cirrhosis and/or hepatocellular carcinoma). Administration of anti-D in the years 1977–1978 and also 1991–1993 was responsible for a number of women developing hepatitis C infection in Ireland (Power *et al.*, 1995). The potential risk of other viral infections being acquired through blood products reduced the desire of many people to avail of a blood transfusion, even if indicated from a clinical point of view. This led to a move towards autologous blood transfusion.

CONGENITAL HEMOLYTIC DISEASE – RHESUS DISEASE

James Ballantyne (1892) observed in his book *The Diseases and Deformities of the Foetus* that the amniotic fluid and vernix caseosa were bile-stained in pregnancies complicated by what we now know to be congenital hemolytic disease (CHD) or rhesus disease. The disease manifested itself in a variety of ways and in the mid-twentieth century the three most widely recognized variants of CHD were known as fetal hydrops, icterus (Greek, jaundice) gravis neonatorum and congenital anemia. The most common clinical findings in CHD were hemolytic anemia, generalized edema or jaundice, splenomegaly, hepatomegaly and an increase in the number of immature red blood cells in the circulation. The most common histologic change was the presence of widespread extramedullary erythropoiesis.

Edith L. Potter, assistant professor of pathology, Department of Obstetrics and Gynecology, University of Chicago and the Chicago Lying-in Hospital, outlined the history of CHD prior to 1941: 'The fact that universal edema of the fetus, icterus gravis neonatorum and anemia of the newborn are different clinical manifestations of a single pathologic process was not generally appreciated until the early 1930s, although each had been individually recognized many years earlier … it was not until after 1910 when Schridde

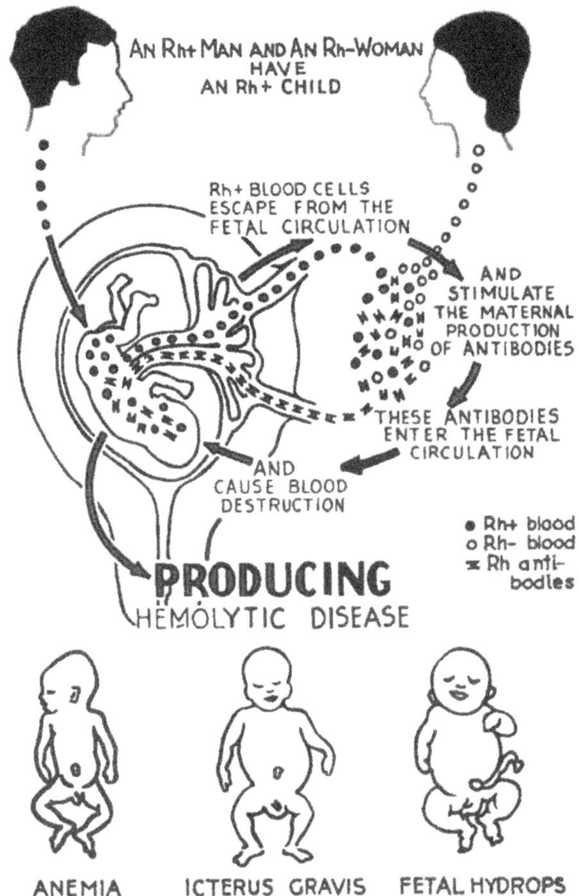

Figure 8 Congenital hemolytic disease. From Potter, *Rh. Its Relation Congenital Hemolytic Disease* (1947)

(1910) described an abnormality of the hemopoietic system as the cause of certain cases of general edema that the relation between edema and an abnormality in erythrocyte formation was generally appreciated'.

Icterus gravis neonatorum was characterized by severe icterus that had a very poor prognosis and the disease often affected several children in a family: 'the term erythroblastosis was introduced by Rautman (1912) to designate the organ changes found in association with icterus gravis and in many cases of universal edema' (Ecklin, 1918–1919). The concept of erythroblastosis fetalis as a single disease with various clinical manifestations, all of which were due to the same underlying pathologic process was presented by Diamond, Blackfan and Baty (1932).

However, it was not until 1956 that Bevis devised the means of avoiding a fetal death by showing that the concentration of bilirubin in amniotic fluid correlated with the severity of erythroblastosis fetalis. Several years later, Liley demonstrated that amniocentesis and amniotic fluid analysis, used in a systematic manner, to aid obstetric intervention, could decrease the perinatal mortality rate in rhesus-immunized patients from 22% to 9% (Queenan, 1971).

Macaca mulatta – the rhesus monkey

In spite of the many precautions taken in preparation for transfusion, serious reactions occasionally occurred. By 1940 it was apparent that almost all the transfusion reactions could not be explained on the basis of ABO incompatibility. An answer to the problem was on hand from the work of Karl Landsteiner and Alexander Wiener. In 1937 they found that rabbits injected with the blood from the rhesus monkey, *Macaca mulatta*, responded by producing agglutinins that were specific for the M substance in human cells. Three years later they reported that 39 of 45 tested samples of human red cells shared an antigen with the red cells of rhesus monkeys (Landsteiner and Wiener, 1940). The antibody in the rabbit serum was called anti-rhesus and the people whose red cells were agglutinated by it were called rhesus positive. Those whose red cells were not agglutinated were called rhesus negative. The first two letters of the word rhesus were used to name the new antibody and it became known as anti-Rh.

Further research revealed that Rh antibodies did not occur naturally in the blood and that they were found only as a result of the introduction of the Rh antigen into the body of a susceptible individual. Soon after the discovery of the new agglutinin, Wiener and Peters studied the blood of patients who had suffered severe transfusion reactions. They demonstrated the presence of antibodies whose action paralleled that of the antibodies in the anti-Rh serum. They thus proved that the substance first revealed by the use of the serum from monkeys actually existed in human blood and that it was capable of exerting an antigenic action. They also discovered that the Rh factor was inherited as a Mendelian dominant (Potter, 1947).

Philip Levine and Rufus Stetson (1939) reported a case of stillbirth in a mother found to have antibodies in her blood. They concluded that the fetus must have inherited an antigen from the father that was responsible for the maternal immunization. In a further review of cases related to pregnancy, Wiener and Peters (1940) determined that maternal antibodies could be caused by incompatible blood transfusions. Of far more importance was the realization that leakage of (paternally determined) Rh-positive red cells from the fetal circulation in the placenta into the circulation of the Rh-negative mother was the commonest and most sinister reason for maternal antibody formation. By late 1941 it was generally recognized that the maternal antibodies, if present in sufficient degree, destroyed fetal red cells in utero and were responsible for the various forms of congenital hemolytic disease of the newborn, if the mother was rhesus negative and the fetus was rhesus positive.

By 1943, in England, R.R. Rees and coworkers accumulated evidence that there were at least three further antigens in addition to the original. Soon afterwards, Sir Ronald Fisher suggested that the original anti-Rh should be called anti-D. The D antigen was found to be responsible for about 95% of the cases in which immunization was due to the Rh antigens. In the USA the anti-D was called Rho, and two further antigens became known as Rh' and Rh". The Rho classification was introduced in 1945.

Investigations

The Rho (D) negative patient was known to be at risk and routine examination of her serum for anti-Rh antibodies was introduced based on a test perfected by Coombs, Mourant and Race (1945) of Cambridge University. They discovered a method for detecting the presence of weak and 'incomplete' Rh antibodies. The test, also known as the indirect globulin method, became the eponymous 'Coombs test'. If antibodies were found in the maternal serum, a quantitative test was carried out to determine the titer of antibody. Many studies reported that the strength and changes in antibody Rh titers could be useful in determining how the pregnancy should be managed and whether preterm delivery could effect a satisfactory outcome for the fetus.

Based on studies by Bevis, amniocentesis and amniotic fluid analysis became the next important diagnostic tools. In his studies Bevis correlated amniotic fluid bilirubin pigments with the severity of fetal compromise due to erythroblastosis: 'Although serological evidence of sensitization in a rhesus-negative woman indicates the possibility of hemolytic disease in her child, the probability of this event is difficult to assess. Changes in titer of the maternal antibodies are unreliable evidence, and biochemical changes in the mother's serum are equivocal'. Bevis originally obtained the amniotic fluid at artificial rupture of the membranes but later introduced what he called 'abdominal paracentesis', now known as amniocentesis. If the Coombs titer exceeded 1:8, or if there was a history of a previous severely affected infant, amniocentesis was carried out at the 28 week of gestation and repeated at fortnightly intervals until delivery. Bevis discovered that the non-hematin iron and the urobilinogen concentrations in the amniotic fluid proved of prognostic value in the management of the compromised fetus (Bevis, 1952, 1956).

A test to detect whether fetal cells had leaked into the mother's blood at delivery was introduced by Kleihauer and colleagues (1957). This was an acid elution technique, in which the fetal red cells could be demonstrated and counted among the population of adult red cells in the mother's blood.

When the predictive nature of amniotic fluid analysis became apparent, numerous methods for analyzing amniotic fluid were reported. Liley (1961) introduced one of the most comprehensive and enduring techniques until Charlie Whitfield (1970) reported from Belfast on the 'action line' method of managing Rh-immunized pregnancies that was based on the optical density of the amniotic fluid.

Treatment

Preterm delivery and delayed cord clamping were the first treatment modalities. Delayed cord clamping, introduced in 1941, allowed placental blood to pass into the fetus as a form of auto-transfusion. Cappell of Glasgow recommended blood transfusion of the anemic infant in 1944 (Potter, 1947 pp. 204–13). Soon afterwards, exchange transfusion (an idea pioneered by Alfred Hart of Canada in 1925), during which the infant's Rh-positive blood was replaced with Rh-negative donor blood, was introduced by Diamond, Allen and Thomas (1951). In Europe, therapy with Phenobarbital and/or exposure to phototherapy were used in the prevention of hyperbilirubinemia due to red cell hemolysis, from the early 1950s, but neither treatment gained acceptance in the USA until 1968.

Occasionally a fetus was so severely affected that it could die before preterm delivery could be safely accomplished. To combat that problem, Liley (1963) introduced intrauterine fetal transfusion. The technique was difficult to perform, and hazardous to both fetus and mother, but successful intraperitoneal transfusion saved many lives. (Experimental intraperitoneal transfusion was carried out on animals in the 1800s and the first occurrence in a humans was documented by Ponfick (1875)).

Charles Rodeck and colleagues (1981) described direct intravascular fetal blood transfusion via fetoscopy in severe rhesus iso-immunisation. Great skill was required to place a catheter in the umbilical cord blood vessels. In time the technique was carried out under ultrasound control. Another therapy of the era was plasmapheresis. The original report of the technique came from John Jacob Abel and colleagues (1914). Blood was removed from a living animal and the corpuscles were returned after washing and separation. In the 1980s John Abel's (modified) technique of plasmapheresis was used to good effect in the treatment of maternal blood and consequent reduction of maternal antibody levels in cases of severe rhesus iso-immunisation.

Flint Porter and colleagues (1997) from the Department of Obstetrics and Gynecology, University of Utah School of Medicine, reported on the use of adjuvant therapy to suppress maternal Rh antibody production: 'although intra-uterine fetal transfusion has improved dramatically perinatal outcome ... Intravenous immune globulin (IVIG) administration has been increasingly used to successfully treat a variety of immune-mediated diseases'. The paper reported a favorable outcome with IVIG treatment of a severe case of rhesus disease: 'IVIG may have an adjunctive role in the treatment of severe Rh iso-immunisation'. The technique may be used in concert with intrauterine transfusion. Combined modes of therapy could help to conserve the affected pregnancy until the third trimester, and increase the prospects for fetal survival.

Prevention of rhesus disease

The prevention of rhesus iso-immunization by administration of RhoGam (Anti-D immunoglobulin) was developed by R. Finn, Cyril Clarke and colleagues of Liverpool (1961) and John Gorman, Vincent Freda and W. Pollack of New York (1962). In an article in *Clinical Obstetrics and Gynecology* Freda (1971) recounted the story of the experimentation on, and introduction of, RhoGam (Anti-D). He related that 'the discovery of the pathogenesis of hemolytic disease of the newborn by Levine and the simultaneous and related discovery of the Rh factor in 1940 by Landsteiner and Wiener together constituted one of the scientific milestones of the century. Rh hemolytic disease of the newborn (erythroblastosis fetalis) exacts a high death toll of almost 10 000 infants per year in the United States alone'.

Freda recalled that in 1960 he and his coworkers and Finn and Clarke in Liverpool carried out trials of Rh immune globulin (RhoGam/Anti-D). The American volunteers were Rh-negative male inmates at Sing Sing Prison at Ossining, New York: 'Reassured by our experience at Sing Sing with Rh-immune globulin, which demonstrated its safety and effectiveness, the first trial in mothers was commenced by our group at Columbia University in April 1964. In this trial, Rh-immune globulin was injected intramuscularly into non-immunized Rh-negative mothers within 72 hours after delivery of a ABO compatible Rh-positive baby'. The RhoGam (Anti-D) successfully protected mothers from becoming sensitized if administered within an arbitrary 72 hour period. Freda wrote in conclusion that the conquest of Rh disease is now a reality'.

A program to prevent rhesus iso-immunization by the administration of anti-D immunoglobulin to Rh-negative women was introduced to the United Kingdom in 1969. The program protected the vast majority of Rh-negative women at risk from pregnancy-induced iso-immunization and the subsequent possibility of congenital hemolytic disease of the newborn. Initial recommendations were updated and it was advised that anti-D should be used after all spontaneous miscarriages and therapeutic abortions (Standing Medical Advisory Committee, 1976). Potential sensitizing events during pregnancy were identified in 1981 for which prophylaxis was also recommended (Standing Medical Advisory Committee, 1981). Current opinion is that all Rh D-negative pregnant women should have prophylactic anti-D in each pregnancy, but cost is still a problem. In the UK it was estimated that deaths attributed to rhesus immunization had fallen from 46 per thousand births before 1969 to 1.6 per thousand in 1990 (Mollison *et al.*, 1997).

And so one of the great discoveries in the immunology of obstetrics was based on the finding that an antibody formed by a rabbit, immunized by the blood of a rhesus monkey, was shown to be the same as an immune antibody found in the serum of a mother. Following the discovery in 1941 of the relationship between the Rh factor and congenital hemolytic disease, it became apparent that CHD existed as a specific clinical disease. It was then determined that the incidence of CHD was approximately one in 150 births, and about half of the infants were severely affected or born as hydropic stillbirths. The development and administration of RhoGam/Anti-D, through monkey business and willing prison inmates, has saved countless lives.

References

Abel, J. J., Rowntree, L. G. and Turner, B. B. (1914). Plasma removal with return of corpuscles (plasmapheresis). *J. Pharmacol.*, 5, 624–41

Agote, L. (1915). Nuevo procedimiento para la transfusion de la sangre. *An. Inst. Mod. Clin. Med.* (Buenos Aires, 1914), 1, 24–31

Ballantyne, J. W. (1892). *The Diseases and Deformities of the Foetus: an Attempt Towards a System of Ante-natal Pathology*, Vol. 1, p. 265. (Edinburgh: Oliver & Boyd)

Bevis, D. C. A. (1956). Blood pigments in haemolytic disease of the newborn. *J. Obstet. Gynecol Br. Common.*, 63, 68–75

Bevis, D. C. A. (1952). The antenatal prediction of hemolytic disease of the newborn. *The Lancet*, **1**, 395–8

Blundell, J. (1818). Experiments on the Transfusion of Blood by the Syringe. *Med. Chir. Trans.*, **9**, 56–92

Blundell, J. (1819). Some Account of a Case of Obstinate Vomiting, in which an Attempt was made to prolong Life, by the injection of Blood into the Veins. *Med. Chir. Trans.*, **10**, 296–311

Blundell, J. (1827/1828). Lectures on the Theory and Practice of Midwifery, Delivered at Guy's Hospital by Dr Blundell. Lecture 27. *The Lancet*, **2**, 161–7

Blundell, J. (1828). Successful Case of Transfusion. *The Lancet*, **1**, 431–2

Blundell, J. (1828–29). Observations on Transfusion of Blood. *The Lancet*, **2**, 321–4

Blundell, J. (1834). *The Principles and Practice of Obstetrics*, pp. 579–80. (London: T. Castle & E. Cox)

Blundell, J. (1839). *Lectures on the Principles and Practice of Midwifery*. (London: J. Masters)

Braxton Hicks, J. B. (1868). On Transfusion and New Mode of Management. *BMJ*, 8,151

Braxton Hicks, J. B. (1869). Cases of Transfusion, With Some Remarks on a New Method of Performing the Operation. *Guy's Hosp. Rep.*, **14**, 1–14

Braxton Hicks, J. B. (1872). On the Contractions of the Uterus throughout Pregnancy. *Trans. Obstet. Soc. London*, **13**, 216–31

Carrel, A. (1907). The Surgery of Blood Vessels. *Johns Hopkins Hosp. Bull.*, **18**, 18–28

Channing, W. (1848). Notes on Anhaemia Principally in Connection with the Puerperal State, and with Functional Disease of the Uterus. *New Eng. J. Med.*, p. 157

Coombs, R. R. A., Mourant, A. E. and Race, R. R. (1945). A new test for the detection of weak and 'incomplete' Rh agglutinins. *B. J. Exp. Path.*, **26**, 255

Denis, J. B. (1667). *Lettre ... Touchant deux experiences de la Transfusion faites sur des hommes*. (Paris: J. Cusson)

Diamond, L. K., Blackfan, K. D. and Baty, J. M. (1932). Erythroblastosis fetalis and its association with universal edema of the fetus, icterus gravis neonatorum, and anemia of the newborn. *J. Pediat.*, **1**, 268

Diamond, L. K., Allen, F. H. and Thomas, W. O. Jr. (1951). Erythroblastosis fetalis, VII: Treatment with exchange transfusion. *New Eng. J. Med.*, **244**, 39

Ecklin, T. (1918–19). A case of anaemia in the newborn. *Monatschr. F. Kinderh.*, **15**, 425

Elsholtz, J. S. (1665). *Clysmatica nova: Oder neue clystier-kunst*. (Berlin: D. Reichel)

Fantus, B. (1937). The therapy of the Cook County Hospital. Blood preservation. *JAMA*, **109**, 128–31

Finn, R., Clarke, C. A., Donohoe, W. T. A., *et al.* (1961). Experimental studies on the prevention of Rh haemolytic disease. *BMJ*, **1**, 1486

Freda, V. J. (1971). Rh immunization-experience with full-term pregnancies. *Clinical Obstetrics and Gynecology*, pp. 594–610. (New York: Harper & Roe)

Gorman, J. G., Freda, V. J. and Pollack, W. (1962). Intramuscular injection of a new experimental gammaglobulin preparation containing high levels of anti-Rh antibody as a means of preventing sensitization to Rh. *Proceedings of the 9th Congress of the International Society of Haematology*, **2**, 545

Graham, H. (1950). *Eternal Eve*, pp. 620–3. (London: Heinemann)

Gronwall, A. J. T. and Ingleman, B. (1944). Untersuchungen uber dextran und sein verhalten bei parenteraler zufuhr. *Acta Physiol. Scandanavia*, **7**, 97–107

Harvey, W. (1651). *Exercitationes de Generatio Animalium*. (London: William Dugard for Octavian Pulluin)

Howkins, J. and Brewer, H. F. (1939). Placental blood for transfusion. *The Lancet*, **1**, 132–6

Hustin, A. (1914). Principe d'une nouvelle methode de transfusion muqueuse. *J. Med., Brux.*, **12**, 436–9

Kimpton, A. R. and Brown, J. H. (1913). A new and simple method of transfusion. *JAMA*, **61**, 117–18

Kinsella, T. (1970). *The Tain. From the Irish Epic Tain Bo Cuailnge*, pp. 211–13. (Oxford: Oxford University Press)

Kleihauer, E., Braun, H. and Betke, K. (1957). Demonstration von fetalem haemoglobin in den Erythrocyten eines Blutausstrichs. *Klin. Wochsch.*, **35**, 637–8

Landsteiner, K. and Wiener, A. S. (1940). An agglutinable factor in human blood recognized by immune serum for rhesus blood. *Proc. Soc. Exp. Biol.*, New York, **43**, 223

Landsteiner, K. (1901). On the phenomenon of agglutination in normal human blood. *Wien Klin. Wochsch.*, **14**, 1132–4

Landsteiner, K. (1900). The first observations of differences in blood of normal human beings. *Zentralbl. für Bakt.*, 27, 357

Lawler, S. D. and Lawler, L. J. (1957). *Human Blood Groups and Inheritance*, pp. 8–9. (London: Heinemann Ltd.)

Levine, P. and Stetson, R. (1939). Unusual case of intra-group agglutination. *JAMA*, **113**, 126

Lewisohn, R. and Rosenthal, N. (1933). Prevention of chills following transfusion of citrated blood. *JAMA*, **100**, 466–9

Liley, A. W. (1961). Liqour amni analysis in management of pregnancy Complicated by rhesus sensitization. *Am. J. Obstet. Gynecol.*, **82**, 1359–70

Liley, A. W. (1963). Intrauterine transfusion of fetus in hemolytic disease. *BMJ*, **2**, 1107–9

Lindeman, E. (1913). Simple syringe transfusion with special cannulas. *Am. J. Dis. Children*, **6**, 28–32

Lower, R. (1665–66). The Method Observed in Transfusing the Blood out of one live animal into another. *Phil. Trans. R. Soc.*, **1**, 353–58

Lower, R. (1667). An Account of the Experiment of Transfusion, Practiced upon a Man in London. *Phil. Trans. R. Soc.*, **2**, 557–64

Lower, R. (1669). *Tractatus de Corde*, p. 200. (Londine: J. Allestry)

Maluf, N. S. R. (1954). History of Blood Transfusion. *J. Hist. Med.*, **9**, 59–107

Mollison, P. L., Engelfriet, C. P. and Contreras, M. (1997). Haemolytic Disease of the Fetus and Newborn. In *Blood*

Transfusion in Clinical Medicine, pp. 543–91. (Oxford: Blackwell Science)

Munro Kerr, J. M. (1954). Obstetric operations. Summary of notable advances 1800–1850. In *Historical Review of British Obstetrics and Gynaecology*, pp. 37–42. (Edinburgh & London: E. & S. Livingstone)

O'Donel Browne, T. D. (1947). *The Rotunda Hospital 1745–1945*, p. 185. (Edinburgh: E. & S. Livingstone)

O'Dowd, M. J. and Philipp, E. (1994). *The History of Obstetrics and Gynaecology*, pp. 87–92. (London, New York: Parthenon Publishing)

Ottenberg, R. (1911). Studies in iso-agglutination. 1. Transfusion and the question of intravascular agglutination. *J. Exp. Med.*, **13**, 425–38

Pepys, S. (1972). *The Diary of Samuel Pepys*, Edited by Nathan, R. and Matthews, W. Vol. 7, p. 70; Vol. 8, p. 554. (London: G. Bell & Sons)

Ponfick, E. (1875). Experimentele beitrage zur lehre von der transfusion. *Virchow Arch. Pathol. Anat.*, **62**, 273–335

Porter, T. Flint, Silver, R. M., Jackson, G. M., Branch, D. W. and Scott, J. R. (1997). Intravenous immune globulin in the management of severe Rh D hemolytic disease. *Obs. and Gyn. Survey*, 52(3), 193–7

Potter, E. L. (1947). *Rh. Its Relation to Congenital Haemolytic Disease and to Intra-group Transfusion Reactions*, pp. 33, 204–13. (Chicago: The Year Book Publishers)

Power, J. P., Davidson, F., O'Riordan, J., Simmonds, P., Yap, P. L. and Lawlor, E. (1995). Hepatitis C infection from anti-D immunoglobulin. *The Lancet*, **346**, 372–3

Queenan, J. T. (1971). The Rh Problem, *Clincal Obstetrics and Gynecology*, pp. 491–3, 505–36. (New York: Harper & Row)

Rautman, H. (1912). On Blood Formation in the Fetus with Universal Oedema. *Beitr. Z. Path. Anat. U. Z. Allg. Path.*, **54**, 322

Rodeck, C. J., Kemp, J. R., Hollman, A., *et al.* (1981). Direct intravascular fetal blood transfusion by fetoscopy in severe rhesus iso-immunisation. *The Lancet*, 1, 625–7

Schridde, H. (1910). Universal Oedema of the Newborn. *Munch. Med. Wochnschr.*, 57, 397

Standing Medical Advisory Committee (1976). *Hemolytic Disease of the Newborn.* (London: Department of Health & Social Security)

Standing Medical Advisory Committee (1981). *Memorandum on Haemolytic Disease of the Newborn.* 1976 Addendum. (London: Department of Health and Social Security)

von Ziemssen, H. W. (1892). Ueber die subcutane Blutinjection und ueber eine neue einfache Methode der intravenosen Transfusion. *Munch. Med. Wochnsch.*, **39**, 323–4

Whitfield, C. R. (1970). A three-year assessment of an action line method of timing intervention in rhesus iso-immunization. *Am J. Obstet. Gynecol.*, **108**, 1239–44

Wiener, A. S. and Peters, H. R. (1940). Haemolytic reactions following transfusions of blood of the homologous group, with three cases in which the same agglutinogen was responsible. *An. Int. Med.*, **13**, 2306

Williams Whitridge, J. (1903). *Obstetrics. A Text-Book for the Use of Students and Practitioners*, pp. 729–30. (Stamford, Connecticut: Appleton & Lange)

Eclampsia 21

INTRODUCTION

The word 'eclampsia' is derived from the Greek *eklampsis*, to flash/shine forth, or, to burst forth violently, and is defined as the occurrence of convulsions in a patient with preeclampsia, and not due to epilepsy or other cause. Alexander Hamilton (1720–1800) of Edinburgh, usually gains the credit for being one of the first writers in English to use the term but according to Fleetwood Churchill of Dublin (1864), it was Carl Braun of Vienna who introduced the term (uremic) eclampsia in the mid-nineteenth century.

Although not known by its modern name, eclampsia has been recognized as a complication of pregnancy since antiquity. In the seventeenth century James Wolveridge (1671) attempted to distinguish between the various types of convulsions which afflicted women in pregnancy: 'fits of the mother ... suffocation of the womb ... hysterical [i.e. uterine], epilepsie, apoplexy and fainting fits' and he attempted to evaluate whether they were an obstetric complication or not. In 1688 François Mauriceau described eclampsia in detail and was aware that the primigravida was at most risk.

Many years later, John Charles Weaver Lever published a paper on 'Puerperal Convulsions' in the *Guy's Hospital* (*London*) *Reports* of 1843. Our subsequent understanding of the causes of fits and the description of preeclampsia and eclampsia owes much to Lever's observations. He described the clinical appearance of edema and was the first to discover that albumin was present in the urine of eclamptics and preeclamptics, but not in normal pregnant women (O'Dowd and Philipp, 1994). James Young Simpson made the same observations almost simultaneously. The realization that hypertension was also present in these cases only occurred after the invention of the sphygmomanometer (from the Greek, *sphugmos*, pulse) with inflatable armband by the Italian physician, Scipione Riva-Rocci in 1896, and its subsequent application to obstetrics.

Our obstetric predecessors found the incidence of eclampsia was approximately 1:500 pregnancies with a maternal mortality of 20–30% and an even higher perinatal mortality. Apart from sepsis, hemorrhage and difficulty in labor, the condition of eclampsia was the worst complication which could befall a pregnant woman. The problem of eclampsia excited much medical and scientific research and debate. O'Donel Browne, of the Rotunda (1947), commented that 'more has been written of eclampsia than of any other obstetrical complication, and between 1909 and 1912 there were no less than 1009 publications on this subject'.

At the dawn of the twentieth century the treatment of eclampsia was enunciated by Henry Jellett, Master of the Rotunda and professor of midwifery at the University of Dublin, and considered under two headings, prophylaxis and curative. Quoting the French writer Ribemont-Dessaignes, Jellet observed that eclampsia occurred almost exclusively in women whose urine had not been checked for albumin. However, according to Etienne Tarnier of the Maternite in Paris, a woman with albuminuria 'almost to a certainty escapes eclampsia', if she has been 'on a milk diet for a week'. Even more necessary was the regulation of the eliminatory functions of the body, particularly that of the bowel.

Curative treatment consisted of 'the arrest of the fits and the staving off of complications'. Fits were controlled by sedatives; by removing toxic substances from the blood and tissues (by bleeding, purgation, and emesis, and the promotion of diuresis via subcutaneous or intravenous administration of saline) and by 'emptying the uterus'. The latter requirement had caused much controversy over the previous two centuries. Complications of eclampsia were avoided 'by means of intelligent nursing ... the use of a gag ... all feeding by mouth must be stopped' and the patient was lain on her side to avoid inhalation of gastric contents (Jellett, 1907).

OLDER TREATMENTS

Conservative

Greco–Roman

The occurrence of convulsions in pregnancy was known to the Greco–Roman physicians. They categorized fits as being due to epilepsy or hysteria, and the uterine affectations 'suffocation' or 'strangulation'. A large number of treatments evolved, one of which was the application of burnt hair or wool to the nostrils of the comatose patient. That remedy was copied many centuries later by making the woman inhale vile-smelling substances such as 'smelling salts' (a preparation with spirits of ammonia).

Some treatments for convulsions. Soranus' gynecology second century AD

Burnt hair, cabbage, castoreum, cedar, fenugreek, mallow, mustard plasters, radish, spikenard, storax.

(Temkin, 1956)

The seventeenth century

Further treatments for convulsions evolved and by the seventeenth century many therapies were available, as demonstrated in the materia medicae of Nicholas Culpeper and James Wolveridge. The latter author in his *Speculum Matricis* (1671) offered a wide range of drugs known to him and passed down from 'the ancients'. His remedies included laudanum (tincture of opium – opium dissolved in alcohol and used as a sedative), hellebore (now known to contain an antihypertensive) and purges (which caused hypotension through loss of body fluids), to treat the fits. Although his rationale for therapy was based on an entirely different concept of disease and its resolution, his recipes, proven by the passage of time, would have helped the eclamptic woman.

Some treatment for convulsions. Culpeper's Complete Herbal of 1653

Alkanet, asafetida, bistort, briony, castoreum, emplastrum hystericum, greater centaury, herb mastich, motherwort, peony.

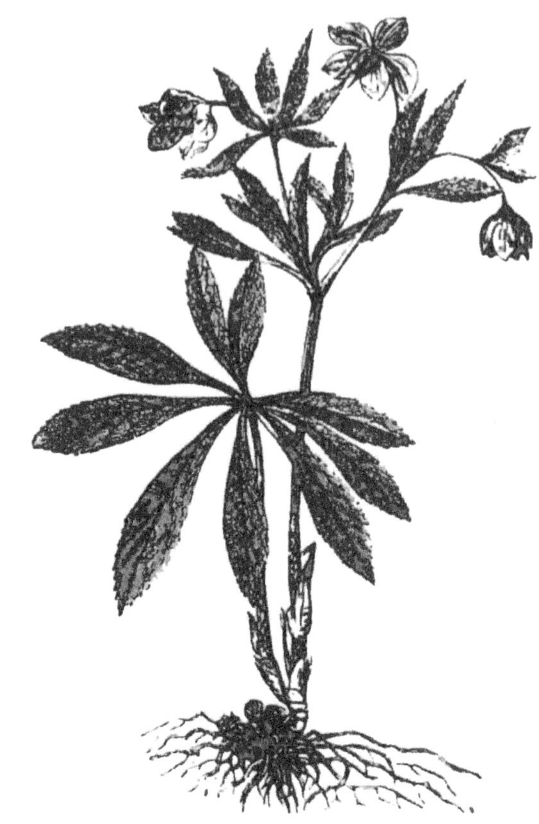

HELLEBORUS VIRIDIS
(*Green Hellebore*)

Figure 1 Hellebore (*Helleborus viridis*)

Some treatment for convulsions. Wolveridge's Speculum Matricis of 1671

Agarick, asafetida, castoreum, dragon tree, hellebore, laudanum, nutmeg, peony, pepper, rue, Saint John's wort, wine.

The eighteenth century

In 1767, John Harvie, the great 'Teacher of Midwifery' at Wardour Street London, advised venesection, application of a stimulating clyster (enema) and forceps delivery if labor was protracted (Spencer, 1927). Venesection remained in vogue right up to the 1940s and its benefit was found to relate to its hypotensive effect.

Alexander Hamilton, the fourth professor of midwifery in Edinburgh, wrote a number of works on obstetrics including his *Outlines of the Theory and Practice of Midwifery* in 1783, which subsequently passed through many editions. He described the premonitory symptoms of eclampsia but regarded treatment with opiates and emetics as being dangerous. He recommended bleeding from the jugular vein and the administration of camphor in doses of 10 grains every 2 hours, while noting that delivery was absolutely necessary as 'the mother's life depends on it' (Spencer, 1927). Camphor, which was soluble in oil or alcohol, could cause drowsiness but if administered in large doses was itself likely to cause convulsions (Ringer, 1888).

Thomas Denman (1713–1815), of London, a renowned man-midwife famed for his *Aphorisms* and his magnum opus the *Introduction to the Practice of Midwifery*, mentioned that François Mauriceau (1637–1709), who conducted an extensive midwifery practice at the Hotel Dieu of Paris, was the originator of the 'active treatment' of eclampsia – the termination of pregnancy and the hastening of labor. Denman disagreed with 'active' treatment and advocated the 'conservative regimen' which he borrowed from Johann Roederer (1727–1763), founder of the Lying-in Hospital at Göttingen, Germany. This employed 'bleeding, occasionally up to 40 or 60 ounces, hot baths, fomentations, and opiates in small quantities, often repeated'. Denman, himself the son of an apothecary, observed that 'Some writers have recommended the speedy delivery of the patient' but he was aware of the dreadful mortality associated with forceful efforts to deliver the convulsing parturient. Making a plea for conservatism he indicated that 'As far as my experience enables me to judge we ought not to attempt to deliver women with convulsions before some progress is made in the labor' (Denman, 1793).

The nineteenth century

William Potts Dewees, professor of midwifery at the University of Pennsylvania, again pleaded against traumatic intervention: 'I had like to have said [it is] murderous to attempt it. Our whole duty in this case consists in proper medical treatment' (Dewees, 1823). Although Denman and Dewees were very influential and their opinions held sway for a time, the management of eclampsia suffered from the introduction of anesthesia in 1847 and the re-application of 'accouchement force' which it allowed. Towards the end of the nineteenth century, Green of the Boston Lying-in Hospital reported that six of ten patients in whom labor had been induced died as a result (Green, 1896). Other centers reported equally bad results for operative intervention.

In the second half of the nineteenth century, conservative treatment consisted of arterial or venesection with removal of 30–50 ounces of blood; application of leeches; cupping to the nape of the neck; strong purgation with calomel and jalap (a purgative root from Xalapa, Mexico); an enema of castor oil, turpentine and asafetida were also used; shaving of the head and application of ice or cold water; application of a blistering plaster to act as a counter-irritant; a tartar emetic; tincture of opium; insertion of a leather or wooden wedge between the teeth to prevent injury to the tongue; and for a time, following the lead of Walter Channing of Boston, ether or chloroform were administered to help control convulsions (Churchill, 1864).

Accouchement force

The term 'accouchement' comes from the French for confinement, delivery, or midwifery. The 'accoucheur' was the man-midwife, and the French term was introduced to English literature in Laurence Sterne's *Tristam Shandy*, the first part of which appeared in 1760. The term 'accouchement force' was introduced by Jacques Guillemeau (1550–1631) of Paris. He was the favorite pupil of Ambroise Paré (1510–1590) who initiated the concept of 'forced delivery', i.e. rapid and forcible dilatation of the cervical canal and immediate extraction of the child by version and traction on the legs (this procedure was replaced in part by forceps delivery in later centuries). Paré was responsible for the re-introduction of podalic version (turning the fetus in utero to a feet-first presentation – as taught by Soranus in the second century AD, for use in difficult deliveries, but then forgotten about for centuries) and for the great revival in midwifery which occurred in the sixteenth century.

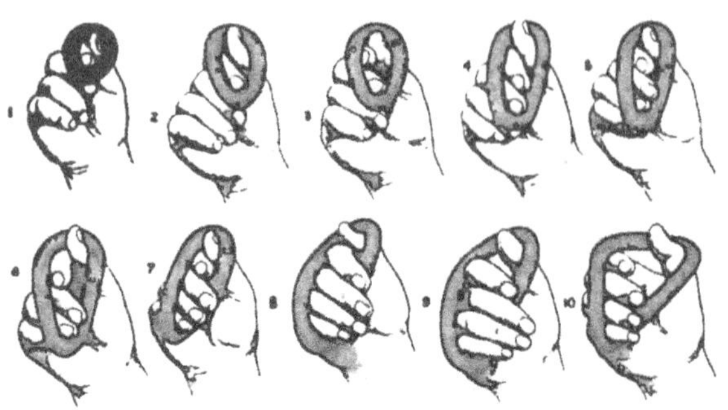

FIG. 342.—DIAGRAMS ILLUSTRATING MANUAL DILATATION OF CERVIX (HARRIS).

Figure 2 Manual dilatation. From Williams, *Obstetric Text-Book for Students and Practitioners* (1911)

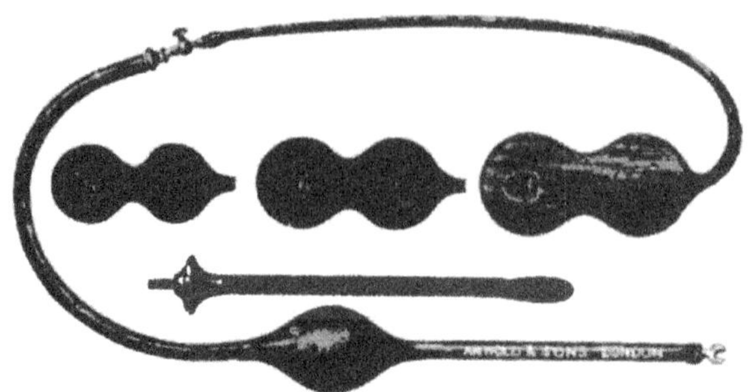

Figure 3 Cervical dilators. From Kerr and Moir, *Operative Obstetrics* (1949)

Paré's own daughter, Anne, was dramatically saved in childbirth by Guillemeau who performed podalic version and extraction of her child.

'Accouchement force', referred to by Celsus (27 BC–50 AD) and Galen (c. AD 130–200), and popularized by Paré and his followers, was initially used in cases of antepartum hemorrhage but was applied as a treatment modality for eclampsia and became popular in the nineteenth and early twentieth century. Obstetricians of the time were aware that delivery of the fetus (and placenta) was the only sure method of halting the eclamptic process. Cesarean section was not an option as the technique had yet to be perfected and the operation resulted in an extremely high maternal mortality rate.

Forcible dilatation of the cervix could be carried out with the hands, rubber bags, expanding metal dilators or by incision. Manual dilatation, the oldest of the methods, was usually carried out with the fingers and thumb of one hand and is eponomously associated with Philander A. Harris (1894). Alternatively, a bimanual approach was possible as described by Bonnaire and also Edgar in 1903. Both techniques were lengthy procedures; they could cause rupture of the cervix with profound shock and rarely succeeded in primigravidae unless the cervix was already somewhat dilated.

Hydrostatic dilatation was originally introduced in 1859 by Keiller and was a method whereby the cervix was dilated by using various rubber or waterproof silk bags which were gradually inflated with water. Famous among the devices were the 'metreurynter of Champetier de Ribes' (1888) and those introduced by Barnes, Muller, Pomeroy and Voorhees – the latter being a modification of the French style and much favored by American obstetricians. Application of the metreurynter remained popular until the early 1950s as a method to accelerate the progress of protracted labor caused by what was then considered to be 'rigidity of the cervix'.

Pronged metal dilators are of ancient date and from time to time were re-introduced for use in labor. A new form of the instrument was introduced by Bossi in 1890. The dilator had three prongs (later four) attached to a handle with a screw device. Dilatation was readily achieved when the device was placed in the cervix but cervical tears or rupture were common. Other metal dilators included the 'ecarteur' of Etienne Tarnier (1828–1897) and the instrument described by de Seigneux in 1905, with its graduated caps and pelvic curve.

Deep cervical incisions were recommended by Alfred Duhrssen (1890), a technique also described by Alfred Velpeau of Paris almost 60 years previously, and from about 1906 this technique of 'accouchement force' became the method of choice, being the subject of reports right up to 1955. The incisions, usually four in number (anterior, posterior and two lateral), frequently became deep cervical tears during extraction of the child, causing profuse hemorrhage.

Vaginal cesarean section (hysterotomy in reality) was first described by Duhrssen in his book on the subject (1896) and popularized by Stamm of America and Munro Kerr of England after their publications of

1903 and 1904 respectively, although well known and used in continental European countries prior to then.

Thomas Eden and Eardley Holland of London, reviewed the maternal mortality rates of the early twentieth century for mild and severe eclampsia. They determined that where labor was natural, assisted or induced, the maternal mortality was 5 to 34%; cesarean section cases had a mortality of 11 to 46%, but with 'accouchement force' rates of 18 to 63% were recorded. The latter rates were so high as 'to place such a method of delivery entirely beyond the pale' (Eden and Holland, 1937) and the various techniques of 'accouchement force' were abandoned. Over half a century later 'accouchement force' was reintroduced under the guises of induction of labor and its acceleration by oxytocics or, alternatively, the performance of cesarean section.

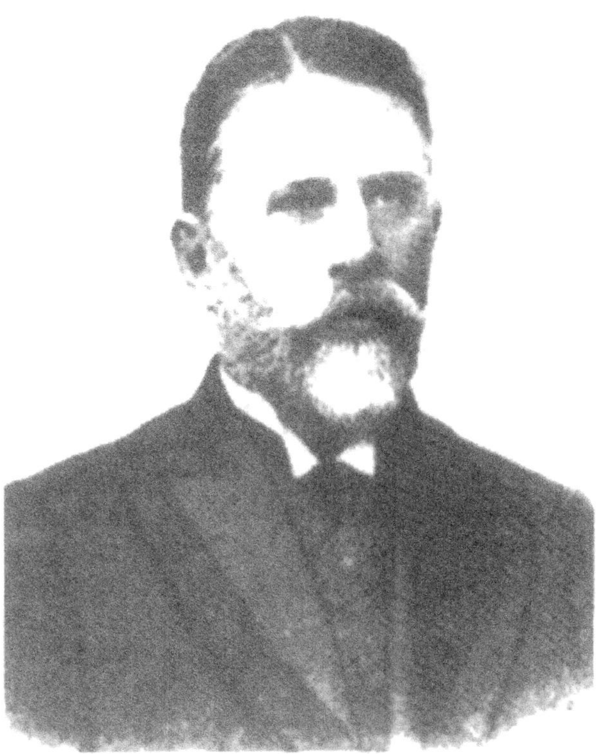

Figure 4 Vasili Vasilievich Stroganov (1857–1938)

MODERN TREATMENTS

Tweedy method

The 'expectant treatment' of eclampsia employed in the early part of the twentieth century was first described by Hastings Tweedy (1896). In his paper, he described the 'modern' management then in use at the Rotunda Hospital Dublin, which included morphia, venesection, purges and oxygen by facemask. No food or oral drugs were allowed throughout the eclamptic attack. The patient was kept in the lateral position and suction was used to decrease the risk of aspiration. Tweedy disagreed with the use of chloroform or bromides and also advised against all unnecessary interference. He condemned the routine induction of labor which was then the usual practice, but did allow the application of forceps to expedite delivery. Tweedy later reported 74 cases of 'expectant management', by then modified by the addition of stomach and bowel washouts (Tweedy, 1911). The maternal mortality of 8.11% from eclampsia with this regime was approximately one third of that reported from many other centers during that same period.

Stroganov regimen

Stroganov began his conservative method for the treatment of eclampsia in 1897 and three years later reported the unprecedented maternal mortality of 5.4% for the regimen to an astounded audience at a congress in Paris (Stroganov, 1900). 'I regard the systematic, prophylactic use of morphine (subcutaneously) and chloral hydrate (rectally)' wrote Stroganov, 'acting concurrently, as a comparatively innocuous measure. In eclampsia, moreover, an effect is necessary both on the sensory centers and the convulsive center. The best agent for the former is morphine; for the latter chloral'. He also advocated that eclamptic patients should be protected from all stimuli and wrote that 'Medical treatment ... eliminated the need for forceful methods, which are dangerous for both mother and child'. The avoidance of inhalation of stomach contents; the improvement of oxygenation and if necessary the use of digitalis to regulate the heart's activities were also part of his treatment. The Stroganov regimen, which differed but little from Tweedy's method, was quickly adopted in most obstetric centers worldwide. Stroganov continued to make minor modifications to his own treatment protocol and by 1935 reported on

1113 cases with a maternal mortality of 3.7% and a fetal mortality of 20% (Stroganov, 1935).

Veratrum viride (Veratrone)

At an international congress of obstetricians and gynecologists held in Dublin during July 1947, Frederick C. Irving, professor of obstetrics at Harvard University, read a paper on the use of *Veratrum viride* and magnesium sulfate in eclampsia and preeclampsia (Irving, 1949). Veratrone, usually given intramuscularly, in a dose of 10 minims (0.6 ml), caused a fall in blood pressure which lasted one to two hours.

Addressing the origin of the *Veratrum* alkaloids, Irving noted that they were derived from three plants belonging to the lily family. The first was *Veratrum album* L., the white or European hellebore; the second was *Schoenocaulon officinalis* Gray., the sabadilla; and the third was *Veratrum viride* Aiton, the green or American hellebore. Veratrone was derived from *Veratrum viride*. Protoveratridine, derived from *Veratrum album* was also employed to treat eclampsia when veratrone was withdrawn from use. Dwelling on the history of hellebore, Irving wrote that the drug had been known since the Middle Ages. He appeared to be unaware that hellebore was used by the ancients, including Soranus of Ephesus in the second century AD, in their treatment of 'hysterical suffocation' and that their medication found its way into the pharmacopoeia of seventeenth century obstetricians, usually administered as a sneezing powder, to treat convulsions (Wolveridge, 1671).

Irving gave credit for the first use of *Veratrum viride* to control the convulsions of eclampsia to P. De L. Baker of Eufala, Alabama, who in 1860 gave it to one patient with a successful result. Reamy, in 1895, founded the veratrum school of Cincinnati. Thirteen years later Mangiagalli of Milan treated one hundred cases of eclampsia with veratrum and recorded a mortality of 12% in the *British Medical Journal* in 1908.

However, it was Bryant (1935) who really popularized the use of veratrum (with magnesium sulfate) recording a maternal death rate of 9.9%. In a later report (Bryant and Fleming, 1940 p. 1333) he reported a maternal mortality of only 1.6% for a purified extract of *Veratrum viride*, marketed as veratrone. In their *Evaluation of Modern Treatments of Eclampsia*

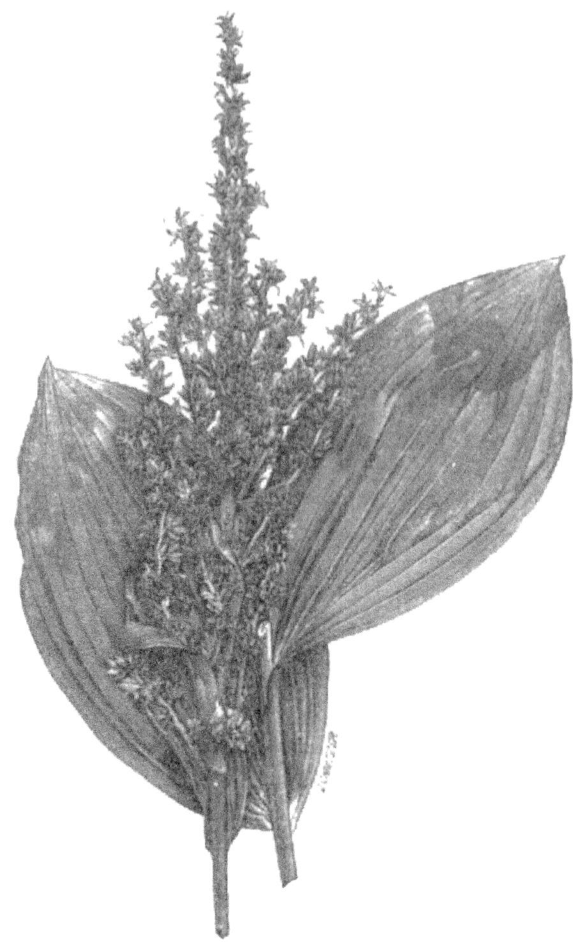

FIG. 159.—Veratrum viride.

Figure 5 *Veratrum viride*

Stern and Burnett (1954 p. 590–601) recorded the results of 1718 cases managed by sedation, sedation and hypotension (bromethol) or hypotension (veratrone) and found that the latter was superior, with a maternal mortality of 1.81% and perinatal mortality of 28%. The drug was later abandoned due to its unpredictable effect on the blood pressure.

Paraldehyde

Paraldehyde was introduced by Cervello in 1882 and found to be a good anticonvulsant. Douglass and Lynn (1942) evaluated its rectal use in eclampsia and reported only one maternal death in 49 cases. The drug caused profound sedation, thus treating convulsions and lowering blood pressure. Bryan Williams (1964 pp. 621–3) reported from Middlesborough, England, on a series of patients treated between 1947 and 1963, with a maternal mortality rate of 4.6% and fetal mortality of 37% but damned the drug with faint praise.

Magnesium sulfate

Magnesium sulfate (Epsom salts), originally obtained from the Epsom Springs in Surrey, was a hydragogue purgative used to treat 'dropsy' and to ward off 'apopleptic' attacks (Squire, 1908). It was prescribed in eclampsia as a laxative or to promote diuresis, and was administered rectally, by subcutaneous injection or via stomach tube. In England, Ballantyne (1910) wrote enthusiastically of its use, combined with venesection and intravenous saline, when reporting nine cases of eclampsia with no maternal death. Ballantyne's paper was largely ignored in his own country and it was in America that magnesium sulfate came into its own. Lazard (1925) pioneered the use of intravenous magnesium sulfate for eclampsia in America and eventually this treatment modality was endorsed by Stroganov himself (Stroganov and Davidovitch, 1937). Particular advantages of magnesium sulfate were that, even though it crossed the placenta, it did not cause sedation and no significant neonatal side-effects were demonstrated.

Many important papers corroborated the early findings of the value of the drug but it was Jack Pritchard (with F.G. Cunningham and Signe A. Pritchard) of the Parkland Memorial Hospital, Dallas, Texas, who was instrumental in demonstrating that magnesium sulfate was the ideal anticonvulsant in preeclampsia and eclampsia. In their paper of 1975, which dealt with 154 consecutive cases of eclampsia, the authors related that 4 g of magnesium sulfate 'at times produced a moderate lowering of blood pressure' and that hydralazine (Apresoline) was administered if the diastolic blood pressure exceeded 110 mmHg. There were no maternal deaths and the perinatal mortality was 15.4% – a unique accomplishment which revolutionized the management of eclampsia in America, and eventually, worldwide (Pritchard, 1955; Pritchard *et al.*, 1975; Pritchard *et al.*, 1984). Writing on his point of view in the management of pregnancy-induced hypertension, Zuspan (1978) described the intravenous magnesium sulfate regimen which is currently used in most centers. The American College of Obstetricians and Gynecologists (1986) recommended magnesium sulfate as standard care in eclampsia but European obstetricians remained skeptical. Hutton *et al.* (1992) reported that the drug was only used by 2% of English obstetricians. The results of the Collaborative Eclampsia Trial (1995), which found in favor of magnesium sulfate over diazepam and/or phenytoin, meant that magnesium sulfate, the humble Epsom salt, was to become the drug treatment of choice in eclampsia.

Tribromethanol (Avertin)

Although first used by Conrad (1927), it was not until Dewar and Morris (1947) reported their use of tribromethanol in a series of 45 eclamptics, in which only two deaths occurred, that the drug became popular. Administered rectally, in a four-hourly dose of 4.5 ml in 250 ml water, the drug controlled convulsions in over 80% of cases but was difficult to use, particularly in the laboring patient. Despite that, the use of Avertin in eclampsia remained popular until the late 1960s.

Thiopentone

Thornley D. O'Donel Browne, Master of the Rotunda Hospital and professor of midwifery to Trinity College Dublin, introduced the use of sodium thiopentone in dextrose to the management of eclampsia and reported a mortality of only 5.55% in his series (O'Donel Browne, 1950). His concept of continuous drug infusion was judged to be 'revolutionary' at the time (Falkiner, 1953) and paved the way for other drug therapies over the subsequent 40 years which would also rely on intravenous titration of drug dosage against convulsions. Browne also developed the scope of antenatal care which itself led to a marked decrease in the incidence of eclampsia.

Lytic cocktail

This mixture of drugs was introduced by Laborit in 1950 and was found to cause hypotension and a depressant effect on the central nervous system. The chlorpromazine–promethazine and/or pethidine–diethazine combinations were found to control eclamptic convulsions (Shears, 1957) and various treatment schedules and dosage regimens evolved. Krishna Menon, professor of obstetrics and gynecology at Madras Medical College, became an acknowledged expert in the use of the 'lytic cocktail'. He wrote an account of *The Evolution of Treatment of Eclampsia* in which he reported details of 402 cases of eclampsia with a maternal mortality of only 2.2% (Krishna Menon, 1961).

Benzodiazepines

This group of psychotropic drugs caused muscular relaxation with sedation and also had anticonvulsive effects. Lean and colleagues (1968) from the Kandang Kerabu Hospital and the University of Singapore reported a maternal mortality rate of 3.3% and the lowest ever perinatal mortality to that date of 11% when using chlordiazepoxide (Librium) and diazepam (Valium) in their treatment of eclampsia. Lean commented that Lecart and Cavenagh had reported favorably on the use of benzodiazepines in 'toxemia of pregnancy' in 1954 and also that Gilbert was first to use chlordiazepoxide (Librium) in a case of eclampsia in 1961. However, it was the definitive study by Lean *et al.* (1968) which launched the benzodiazepines, particularly diazepam (Valium), in the control of eclamptic convulsions.

The main disadvantage of the benzodiazepines was found to be their rapid transplacental transfer. Cree and colleagues (1973) discovered that low Apgar scores, respiratory depression, poor feeding, and hypothermia were prominent neonatal side effects when maternal doses exceeded 30 mg of diazepam. Despite the risk of side effects, diazepam, plus an antihypertensive (usually hydrallazine), became the favorite and standard drug treatment for eclampsia in much of the world outside of North America until the renewed challenge of magnesium sulfate in the late 1990s.

Diphenylhydantoin (Phenytoin)

Diphenylhydantoin, a synthetic organic chemical, was introduced for the treatment of epilepsy in 1938. Slater and associates (1987) proposed its use for eclampsia as it did not cause the sedation and respiratory depression which occur with diazepam and chlormethiazole. The potential of the drug was never fully realized as the Collaborative Eclampsia Trial of 1995 found in favor of magnesium sulfate over phenytoin.

Antihypertensives

Hydrallazine (apresoline), hydrazinophthalazine (nepresol), nifedipine, methyldopa, clonidine, diuretics and other antihypertensive agents such as reserpine, diazoxide, and labetalol were all resorted to, sometimes singly or in combination. Diazoxide and (di)hydrallazine were a potent mixture which caused extreme lowering of blood pressure leading to maternal collapse. Such drug interactions, with their uncertain synergistic effects, led to maternal deaths. Only hydrallazine, reported on by Assali (1954) and also by McCall (1954), remained popular and was combined with magnesium sulfate to form the drug therapy of choice.

Caudal analgesia and other methods

Continuous caudal or spinal anesthesia, with or without magnesium sulfate, was proposed by Whitacre, Hingson and Turner (1948) who reported only three maternal deaths in 74 cases of eclampsia.

Apart from drugs, operative delivery, and the avoidance of complications, a number of novel methods of therapy were considered. Renal decapsulation was introduced by Edebohls in 1903 and reported in the *American Journal of Obstetrics and Gynecology*. Another treatment, which also did not catch on, was that of Helme in Manchester who introduced the use of lumbar puncture in 1903 – he reported his findings in the *British Medical Journal* the following year (Jellett, 1907).

Induction of labor

The ancients attempted to induce or accelerate labor in women when 'difficult labor' was expected or already in progress. Purgation, various ecbolics and manual dilatation of the vagina and cervix were resorted

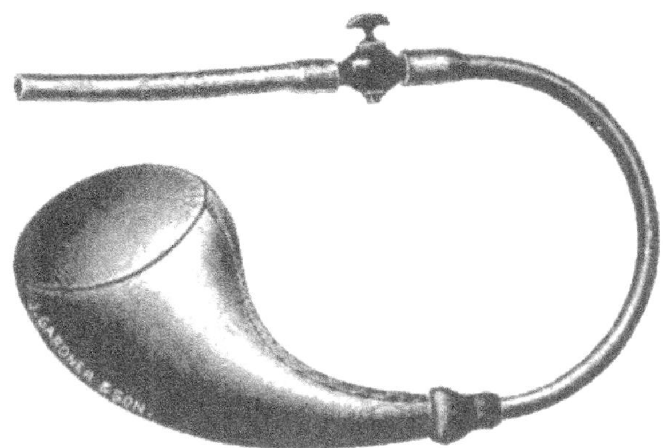

Figure 6 Champetier de Ribes bag for induction of labor. From Kerr and Moir, *Operative Obstetrics* (1949)

to. Artificial rupture of the membranes was found to be relatively successful in inducing labor and was endorsed at a meeting held in London in 1756, thus giving rise to its name – the 'English method'.

Many other methods evolved, including separation of the membranes; massage of breasts or uterus; insertion of sponge tents, Kraus bougies, catheters, bags and dilators; injection of Aretus paste or various fluids under the membranes; electrical stimulation; paracentesis of the amniotic sac; and other methods.

The subject of 'induction of labor' in the treatment of eclampsia gave rise to great debate and the great 'men-midwives and obstetricians' of previous eras were divided on the subject. The conservatives urged caution, and their management of control of the convulsions with induction of labor in favorable cases reflects modern practice.

Cesarean section

John Whitridge Williams (1911) of Baltimore, wrote that the German, Halbertsma, was the first to advocate cesarean section delivery for eclamptic women in his paper of 1899. In 1904, Montuoro of Italy published a list of 62 cases in which 'conservative' cesarean section was performed (the Porro method was used in four cases) with a maternal mortality of 35 (56%) and neonatal mortality of 36.3%. Four years later, John M. Munro Kerr of Glasgow advocated the operation for cases where the eclamptic seizures 'are of great severity' and when the cervix was 'very rigid and undilatable' (1908) and, over 40 years later, he still cautiously advised that 'opinion is divided as regards cesarean section in cases of eclampsia. Here great discrimination is needed in selecting cases for this very radical treatment' (Munro Kerr and Chasser Moir, 1949). Although radical no more, and with a proven record of safety due to many advances, cesarean section is currently retained for eclamptic cases where convulsions are treated but the cervix is very unfavorable for induction of labor; in failed induction; in failure to progress in labor or when fetal distress supervenes.

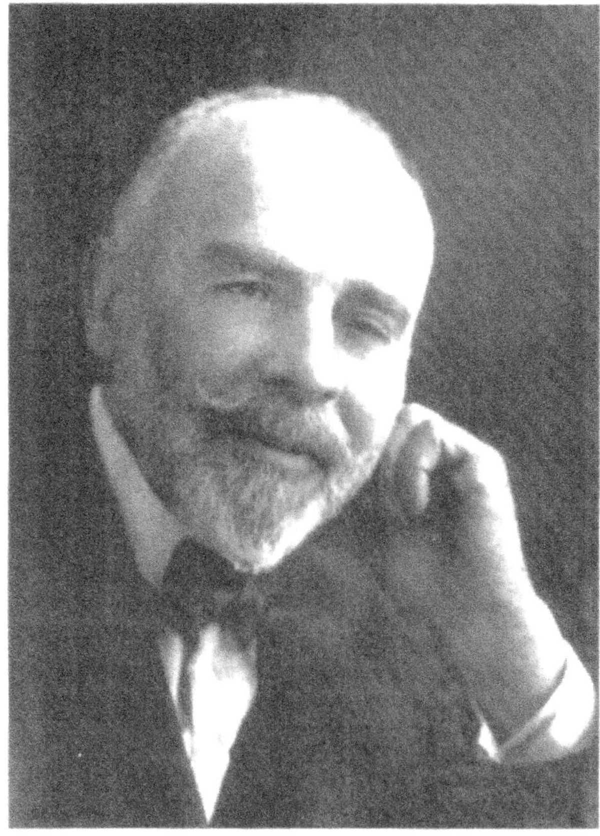

Figure 7 Ernest Hastings Tweedy (1862–1945). From O'Donel Browne, *The Rotunda Hospital* (1947)

Epilogue

Nowadays the principle steps in managing eclampsia are to treat the convulsions and hypertension while stabilizing the mother and then using drug or other therapies to achieve delivery of the infant. The avoidance of eclampsia by carefully monitoring of pregnant women for evidence of preeclampsia has a major role to play. The question arose as to whether preeclampsia itself could be prevented. Theoretically, aspirin, which suppresses thromboxane synthesis and reduces platelet aggregation, could be helpful. Reporting on the collaborative low dose aspirin (CLASP) study in pregnancy, Lawrie Beilin of Perth wrote that routine prophylaxis of 'at risk' women could not be justified as the benefits appeared uncertain and concluded that 'we still have a long way to go before we have a really effective means of preventing or controlling this complex condition' (Beilin, 1994).

BIOGRAPHIES

Ernest Hastings Tweedy (1862–1945)

Born in 1862 and educated in Dublin, Ernest Tweedy qualified from the Royal College of Surgeons in Ireland and then worked in Birmingham and London before becoming Master of the Rotunda Hospital Dublin, a position he held from 1903 to 1910. He wrote extensively and his *Practical Obstetrics* which first appeared in 1908 went into many editions. Tweedy introduced the 'Tweedy' or 'Dublin' method of treatment for eclampsia and during his seven years as Master the maternal mortality for the condition was 9.1% compared to Stroganov's figure of 8.9% in 1912. He became professor of midwifery of the RCSI in 1917 and retired in 1926. Bestowed with many honors for his contributions to obstetrics and gynecology, he was elected a Fellow of the RCOG in London in 1944, the year before his death (O'Donel Brown, 1945; Peel, 1976).

Vasili Vasilievich Stroganov (1857–1938)

Stroganov was born in December, 1857, in Viaz'ma, Russia. After graduation he worked for a period as a district doctor but became interested in midwifery and, in 1885, joined the Povival'nyi Institute, the central governmental research institute for obstetrics and gynecology, and became professor there 12 years later. He was regarded as an excellent teacher and writer. In all, he penned 150 medical articles, three books on eclampsia and a book on practical obstetrical problems. Stroganov was elected an honorary member by many foreign and local medical societies. After his death in 1938 the Russian Ministry of Health created a special prize, named in his honor, for the best published work on eclampsia (Speert, 1958).

References

Assali, N. S. (1954). Hemodynamic effects of drugs used in obstetrics. *Obstet. Gynecol. Survey*, 9, 776–94

American College of Obstetricians and Gynecologists (1986). Management of pre-eclampsia. *ACOG Technical Bull.*, 91, 1–6

Ballantyne, J. W. (1910). The treatment of eclampsia: A resume of eighteen months' experience. *J. Obstet. Gynecol. Br. Emp.*, 18, 378–83

Beilin, L. (1994). Aspirin and pre-eclampsia. Editorial. *BMJ*, 308, 1249–50

Bryant, R. D. (1935). *Veratrum viride* in the treatment of eclampsia. *Am. J. Obstet. Gynecol.*, 30, 46–52

Bryant, R. D. and Fleming, J. G. (1940). *Veratrum viride* in the treatment of eclampsia. *JAMA*, 115(16), 1333–8

Churchill, F. (1864). *On The Diseases of Women*, 5th ed., pp. 866–88. (Dublin: Fannin and Co.)

CLASP Collaborative Group (1994). CLASP: A randomized trial of low-dose aspirin for the prevention and treatment of pre-eclampsia among 9364 pregnant women. *The Lancet*, 343, 619–29

Conrad, G. (1927). *Zbl. Gynak.*, 51, 2222, quoted by Stern, D. M. and Burnett, C. F. W. (1954). An evaluation of modern treatments of eclampsia. *J. Obstet. Gynecol Br. Emp.*, 61(1), 590–601

Cree, J. E., Meyer, J. and Hailey, D. M. (1973). Diazepam in labour: its metabolism and effect on the clinical condition and thermogenesis of the newborn. *BMJ*, 4, 251–5

Culpeper, N. (1653). *The Complete Herbal*, Wordsworth Edition of 1995. (London: Wordsworth)

Denman, T. (1793). *Aphorisms on the Application and uses of Forceps and Vectis; on Preternatural Labours, on Labours Attended with Hemorrhage, and with Convulsions*, 4th edition, pp. 102–3. (London: Johnson)

Dewar, J. B. and Morris, W. I. C. (1947). Sedation with rectal tri-brom-ethanol (Avertin Bromethal) in the management of eclampsia. *J. Obstet. Gynecol Br. Emp.*, 54, 417–25

Dewees, W. P. (1823). *Essays on Various Subjects Connected with Midwifery*, pp. 169–70. (Philadelphia; Carey and Lea)

Douglass, L. H. and Linn, R. F. (1942). Paraldehyde in obstetrics, with particular reference to its use in eclampsia. *Am. J. Obstet. Gynecol.*, 43, 844–8

Duhrssen, A. (1896). *Der Vaginale Keiserschnitt*. (Berlin: Karger)

Duhrssen, A. (1890). Ueber den Werth der tiefen Cervix- und Scheiden-Damm Einschnittein der Geburtshulfe. *Archiv. f. Gynecol.*, 37, 27–66

Eclampsia Trial Collaborative Group (1995). Which anticonvulsant for women with eclampsia? Evidence from the Collaborative Eclampsia Trial. *The Lancet*, **345**, 1455–63

Eden, T. W. and Holland, E. (1937). *A Manual of Obstetrics*, p. 130. (London: J. and A. Churchill)

Falkiner, N. (1953). Obituary. O'Donel Thornley Dodwell Browne. *J. Obstet. Gynecol. Br. Emp.*, **60**(1), 133–4

Green, C. M. (1896). Puerperal eclampsia: The experience of the Boston Lying-in Hospital during the last eight years. *Am. J. Obstet.*, **28**, 18–44

Harris, P. A. (1894). A method of performing rapid dilatation of the os uteri. *Am. J. Obstet. Gynecol.*, 29, 37–49

Hutton, J. D., James, D. K., Stirrat, G. M., Douglas, K. A. and Redman, C. W. G. (1992). Management of severe pre-eclampsia by UK consultants. *B. J. Obstet. Gynecol.*, **99**, 554–6

Irving, F. C. (1949). The treatment of eclampsia and pre-eclampsia with *Veratrum viride* and magnesium sulphate. *Rotunda Hospital Bicentenary. Transactions of the International Congress of Obstetricians and Gynaecologists*, pp. 83–90. (Dublin: The Parkside Press)

Jellett, H. (1907). Eclampsia. In *Green's Encyclopedia and Dictionary of Medicine and Surgery*, Vol. 3, pp. 3–11. (Edinburgh and London: William Green and Sons)

Krishna Menon, M. K. (1961). The evolution of the treatment of eclampsia. *J. Obstet. Gynecol. Br. Common.*, **68**(3), 417–26

Lazard, E. M. (1925). A preliminary report on the intravenous use of magnesium sulfate in puerperal eclampsia. *Am. J. Obstet. Gynecol.*, **9**, 178–88

Lean, T. H., Ratnam, S. S. and Sivasamboo, R. (1968). Use of benzodiazepines in the management of eclampsia. *J. Obstet. Gynecol. Br. Common.*, **75**, 856–62

Munro Kerr, J. M. (1908). *Operative Midwifery*, p. 404. (London: Balliere, Tindall and Cox)

Munro Kerr, J. M. and Chasser Moir, J. (1949). *Operative Obstetrics*, p. 512. (London: Balliere, Tindall and Cox)

McCall, M. L. (1954). Continuing vasodilator infusion therapy. Utilization of a blend of 1- hydrazinophthalazine (Apresoline) and cryptenine (Unitensin) in toxaemia of pregnancy. *Obstet. Gynecol.*, **4**, 403–10

O'Donel Browne, T. D. (1947). *The Rotunda Hospital 1745–1945*, pp. 236, 279–80. (Edinburgh: E. & S. Livingstone)

O'Donel Browne, T. D. (1950). The treatment of eclampsia. *J. Obstet. Gynecol. Br. Emp.*, **57**, 573–82

O'Dowd, M. J. and Philipp, E. E. (1994). *The History of Obstetrics and Gynaecology*, p. 94. (London & New York: Parthenon Publishing)

Peel, Sir J. (1976). *The Lives of the Fellows of the Royal College of Obstetricians and Gynaecologists, 1929–1969*, pp. 45–6. (London: Heinemann Medical)

Pritchard, J. A. (1955). The use of the magnesium ion in the management of eclamptogenic toxaemias. *Surg. Obstet. Gynecol.*, **100**, 131–40

Pritchard, J. A. and Pritchard, S. A. (1975). Standardized treatment of 154 cases of eclampsia. *Am. J. Obstet. Gynecol.*, **123**, 543–52

Pritchard, J. A., Cunningham, F. G. and Pritchard, S. A. (1984). The Parkland Memorial Hospital protocol for treatment of eclampsia: evaluation of 245 cases. *Am. J. Obstet. Gynecol.*, **148**, 951–63

Ringer, S. (1888). *A Handbook of Therapeutics*, pp. 367–70. (London: H. K. Lewis)

Shears, B. H. (1957). Combination of chlorpromazine, promethazine, and pethidine in the treatment of eclampsia. *BMJ*, **2**, 75–8

Slater, R. M., Smith, W. D., Patrick, J., Mawer, G. E., Wilcox, F. L., Donnai, P., Richardson, T. and D'Souza, S. (1987). Phenytoin infusion in severe pre-eclampsia. *The Lancet*, **i**, 1417–20

Speert, H. (1958). *Essays in Eponomy*, pp. 604–11. (New York: Macmillan)

Spencer, H. R. (1927). *The History of British Midwifery from 1650 to 1800*, pp. 65–6, 96–7. (London: John Bale, Sons and Danielsson)

Squire, P. W. (1908). *Squire's Companion to the latest edition of the British Pharmacopoeia*, 18th edition, p. 752. (London: J. & A. Churchill)

Stern, D. M. and Burnett, C. F. W. (1954). An evaluation of modern treatments of eclampsia. *J. Obstet. Gynecol. Br. Emp.*, 61(1), 590–601

Stroganov, V. V. (1900). Lecheniyu Eklampsii. *Vrach. delo.*, 21, 1137–40

Stroganov, V. (1935). *Traitment de l'Eclampsie: Technique Actuelle du Traitement Prophylactique*. (Paris: Masson et Cie)

Stroganov, V. V. and Davidovitch, O. (1937). Two hundred cases of eclampsia treated with magnesium sulphate. *J. Obstet. Gynecol. Br. Emp.*, **44**, 289–99

Temkin, O. (1956). *Soranus' Gynecology*. (Baltimore and London: The Johns Hopkins University Press)

Tweedy, E. H. (1911). The cause and cure of eclampsia. *BMJ*, 2, 990–3

Tweedy, E., H. (1896). Eclampsia. *Trans. R. Acad. Med. Ireland*, 14, 272–84

Whitacre, F. E., Hingson, R. A. and Turner, H. B. (1948). The treatment of eclampsia by regional nerve block. *Southern Med. J.*, 41, 920–2

Whitridge Williams, J. (1911). *Obstetrics*, p. 444. (New York: Appleton and Co.)

Williams, B. (1964). Paraldehyde in the treatment of eclampsia. *J. Obstet. Gynecol. Br. Common.*, 70(4), 621–3

Wolveridge, W. (1671). *The Speculum Matricis*, pp. 155–61. (London: E. Oakes)

Zuspan, F. P. (1978). Problems encountered in the pretreatment of pregnancy-induced hypertension. A point of view. *Am. J. Obstet. Gynecol.*, 131, 591–7

Family planning 22

INTRODUCTION

The two areas of great controversy in the materia medica of women were analgesia in labor and contraception. The religious and social objections to analgesia were all but eradicated in the twentieth century. The same is not true of contraception. Some religions, particularly the Roman Catholic Church, teach that only 'natural' family planning is allowed for their flock and there are social groups who adhere to the same belief. In opposition are those who uphold the principle that the freedom to choose their particular method of family planning is a basic human right.

The evolution of birth control in the early part of the century was heavily influenced in America by Margaret Higgins Sanger, of an Irish immigrant family. From the 1950s onwards she played an important supportive role in the development of the oral contraceptive pill. At the same time in England the campaigner for birth control was Marie Carmichael Stopes. Both women, and their supporters, facilitated the move from ignorance and prejudice against birth control to knowledge and enlightenment. Both were motivated by the desire to help the most needy families in society but their efforts enriched society as a whole.

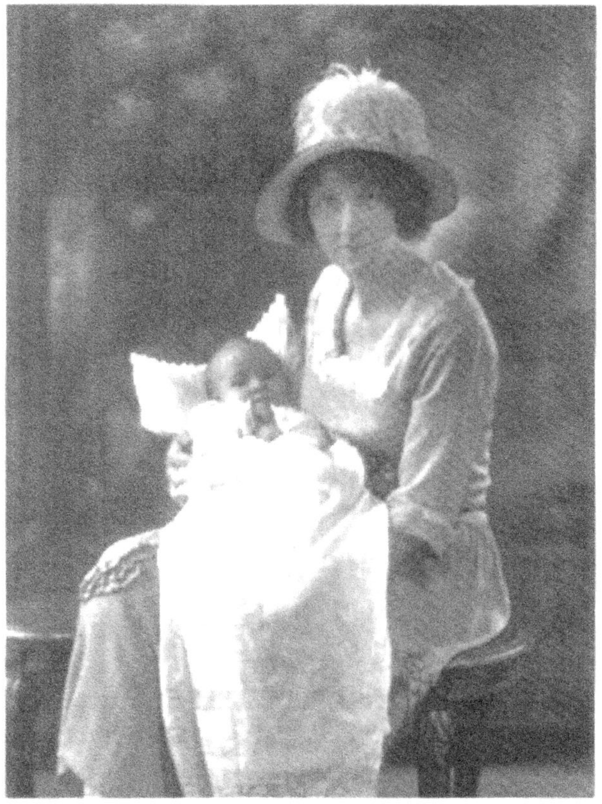

Figure 1 Marie Charlotte Carmichael Stopes (1880–1958)

The conflict of interests as they appeared in the first quarter of the twentieth century were dealt with in great detail by Marie Carmichael Stopes (1923) in her book *Contraception (Birth Control) It's Theory and History and Practice*. Marie Stopes, Doctor of Science, Doctor of Philosophy, Munich, and Fellow of University College, London, played a major role in the story of contraception and the liberation of women's sexuality. Stopes, a lecturer in fossil plants, also wrote the book *Married Love* in 1918 that sold over a million copies and was translated into 13 languages, much to the horror of the establishment. She went on to open the first free birth control clinic in the British Empire and was acclaimed internationally for her work on family planning. Stope's book on birth control is a fascinating read and the extracts in this chapter highlight the radical changes in attitudes to contraception that occurred worldwide in the past three-quarters of a century.

The *Medical History of Contraception* (1936) was related by Normal E. Himes, economist and sociologist, of Colgate University, Hamilton New York. Written at the request of the National Committee on Maternal Health, it remains the definitive work on the early history of the subject, and was so popular that it was reprinted in 1963. In his heavily referenced book, Himes dealt with the contraceptive techniques from before the dawn of written history and investigated the various forms of birth control used by the ancient Egyptians, Greeks and Romans, and those available in

China, India, Japan and the Islamic world. European folk beliefs and the history of the condom and sheath were also related. Himes included a tract on the democratization of contraception in England and in the United States. Evidenced by the details in Himes book, and the many references compiled in the research for *A History of Medications for Women*, and despite governmental, religious and social objections, contraception was a reality from antiquity.

CONTRACEPTION THROUGH THE AGES

Egypt

The oldest contraceptive prescriptions are contained in the Petri or Kahun Papyrus c. 1850 BC.

Prescription No XXI. To prevent (conception) ... crocodiles dung cut up on auyt-paste.

Prescription No XXII. Another medicine: one pint of honey, sprinkle on her uterus with natron.

Prescription No XXIII. Another: sprinkle auyt-gum on her uterus.

The Ebers Papyrus c. 1550 BC contains a reference to tampons impregnated with tips of acacia moistened with honey and placed in the vagina. Such a prescription should release lactic acid which has a contraceptive effect, while the honey had adhesive and barrier properties. The Berlin Papyrus, c. 1300 BC, advised fumigation with medicinal herbs or an oral prescription of grease, herbs, and sweet ale to be cooked, and taken on four mornings.

Greece

The Greeks used a variety of pastes and pessaries for local application and it appears that coitus interruptus was practiced. A form of post-coital contraception was practiced by digitally clearing the vagina of seminal deposit or by squatting to increase pelvic pressure and seminal outflow. Medicinal herbs were used as anaphrodisiacs and hemp seed was thought to render males impotent. Aristotle (384–322 BC) was the first Greek writer to mention contraceptive measures. His prescription included cedar oil, lead or frankincense mixed with olive oil as an intravaginal application. Olive oil is now known to reduce sperm motility and the other components acted as mechanical barriers. Dioscorides (second century AD) recommended the wearing of amulets, the use of medicated pessaries and anointing of the genitals with sticky substances. Soranus of Ephesus, of the same era, wrote *On the Use of Abortifacients and of Measures to Prevent Conception* and included it is his famous text of antiquity, the *Gynecology*. Soranus described astringent solutions, fruit acids, occlusive pessaries, wool impregnated with gum, and vaginal plugs for use by the female but warned against the use of oral preparations as they caused indigestion, vomiting and other side effects.

Hebrew

The Bible, Genesis 38: 7–10, related the story of Onan who practiced coitus interruptus when asked to perform the duty of a husband with the wife of his deceased brother. Coitus interruptus was allowed during the 24 months that a mother nursed her infant, the interval during which the husband must thresh inside, and winnow outside. On occasion, the Hebrew women placed a sponge or mokh in the vagina to cover the cervical opening and to absorb the semen. Violent jumping movements were made to dislodge the semen after intercourse. Mentioned in the Talmud was 'The Cup of Roots', a medicine to induce temporary sterility in women. The components, Alexandrian gum, liquid alum and garden crocus were mixed with two cups of beer to form the love cup.

Islamic culture

Rhazes (AD 860–932) included 24 different contraceptive prescriptions in his text the *Quintessence of Experience*. To prevent semen entering the vagina he advised that coitus interruptus take place. Alternatively, the man should prevent ejaculation. A third method was to apply pills or pessaries to block the uterine aperture or to expel the semen and prevent conception. In another method, the woman was advised oxytocic drugs which were normally used to hurry on labor. Rhazes finally suggested that a prepared piece of mallow root be introduced into the

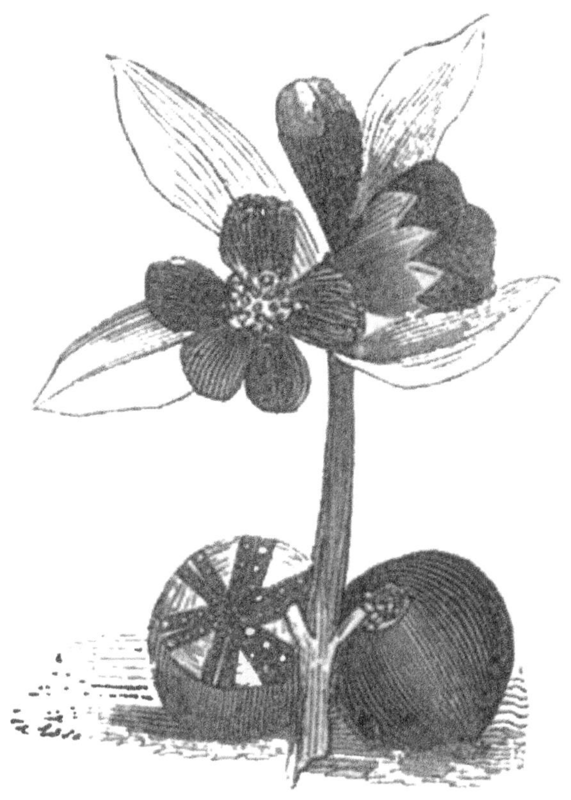

Figure 2 Pomegranate tree

cervical canal to induce menstruation if the contraceptive measures had failed.

Rhazes' contraceptive remedies

Almond oil, bamboo concretions, broth of onions, bryony, cabbage, coloconth pulp, eggs, elephant dung, fowl fat, ginger, leeks, mallows, melon, mulberry, ox-gall, peach, pitch, pomegranate, potash, sal ammoniac, saffron, scammony, sugar candy, tamarisk.

In his *Royal Book* Avicenna (AD 980–1037) wrote that conception could be prevented if women inserted rock salt in the vagina prior to coitus. He also advised the use of cabbage seed, rue juice and leaves or fruits of the weeping willow. Daily intake of three pints of an infusion of sweet basil or eating beans on an empty stomach were thought to prevent conception. Amulets with rabbit rennet, weeping willow leaves or fruits were also thought to act as contraceptives. Coitus interruptus, violent body movements, prolonged sneezing or smearing tar on the vagina or penis were alternative means. Avicenna, in his *Canon of Medicine*, increased the number of contraceptive remedies, some of which are included in the tables.

Constituents of Avicenna's contraceptive pessaries

Balm oil, elephant dung, hellebore, iron dross, mandrake, myrrh, opopanax, ox-gall, pennyroyal, pepper, scammony, sulfur, tar, white lead

Avicenna's contraceptives to anoint the penis

Balm oil, expressed juice of onion, olive oil, rock salt, sesame oil, sweet oil, tar, white lead

Byzantium

Aetius, Greek physician in the first half of the sixth century, was born in Amida, Mesopotamia, and flourished under Justinian 1, Emperor of the East (AD 527–565). He was a physician at the Byzantine Court and is known chiefly as the author of a medical encyclopedia, *On Medicine in Sixteen Books or Discourses*, an eclectic compilation of great historical value because it quotes many medical works of antiquity. Book XVI contains two chapters on contraceptive technique, the full text of which is contained below as the English version from a French translation of Aetius by M. Moissides of Athens and contained in Himes (1936). James Ricci (1950) of York translated the entire gynecology and obstetrics of Aetius from the 1542 Latin edition of Cornarius and the section on contraception is similar, but more lucid.

'On contraceptives and abortifacients'

'Contraception differs from abortion. The first prevents conception, the second destroys the product of conception and drives it out of the uterus. In order to avoid conception it is necessary to abstain from coitus during the days favorable to conception, for example, at the beginning or end of menstruation. During coitus, when the man is about to ejaculate, the woman ought to hold her breath and withdraw a little in order that the sperm might not penetrate the uterine cavity; she ought to get up immediately and squat down on her haunches, provoke a sneeze, and carefully clean the vagina.

Smearing the cervix before coitus with honey or opobalsam or cedar rosin alone or in combination with lead ointment with myrtle and lead or liquid alum or galbanum with wine aids contraception. These medicaments, when they are stringent, unctuous and refrigerant, close the orifice of the womb before coitus and prevent the sperm of the man from entering the uterus. When they are cold they irritate; and they not only prevent the sperm of the man from remaining in the uterine cavity but they draw a liquid from the uterus. All these medicaments belong to the anti-conceptional class.'

'Anti-conceptional pessaries'

'Pine bark, *Rhus cotinus* in equal quantities: Triturate with wine and make a pessary of wool. Place it (before the os) prior to coitus, withdraw it after two hours and then have coitus.

Or else: The inside of young pomegranates: mix with water and prepare pessaries to introduce into the vagina.

Or else: Pomegranates, 2 parts, gallnut, 1 part: triturate and make into small suppositories. Introduce into the vagina after the end of menstruation.

Or else: 3 drachms gallnut, 2 drachms myrrh: prepare some pessaries with wine of the size of peas. Dry in the shade and introduce into the vagina before coitus.

Or else: Make pessaries with the pulp of dried figs and mix with nitre and put into the vagina.

Or else: 2 drachms pomegranate, 2 drachms gallnut, 1 drachm absinthe: after having pulverized these, mix with cedar rosin, and prepare barley-sized pessaries, and put on the cervix for two days immediately after the end of menstruation. The woman ought to remain quite tranquil for a day, and then have sexual congress, not before. This contraceptive is infallible.'

'Anti-conceptional potion'

'Cyrenaic sap, of the size of a pea in two glasses of winy water: to be drunk once a month. This also causes onset of menstruation.

Or else: Cyrenaic sap, opopanax, rue leaves to equal parts; triturate, mix with some sap. Take an amount the size of a bean and drink with winy water. This potion is also an emmenagogue.

Or else: 1 drachm aloes, 3 obols of stock seed, 3 drachms ginger, 2 grains of pepper, and saffron: give it to the woman to drink with wine in three doses immediately after the end of menstruation. Copper water in which one extinguishes (hot) iron, drunk continually, and above all immediately after the end of menstruation is anti-conceptional. One drachm of root of poplar, with a seventh of a small glass of water; give it to the woman to drink once a month during menstruation.'

'Anti-conceptional' (Amulets)

'Wear cat liver in a tube on the left foot, or wear the testicles of a cat in a tube around the umbilicus.

Or else: Wear part of the womb of a lioness in a tube of ivory. This is very effective. Or lead with oil in a pessary; put in the vagina before coitus or sooner. Pomegranate and gallnut and 2 drachms sour fruit juice [usually grape?], 1 drachm absinthe: mix with cedar rosin and prepare pessaries of the size of barley, and put into the vagina for two days after menstruation.

Mix with the milk of a she ass, a little myrtle and a berry of black ivy or some corymb: to be worn after having been wrapped in the skin of the hare or the mule or stag. The amulet ought not to touch the ground at all.

Or else: The woman should carry as an amulet around the anus the tooth of a child or a glass from a marble quarry.

Another experiment: Wrap in a stag skin the seed of henbane diluted in the milk of a mare nourishing a mule. Carry that as an amulet on the left arm, and take care that it does not fall to the ground. And give the woman the seed of Artemisia to drink. These prevent conception for a year.'

'Another contraceptive' (Oral)

'As long as a woman desires to remain sterile, she ought to drink during this time a quantity of black ivy berries in winy water after menstruation; or the seeds of henbane gathered from the plant before they have fallen to the ground.

Or give the woman cold copper water [Is this the Hippocratic 'misy'?] to drink on an empty stomach after menstruation.

Or else: Give the woman a decoction of willow bark with honey to temper its bitterness. To be drunk continually.'

'For the man'

'Or else: The man ought to smear his penis with astringents, as for example, with alum or pomegranate or gallnut triturated with vinegar; or wash the genital organs with brine, and he will not impregnate. The burned testicles of castrated mules drunk with a decoction of willow constitute contraception for men.'

THE CONDOM

The gap between the herbal medications of antiquity and birth control methods of the nineteenth century was bridged by the introduction of the condom by Gabriele Falloppius (1564) in his *De Morbo Gallico*, in a chapter entitled 'De praeservatione a carrie gallica'. Eponymously related to the Fallopian tubes, he described a linen sheath, cut to shape, to protect against the ravages of syphilis. In the following year Albertus Magnus (1565) mentioned the condom as a contraceptive measure in his *De Secretis Mulerium*. In his book on syphilis, the eighteenth century English physician, Daniel Turner (1732), wrote, 'The Condum being the best, if not the only Preservative our Libertines have found out at present; and yet by reason of its bluntiness sensation, I have heard some of them acknowledge, that they have often chose to risk a Clap, rather than engage cum Hastis sic clypeatis' [with spears sheathed].

In the eighteenth century Casanova referred to his condoms as his 'English riding coats' and also called them 'preservative sheaths' or 'assurance caps'. Although initially made from linen or silk, condoms were later available as animal intestine or fish skin. In 1839 Goodyear introduced vulcanization of rubber and rubber condoms soon became available. In the 1930s the introduction of the latex process improved both quality and efficacy of condoms. Apart from acting as family planning contraceptives, it was proven that the condom was effective against the spread of sexually transmitted disease, the original reason for the invention of the device.

In mythology the story is told that the first portion of the semen of Minos, the King of Crete, contained serpents and scorpions, and that all the women who cohabited with him were injured. He married Pasiphae who was immune against such hurt as she was the daughter of the Sun King. However, the couple failed to become pregnant. On the advice of Prokris the sage, Minos had intercourse with a woman who wore a protective goat bladder in her vagina. Once cleared of noxious (infertile) semen, he cohabited with Pasiphae. The couple became parents of eight children.

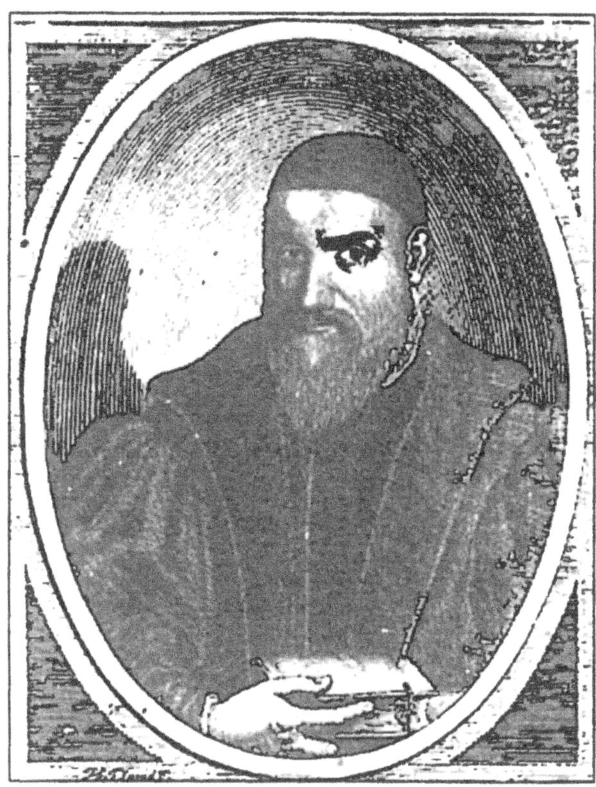

Figure 3 Gabriele Falloppius (1523–1562)

THE 'BIRTH CONTROL' MOVEMENT

The British economist, Thomas Robert Malthus published his *Essay on the Principle of Population* (1798), restating the widespread idea that the world would long ago have been completely populated if it had not been for the population-reducing factors – disease, epidemics, wars and misery, but offered no solution to the problem. In a later edition, Malthus introduced the idea of late marriage as a birth control measure designed to keep the population within

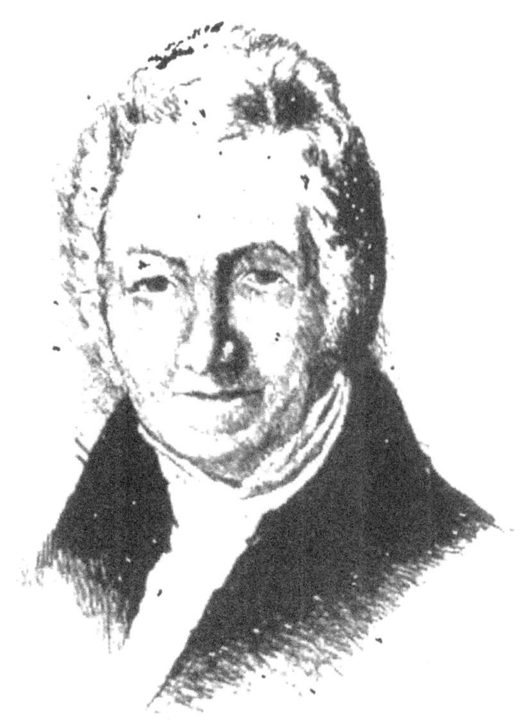

Figure 4 Thomas Robert Malthus (1766–1834)

bounds, but did not advocate any contraceptive means. (The second edition of Malthus appeared in 1803 and revised editions continued until the sixth in 1826.)

Francis Place (1822) boldly attacked Malthus and reasoned that the unnatural birth control remedy of deferred marriage proposed by him was unworkable. Place was the first important proponent of family planning in the English-speaking countries and was associated with the phrase, later to become a household word, concerning the difficulties of over-breeding: 'The remedy can alone be found in 'preventives', as will be further shown in the following section'. According to Marie Stopes there were two contraceptive measures recommended at the time. The female mode consisted of a piece of moist sponge, attached to a twisted thread and inserted into the vagina prior to coitus. The alternative was coitus interruptus, often referred to as 'la chamade', the retreat, also called 'la prudence or la discretion', the preferred method on the Continent, especially in France in the early 1840s.

In England, the next event of special interest was the publication of *The Wives Handbook* (1887) by Henry Arthur Allbutt. The book contained a short chapter dealing with 'How to Prevent Conception' in which Allbutt described withdrawal, the 'safe period', injections of permanganate, boric acid or other disinfectant, the sponge, French letter, Mensinga's pessary, and also Rendell's soluble quinine pessaries and contraceptive powders for introduction with an insufflator. Allbutt was arraigned before his colleagues and struck off the Medical Register ostensibly because he had published his book 'at so low a price'. The Royal College of Physicians of Edinburgh charged him with having published and exposed for sale 'an indecent publication, titled *The Wives Handbook*, and having published, as attached thereto advertisements of an unprofessional character, titled *Malthusian Appliances*' (Stopes, 1923). Allbutt brought his case to the Law Courts but failed in his appeal.

In America, a number of books were published on sexuality and contraception, the most famous of which was *Sexual Physiology* by R.T. Trall (1866). The illustrated book dealt with many aspects of intimate sex life and contained practical information on birth control. Early advocates of the use of contraception in the USA were Robert Dale Owen of Indiana and Charles Nowlton, who spent three months in jail for his work on birth control. The strict European approach to contraception of the era was carried to the New World. Those who adopted an antibirth control stance found a champion in Anthony Comstock. One of ten children, he was born in Connecticut in 1844, and was said to have been influenced by his mother who was a strict Puritan. Comstock spent a large part of his life waging war on the emerging birth control movement in America, which he saw as an evil force. Many influential and wealthy people were attracted to his cause, and legislators introduced strict anticontraceptive laws in many of the States. The last of the so-called 'Comstock' laws prohibiting contraception was only finally struck out in 1973.

During the early part of the twentieth century the birth control movement in America found its champion in Margaret Higgins Sanger. Her father was an Irish agnostic immigrant and her mother, who gave birth to eleven children, died of tuberculosis at the age of forty-eight. Sanger trained as a nurse and worked in the slums of New York among the immigrant community. The women were ignorant of birth control and had large families. An event that had a profound effect on her occurred when she witnessed the final

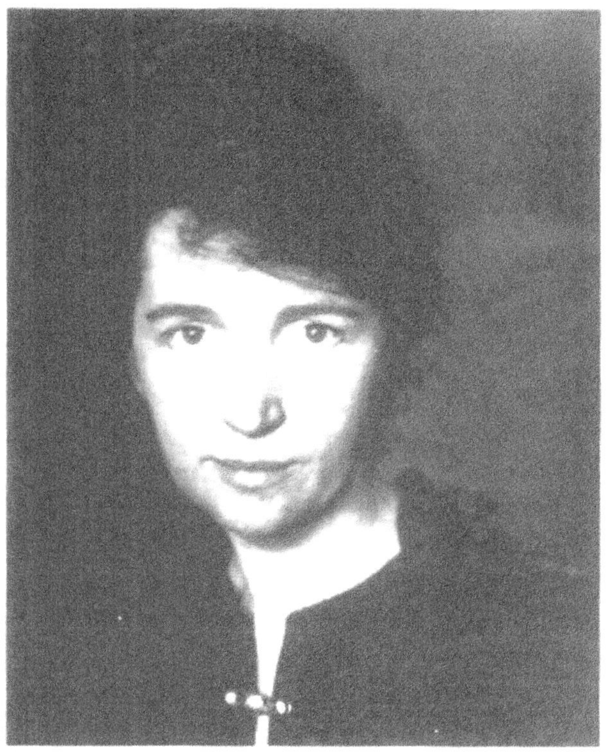

Figure 5 Margaret Sanger (1883–1966)

illness and death of a woman called Sadie Sacks following an attempted illegal abortion. Sanger wrote in her biography that on her arrival home 'I looked out of my window and down upon the dimly lighted city. It's pains and griefs crowded in upon me ... women writhing in travail to bring forth little babies; the babies themselves, naked and hungry, wrapped in newspapers to keep them from the cold ... as I stood there the darkness faded, the sun came up and threw its reflection upon the roof-tops. It was the dawn of a new day in my life also. I was resolved to seek out the roots of the evil, to do something to change the destiny of others to whom miseries were as vast as the sky' (Sanger, 1931; Gillmer, 1998).

Sanger researched the available literature on contraception in both America and Europe. She wrote books and produced pamphlets, and lectured extensively on the benefits of contraceptive methods and their potential to decrease abortion rates. Her first birth control clinic opened in Brownsville, Brooklyn in 1916. Sanger enlisted the help of Dr Robert Dixon, President of the American Gynecological Society who in turn influenced the medical profession to become involved in family planning. In 1915 Marie Stopes met Margaret Sanger and later developed a lifelong commitment to the birth control movement. In a recent article Michael Gillmer wrote that while Gregory Goodman Pincus 'is widely accepted as the 'Father of the Pill' ... few are aware that the pill also has a mother. She was Margaret Higgins Sanger, a pioneer of the birth control movement and founder of the Planned Parenthood Federation' (Gillmer, 1998)

MARIE STOPES' *CONTRACEPTION*

'The Problem Today'

In the first chapter of her book, Marie Stopes (1924) wrote of 'The Problem Today', and informed the reader that 'The death-rate of women in childbirth remains approximately what it was 25 years ago, and we lose by death every year upwards of 3000 mothers ... a substantial number of the 700 000 who gave birth to children in 1919 were so injured or disabled in pregnancy or childbirth as to make them chronic invalids. Individual practitioners, therefore, all over the country are taking an unprecedented interest in contraceptive methods, and many are feeling justly aggrieved that no information on the subject is included in their academic courses of training ... It is the medical man's business to tame and control the stork'. Case histories were offered to support the desirability of birth control in some instances:

'Case C. 866. Age 40, looks older, sight very bad. Hates and loathes the sight of her husband who gives her no peace'. The woman had 17 pregnancies between 1903 and 1922, of which only seven living children resulted.

'Case C. 1167. Fifteen times pregnant since 1900. Eight living children; three who died as imbeciles in the second year, and three miscarriages'.

Contraceptives in use, classified

Marie Stopes recognized three forms of true contraceptives and, as detailed below, her text encapsulates the known birth control techniques of the early twentieth century. The many herbal medications of previous centuries, from ancient Egypt to the nineteenth

CONTRACEPTION

(BIRTH CONTROL)

ITS THEORY, HISTORY AND PRACTICE

A Manual for

The Medical and Legal Professions

BY

MARIE CARMICHAEL STOPES,

Doctor of Science, London; Doctor of Philosophy, Munich; Fellow of University College, London; Fellow of the Linnean and Geological Societies, and The Royal Society of Literature; Author of "Married Love."

With an Introduction by

PROF. SIR WILLIAM BAYLISS, M.A., D.Sc., F.R.S.

and Introductory Notes by

SIR JAMES BARR, M.D., LL.D., F.R.C.P.

DR. C. ROLLESTON, DR. JANE HAWTHORNE & OBSCURUS

LONDON

JOHN BALE, SONS & DANIELSSON, LIMITED,

83-91, GT. TITCHFIELD STREET, OXFORD STREET, W. 1.

1924

Figure 6 Frontispiece from Stopes *Contraception, Its Theory, History and Practice* (1924)

century, were either ignored or not included in the texts she had used as her reference material.

With regard to the very widespread method of contraception known as coitus interruptus or 'masculine prudence', Marie Stopes and other researchers were of the opinion that the method would have harmful effects on both men and women, leading to functional disorders and even insanity. Stopes referred to the work of John Hunter in 1861 who found that 'The semen would appear, both from the smell and taste, to be a mawkish kind of substance; but when held some time in the mouth it produces a warmth similar to spices, which lasts some time'. She quoted further from Havelock Ellis on the value of the seminal fluid for women, 'If semen is a stimulant when ingested, it is easy to suppose that it may exert a similar action on the woman who receives it into the vagina in normal sexual congress'. Stopes was disapproving of coitus interruptus because of its unreliability and possible emotional and physical effects on the couple.

Marie Stopes wrote briefly on sterilization by vasectomy and double tying of the Fallopian tubes. In regard to termination of pregnancy, she reasoned that 'Methods of abortion are most frequently used by poor and ignorant women who are denied the necessary contraceptive knowledge ... all can fairly be described as physiologically harmful as well as legally criminal', although she mentioned medically necessary 'evacuation of the uterus'. The various methods of birth control tabulated below fell under the three main headings of her 'true contraceptives' and were the subject of detailed discussion by Stopes in the fifth chapter of her book.

A. Actions or modes of procedure by either sex not involving chemical substances or appliances of any sort: many of these are mistakenly described as 'natural' by persons prejudiced against the application of science to human breeding:

Actions by the Female

- Extreme passivity in order to control her own orgasm so that it does not take place.
- Placing the body in positions likely in her individual case to prevent contact of the penis with the cervix.
- Sitting upright the moment after ejaculation has taken place and coughing violently, or taking some other exercise to contract the pelvic muscles.
- Prolonged suckling an infant or child.

Action of the Male

- Extra-vaginal union without normal penetration.
- Vaginal stimulation consummating the ejaculation after withdrawal, commonly called 'coitus interruptus', sometimes called 'onanismus conjugalis'.

By both Parties

- Control of the coital act so that ejaculation shall not take place even after prolonged union, known as 'male continence' or 'karezza'.
- Seasonal fertility.

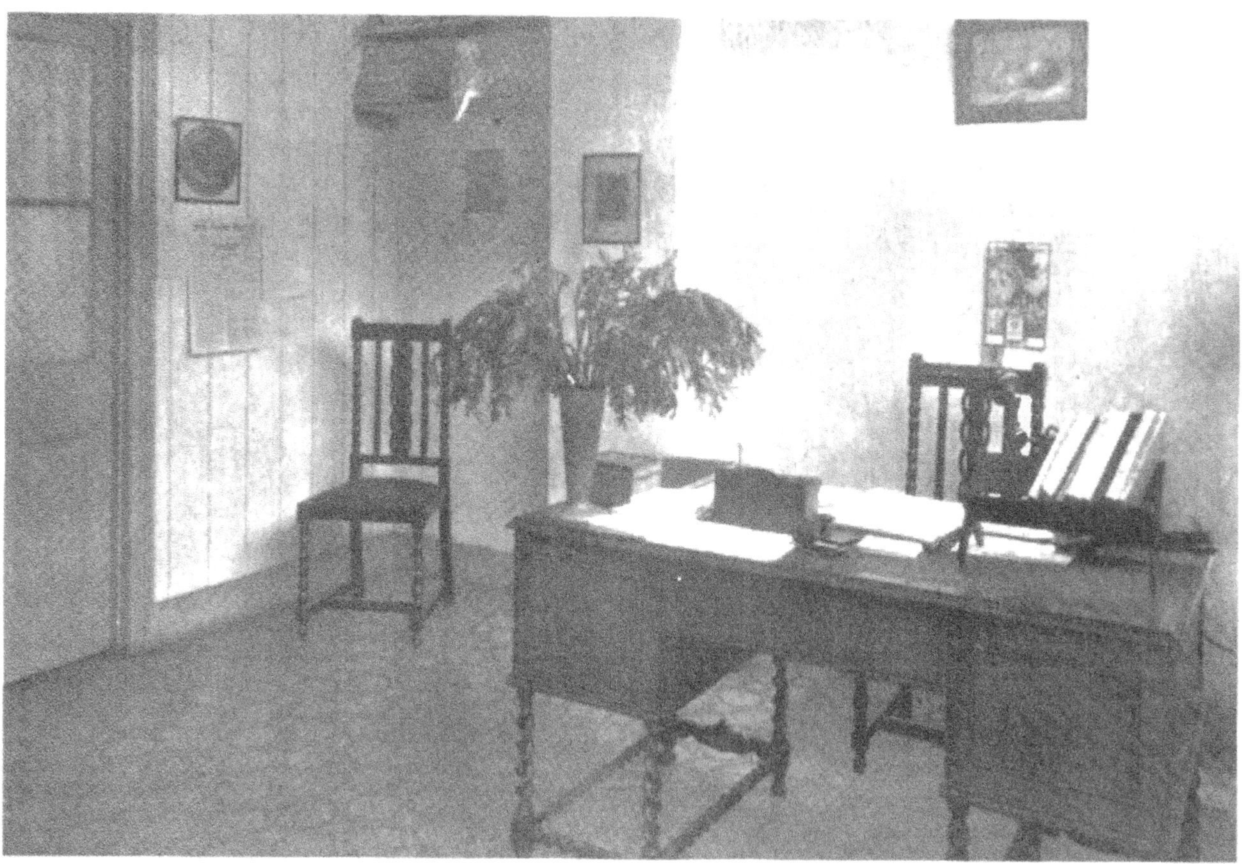

Coitus intermenstruous or restriction of the coital act to certain specified dates in the month, commonly called the 'safe period' or 'tempus ageneseos'.

Mutual and complete abstention from the coital act.

B. Actions or modes of procedure involving the introduction of chemical substances with the supposed intention of incapacitating the spermatozoa so that they do not fuse with the ovum ... The commonest chemical substances introduced into the vagina are:

Quinine compounds in a variety of forms, as a powder, as ointment on a sponge, plug, cap or merely rubbed around the cervix; in a pessary or suppository contained in a matrix of low-melting point wax, such as cocoa butter or gelatin; dissolved in or mixed with oil which is injected by a small specially constructed syringe; various suppositories. (quinine pessaries contained boric acid, cocoa butter or gelatin, salicylic acid and quinine).

Alum in powdered form.

Common salt in solution as a douche.

Vinegar and water, or lactic acid, etc. as a douche.

Disinfectants of one sort or another in the form of a douche.

Plain cold water in the form of a douche.

C. Appliances used by either sex to prevent the spermatozoa coming in contact with the ovum.

By the Male

Condoms (popularly called French letters).

Pin or stud-like apparatus supposed to close the urethra in case unpremeditated ejaculation took place before coitus interruptus was accomplished.

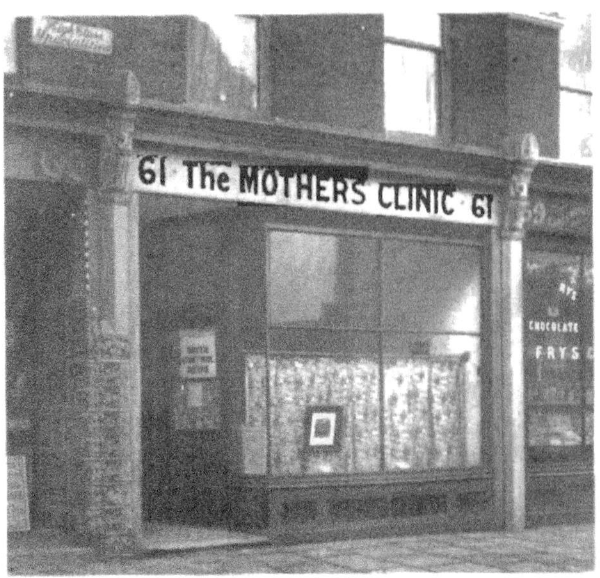

Figure 8 Front of Stopes' birth control clinic

THE
AUTHORIZED LIFE
OF
MARIE C. STOPES

BY
AYLMER MAUDE

AUTHOR OF
Life of Tolstoy.
Editor of the "Maude Tolstoy" in the World's Classics Series.

LONDON:
WILLIAMS & NORGATE, LTD.
14, HENRIETTA STREET, COVENT GARDEN, W.C.2
—
1924

Figure 9 Frontispiece from Stopes biography by Maude (1924)

By the Female

- The sponge, used with or without chemical solutions, soap powder or other potential spermaticide.
- Soft plug; special tampons;
- Dome-shaped cap-like pessaries designed to fit over the cervix;
- Cap-like pessaries similar to above but covered with sponge on the convex surface;
- Flat lens-shaped cap (Dumas) designed to close the end of the vaginal canal;
- Hemispherical-shaped caps with spring designed to close the end of the vaginal canal: the 'Dutch cap'.
- Cap-shaped pessary with separate ring and soft detachable cap, called the 'Mizpah'.
- 'Matrisalus' pessary, rubber cap or turtle-back shaped.
- Balls of soft rubber.
- Large membranous or rubber sheath, or 'capote Anglaise' calculated to cover the internal female organs completely, acting like the male sheath in preventing contact of the seminal fluid with the vaginal surface.
- Springs, studs, metal buttons, the 'gold spring' or 'wishbone' pessary, metal cigar-like structures in a great variety of shapes and forms, designed to enter the cervical canal, and some also to fill the cavity of the uterus'.

THE LEGAL 'POSITION' OF CONTRACEPTION IN BRITAIN, FRANCE AND AMERICA

'In Great Britain there is not and there never has been any law against contraception or the publication and distribution of contraceptive knowledge'.

America

As might have been expected from a progressive community of persons of intelligent mind, America was one of the leading pioneers in the earlier dissemination of modern contraceptive methods. This, I think, will be apparent in the chapter on the history of the nineteenth century. Knowlton's pamphlet itself emanated from America as did the great work of Dr Trall in 1866 which, though a serious book, had an immense and popular success. Then in the year 1873 into Anthony Comstock's law regulating obscenity, the words 'prevention of conception' were slipped which led to very serious results in the USA. The Comstock Bill was introduced on February 11 1873, passed by both Houses and signed by the President before close of the session on March 4. It appears that the measure was enacted without discussion, in the last few days of the expiring Congress, and that contraceptive knowledge was not once mentioned by any member of Congress during the session.

The Federal Law was passed in 1873 and the now notorious Section 211 of the Penal Code reads as follows: 'Every article or thing designed, adapted or intended for preventing conception or procuring abortion, or for any indecent or immoral use ... or notice of any kind giving information directly or indirectly ... and every letter, packet or package, or other mail matter containing any filthy, vile, or indecent thing ... for preventing conception ... is hereby declared to be non-mailable matter ... whosoever shall knowingly deposit or cause to be deposited for mailing or delivery, anything declared by this section to be non-mailable ... shall be fined not more than $5000, or imprisoned not more than five years, or both'. Further restrictions were passed in 1909 that made it illegal for any non-American citizen to carry any form of contraceptive, or contraceptive knowledge, into the United States.

Planned Parenthood

Margaret Sanger founded the American Birth Control League in 1921 but the name was changed to the Planned Parenthood Federation of America in 1942. The Family Planning Association of Great Britain was founded in 1930. The International Planned Parenthood Federation was launched in 1952 in New Delhi under the leadership of Margaret Sanger and Lady Rama Rau of India, with 20 nations represented. In 1960 The World Population Emergency Campaign was organized in the United States and merged with the Planned Parenthood Federation of America in 1961.

Alan F. Guttmacher, 1963

In the preface to Norman E. Himes' *Medical History of Contraception* (Reprint, 1963 pp. ix–xxx), Alan F. Guttmacher related that in 1936 a Dr Hannah Stone imported vaginal diaphragms from Japan to America. They were seized by the Customs Authority. Stone sought to test the validity of this application of the Customs Law and the test case became known as 'The United States versus one package'. The case finally went to the Court of Appeals and Justice Augustus Hand read into the Federal Statute that it was permitted, that the 'importation, sale or carriage by mail of things which might intelligently be employed by conscientious and competent physicians for the purpose of saving life or promoting the well-being of their patients'. At the time of writing in 1963, Guttmacher noted that there were still restrictive statutes in a number of states, but only the laws in Massachusetts and Connecticut were still drastic. In Guttmacher's view the three most important developments in contraception since 1935 were the more extensive and accurate use of the rhythm method; the development of modified intrauterine rings, and the first truly physiologic method of contraception – the inhibition of ovulation by oral medication'. Guttmacher, who was President of the Planned Parenthood Foundation of America died in 1974.

Contraception in 1955 (Guttmacher, 1963):

Condom	26%
Diaphragm	24%
Rhythm	21%
Douche	7%
Withdrawal	7%
Other methods (or combinations of)	15%

France

In the year 1929 an extraordinary bill was passed making even scientific consideration of contraception a criminal offense with punishment of a term of imprisonment varying from six months to three years or a fine from 100 to 3000 francs.

Contraception and teaching in medical schools in Britain

'The majority of doctors who are now qualified and practicing have received nothing in the form of training or instruction in contraception in the whole of their college courses'. Stopes circulated the leading medical schools in Great Britain in March 1922 and had replies from the deans or secretaries of all. With one exception, they replied with a categorical negative to the question on whether they were offering lectures or classes on contraception to their medical students.

Birth control clinics

Stopes reported that, in 1885, Aletta Jacobs opened the first birth control clinic in the world, in Holland, where a Dutch Birth Control League was founded. In 1916 an American attempt to imitate the Dutch experience was stopped by the police. The first British Birth Control Clinic, known as 'The Mothers' Clinic', was founded by Marie Stopes and her aviator husband, Humphrey Verdon Roe, at 61 Marlborough Road, Holloway, London N 19 in 1921. Marie Stopes died of cancer at the age of 77 in 1958.

HORMONAL CONTRACEPTION

Joseph W. Goldzieher of San Antonio, Texas and Harry W. Rudel of the Brookdale Hospital Center, New York (1974) wrote an entertaining history of hormonal contraception in their paper *How the Oral Contraceptives Came to be Developed.* They were of the opinion that 'The development of hormonal contraceptives is one of the epochal events of the twentieth century' although it's impact on the 'ultimate state of the human condition remain(s) for future historians to assess'.

Early observations

- Professor Zschokke, a Zurich veterinarian, stated in 1898 that it was the practice to manually crush persistent corpus lutea in sterile cows, a procedure that was in vogue for at least 50 years. It was clear to Zschokke that while the corpus luteum persisted further development of the graffian follicles (and ovulation) were inhibited.
- John Beard (1897), an anatomist at the University of Edinburgh, surmised that ovulation was suppressed in higher mammals during pregnancy. He indicated that the increasing size of the corpus luteum was the reason for prevention of normal ovulation.
- In France, Prenant (1898), a histologist at the University of Nancy, proposed an endocrine function for the corpus luteum.
- By 1909, Leo Loeb of Philadelphia, observed that removal of corpora lutea in pigs hastened the onset of ovulation and concluded that ovulation was suppressed by the growing corpus luteum.
- In 1916, Herrmann and Stein of the Institute of Anatomy in Vienna suppressed ovulation in rats with lipid extracts of corpora lutea.

Early studies on hormonal contraception

- Ludwig Haberlandt, professor of physiology of Innsbruck, Austria 'formulated these observations and inferences into a concept of purposeful contraception'. In March 1919 he transplanted ovaries from pregnant rabbits under the skin of fertile adult does and rendered them infertile. Over the following 13 years he experimented with extracts of corpora lutea and in 1927 reported that ovarian extracts given orally to mice produced temporary sterility.
- In 1921, Otfried Fellner of Vienna reported that liquid extract of pregnant sows ovaries had potent biological (estrogenic) effects. Fellner prepared injectable extracts and an oral preparation called Feminin which produced sterility in rabbits and mice. He concluded in 1927 that his ovarian (estrogenic) extract prevented pregnancy by destruction of ova and by inhibition of corpus luteum formation.
- Unaware of Fellner's work, Loeb and Kounitz in St Louis, obtained similar results working with guinea pigs.

Isolation of estrogen and progesterone

- Allan and Doisy (1923) reported the localization, extraction, and partial purification of estrogen.
- Doisy in 1929 reported the isolation of estrogen. The structure of estrone was elucidated in the 1930s as a result of the work of Doisy and also Marrian and Butenandt. Ethenol estradiol was synthesized in 1938.
- Corner and Allen (1929) developed a bioassay for progestational activity in 1929 and progesterone was isolated as the active component of the corpus luteum soon afterwards. Then it was reported that pure progesterone inhibited post-coital ovulation in the rabbit and guinea pig.
- In 1935, Russell Marker went to Penn State College and began a career in sterol chemistry. He converted plant sterols (sapogenins) into progesterone and began a search for a good botanical source as, until then, progesterone was obtained from sow's ovaries with a yield of 1 mg per 2500 sows. In 1943, Marker ran into funding difficulties and moved to Mexico City where he continued his research in an old pottery shed. Within two months he had produced 2000 gm of progesterone which at that time was worth $80 a gram. Shortly afterwards he formed an association with Emeric Somlo and Frederico Lechman. Together they founded a company named Syntex (synthesis and Mexico) and produced the Diosgenin (isolated from the root of the *Dioscorea*) from which progesterone was obtained. Some time afterwards it was discovered that the barbasco root was a richer source of the desired sterol.
- Marker departed from Syntex who, in turn, hired George Rosenkranz, a Swiss chemist, and he continued with progesterone production.
- In 1951 while carrying out further research on steroid hormones, Carl Djerassi developed norethindrone.
- In the following year Colton synthesized norethynedrol.

Clinical practice

- In clinical practice Sturgis and Albright reported in 1940 that injections of estradiol benzoate prevented the cramps of dysmenorrhea and also successfully inhibited ovulation.
- In 1945 Albright specified the potential of ovulation-inhibiting doses of estrogen as a contraceptive method.

Funding and trials

In 1950 Margaret Higgins Sanger and her wealthy friend Mrs Katherine McCormick decided that contraceptive technology required advancement. They enlisted the aid of Gregory Goodman Pincus, a reproductive biologist at the Worcester Foundation in Massachusetts. Pincus and associates decided to examine the potential of progesterone. Soon afterwards he secured the collaboration of John Rock, a gynecologist with an interest in infertility and endocrine treatments. The first reported studies of norethynodrel (contaminated with estrogen, mestranol) appeared in 1956. With financing made available through Mrs McCormick, a clinical contraceptive trial was undertaken in Puerto Rico by C.R. Garcia. The first British trial commenced in Birmingham in March 1960 and in early 1961 Conovid, containing 5 mg norethynodrel and 0.075 mg mestranol, was introduced.

Dose-related side effects

The early brands of the contraceptive pill contained 10 mg of progesterone and 150 μg of estrogen. Many women experienced unwanted side effects and this provided a stimulus to reduce the dose of both progesterone and estrogen. A 30 μg estrogen pill was introduced in 1972 and, by 1979, the progesterone dose had been reduced from 10 mg to 0.15 mg.

The first major adverse effect of the pill was documented by a family doctor, W.M. Jordan (1962) of Suffolk, England, who reported the occurrence of thrombosis and embolism in a patient using Enovid as treatment for endometriosis. Soon afterwards, Boyce *et al.* (1963) reported thrombotic effects of Conovid. Further reports implicated the oral contraceptive with hypertension and alterations in blood lipid levels. It was discovered that the complications directly related to the quantity of both estrogen and progesterone. Low-dose formulations were produced that had very low complication rates and were safe to use. Studies revealed that the oral contraceptive also had beneficial side effects.

OTHER FORMS OF CONTRACEPTION

Occlusive means

The diaphragm was introduced in 1882 by a German physician, Wilhelm P.J. Mensinga of Flensburg.

Sterilization

James Blundell of London was the first to recommend sterilization as a means to prevent the hazards of disproportion in women with contracted pelves (1834). 'I would advise an incision of an inch in length in the linea alba above the symphysis pubis; I would advise further, that the fallopian tube in either side should be drawn up to this aperture; and lastly I would advise, that a portion of the tube should be removed, an operation easily performed when the woman would, forever, be sterile.' The first sterilization in America was carried out by S.S. Lungren, of Toledo, Ohio (1881), in a woman during her second cesarean section. Max Madlener of Germany, Ralph Pomeroy of New York, and Frederick Carpenter Irving also of New York, are all eponymously related to their sterilizing techniques from the early twentieth century (Speert, 1958). Power and Barnes (1941) introduced laparoscopic sterilization with tubal fulguration. During the 1970s various fallopian tube occlusion devices were introduced for use during laparoscopy. A number of the inventors achieved eponymous fame, including Marcus Filshie (1983).

Intrauterine contraceptive device

In 1909, Richter of Waldenburg, Germany, described a thread pessary for contraceptive use. Intrauterine contraceptive devices were popularized by the German gynecologist Ernst Grafenberg in the 1920s. His first IUDs were made from silkworm gut and were frequently expelled, but he later developed a ring made of silver wire, the so-called Grafenberg ring (1931). Over the years a large number of devices were patented and referred to as the 'children of Grafenberg's ring'. One form of IUD, the Dalkon Shield, was associated with serious pelvic infection and fatality. The Mirena IUCD was introduced in the 1990s. It contained Levonorgestrel 52 mg and about 20% of users developed oligo- or amenorrhea. As a result, the device was not only contraceptive but had the benefit of treating menorrhagia in some women.

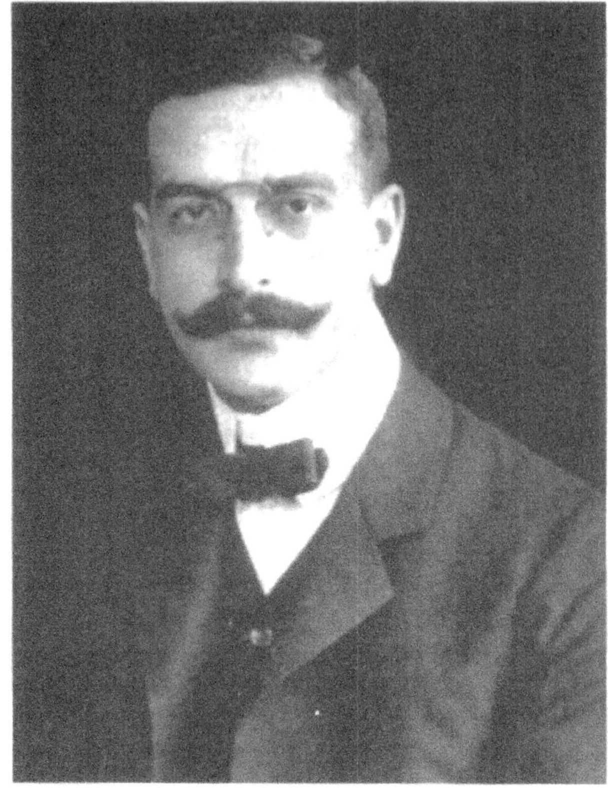

Figure 10 Ernst Grafenberg (1881–1957)

Depot hormonal preparations

Depo-provera was introduced in 1967 and since that time various injectable or implanted contraceptives that contained estrogen or progesterone were developed.

Natural family planning

Since Squire (1868) described an increase in the basal body temperature in the second half of the cycle, it became apparent that ovulation could be detected. Avoidance of intercourse at that time led to the concept of 'natural family planning'. Ogino (1930) of Japan, estimated a method of determining the fertile period later known as the 'calendar method'. Seguy and Simmonet (1933) related cervical mucous change to ovulation. Their research prompted John Billings (an Australian ear, nose and throat surgeon) and his wife Evelyn to investigate the use of cervical mucous changes in the prediction of ovulation as a method of family planning (Billings *et al.*, 1972).

Vasectomy

Sir Astley Cooper (1830) carried out experimental vasectomy in dogs in 1823. Later in the century Harrison (1899) recommended its use in men as a 'cure' for prostatic enlargement. The method only became popular as a contraceptive device in the 1960s.

The male pill

The possibility of a male 'pill' was mooted with the advent of gossypol or by using combinations of cyproterone acetate with testosterone enanthate. Extract of the Chinese plant, *Tripterygium* (Zhen, Ye and Wei, 1995) was found to have infertility effects in the male but further developments are awaited.

References

Allan, E. and Doisy, E. A. (1923). An ovarian hormone. Preliminary report of its localization, extraction, and partial purification and action in test animals. *JAMA*, 81, 819–21

Allbutt, H. A. (1887). *The Wife's Handbook: How a Woman should order herself during pregnancy, in the Lying-in Room, and after Delivery, with Hints on the Management of the Baby, and on other matters of importance, necessary to be known by married women*, 46th ed. 1916 p. 59. (London: George Standring)

Beard, J. (1897). *The Span of Gestation and the Cause of Birth.* (Jena: Fischer)

Boyce, J., Fawcett, J. W. and Noall, E. W. O. (1963). Coronary thrombosis and conovid. *The Lancet*, 2, 111

Billings, E. L., Billings, J. J., Brown, J. B. and Burger, H. G. (1972). Symptoms and hormonal changes accompanying ovulation. *The Lancet*, 1, 282–4

Blundell, J. (1834). *The Principles and Practice of Obstetrics*, pp. 352, 360. (Washington: Duff Green)

Cooper, A. (1830). *Observations on the structure and disease of the testes.* (London: Longman)

Corner, G. W. (1943). *Hormones in Human Reproduction*, Rev. (ed.) (New York: Princeton University Press)

Corner, G. W. and Allen, W. M. (1929). Physiology of the corpus luteum: 2. Production of a special uterine reaction (progestational proliferation) by extracts of the corpus luteum. *Am. J. Physiol.*, 88, 826

Falloppius, G. (1564). *De Morbo Gallico: Liber Absolutissmus*, Chapter 89, p. 52 'De Praeservatione a Carrie Gallica'. (Patavia: C. Gryphum)

Filshie, G. M. (1983). The Filshie Clip. In Van Lith, D. A. F., Leith, L. G. and Van Hall, E. V. (eds) *New Trends in Female Sterilization*, pp. 115–24. (Chicago, London: Medical Year Book)

Gillmer, M. D. G. (1998). The oral contraceptive pill – A product of serendipity. *The Diplomate*, pp. 231–5

Goldzieher, J. W. and Rudel, H. W. (1974). How the oral contraceptives came to be developed. *JAMA*, 230(3), 421–5

Grafenberg, E. (1931). Intrauterine methods: An intrauterine contraceptive method. In Sanger, M. and Stone, H. M. (eds) Procs. of the 7th International Birth Control Conference: *The Practice of Contraception*, pp. 33–47. (Baltimore: Williams & Wilkins)

Harrison, R. (1899). *Selected Papers on Stone, Prostate and other Urinary Disorders.* (London: Churchill)

Himes, N. E. (1936). *Medical History of Contraception*, Reprinted 1963. (New York: Gamut Press)

Jordan, W. M. (1962). Pulmonary embolism. *The Lancet*, 2, 1146

Lungren, S. S. (1881). A Case of Cesarean Section Twice Successfully Performed on the Same Patient, with Remarks on the Time, Indications, and Details of the Operation. *Am. J. Obstet.*, 14, 78–94

Magnus, A. (1565). *De Secretis Mulerium Item De Virtutibus Herbarium Labidum et Animalium*, p. 329. (Amsterdam)

Malthus, T. R. (1798). *An essay on the principle of population, as it affects future improvement of society.* (London: J. Johnson)

Ogino, K. (1930). Ovulationstermin und Konzeptionstermin. *Zbl. Gynakol.*, 54, 464–79

Place, F. (1822). *Illustrations and Proofs of the Principle of Population; Including an examination of the proposed remedies of Mr. Malthus and a reply to the Objections of Mr Godwin and others*, p. XV, 280. (London: Longman)

Power, F. H. and Barnes, A. C. (1941). Sterilization by means of peritoneoscopic tubal fulguration. *Am. J. Obstet. Gynecol.*, 41, 1038–43

Prenant, A. (1898). La Valeur Morphologique du Corps Jaune. Son Action Physiologique et Therapeutique Possible. *Rev. Gen. Sci. Pure Appel.*, 9, 646–50

Ricci, J. V. (1950). *Aetios of Amida. The Gynecology and Obstetrics of the VIth Century AD*. Translated from the Latin Edition of Cornarius, 1542. (Philadelphia: Blakiston Co.)

Sanger, M. H. (1931). *My Fight for Birth Control*. (New York: Farrar and Rinehart)

Seguy, J. and Simonnet, H. (1933). Recherche de signes directs d'ovulation chez la femme. *Gynecologie et Obstetrique*, **28**, 656–63

Speert, H. (1958). *Essays in Eponomy. Obstetric and Gynecologic Milestones*, pp. 619–29. (New York: Macmillan Co.)

Stopes, M. C. (1924). *Contraception (Birth Control) It's Theory and History and Practice. A Manual for The Medical and Legal Professions*. (London: John Bale, Sons, and Danielsson)

Squire, W. (1868). Puerperal temperatures. *Trans. Obstet. Soc., London*, **9**, 129

Trall, R. T. (1866). *Sexual Physiology: A Scientific and Popular Exposition of the Fundamental Problems in Sociology*, pp. 14, 312. (New York & London: Wood and Holbrook)

Turner, D. (1732). *Syphilis. A Practical Treatise on the Venereal Disease*, 4th ed. p. 107. (London)

Zhen, Q. S., Ye, X. and Wei, Z. J. (1995). Recent progress in research on *Tripterygium*: A male anti-fertility plant. *Contraception*, **51**, 121–9

The menopause 23

INTRODUCTION

The word 'menopause' signifies the cessation of menstruation and was derived from the Greek, *men*, month and *pausis*, cessation. The term was introduced as 'menespausie' by the Frenchman, Gardanne (1816), and shortened by him to 'menopause' in 1821 (Wilbush, 1979, 1981a). This transition in the life of women is also referred to as the 'climacteric', a term from the Greek, *klimakter* or *klimax*, a rung of a ladder, a critical period in human life. The 'ladder of life' is usually divide into periods of seven years, each multiple of seven being characterized by alterations in the health and constitution of the individual; the ninth period, or 63rd year, being the 'grand climacteric'. The climacteric was also used to signify puberty but now refers exclusively to the peri-menopause.

The short-term symptoms of the menopause affect 25–50% of women. There may be vasomotor instability with hot flushes/flashes and with sweats, palpitations and headaches which severely impede well-being and quality of life. Symptoms commonly wane after 3–5 years but may persist for 10 years or more. The long-term sequelae of osteoporosis and cardiovascular disease may cause mortality or disabling morbidity and have a major deleterious impact on women's health. Under the circumstances, it is difficult to comprehend that the first medical conference devoted exclusively to the menopause was organized by the International Health Foundation in Geneva as late as 1971 (Rekers, 1990).

Although the ancients were aware of the menopause and used menstrual inducers in a vain effort to restore normal menstruation, the subject of the 'change of life' received scant attention from the medical profession until the eighteenth century. It was then that European physicians undertook their initial researches on the subject. In the following century the Frenchman, Gardanne (1816), wrote the first book about the menopause. The first English text on the subject by Edward J. Tilt (1857) raised awareness of the issue on a wider scale and his book was particularly popular among American physicians.

With the development of reproductive endocrinology, a crude form of ovarian replacement therapy was available from the early twentieth century, but Hormone Replacement Therapy (HRT) as we understand it only became available as estrogen treatment from about 1966, and as combined estrogen and progesterone therapy from 1971. The introduction of HRT involved risk-taking but found its champion in Robert Wilson (1966), a New York gynecologist. His book, *Feminine Forever*, brought the topic of HRT to the attention of the lay public and the medical profession slowly responded in positive fashion. HRT was not without its problems and there were suspicions about serious side-effects, some of which were well founded. Fortunately, the issues of HRT and its relationship to the possible side effects of breast cancer, cardiovascular disease, hypertension, thrombosis, ischemic heart disease, and stroke appear to be resolved.

THE MENOPAUSE AND LIFE EXPECTANCY

Amundsen and Diers (1970) estimated that the age of menopause in classical Greece and Rome was typically between 40 to 55 years – but how many women actually entered the 'change of life'? John Riddle (1997) indicated that life expectancy remained around 30 years (average) from 11 000 BC until 650 BC and the advent of the Greco–Roman era. During the latter period, and until AD 200, the average age at death of women, as determined from skeletal remains in ancient cemeteries, was 35 to 37 years. Robert Garland (1990) agreed with those estimates and pointed out that, despite wars and aggression, men lived an average of 10 years longer. At the dawn of the twentieth century the average life expectancy in the USA was 47.3 years, with women living two years longer, and by 1978 the average was 73.3 years. At the same time, women in developing countries such as Upper Volta and Chad had average life expectancy of 31 and 35 years, respectively, in 1979.

The expectation of life to a certain age helps us to focus more clearly on the percentages, and thus the numbers of women who will achieve menopause and older age. From the Middle Ages until the late nineteenth century, less than 30% of women reached the menopause. In the 140 years from 1841–1980, the number of Irish women reaching 55 years almost doubled. By the late 1980s, 90% of women in Western industrialized countries experienced menopause; almost 60% lived to age 75. It was estimated at that time that the average woman could expect to spend one third of her life, some 30 years, in the post-menopausal state. At the time there were 10 million post-menopausal women in the United Kingdom and West Germany. In the USA the 40 million such women totaled almost 20% of the population (Schneider, 1986).

By the year 2015, approximately 46% of the female population may be of climacteric age or older. It is estimated that in 2020, over one billion individuals will be over the age of 60, and two thirds of them will be living in affluent countries. Population aging has thus become a major public health challenge for the new millennium, with specific concerns for womens' long-term health. An editorial in the *World Medical Journal* indicated that around 30% of people in developed nations will exceed 60 years of age by the year 2020 (Gillibrand, 1997).

MENOPAUSE THROUGH THE AGES

Stone Age menopause

There is a Stone Age funerary mound, known as Newgrange, not far from Dublin, that dates from c. 2500 BC and antedates the first Egyptian pyramid constructed by the Pharaoh Djosser. Newgrange, known until recent times as Bruigh Na Boinne, was also the home of Aonghus, Ireland's god of love. At the entrance to the funeral mound there is a carved stone that bears Ireland's third most famous symbol (after the harp and shamrock) commonly referred to as 'The Three Spirals'. Archeologists, historians and those who deal in myth and legend have determined that 'The Three Spirals' signify, birth, death and regeneration, or the young lady, the reproductively mature, and the older woman. It appears that we are not the first to dwell on the topic of the three ages of women.

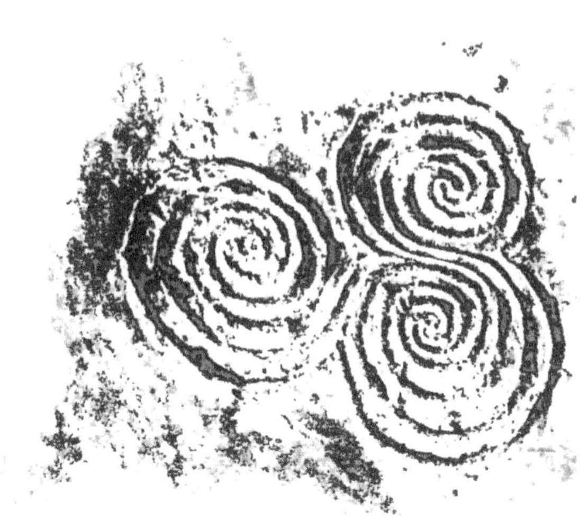

Figure 1 Irish triad representing female fertility

Triads, or groups of three, were common in the ancient world and the concept entered midwifery as the 'Three Goddesses of Childbirth'. Triads were usual in oral traditions, literature, and music. Triads are part of the ancient philosophy of numerology which evolved from Assyrian culture some 5000 years ago. Numerologists divide life into three stages. The first stage lasts for 27 years and is concerned with physical and emotional development. The second of 27 years are a transitional period moving toward the more contemplative nature of mid- to later life. The third stage lasts from the age of 54 until death and is a period of love, spirituality and wisdom.

The concept of numerology and its relationship to women and the menopause continues to the present. In his 'Prologue' to a scientific meeting on the menopause, later published as *A Modern Approach to the Perimenopausal Years*, Hannse (1986) wrote that 'Each woman passes through three epochs in her progression through life'. The first, from birth to adolescence is in preparation for the second, the years of fecundity. The third ends her potential for reproduction. Thus, she enters the menopause, the permanent cessation of menstruation.

Ancient Egypt

According to David Sturdee and Mark Brincat the hot flush 'recognized ... as the most characteristic manifestation of the climacteric ... was first referred to in the Ebers Papyrus c. 1500 BC'. They quoted from Bryan's (1930) translation 'When thou examinest a woman who has lived many years without her menstruation having appeared ... her body is as though a fire were under it'.

The Bible

The menopause was alluded to in the Bible when 'It [menstruation] ceased to be with Sarah after the manner of women'. As with other events, we can discover other Biblical precedents, when we recall Elizabeth, cousin to Mary, the mother of Jesus who conceived in her elderly barren state (post-menopausal), and gave birth to John the Baptist. Her pregnancy meant that newspaper headlines of 'Naturally occurring Pregnancy in a 60 year old' and 'IVF for Grandmothers' would not unduly shock us.

Ancient Greece and Rome

In Ancient Greece the menopause heralded a time of great social change for women. They were allowed, for the first time, to appear unattended in public. They could become midwives and mourners at funerals, functions for which they were paid. Of course, as they were no longer capable of childbearing, they did not need the same degree of protection against the amorous advances of the indiscriminate Greek males of the time (Garland, 1990).

Compared to other gynecological problems, little was written in the ancient texts about the symptoms or signs of the menopause. However, the conditions likely to occur at that age, such as uterine growths and prolapse, were discussed in great detail. Hippocrates c. 430 BC made the interesting observation in his *Aphorisms* or 'medical truths' that 'gout does not occur in women except after the menopause' (Chadwick and Mann, 1950). Was that a reference to osteoporosis?

Soranus (AD 98–138), the foremost authority on obstetrics and gynecology in antiquity, came from the ancient city of Ephesus, home to the female deity Artemis, also known as Diana, the goddess of fertility and hunting. Soranus detailed the knowledge of Greco–Roman physicians about menstruation and the menopause. In a tract entitled *On the Catharsis of the Menses* he wrote that 'the menstrual flux, since it occurs monthly, is also called 'katamenion'; and 'epimenion' as well because it becomes the food of the embryo, just as we call the food prepared for seafarers 'epimenia'. It is also called 'katharsis', since, as some people say, excreting blood from the body like excessive matter, it affects a purgation of the body'. (It was long believed that the 'menstruum', or menstrual fluid, had a solvent quality. The term 'menstruum' was thus used in alchemy and chemistry to denote a solvent.)

'Menstruation, in most cases, first appears around the fourteenth year, at the time of puberty and swelling of the breasts ... it diminishes again, and so it finally comes to an end, usually not earlier than 40 nor later than 50 years. In women who are about to menstruate no longer, their time for menstruation having passed, one must take care that the stoppage of the menses does not occur suddenly ... The methods we employ at the approach of the first menstruation [emmenagogues] must now be marshaled forth during the time when menstruation is about to cease ... In addition, vaginal suppositories capable of softening and injections which have the [same] effect should be employed, [together] with all the remedies capable of rendering hardened bodies soft' (Temkin, 1956). Passive exercise, massage, daily baths and 'diversion of the mind' all had a role to play for those entering the 'change of life'. No additional information on the menopause came to light for many centuries.

The sixteenth and seventeenth centuries

The medical texts of the era devoted to women contented themselves with discourses on midwifery and normal or abnormal menstruation in the child-bearing woman. The herbals and pharmacopoeias offered no treatments except menstrual inducers. William Turner (1568) did not mention either the 'change of life' nor the 'menopause' in his famous herbal of medicinal plants. Nicholas Culpeper (1653) was equally silent on the topic in his *London Dispensatorie*, the translation of the *Pharmacopoeia Londinensis*.

William Shakespeare, the playwright of the age, had a keen eye for women and appeared to offer them equality in his play *As You Like It*: 'All the world's a stage, and all the men and women merely players: they all have their exits and their entrances' but continued in manly fashion: 'and one man in his time plays many parts, his acts being seven ages'. Thus, Shakespeare (1599) reflected the current knowledge of numerology based on the 'Seven Seas' etc. and recounted the relationship between seven and the 'Ages of Man'. Shakespeare's seven ages accurately defines the human cycles of maturation as they related to men but with mea culpa and due respect I extend the bard's possible thought processes to the female gender:

The Seven Ages of 'Man'	
The infant	The infant
Schoolboy	Schoolgirl
Lover	Lover
Soldier	Mother
Justice	Grandmother/menopausal
Lean old man	Bowed/osteoporotic
Second childhood	Second childhood

The eighteenth century

Joel Wilbush (1988) displayed his extensive knowledge of the menopause in the eighteenth and nineteenth centuries in an *Historical Perspective* contained in *The Menopause*, a celebration of the climacteric, and edited by John Studd and Malcolm Whitehead. His numerous publications, including those listed here, form essential reading for the history of the menopause (Wilbush, 1979, 1980, 1981a, 1981b, 1982, 1984). According to Wilbush (1988) the first reference in the English language to the symptoms of the menopause was contained in an anonymous medical guide for women, published in 1727. The author offered treatments of venesection and removal of 8 ounces of blood, or with purging pills and uterine drops. About the same time, the problems of the climacteric were investigated in France and Germany and the menopause was the subject material of university theses and books.

Furor Uterinus

A review of the tracts on 'Midwifery' and also 'Of Women's Diseases' contained in the first edition of

Encyclopædia Britannica;

OR, A

DICTIONARY

OF

ARTS and SCIENCES,

COMPILED UPON A NEW PLAN.

IN WHICH

The different SCIENCES and ARTS are digeſted into diſtinct Treatiſes or Syſtems;

AND

The various TECHNICAL TERMS, &c. are explained as they occur in the order of the Alphabet.

ILLUSTRATED WITH ONE HUNDRED AND SIXTY COPPERPLATES.

By a SOCIETY of GENTLEMEN in SCOTLAND.

IN THREE VOLUMES.

VOL. I.

EDINBURGH:

Printed for A. BELL and C. MACFARQUHAR;

And ſold by COLIN MACFARQUHAR, at his Printing-office, Nicolſon-ſtreet.

M.DCC.LXXI.

Figure 2 Frontispiece from the *Encyclopedia Britannica*

the *Encyclopaedia Britannica* (1771) reveals that the writings may fairly be taken to reflect the knowledge of the era. In the tract 'Of Women's Diseases' there is a piece on 'Of the Suppression of the Menses'.

There was no specific mention of the menopause or 'Change of Life', as it was known at the time, but there was a reference to 'old subjects' in a segment entitled 'Of the Furor Uterinus'. The Society of Gentlemen in Scotland, who were responsible for the *Encyclopaedia Britannica* of 1771, wrote that the furor uterinus was 'Salacity in Women, attended with impudence, restlessness, and a delirium, [and] is called the Furor Uterinus. In the delirium maniacum, the patient is entirely shameless; ... in old subjects. The indications of cure ... [are] answered by frequent and copious bleedings, as in an incipient madness; even to eight times a day, if nothing forbids; if she faints, there is no danger. She must likewise be purged, as mad folks are, with Jalap,

Table 1 Aetius' sixth century treatment for uterine fury

Castorium, coriander, crocomagma, cypheos aromatic
Diacodion
Myrtle wax
Nightshade plant juice
Poppy juice
Rosewater
Saffron, smyrnion (similar to myrrh), sodium cardamom, spikenard
Trigonus lozenge
Vinegar
Wax

Scammony, Diagrid. The dose must be increased one third, as being hard to purge. Emetics are also good; for they evacuate the bile, which abates the acrimony of the humors. In the intervals, order frequent emollient clysters; to which add half a dram of Sal Prunella, or a little vinegar morning and night, baths and semi-cupia; ... moderate the heat, irritation, and sensibility of the parts effected: as also emollient injections into the vagina, and fomentations or pessaries of cotton may be steeped therein; Sal Prunella may also be mixed therein'.

The Scottish Gentlemen's tenuous notion of 'uterine furor' or 'uterine fury' and it's relationship to menopausal women had it's origin in Greco–Roman medicine. Soranus of Ephesus of the early second century AD defined uterine fury as satyriasis, a condition of overpowering sexual desire that could occur in men or women (Temkin, 1956).

Paul of Aegina, in the seventh century AD, also wrote on satyriasis. He was of the impression that it rarely affected women but those who did contract the condition were likely to die from convulsions. In his commentary on *The Seven Books of Paulus of Aegineta*, Francis Adams opined that satyriasis presented a 'disgusting picture' and he hoped that the 'march of improvement in morals has now rendered [it] of rare occurrence' (Adams, 1844).

Aetius of Amida, in the sixth century AD, also dealt with uterine fury (Table 1). His work was translated into Latin by Cornarius in 1542 and subsequently to English by James Ricci (1950). Aetius was of the opinion that 'those [subject to uterine furor] become completely mad in sex matters ... this disease attacks [those] with a warm body temperature, girls of twenty, virgins and chaste [?older] women'. Aetius offered a large number of remedies to treat uterine fury, some of which were prescribed as components of medicated vaginal pessaries.

The notion of 'furor uterinus' was still alive and well in the twentieth century. Havelock Ellis (1936) in his *Studies in The Psychology of Sex* wrote of a 48-year-old school mistress who had failed to complete intercourse due to vaginismus. Ellis related that it was not 'until the period of the menopause that the long repressed desires broke out ... and ... due probably to troubles of the climacteric, led to [sexual] indulgence, under abnormal conditions' that led to her requiring psychiatric treatment.

The nineteenth century

At the beginning of the nineteenth century Gardanne (1816) of France wrote the first book entirely dedicated to the menopause and made the condition the focus of medical and lay attention. Gardanne introduced the term 'menespausie' and shortened the name to 'menopause' in a publication in 1821 (Wilbush, 1988). In England, Tyler Smith (1849) wrote an article for the *London Journal of Medicine*, entitled 'The climacteric disease in women' and referred to 'heats and chills' that accompanied the menopause. Sturdee and Brincat (1988) referred to the paper and wrote that 'Treatments for the hot flush have provoked controversy throughout the ages, and the multitude of remedies that have been tried are proof of the lack of a satisfactory explanation for the mechanism of flushing. The application of leeches and phlebotomy were advocated by Tyler-Smith (1849) and other remedies of this time included the sedatives bromide and valerian and tepid bathing of the skin to diminish the excess sensibility'.

Menopausal women had to wait until 1857 when they found an advocate in Edward Tilt (1857) who wrote the first English book dealing with disorders of the climacteric. Tilt suggested that the symptoms of the change of life were due to ovarian involution and he was the first to publish a statistical analysis of symptoms. Tilt's book was ignored for almost 20 years but, towards the end of the nineteenth century, his work became popular on the European continent and also

PRACTICAL MANUAL

DISEASES OF WOMEN

AND

UTERINE THERAPEUTICS.

For Students and Practitioners.

BY

H. MACNAUGHTON-JONES, M.D., M.CH., M.A.O. (HON. CAUS.),

FELLOW OF THE ROYAL COLLEGES OF SURGEONS OF IRELAND AND EDINBURGH;
FORMERLY
UNIVERSITY PROFESSOR OF MIDWIFERY AND DISEASES OF WOMEN AND CHILDREN IN
THE QUEEN'S UNIVERSITY,
EXAMINER IN MIDWIFERY AND DISEASES OF WOMEN AND
CHILDREN IN THE ROYAL UNIVERSITY OF IRELAND,
AND
LECTURER ON SURGICAL AND DESCRIPTIVE ANATOMY, QUEEN'S COLLEGE,
CONSULTING SURGEON TO THE MATERNITY AND TO THE WOMEN AND CHILDREN'S
HOSPITAL, CORK.

SIXTH EDITION,
REVISED AND ENLARGED.

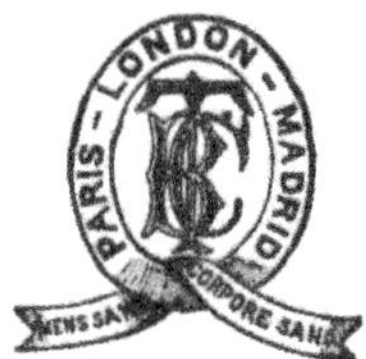

LONDON:
BAILLIÈRE, TINDALL AND COX
20 & 21, KING WILLIAM STREET, STRAND.
1894.

Figure 3 Frontispiece from MacNaughton Jones' *Diseases of Women and Uterine Therapeutics* (1894)

in America. The third edition of his book (Tilt, 1870) ascribed 135 different conditions to the 'change of life', including aortic pulsation, hysterical flatulence, blind piles and boils in the seat, and hot flushes.

Towards the end of the nineteenth century, MacNaughton Jones (1885) of Cork wrote in his *Diseases of Women and Uterine Therapeutics* that the menopause 'the critical autumn time [of life]' was recognised as a time 'when the active discharge of the function of ovulation is ceasing, and the child-bearing epoch is about to end ... sometimes culminating in local apoplexies, congestion of the ovaries, menorrhagia, the growth of uterine fibroids or polypus and the commencement of malignant disease'.

In the sixth edition of his book, MacNaughton-Jones (1894) wrote of the insanity of the menopause: 'During the climacteric, women may be troubled with ... important disturbances of the nervous system, as convulsions or paralysis. Climacteric insanity manifests itself in taciturnity, melancholia with or without delusions, and hypochondriasis ... all such cases during the climacteric require exceptional watching and care. They are typically cases for nursing and supervision in a medical home, and save in rare instances, they are not to be treated as insane women. A very large proportion recover when the climacteric period has passed by'.

Towards the end of the nineteenth century, Sidney Ringer (1888), Professor of Medicine in University College, London, in his *Handbook of Therapeutics* advised some or all of the following treatments for the 'change of life':

Actaea derived from *Cimifuga racemosa*, or American black cohosh, is a powerful uterine stimulant, similar to ergot. It was said to relieve headache, and to be useful for the distressing mental symptoms which occur at the 'change of life'.

Ammonia derived from the resinous gum of *Dorema ammoniacum*, was taken by mouth or applied to the scalp, as advised by Tilt for 'change of life' headaches and as a sedative.

Bromide of potassium was the first agent to be specifically introduced as a sedative (others were chloral hydrate, paraldehyde, urethan, and sulfonal), and replaced laudanum, alcohol and herbal potions. Bromide was prescribed for irritability and insomnia and it remained the leader in the field until the introduction of Barbital (a barbiturate) in 1903. Bromides were still prescribed for menopausal symptoms in the mid-twentieth century.

Calabar bean the dried ripe seed of the *Physostigma venosum* Balfour, was the source of physostigmine, an anticholinesterase, which can cause cholinergic stimulation. In toxic doses it is used as an insecticide and a chemical warfare nerve gas. It was recommended for relief of the flatulence of the climacteric period.

Camphor is derived from *Cinnamomum camphora*. It is a sedative and was also used in eclampsia, but in large doses camphor could itself cause convulsions. It was prescribed for drowsiness and headaches.

Change of scene or traveling for three to six months, was also advised.

Eucalyptol derived from the leaves of the *Eucalyptus globulus*, is an antiseptic and irritant. It increases secretions and stimulates the bowel. It was advocated for menopausal flatulence, palpitations, and flushings.

Hot sponges as hot as could be borne, followed by cold, to the spine were said to prevent 'the fidgets'. Water, or water and white vinegar were best, applied morning and evening for 10 minutes.

Iron for frequent flushings and hot and cold perspirations, and for flutterings of the heart, was prescribed alone or combined with *Strychnos nux-vomica* (which contains strychnine), belladona (the source of atropine), and opium.

Nitrite of amyl was advised for hot sweats and flushing; to relieve nervousness and depression, and to promote sleep. Derived from the action of nitric and nitrous acids upon amylic alcohol, nitrite of amyl is a powerful central nervous system depressant which was also used in eclampsia.

Valerianate of zinc was thought to relieve all symptoms, but not sleeplessness. Zinc stimulates the central nervous and cardiovascular systems and is an astringent. Valerian is the rhizome of *Valeriana officinalis*, and causes mild depression of the nervous system. It was mainly used for 'nervous hysteria' in females, but was also useful for delirium tremens.

Vinegar + water sponging every morning to the spine.

Warm bath once a week. Presumably the 'sweats' took care of any ablutions required in the interim.

An American Text Book of Gynecology (1894)

On the opposite side of the Atlantic ocean, J.M. Baldy (1894) of the Philadelphia PolyClinic and the Pennsylvania Hospital, included a tract on the menopause in the renowned *An American Text Book of Gynecology*. With regard to therapy, he was of the

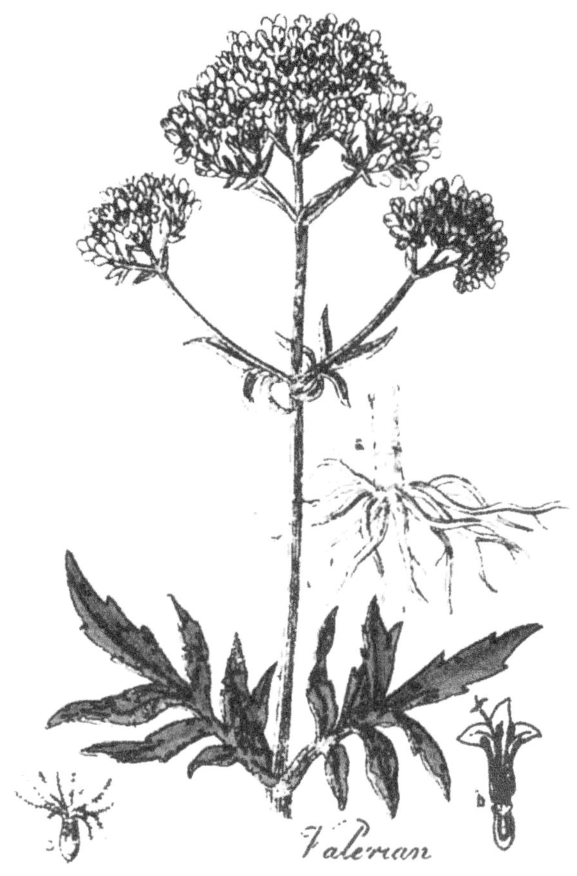

Figure 4 Valerian (*Valeriana* sp.)

opinion that 'The axiomatic principle of the treatment of all disorders follows through in the management of the menopause, and that is to make waste and repair as nearly equal as professional skill will permit. This involves a most careful attention to the secretions, the excretions, and the blood state'.

Alimentary tract 'The state of the alimentary tract demands particular attention ... gastric lavations, creosote, salicyne, corrosive sublimate and other antiseptic remedies are indicated. A tender liver and chronic constipation call for daily laxatives. Cascara, compound liquorice powder, Hunyadi salts, Rochelle salts, and other salines are highly useful ... daily defecation should be insisted upon. Constipation, producing numberless reflexes in leading to fecal anemia, is a most deplorable condition and should not be tolerated'.

Renal system 'Renal insufficiency must be corrected. Lithemia may be eliminated by the free use of lithic acid solvents, as the citrate of potassium or lithium'.

Cutaneous system 'Frequent warm baths are useful. Above all, the skin should be protected from changes of temperature by suitable underwear ... general massage and Turkish baths'.

Heart 'One of the most common complaints is paroxysmal tachycardia ... these attacks generally do not depend upon organic cardiac disease, but upon local congestion of the heart-center in the medulla oblongata, doubtless a reflex, in the majority of cases, from the alimentary tract'.

Blood state 'Anemia is often caused by the dyspepsias and constipation ... Where plethora exists venesection is in many cases most urgently demanded ... Bleeding from the arm or from the cervix uteri gives more speedy and protracted relief than any other measure; it rarely does harm. Leeches can be used over the region of the round ligament at the external abdominal ring, or at the anus, in cases of ovarian or uterine congestion'.

Nervous system The flushes, headaches and other problems were 'best relieved with bromides ... they are all cardiac depressants ... the tendency to produce acne can largely be averted by the use of arsenic ... used in combination with camphor, their anaphrodisiac action, where needed, is most gratifying'.

'It is understood that uterine, tubal, and ovarian congestions, when found, are to be treated 'secundum artem'. The remainder of the treatment of women at the climacteric is purely symptomatic. There is no specific treatment of the menopause'.

A SELECTION OF TREATMENTS TO INDUCE MENSTRUATION

Over the centuries, many herbal remedies were prescribed to women to induce menstruation, when the 'courses' or 'flowers' failed to flow. It is not clear from the ancient texts whether pregnant women or those entering the menopause were excluded from treatment but, as both were difficult to diagnose, many women in both categories were treated with emmenagogues. Soranus of Ephesus offered menstrual inducers to perimenopausal women and it appears that emmenagogues were still used to treat the oligo/amenorrhea of the climacteric during the twentieth century.

Assyria c. 400 BC

Bay, caper, cypress, galbanum, marigold, papyrus, storax.

(Campbell-Thompson, 1924)

Soranus second century AD

Cucumber, cyrenaic balm, hellebore, panax.

(Temkin, 1956)

Pseudo-Aristotle (c. 1830) for 'obstruction' of menstruation

Anise, atriplex, asparagus
Bay, betony, betony flowers
Calamint, chamomile, castus, chalybeat medicines, cinnamon, water of calamint
Diacatholicon, dictam, dill
Fennel, fenugreek, syrup of feverfew, syrup of flachus
Galengal, gili flowers, groundsel
Hierae, honey, hyssop
Laxative, letting of blood in ankles or arm, lilies, linseed
Mallows, marjoram, matrimonial conjunction, melilot, mercury, syrup of mugwort
Nutmeg
Oil of rue, oil of sweet almonds
Parsley, pennyroyal
Rose, rosemary, syrup of roses
Saffron, sage
Venice treacle
Wallflower, wine.

Pharmacopoeia of The People's Republic of China (1992)

Chishao (red peony root), chuanxiong (Szechwan lovage rhizome)
Dahuang (rhubarb), danggui (Chinese angelica), danshen (danshen root)
Guanmutong (Manchurian Dutchman's pipe stem), guizhi (cassia twig)
Heizhongcaozi (fennel seed)
Jianghuang (turmeric), jixingzi (garden balsam seed)

Lulutong (beautiful sweetgum fruit)
Qiancao (India madder root), qumai (lilac pink herb)
Rougui (cassia bark)
Shuizhi (leech), sumu (sappan wood)
Taoren (peach seed), tubiechong (ground beetle)
Yimucao (motherwort herb), yuzhizi (akebia fruit).

THE TWENTIETH CENTURY

To the Ringer's list of therapeutic agents of 1888, Hobart Amory Hare, professor of therapeutics and materia medica in the Jefferson Medical College of Philadelphia, could add in 1901:

Aloes derived from *Aloe perryi* or *Aloe vera*, apart from being emollients act as a strong purgative.

Cannabis indica or *C. sativa* were prescribed to relieve nervousness and to promote sleep. According to Hare, cannabis also caused sexual stimulation, and to quote from his text 'The drug, as prepared by Parke Davis and Co., has proved efficacious in the author's hands for years'.

Eau de Cologne a perfumed spirit, first manufactured by Johann Farina in 1709, and combined with camphor (recommended by Ringer and Tilt) 'was applied to the painful or hyperesthetic spots at the top of the head, so commonly felt by nervous women at the 'change of life''.

Ovarian extract as the new century dawned, hormone replacement treatment became a possibility for menopausal women. Hare, in 1901, advised dried ovarian gland substance, or extract of it, in compressed tablets or capsules. He was unaware that the medication would have no effect as an oral preparation. In a separate section of his *Textbook of Therapeutics* devoted to 'Glandular Treatment', Hare wrote a note of caution that 'given to dogs in overdose the ovary causes erections, with ejaculations of semen, and, if the dose is large, death with hemorrhage into the spinal cord'. Such information would surely take a woman's mind off her hot flushes!

Thomas D. Savill (1903), a London physician wrote of the 'flush storms, which consist of a hot stage, a cold stage with or without shivering, and sometimes a stage of perspiration'. He wrote of the nervous phenomena which occurred at the time 'there is generally an irritability and restlessness, and generally also a marked tendency to depression of spirits, and to burst into tears at the slightest provocation. This may amount, especially when there is mental heredity, to definite melancholy. Sexual perversions, with a marked tendency to excesses of all kinds, are apt to occur'. No treatment was offered.

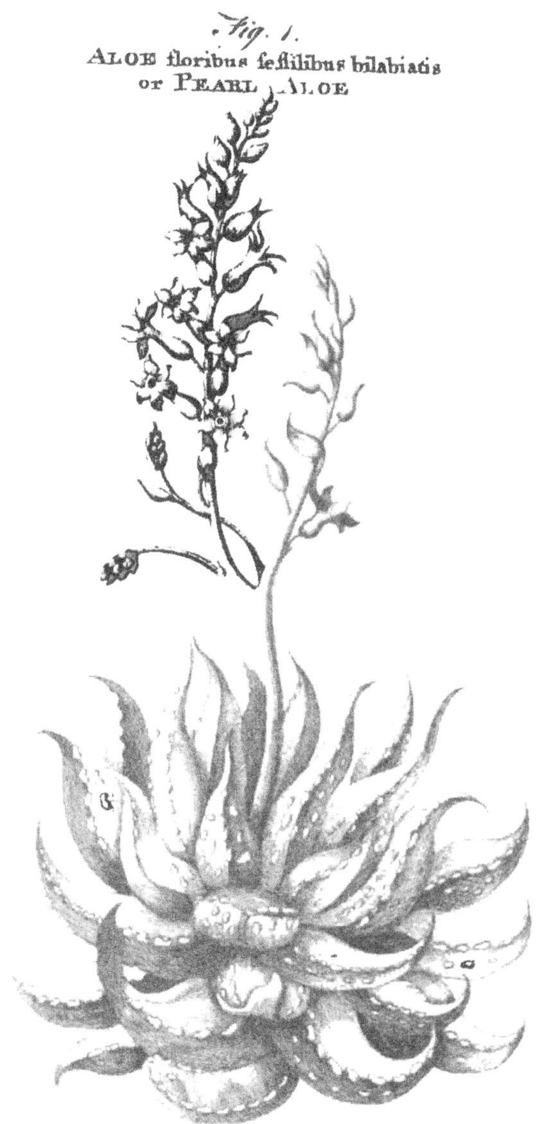

Figure 5 Aloe (*Aloë* sp.)

Mrs Garrett Anderson (1907) held the opinion that 'There seems to be no clear evidence that the ovaries form any internal secretion of great nutritive value. The disturbance seen at the menopause is nervous rather than nutritional or chemical'. The patient was advised that the 'organs of elimination must be kept well up to their work'. Warm bathing, flesh-glove rubbing, mild laxatives, an occasional blue pill (mercury) 'and a little patience, are in ordinary cases all that is wanted ... When a stimulant is really indicated, quinine and strychnia with hydrobromic acid answer the purpose adequately. In cases of more severity ... mild purgation followed by a short course of Bromides and a fairly long one of Liq. Ferri. Perchlor., combined with Liq. Amm. Acet., will usually give quick relief. In climacteric melancholy good results seem to follow ... from pil. Hydrar ... a month at Buxton or any similar place, under conditions of absolute rest, is of the greatest value'.

Howard A. Kelly (1909) of Johns Hopkins, Baltimore, found that he had 'been able to give a great deal of relief in these cases by the administration of lutein in 20 grain doses, three times a day ... the lutein is made by squeezing out the corpora lutea from the ovaries of the pig obtained at the slaughter-house. The corpora are then rapidly dried, powdered and compressed into tablets ... There is one prescription, which I give here, that I have found to be most beneficial in the class of women now under discussion,

Rx.

Strychnine sulfate,
Atropine sulfate,
Extract of calumba (*Frasera walteri*)'.

Margaret Moore-White (1946) outlined the various changes that occurred during the climacteric and menopause. She was of the opinion that 'Since most of the symptoms at the menopause depend on changes in the endocrine ratio, replacement by injection or by mouth of those ovarian hormones which are produced in smaller quantities than before, is most likely to benefit the patient ... Oestrin may be given in its synthetic form, diethylstilboestrol ... hexoestriol, which has lower potency than stilboestrol, has being found less toxic ... thyroid gland may be given with benefit ... sedatives, small doses of phenobarbitone, bromovalerianate or bromide and chloral ... a pill containing phenobarbitone and atropine sulfate ... dramatic improvement ... results from small doses of X-rays to the pituitary gland'.

Table 2 The symptoms and signs of the menopause (Moore-White, 1946)

Vasomotor	Hot flushes, feeling of sudden chill, changes in blood pressure, sweating, giddiness, and headaches
Metabolic	Increase or loss of weight, lethargy
Nervous	Emotional instability, depression, anxiety states, hypochondria, insomnia
Alimentary	Anorexia, dyspepsia, flatulence, constipation
Tegumentary	Pruritus, falling hair
Breasts	Breast pains, atrophy, or deposition of fat
Joints	Pains in the joints (particularly in the knees) and aching in the limbs
Sexual	Increase or diminution of libido

Wilfred Shaw (1946), physician–accoucheur of St Bartholomew's Hospital, London, was of the opinion that 'most patients with severe menopausal symptoms are psychically disturbed, and such patients are not satisfied by simple pills and medicines ... the old fashioned remedy of giving a gentian and rhubarb mixture combined with thyroid is suitable for the average case ... it has been shown in recent years that the common menopausal symptoms of flushings, irritability and depressions are cured almost specifically by the administration of oestrin. It is usual to give the hormone in the form of tablets of stilboestrol by mouth ... in view of the psychological disturbances, such stimulants as alcohol and coffee are contra-indicated'.

The mid-1960s

Incredible as it may seem, little had changed by the mid-1960s when T.L.T. Lewis of Guy's and Queen Charlotte's Hospitals, London (1964), reported that 'About 5% of women need no more than reassurance. Phenobarbitone half grain (32 mg) daily may be indicated for irritability or emotional upset. A tranquilizer, promezathine 10 to 25 mg or meprobromate 400 to 800 mg, may be taken at night. Amphetamine or dextroamphetamine sulfate, 5 to 10 mg, is helpful when the patient is lethargic or depressed ... although many patients are quite content with sympathy and reassurance and a small dose of phenobarbitone, some are not well until endocrine therapy is added ... low doses of estrogen are adequate ... the smallest effective dose should therefore be found by trial and error ...

treatment should not be continued for longer than six months to a year ... combined estrogen–androgen preparations ... are said to be more effective than estrogen alone ... however, facial hirsutes occurs in some women'.

SEX ORGAN THERAPY, OLD AND NEW

The idea of sex organ therapy has a long history. Min, the Egyptian god of fertility, was fed large quantities of lettuce, the wild variety of which contained lactucarium (similar to a mild form of opium) to increase his potency and performance. Although the sex organs of animals were used rather non-selectively in ancient Egypt, the Ebers Papyrus specifically mentions the use of placenta as a medication, to stop hair going gray (Nunn, 1996), and thus placental product must have been regarded as an anti-aging device. In recent times, until the advent of the HIV crisis, human placental products were frozen and sold to pharmaceutical firms for use in cosmetics and for hormonal extraction, and often without the patient's knowledge or consent.

The testicles of ass, deer, horse and wolf, all of whom were thought highly potent, were used as aphrodisiacs in ancient Greece and Rome, and the custom spread throughout the known world. Animal pissle (penis) and ovaries were also prescribed but the uterus was rarely resorted to as a treatment modality. As time went by, the gonadal tissue, eventually known with pancreas as 'sweetbreads', was also used by women to increase their fertility. Even the dear old Emerald Isle became involved in gonadal therapy, and William R. Wilde FRCS (1849), father of Oscar Wilde, reported in the *Monthly Journal of Medical Science*, that animal testicles were used as fertility agents among 'Mna na hEireann', the women of Ireland!

The scientific approach to sex hormone replacement therapy for non-fertility indications was signaled in 1889 by Charles Edouard Brown-Sequard, the so-called founder of endocrinology, of the National Hospital, Queen's Square, London, when he reported the rejuvenating effects of self-administered injections of pasteurized testicular extract (Brown-Sequard, 1889). He later theorized that ovarian extract could have a beneficial effect in women (Brown-Sequard,

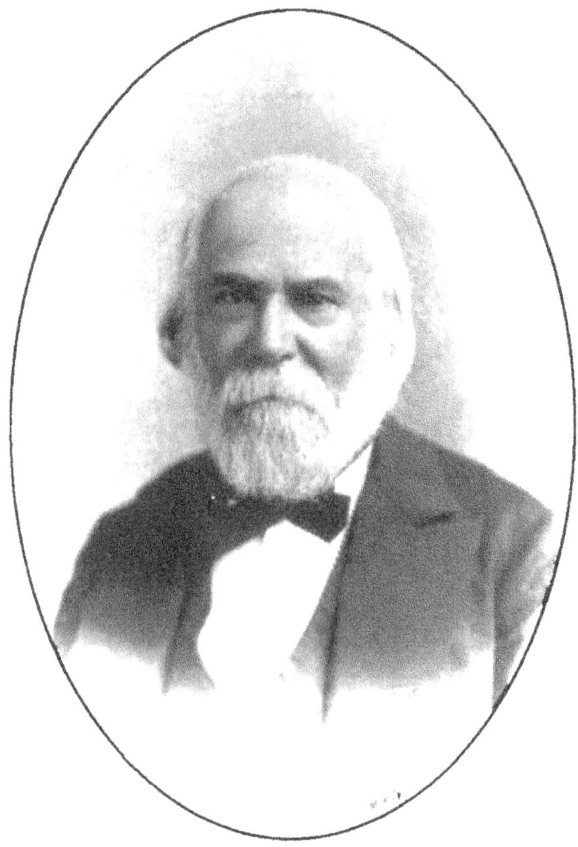

Figure 6 Charles Edouard Brown-Sequard (1817–1894)

1890). 'Brown Sequard was reported to have prescribed two sheep's ovaries a day sandwiched between slices of unleavened bread.' Injections of ovarian extract proved more acceptable and were given initially at the Landau Clinic in Berlin from 1896 and also in Paris (Sturdee and Brincat, 1988). In 1894, Regas injected ovarian extracts into a patient with menopausal psychosis and a cure was effected.

In 1899 Glass grafted ovarian tissue for women who had previously undergone premature menopause due to oophorectomy. The women re-established menstruation, and their sense of well-being and sexual desire. Sliced ovarian tissue was implanted under the abdominal muscles in an effort to relieve menopausal symptoms. Dried ovarian tissue was prescribed for oral administration in the early twentieth century but any beneficial effect appeared to be placebo in nature (Greenblatt, 1986). Fraenkel (1903) relieved climacteric symptoms with dried extracts from corpora lutea of cows, sheep or pigs, administered three times per day. According to Eskes of The Netherlands, and Longo of California (1994), Ludwig Fraenkel was one of the first clinicians to use ovarian extracts to treat the physical complaints associated with the menopause. Over the next half century the various sex hormones were identified and synthesized.

During the 1940s and 1950s there was a great increase in experimental and therapeutic hormone therapy, including the treatment of climacteric disturbances. The *Physicians Desk Reference* of 1950 contained 67 preparations for menopausal disorders, mainly estrogen's and testosterone (Morgan Jones, 1950), and that of 1976 contained 17 combined androgen/estrogen combinations and 23 estrogen products (Huff, 1976). Hunt and Vessey (1986) reported that there was a considerable increase in the number of prescriptions for HRT from the early 1970s up to the peak year of prescribing in 1977. Thereafter, use declined in response to the publication of papers that showed an increased risk of endometrial cancer among post-menopausal women taking unopposed HRT. Estrogen–progesterone HRT was prescribed from 1971.

OTHER LANDMARKS IN HORMONAL THERAPY

Estrogen

Allen and Doisy (1923) isolated an ovarian hormone, later called estrogen. Dodds and Robertson (1930) described the use of 'estrin', a substance derived from human placental sources, in the treatment of women with menopausal complaints. Oral estrogen therapy became widely available after the development of the semi-synthetic estrogen, stilboestrol, by Dodds and associates (1938). The semi-synthetic estrogens, ethinyl estradiol and mestranol were produced for oral contraception but also used for menopausal therapy. Natural estrogens were mainly used thereafter.

Bishop (1938) reported his clinical experience of subcutaneous estrogen implants in estrogen replacement therapy (thus avoiding the 'first-pass' liver effect), and that treatment modality was later popularized by Greenblatt (1949). Eventually, estrogen was available in tablet form; transdermally as a patch; parenterally as a cream; percutaneously; or directly to the vagina; and as a subcutaneous implant. Estrogen therapy remains the best treatment for the menopause and progestogen (oral norethisterone) administration was found to be the next most effective (Appleby, 1962).

Table 3 Hannse's (1986) chronology of the discovery and use of the female sex hormones

1925	The Allen–Doisy test
1928	Progynon, the first estrogen preparation from placenta
1928	Folliculin, from follicular fluid and urine of pregnant women and mares
1929	Follicular hormone-isolated estrone
1929	The Allen–Corner test
1933	Estradiol synthesized by hydrogenating estrone
1938	Estradiol synthesized from cholesterol
1938	Ethinyl estradiol synthesized
1938	Ethisteron, the first orally active progestogen
1932	Artificial menstruation induced in a castrate using sequential estrone benzoate and purified corpus luteum extract

Progesterone and Russell Marker

In the early days, estrogen and progesterone were obtained from cattle, horses, pigs and sheep ovaries. Progesterones were produced, in particular from sows ovaries, with a yield of 1 mg per 2500 sows. Meanwhile, a whole ton of bulls' testicles were required to obtain just 300 mg of testosterone. Hormonal preparations were thus extremely expensive and difficult to obtain and hormonal therapy was but a dream.

Onto the scene came Russell Marker, a research chemist at Pennsylvania State College who was funded by the Parke-Davis Company. He was aware that some plants contain saponins, used in many parts of the world for their detergent properties. Marker submitted the radical idea that saponins had the potential to be altered and synthesized into hormones, at a low cost. Executives of the Parke-Davis Company were unimpressed and refused to fund his further research and so Marker was forced to go it alone. He moved to Mexico. There, in a crude laboratory in a garage, he investigated over 400 local plants.

In his unlikely surroundings, Marker made the major discovery that the humble Mexican yam, *Dioscorea mexicana*, contained diosgenin, which had a steroid nucleus similar to cholesterol, and from which he soon obtained 3000 g of progesterone, with a market value of up to $800 per gram. Marker failed to take out any patents. His chemical methods were copied, and soon afterwards the drug companies produced massive amounts of cheap progesterone (Robertson, 1990), but the chemical had little effect when taken by mouth.

The next chemical advance was the discovery in the early 1950s of the orally active progestins, norethindrone by Carl Djerassi at Syntex, and norethynodrel by Frank Colton at Searle. In his book on the evolution of the oral contraceptive pill, and other topics, Djerassi wrote that Syntex filed their patent for norethindrone in November 1951 while Searle did not submit their patent application until August 1953 (Djerassi, 1992). Field trials were put in place which led to the birth of the oral contraceptive pill. Robert Wilson applied the concept of cyclical hormonal therapy as treatment for the menopause and it became known as hormone replacement therapy.

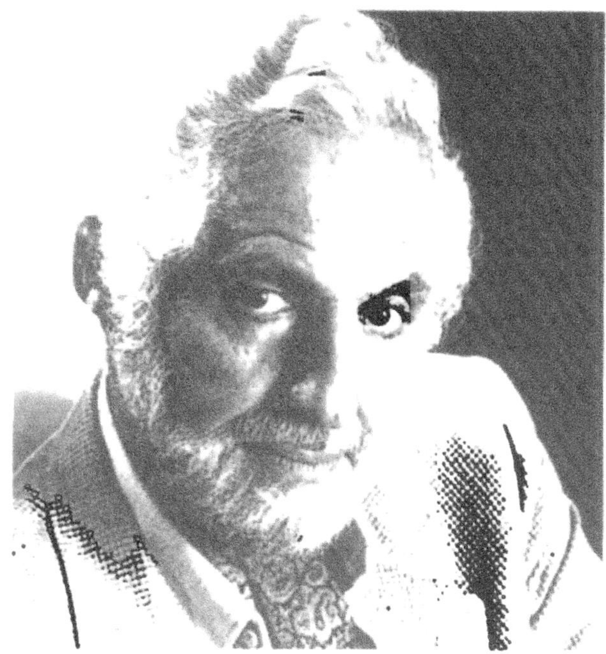

Figure 7 Carl Djerassi

Androgens

Until the late 1970s many clinicians and investigators included androgens in HRT for their beneficial effects on libido and bone conservation. Although out of favor for a decade, testosterone made a brief comeback in the late 1980s. Robert Greenblatt (1986) referred to the role of androgens in women and advocated their administration 'in judicious amounts' and opined that 'the male canary normally sings; when testosterone is administered to the female canary, she too will sing'.

Robert Wilson's *Feminine Forever* (1966)

Onto the mid-1960s menopause scene came Robert Wilson of the Methodist Hospital, Brooklyn, New York. In his *Feminine for Forever* (1966), a book aimed at a general audience, he advocated the use of HRT in the menopause.

In a brief look at the hormonal therapy for the 'change of life' Wilson wrote that 'Investigation of the therapeutic uses of estrogens followed close upon Doisy's historic discovery of these hormones in 1923. Curiously, the initial research was carried out largely in agricultural colleges with a hopeful view towards encouraging the sex life of chickens'. Wilson's own initial experiments, in the late 1920s, were carried out with a crude extract made from dried sheep ovaries. Estrogen became available in the early 1930s and the German preparation, estradiol benzoate, that was relatively side-effect free, allowed patients to enjoy the benefits of estrogen therapy without discomfort. Some clinicians nicknamed it the 'cadillac of hormones', but unfortunately the preparation had to be given on an on-going basis by intramuscular injections. Natural conjugated estrogens became available shortly after the outbreak of World War Two. They were prepared from mares' urine and soon the conjugated estrogens became available in convenient tablet form.

On 13 February 1963, Wilson carried out a routine medical check-up on a 52-year-old woman and was amazed at her physical and emotional condition. As it happened, the woman was taking the birth control pill. It struck Wilson that some forms of birth control pills could prove to have an even more important function than their principal purpose of contraception. Wilson initiated studies and found that the menopause was effectively prevented or cured by the use of estrogenic oral contraceptives. Wilson's response to the findings were: 'We stand at a threshold. Like Moses glimpsing the Promised Land'.

HORMONAL THERAPY: BENEFITS AND RISKS?

Post-menopausal osteoporosis

The problem of post-menopausal osteoporosis was first described by Albright and colleagues (1940). It is estimated that there may be up to 15 million women with evidence of osteoporosis in the USA. Risk factors for the development of osteoporosis were: female sex, loss of ovarian function, European or Asian race, nulliparity, low body weight, poor diet in childhood, alcohol abuse, and heavy smoking. Secondary causes of bone loss were related to steroid intake, thyrotoxicosis, and hyperparathyroidism.

The fractures consequent upon osteoporosis were a major clinical problem. During the years 1970–1980 there was an overall increase of 40% in annual fracture of the hip reporting in the USA. Such fractures caused considerable morbidity and a 10–15% mortality within six months. Only a third of the survivors of hip fracture regained normal activity. Estrogen therapy was the single most effective approach to the prevention of bone attrition. Exercise, calcium supplements, less caffeine, cessation of smoking, and the adoption of a 'Mediterranean' diet were also helpful.

Coronary heart disease

Reports from the early 1970s were supported by the findings of the Framingham Study of Kannel and associates (1976) who reported that post-menopausal women had an increased risk of coronary heart disease in comparison to pre-menopausal women of the same age. Ross and coworkers (1981) discovered that the administration of conjugated estrogens to post-menopausal women over a period of five years reduced the relative mortality rate from ischemic heart disease.

The bladder

Everett (1941) reported to the *American Journal of Surgery* that the vaginal and urethral epithelium were both subject to estrogenic action. Estrogen receptors were detected in the human female urethra by Iosif and colleagues (1981).

Endometrial cancer

Fremont Smith and colleagues (1946) in a case report indicated that a key factor in the development of endometrial cancer was estrogen stimulation. Smith *et al.* (1975) confirmed the link between estrogen therapy and endometrial cancer. Further studies demonstrated there was almost no risk of endometrial carcinoma if progestogen was added to the oral estrogen for at least 10 days of each cycle (Sturdee *et al.*, 1978).

Breast cancer

Breast cancer accounts for 26% of cancers but is the leading cause for death from malignancy in women. Breckwoldt (1996) related that there was no compelling evidence as to 'cause and effect' relationships between HRT and breast cancer.

MEDICAL, NONHORMONAL TREATMENT

Clonidene was found to reduce hot flushes in a significant number of women in a double-blind crossover study by Clayden and colleagues (1974). Many other nonhormonal treatments became available on prescription after that time. Henri Rozenbaum (1996), President of the European Menopause Society, reported that non-hormonal treatments were used by 2–13% of women surveyed, depending on the country. West Germany was the leader in this type of treatment, with 13% of women being listed as users, of which 30% were perimenopausal women. Tranquilizers were availed of by 6–28% of the women surveyed. 'Self-help' included a diet containing adequate amount of calcium; the avoidance of high caffeine intake; smoking and alcohol excess; exposure to sunlight to aid synthesis of vitamin D; and general fitness, with increased exercise to avoid osteoporosis.

Nonhormonal medication for the climacteric

Anti-depressants
Sedatives
Tranquilizers

Nonhormonal treatment for hot flushes

Clonidine, Ethamsylate, Lofexidine,
Naloxone, Naproxen, Opipramol,
Propranolol, Vitamin B6 (Pyridoxine)

(Utian, 1986)

THE MENOPAUSE IN VARIOUS CULTURES

Payer (1990) of New York, evaluated the studies relating to the menopause in various cultures. He noted that 'In England, perimenopausal women have hot flushes; in America they have flashes, a word the English do not use in polite society. In both countries climacteric women are made to swallow extracts of the urine of pregnant mares, a custom some cultures might find quaint ... Studies from around the world have found the prevalence of hot flushes for example, to range from 0% in Mayan women, to 80% in Dutch women. Do women from one culture report fewer hot flushes because of their diets, as Beyene suggested, or simply because the menopause is considered to be a natural phenomenon that brings with it certain privileges? Or do they simply report fewer symptoms because they may be embarrassed, or because their society places a high value on stoicism?'.

Payer reported that the attitude of women in Asia differed from that of Western society. The menopause was perceived by Asian women as a reward rather than a punishment. Sixty-five percent of Japanese women reported 'the menopause to be an event that was of little or no importance to them. Moreover, there was no word in Japanese to describe hot flushes'. Apart from dietary differences, Payer noted that Asian women had more regular exercise than their Western counterparts and concluded that 'exercise ... could be a major factor in alleviating climacteric symptoms. Exercise could be the key'.

COMPLEMENTARY MEDICINE

There has been a rapid growth in complementary medicine over the past 20 years and many of our patients are aspiring towards what they consider to be 'natural' remedies in the quest for better post-menopausal health. From an historical point of view, the remedies on offer were based mainly on discoveries in conventional medicine and science which were made in this century. Complementary therapists refer to the importance of diet and point out that Japanese women suffer less menopausal symptoms due to a diet that is rich in soy (*Glycine soja*), a good source of plant estrogens. A major part of complementary medicines consists of vitamin and mineral supplements and therapists claim that nutritional deficiencies occur in the majority of the population and so the administration of supplemental calcium and vitamin D must have positive benefits. Part of the complementary medicine approach is to use herbal remedies, some of which are dealt with below. Among the many other plant/herbal products claimed to regulate female sex hormone production are the medicinal herbs, fenugreek, ginseng and yam.

Phytohormones

It is known that certain plants contain phytohormones or chemical precursors of female hormones, including the nonsteroidal coumestans, flavones and the isoflavones but related mainly to the steroidal saponin content (remember the yam and progesterone). Two kinds of saponins are recognized, the steroidal saponins which are commonly tetracyclic triterpenoids and the pentacyclic triterpenoid types (Evans, 1996). Steroidal saponins are related not only to the sex hormones, but also to compounds such as cortisone, diuretic steroids, vitamin D and the cardiac glycosides, and many are, or were, used as starting points for the synthesis of these compounds. Each of the following plants has a large number of active constituents, some of which may induce hormonal effects.

Vitex agnus castus

The *Vitex agnus castus*, or chaste tree, is a native of the Mediterranean and Western Asia. This fragrant plant has a long association with women's health. In ancient Greece it was dedicated to the mother goddess, Demeter, and the Greek name for the plant is 'Agnos', meaning pure or chaste. Pliny in first century AD Rome dubbed it 'Vitex' meaning to twine (Mills, 1992). Ingestion of the plant was thought to reduce sexual desire in men and the ground berries were used

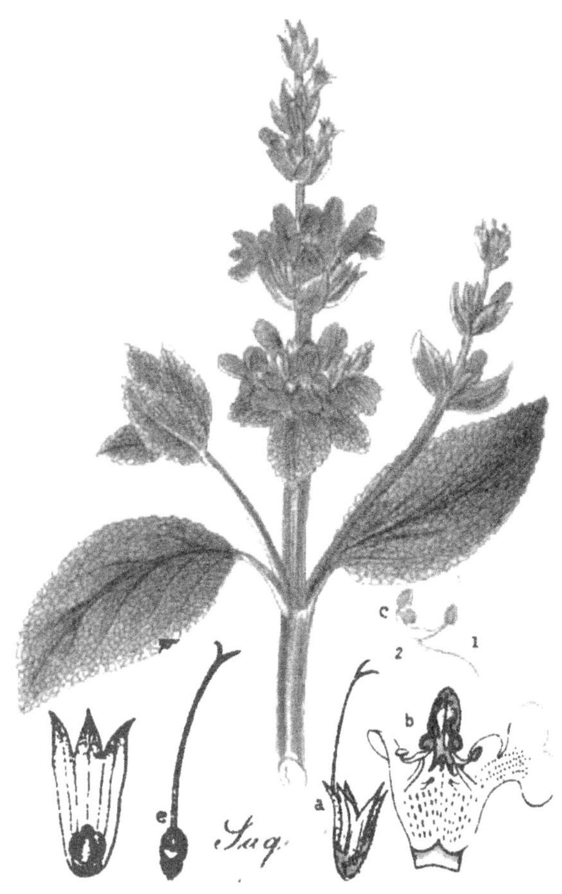

Figure 8 Sage (*Salvia* sp.)

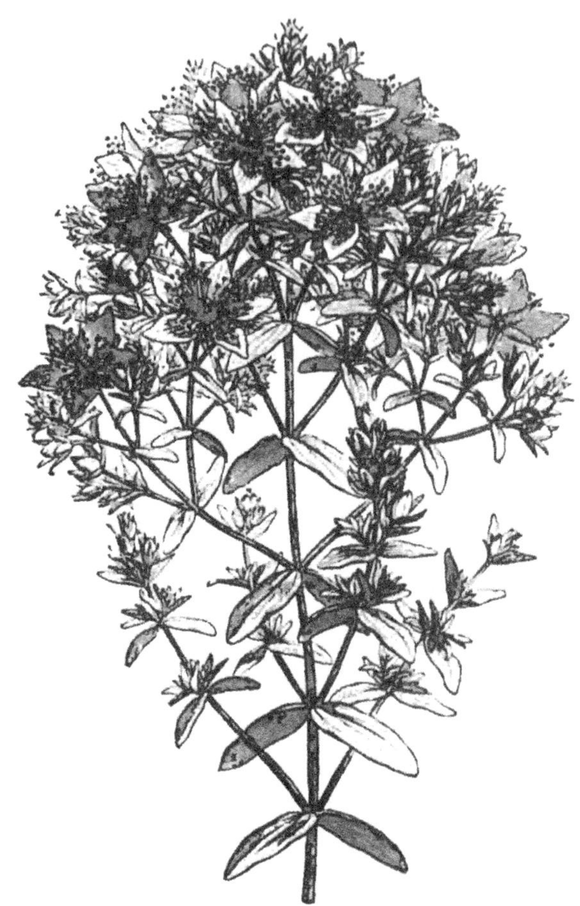

Figure 9 St John's wort (*Hypericum perforatum*)

as condiments in monasteries to reduce libido, thus giving rise to the alternative name for the plant of 'monks' pepper'. The herb has distinct hormonal effects, but the responsible constituents have not yet been isolated. Vitex has been used as a galactagogue for many centuries. It is proposed that the plant has tonic effects on the pituitary gland, causing release of luteinising hormone, and that its overall effect is progesterogenic (Chevallier, 1996).

Sage

Salvia officinalis, or sage, has been cultivated for millennia. The word 'salvia' derives from the Latin, *salvare*, to cure. Known as 'salvia salvatrix' (sage the savior), it developed its reputation as a medicinal drug in classical times. In particular, sage is known to suppress perspiration, and is also said to have estrogenic effects (Ody, 1993).

St John's wort

Hypericum perforatum, or St John's wort, was named 'hyperion' by the ancient Greeks. Hyperion, a Titan and son of Uranus (later to be castrated and thus stripped of his powers), married Thea who gave birth to the sun and the moon. The yellow flowers of St John's wort, turn red when crushed, due to the release of hypericin, a red pigment, said to signify the blood of the beheaded St John, whose feast day is 24 June, the time of year when the plant is in full bloom. The herb became known as 'herbi sancti Joannis' and thus St John's wort. Plant extract has antidepressant effects (Linde *et al.*, 1996).

Herbal remedies for the menopause

British Herbal Pharmacopoeia (1991)
Beth-root, life-root, St John's wort.

The Complete Woman's Herbal (McIntyre, 1994)
Blue cohosh, marigold, dandelion, false unicorn root, ginseng, hops, horsetail, licorice, nettle, rosemary, wild yam, wormwood.

TRADITIONAL CHINESE MEDICINE

Okamura, Yoshida and Oikawa (1989) related the effects of Oriental medicine in the treatment of climacteric patients at a conference entitled 'The Free Woman' held in Amsterdam. They related the effects of Kampo in 58 women with climacteric symptoms who were treated with Goshaku-San: prescription of Tsumura Pharmaceutical Company. It was the mixed powder of 16 drugs. A good response was attained in 56 of the women but in two patients the drug was ineffective. The preparation was given two or three times daily, with a total dose not exceeding 7.5 g. Acupuncture has also appeared to be effective (Yamomoto, 1989).

Table 4 Rx of menopausal night sweats (Pharmacopoeia of The People's Republic of China, 1992)

Baishao (white peony root), baiziren (Chinese arbor vitae kernel)
Guijia (tortoise shell)
Huangbai (amur cork tree)
Mahuanggen (*Ephedra* root), muli (oyster shell)
Wubeizi (Chinese gall), wuweizi (Chinese magnolia vine fruit)
Ziheche (human placenta)

CONVENTIONAL MEDICINE AND RECENT PROGRESS

Nowadays it is recognized that an increasing number of women will live half of their adult lives after the menopause. About 25–50% of women in English-speaking countries experience troublesome symptoms during the menopause transition. Hormone replacement treatment became indicated for symptoms that involved the central nervous system; the cardiovascular and genitourinary systems; hypogonadal conditions, and osteoporosis. Fuller Albright *et al.* (1940, 1941) demonstrated a clear relationship between menopause, estrogen deficiency and osteoporosis. Alendronate sodium (Fosimax) became the first effective treatment to rebuild bone at all sites affected by osteoporosis, consequently reversing the progression of the disease, and was introduced in 1998.

SERMs

Many therapeutic options became available for HRT in the late twentieth century, including the selective estrogen receptor modulators (SERMs), which included the drug Raloxifen. SERMs offered a treatment option to preserve bone mass and prevent vertebral fractures while lowering cholesterol levels without increasing the risk of breast cancer or uterine bleeding. Raloxifen did not, however, relieve the cardiovascular symptoms of hot flushes and sweats. Although many women were reluctant to take HRT because of concerns about breast cancer, SERMs appeared to protect against breast cancer while preventing osteoporosis and having a beneficial effect on plasma lipids.

EPILOGUE

Robert Greenblatt (1988), of Georgia, wrote that 'The proper use of gonadal steroids may enable her (the woman) to obtain fulfillment without interrupting her quest for a continuum of physical and mental health. She can grow old with grace and human worth, glowing with the radiance of the turning leaves of fall. Such was the vision of John Donne, sixteenth century poet and Dean of St Paul's Cathedral in London, when he wrote:

> No spring nor summer hath such grace,
> As I have seen in one autumnal face.

Many years ago, emboldened by these very lines, I wrote in one of my essays 'a woman in the autumn of her life, deserves an Indian summer rather than a winter of discontent'. We can aim for that goal and serve mankind the better if we realize that the cessation of the menses – the menopause – is but the beginning of an epoch in a woman's life which continues to 'the last of life".

It appears that Robert Wilson (1996) and those who followed his crusade made us all realize the true potential of women in the post-menopausal era. What better way to end this chapter than to quote from *Feminine Forever*: 'We stand at a threshold. Like Moses glimpsing the Promised Land'.

References

Adams, F. (1844). *The Seven Books of Paulus Aegineta*, Translated from the Greek. Vol. 1, pp. 596–7. (London: The Sydenham Society)

Albright, F., Bloomberg, E. and Smith, P. H. (1940). Post-menopausal osteoporosis. *Trans. Assoc. Am. Phys.*, 55, 298–305

Albright, F., Smith, P. H. and Richardson, A. M. (1941). Post-menopausal osteoporosis. Its clinical features. *JAMA*, 116, 2465–74

Allen, E. and Doisy, E. A. (1923). An ovarian hormone. A preliminary report on its localization, excretion and partial purification and action in test animals. *JAMA*, 81, 819–21

Amundsen, D. W. and Diers, C. J. (1970). The age of menopause in classical Greece and Rome. *Human Biol.*, 42, 79–86

Anderson, G. (1907). Menopause. In *Green's Encyclopaedia and Dictionary of Medicine and Surgery*, Vol. 6, pp. 332–5. (Edinburgh and London: William Green & Sons)

Appleby, B. (1962). Norethisterone in the control of menopausal symptoms. *The Lancet*, 1, 407–9

Baldy, J. M. (ed.) (1894). *An American Text-Book of Gynecology, Medical and Surgical, for Practitioners and Students*, pp. 83–91. (London: F. J. Rebman)

Bishop, B. M. F. (1938). A clinical experiment in oestrogen therapy. *BMJ*, 1, 939–41

Breckwoldt, M. (1996). Can women with previous oestrogen-dependent cancer receive HRT? In Martin H. Birkhauser and Henri Rozenbaum (eds) *European Consensus Development Conference on Menopause*, pp. 225–8. (Paris: Editions ESKA)

The British Herbal Medicine Association (1991). *British Herbal Pharmacopoeia*. (Bournemouth: The British Herbal Medicine Association)

Brown-Sequard, C. E. (1890). Remarques sur les effets produits sur la femme par des injections sous-cutanees d'un liquide retire d'ovaries d'animaux. *Arch. Physiol. Norm. Pathol.*, 2, 456–7

Brown-Sequard, C. E. (1889). Des effects produits chez l'homme par des injections sous-cutanee d'un liquide retires des testicules frais des cobaye et de chien. *Comptes rendus Soc. Biol.*, 1, 415–9

Bryan, C. P. (1930). Diseases of Women. In Joachim, H. (ed.) *The Papyrus Ebers*, Translation, pp. 82–7. (Herts, UK: Garden City Press)

Campbell, S. and Whitehead, M. (1977). Oestrogen therapy in the menopausal syndrome. In Greenblatt, R. G. and Studd, J. W. W. (eds) *Clinics in Obstetrics and Gynaecology*, pp. 4, 31–48. (London: W. B. Saunders)

Campbell-Thompson, R. (1924). *The Assyrian Herbal*. (London: Luzac & Co.)

Chadwick, J. and Mann, W. N. (1950). *Hippocratic Writings*, G. E. R. Lloyd (ed.) Penguin Classic edition, 1983 p. 229. (London: Penguin Books)

Chevallier, A. (1996). *The Encyclopedia of Medicinal Plants*, p. 149. (London: Dorling Kindersley)

Clayden, J. R., Bell, J. W. and Pollard, P. (1974). Menopausal flushing: Double-blind trial of a non-hormonal medication. *BMJ*, 1, 409–12

Culpeper, N. (1653). *Pharmacopoeia Londonensis*, or the London Dispensatorie, further adorned by the studies and collections of the Fellows, now living at the said College. (London: Peter Cole)

Djerassi, C. (1992). *The Pill, Pygmy Chimps, and Degas' Horse*, p. 60. (New York: Basic Books)

Dodds, E. C. and Robertson, J. D. (1930). Clinical experiments with oestrin. *The Lancet*, 1, 1390–2

Dodds, E. C., Goldberg, L., Lawson, W. and Robinson, R. (1938). Oestrogenic activity of certain synthetic compounds. *Nature*, 141, 247–8

Ellis, H. (1936). *Studies in the Psychology of Sex*, Vol. 2, Part 1, pp. 13–14. (New York: Random House)

Encyclopaedia Britannica (1771). A Dictionary of Arts and Sciences, compiled upon a New Plan. In which The Different Sciences and Arts are digested into distinct Treatises or Systems; and The various Technical Terms, etc., are explained as they occur in the order of the alphabet. Vol. 3, pp. 205–45, 162–7. (Edinburgh: A. Bell and C. MacFarquhar)

Eskes, T. K. A. B. and Longo, L. D. (1994). The Perimenopause. *In Classics in Obstetrics and Gynaecology*, pp. 361–87. (London and New York: Parthenon Publishing)

Evans, W. C. (1996). *Trease and Evan's Pharmacogmosy*, p. 293. (London: W. B. Saunders Company)

Everett, H. S. (1941). Urology in the female. *Am. J. Surg.*, 52, 521

Fraenkel, L. (1903). Die funktion des corpus luteum. *Arch. Gynaekol.*, 68, 438–97

Fremont-Smith, M., Meigs, J. V., Graham, R. M. and Gilbert, H. H. (1946). Cancer of endometrium and prolonged estrogen therapy. *JAMA*, 131, 805

Gardannen, C. P. L. de (1816). *Avis aux Femmes qui Entrent dans L'age Critique*, p. vi. (Paris: Gabon)

Garland, R. (1990). *The Greek Way of Life from Conception to Old Age*, pp. 243–4, 245–7. (London: Duckworth)

Gillibrand, I. (1997). Population Ageing: A Public Health Challenge. (Editorial). *World Med. J.*, 43(5), 75–7

Greenblatt, R. B. and Duran, R. R. (1949). Indications for hormone pellets in the therapy of endocrine and gynaecological disorders. *J. Obstet. Gynecol. Br. Emp.*, 51, 294–301

Greenblatt, R. B. (1986). Prologue. In Greenblatt, R. B. and Heithecker, R. (eds) *A Modern Approach to the Perimenopausal Years*, pp. 3–8. (Berlin, New York: Walter de Gruyter)

Greenblatt, R. B. (1988). Foreword. In Studd, J. W. W. and Whitehead, M. I. (eds) *The Menopause*, pp. vii–viii. (Oxford, London: Blackwell Scientific)

Hannse, H. (1986). Opening Remarks. In Greenblatt, R. B. and Heithecker, R. (eds) *A Modern Approach to the Perimenopausal Years*, pp. 1–2. (Berlin, New York: Walter de Gruyter)

Hare, H. A. (1901). *A Text-book of Practical Therapeutics*, p. 782. (London: Henry Kimpton)

Huff, B. B. (1976). *Physician's Desk Reference*, pp. 216–7. (Oaradell, N. J.: Medical Economics Co.)

Hunt, K. and Vessey, M. (1986). Prospective Study on Long Term Risk of Hormone Replacement Therapy. In Greenblatt, R. B. and Heithecker, R. (eds) *A Modern Approach to Perimenopausal Years*, pp. 157–62. (Berlin, New York: Walter de Gruyter)

Iosif, C. S., Batra, S., Ek, A. and Astedt, B. (1981). Estrogen receptors in the human female lower urinary tract. *Am. J. Obstet. Gynecol.*, 141, 817–20

Kannel, W. B., Hjortland, M. C., McNamara, P. M. and Gordon, T. (1976). Menopause and risk of cardiovascular disease. The Framingham Study. *Ann. Int. Med.*, 85, 447–52

Kelly, H. A. (1909). *Medical Gynaecology*, pp. 89, 87–90, 169–80, 231–2, 604–6. (London: Appleton & Co.)

Lewis, T. L. T. (1964). *Progress in Clinical Obstetrics and Gynaecology*, pp. 463–4. (London: J. and A. Churchill Ltd.)

Linde, K., Ramirez, G., Mulrow, C. D., Pauls, A., Weidenhammer, W. and Melchart, D. (1996). St John's wort for depression – an overview and meta-analysis of randomised clinical trials. *BMJ*, 313, 253–8

MacNaughton Jones, H. (1885). *Practical Manual of Diseases of Women and Uterine Therapeutics*, pp. 27–8, 98–9. (London: Bailliere, Tindall & Cox)

MacNaughton Jones, H. (1894). *Practical Manual of Diseases of Women and Uterine Therapeutics*, pp. 37–8. (London: Bailliere, Tindall & Cox)

McIntyre, A. (1994). *The Complete Woman's Herbal*. (London: Gaia Books)

Mills, S. (1992). *Woman Medicine: Vitex Agnus Castus*, pp. 10–11. (Dorset, UK: Amberwood Publishing)

Moore-White, M. (1946). *The Symptomatic Diagnosis and Treatment of Gynaecological Disorders*, pp. 172–7. (London: H. K. Lewis)

Morgan-Jones, J. (1950). *Physician's Desk Reference to Pharmaceutical Specialities and Biologicals*, p. 353. (Rutherford, N. J.: Medical Economics)

Nunn, J. F. (1996). *Ancient Egyptian Medicine*, p. 149. (London: British Museum Press)

Ody, P. (1993). *The Herb Society's Complete Medicinal Herbal*, p. 95. (London: Dorling Kindersley)

Okamura, Y., Yoshida, K. and Oikawa, K. (1989). Effects of Oriental Medicine in Gynaecological Diseases. In van Hall, E. and Everaerd, W. (eds) *The Free Woman. Women's Health in the 1990s*, pp. 844–8. (London and New York: Parthenon Publishing)

Payer, L. (1990). The Menopause in Various Cultures. In Burger, H. and Boulet, M. (eds) *A Portrait of the Menopause*, pp. 3–22. (London and New York: Parthenon Publishing)

Pharmacopoeia of the People's Republic of China (1992). English edition. Compiled by The Pharmacopoeia Commission of People's Republic of China. Temple of Heaven. (Beijing, China: Gaungdong Science and Technology Press)

Pseudo-Aristotle (c. 1830). *The Works of Aristotle, The Famous Philosopher*. (London: Miller, Law & Cater)

Rekers, H. (1990). Mastering the Menopause. In Burger, H. and Boulet, M. *A Portrait of the Menopause*, pp. 23–40. (London and New York: Parthenon Publishing)

Ricci, J. V. (1950). *Aetios of Amida. The Gynaecology and Obstetrics of the 6th Century AD*, Translated from the Latin edition of Cornarius, 1542 and fully annotated. p. 78. (Philadelphia & Toronto: Blakiston Co.)

Riddle, J. M. (1997). *Eve's Herbs. A History of Contraception and Abortion in the West*, pp. 19–20. (Cambridge, MA: Harvard University Press)

Ringer, S. (1888). *A Handbook of Therapeutics*, pp. 87–90, 604–6. (London: H. K. Lewis)

Robertson, W. H. (1990). *An Illustrated History of Contraception*, pp. 123–9. (London: Parthenon Publishing)

Ross, R. K., Pagnini-Hill, A., Mack, T. M., Arthur, M. and enderson, B. E. (1981). Menopausal oestrogen therapy and protection from death from ischaemic heart disease. *The Lancet*, 1, 858–60

Rozenbaum, H. (1996). Menopause in Europe: The State of the Art. In Birkhauser, M. H. and Rozenbaum, H. (eds) *European Consensus Development Conference on Menopause*, pp. 13–19. (Paris: Editions ESKA)

Savill, T. D. (1903). *A System of Clinical Medicine*, pp. 551–2. (London: J. and A. Churchill)

Schneider, H. P. G. (1986). The Climacteric Syndrome. In Greenblatt, R. B. and Heithecker, R. (eds) *A Modern Approach to the Perimenopausal Years*, pp. 39–55. (Berlin, New York: Walter de Gruyter)

Shakespeare, W. (1599). *As You Like It*, 1994 Penguin Classic ed. p. 58. (London: Penguin)

Shaw, W. (1946). *Textbook of Gynaecology*, pp. 96–7. (London: J. and A. Churchill)

Smith, D. C., Prentice, R., Thompson, D. J. and Herrman, W. L. (1975). Association of exogenous estrogen and endometrial carcinoma. *New Engl. J. Med.*, 293, 1164–7

Sturdee, D. and Brincat, M. (1988). The Hot Flush. In Studd, J. W. W. and Whitehead, M. I. (eds) *The Menopause*, pp. 24–42. (Oxford and London: Blackwell Scientific)

Sturdee, D. W., Wade-Evans, T. and Paterson, M. E. L. *et al.* (1978). Relationship between bleeding patterns, endometrial histology and oestrogen treatment in menopausal women. *BMJ*, **1**, 1575–7

Temkin, O. (1956). *Soranus' Gynecology*, pp. 22, 16–22, 148, 149–54. (Baltimore: The Johns Hopkins University Press)

Tilt, E. J. (1857). *The Change of Life in Health and Disease*, A Practical Treatise on the Nervous and Other Affections Incidental to Women at the Decline of Life. (London: John Churchill)

Tilt, E. J. (1870). *The Change of Life in Health and Disease*, 3rd ed. (London: J. Churchill)

Turner, W. (1568). *The Herbal.* (Collen: Arnold Birckman)

Tyler-Smith, W. (1849). The Climacteric Disease in Women. *London J. Med.*, vii, 601–9

Utian, W. H. (1972). The true clinical features of post-menopause and oophorectomy and their response to oestrogen therapy. *S. African Med. J.*, 46, 732–7

Utian, W. H. (1986). Non-Hormonal Medication. In Greenblatt, R. B. and Heithecker, R. (eds) *A Modern Approach to the Perimenopausal Years*, pp. 117–28. (Berlin, New York: Walter de Gruyter)

Wilbush, J. (1979). Le Menespausie – the birth of a syndrome. *Maturitas*, 1, 145–51

Wilbush, J. (1980). Tilt EJ and the *Change of Life* (1857), the only work on the subject in the English language. *Maturitas*, **2**, 259–67

Wilbush, J. (1981a). What's in a name? Some linguistic aspects of the climacteric. *Maturitas*, **3**, 1–9

Wilbush, J. (1981b). Climacteric symptom formation: Donovan's contribution. *Maturitas*, **3**, 99–105

Wilbush, J. (1982). Climacteric expression and social context. *Maturitas*, **4**, 195–205

Wilbush, J. (1984). Clinical information – Signs, semeions and symptoms: Discussion paper. *J. R. Soc. Med.*, 77, 766–73

Wilbush, J. (1988). Climacteric Disorders – Historical Perspectives. In Studd, J. W. W. and Whitehead, M. I. (eds) *The Menopause*, pp. 1–14. (Oxford, London: Blackwell Scientific)

Wilde, W. R. (1849). A Short Account of the Superstitions and Popular Practices relating to Midwifery, and some of the Diseases of Women and Children in Ireland. *Monthly J. Med. Sci.* May, 711–26

Wilson, R. A. (1966). *Feminine Forever*, pp. 11–19. (Philadelphia and New York: M. Evans & Co. Inc.)

Yamomoto, T. (1989). About acupuncture, and possible uses in gynaecology and obstetrics. In van Hall, E. and Everaerd, W. (eds) *The Free Woman. Women's Health in the 1990s*, pp. 851–6. (London and New York: Parthenon Publishing)

Uterine stimulants 24

INTRODUCTION

Uterine stimulants are known as ecbolics (Greek, *ekbole*, throwing out) or oxytocics (Greek, *oxys*, sharp + *tokos*, birth). The introduction of the oxytocic drug ergot was the most important event in maternity care for many centuries, and the drug was without equal in the obstetric pharmacopoeia. Ergot was used to stimulate the uterus and thus to shorten 'tedious labor', a well known cause of maternal and fetal mortality and morbidity (See Chapter 3). If used too early or in too high a dose, it could cause excessive uterine contractions leading to fetal asphyxia and uterine rupture. Experience showed that it could be used successfully to hasten the second stage of labor and that it helped to shorten the third stage by aiding placental detachment and expulsion. Its main benefit was in reducing the incidence of uterine hemorrhage after childbirth, by causing spasm of the uterine musculature. This action alone was responsible for a major reduction in maternal mortality.

The materia medica before ergot

In the second century AD, Soranus of Ephesus wrote about the problem of prolonged labor and correctly deduced that primigravidae were at most risk, but that women in subsequent labors could also be affected. He divided the causes of prolonged labor into maternal, fetal and pelvic. Soranus also correctly identified that atonia of the uterus was implicated and he ordered various remedies to strengthen uterine contractions – including decoctions of fenugreek, linseed and mallow, with local application of warm olive oil, administration of an enema, emptying of the bladder and adequate dietary intake (Temkin, 1956). Other uterine 'tonics' have been used throughout the ages but many were found to be unreliable, so a code of 'masterly inactivity' (non-intervention) prevailed. Despite that, the medicinal herbs rue (*Ruta graveolans*) and savin (*Juniperus sabina*) had a great reputation as uterine stimulants in early and late pregnancy.

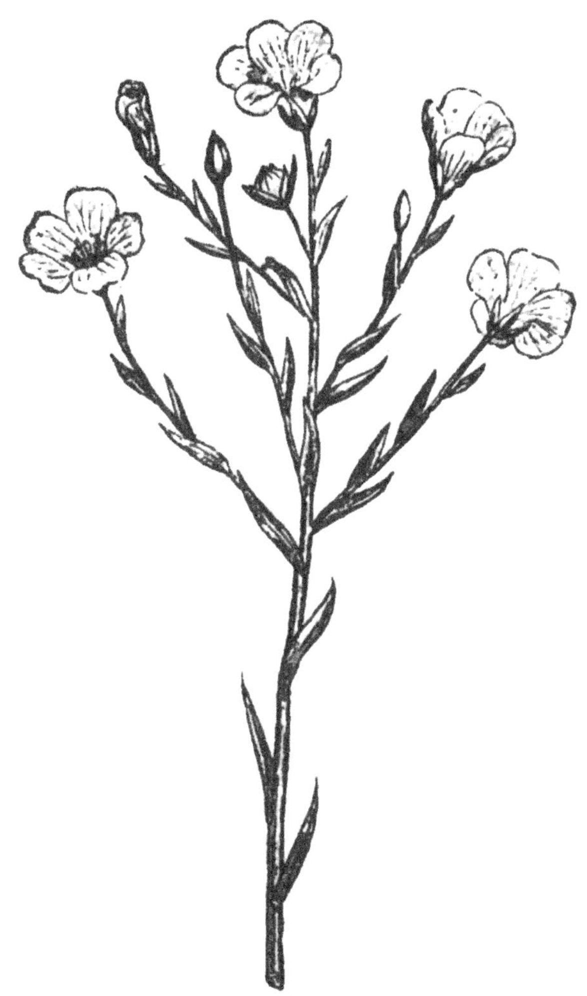

Figure 1 Linseed (*Linum* sp.)

UTERINE STIMULANTS FOR LABOR

Soranus second century AD

To start labor

Fomentations, goose fat, hydromel, linseed (flax), mallow, marrow, oily sitz bath, olive oil, sea sponges, sitz bath of warm water.

In labor

Anise, cedar resin, cucumber, dates, dittany, dried leaves, southernwood, sweet bay (laurel), sweet olive oil.

To deliver the placenta

Black cummin, cantharides, cassia, celery, dittany, galbanum, honey, illyrian iris, myrrh, oil of lilies, oil of roses, salvia, soapwort, spikenard, wormwood.

Rosslin's *The Byrth of Mankynde* (1545)

Aristolochia rotunda, asafetida, amoniacum, madder, asarum, barley meal, benzoin, berries of galbanum, berries of juniper, bothor martis, bran, broth cicercula, canell, cassia lignea, castoreum, cicer, colloquintida, cyclamen, diachylon, dricroceu, fenugreek, gentian, hellebore, hollyhock, hollyhock and bearsfoot, juniper berries, maidenhair, mallows, malum terre root, meliot, myrrh, oil of blue flower de luce, opopanax, pennyroyal, pepper, pyrethium, rhubarb, rose, rue, saffron, savin, pennyroyal, saxifrage, seraphinum, silver montanum, southernwood, water and wine, wild gourd, wild neppe, wine.

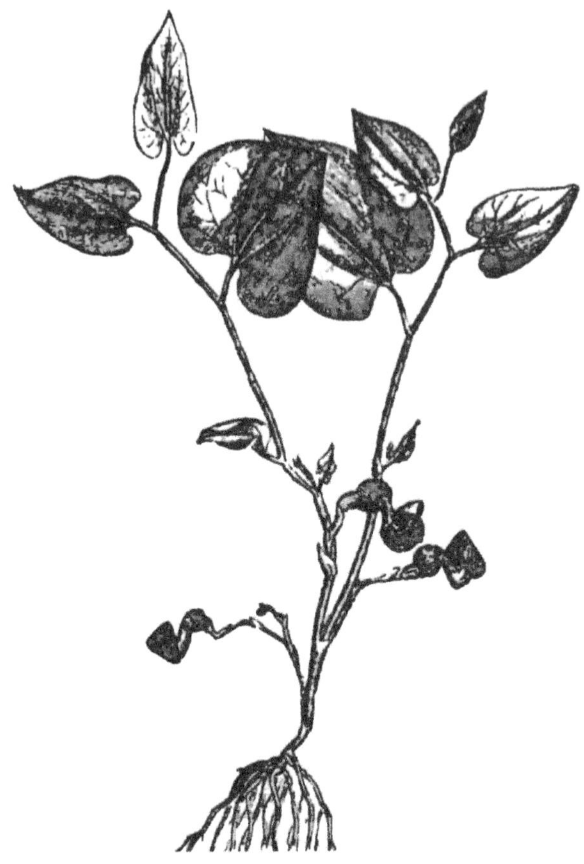

Figure 2 *Aristolochia* sp.

OXYTOCIN

The story of oxytocin dates back to the discovery by Oliver and Schafer (1895) who experimented with extracts of posterior pituitary gland and demonstrated the presence of a vasopressor substance, thus confounding the world of physiology, ably represented by Sir Michael Foster who, in his *Textbook of Physiology* of 1891, remarked that 'absolutely nothing was known at the time with regard to the purpose of this organ [the pituitary]'.

In 1906, Henry Dale, then a young research worker, tested extracts of posterior pituitary and confirmed that the substance caused a significant effect on blood pressure of the female cat. By coincidence, Dale noted that the pituitary extract caused intense spasm of the cat's uterine horns. This remarkable discovery appeared as a note in a paper which dealt primarily with the properties of ergot extracts (Dale, 1906) but Dale confirmed his findings after further experimentation (Dale, 1909). Years later he recounted the story in his *Adventures in Physiology with Excursions into Autopharmacology* of 1950. Dale's papers did not go unnoticed as soon after William Blair Bell (1909), co-founder of the British College of Obstetricians and Gynaecologists in 1929, published the first account of the use of pituitary extract in obstetrics.

In 1917, Stein of Germany reported the use of low dose posterior pituitary extract (pituitrin), by intramuscular injection, for the induction of labor (Eskes and Longo, 1994). However, all did not go well. In his short history on the *Posterior-pituitary Gland Principles* Moir (1964) wrote that: 'Before long the use of pituitary extract was the foremost topic of discussion in obstetrical circles the world over ... then history repeated itself... Ergot had been abused ... now it was the turn of pituitary extract ... recklessly used ... [it] was at least as dangerous as the older drug ... and when used to hasten the progress of lingering labor it ... caused the death of many a woman from uterine rupture, and many a fetus had perished because of intrauterine asphyxia'.

During those early days the posterior pituitary extract varied as much as 80 fold in strength and the substance was only satisfactorily standardized by J.H. Burn of the National Institute for Medical Research, Hampstead, in the early 1930s. Pituitrin, administered by intramuscular injection, had a remarkable effect on the uterus causing powerful spasm for about 8 minutes, followed by strong contractions at frequent intervals. Occasionally, patients showed signs of shock and collapse because of a generalized vasomotor effect.

Posterior pituitary extract was split into its two component fractions by Kamm and coworkers in American (Kamm, 1928) and named pitressin/vasopressin (the vasopressor fraction) and pitocin/oxytocin (the oxytocic fraction) by him. Theobald *et al.* (1948) introduced the concept of the low-dose intravenous drip (i.e. physiological) for induction of labor. Later, in an article entitled 'The pitocin drip', Theobald wrote that in Bradford he and his colleagues had used the technique 'on well over a thousand occasions' not only for inducing labor but also for treating uterine inertia. Theobald reported their triple procedure, 'which consists of low rupture of the membranes, deep sedation and the pitocin drip ... in a dilution never exceeding a concentration of 1:5000 ... if these precautions are strictly adhered to the routine use of the pitocin drip is safe in all patients who are allowed to go into labor' (Theobald, Kelsey and Muirhead, 1956). Theobald's (1959) further assertion that this 'physiological drip is so safe that it can be used in any cottage' did not go unchallenged for long.

Major advances came from du Vigneaud who, in 1951 (after 40 years of experimental work on the subject), isolated pure oxytocin and vasopressin and then went on two years later to produce a synthetic version of oxytocin, known as syntocinon (du Vigneaud *et al.*, 1953). Boissonas and colleagues (1955) also reported their synthesis of oxytocin. A period of intense research activity followed and momentous works on uterine activity and the process of labor flowed from the researches of Friedman of America in 1954, Alvarez and Caldeyro-Barcia of Uruguay in 1957, Philpott of Rhodesia in 1972, and many others.

The effects of oxytocin on uterine contractility and the duration of labor were intensely scrutinized. The method of oxytocin administration was also studied and the intramuscular, intranasal and oral (buccal linguets, oxytocin citrate, reported on by Dillon in 1960) routes were tried but intravenous infusion was found best. The hazards of inappropriate use of oxytocin were described – uterine hyperstimulation, uterine rupture, fluid retention with water intoxication, neonatal jaundice, iatrogenic prematurity and failed induction.

The benefits of correctly used oxytocin were highlighted by Kieran O'Driscoll of the National Maternity Hospital, Dublin who, following extensive clinical trials, included the oxytocic drip in what became known as 'The Active Management of Labour' from January 1968 (O'Driscoll and Stronge, 1975). This brought to an end one of the main scourges of women (and obstetricians alike) through the ages, the problem of 'tedious labor'.

Oxytocin, employed for induction and augmentation of labor, had another benefit. Used alone or in combination with ergometrine, oxytocin became an integral part of the active management of the third stage of labor. The debate arose as to whether the single or combined drug(s) was more effective in the reduction of postpartum hemorrhage. Diana Elbourn, a social statistician at the National Perinatal Epidemiology Unit, Oxford published a meta-analysis on the subject with clinical colleagues from Bristol but found that 'the quality of evidence [in support of either regimen] is not satisfactory' (Elbourne *et al.*, 1988). A randomized controlled trial of oxytocin alone versus oxytocin and ergometrine was carried out by Susan McDonald and colleagues in Perth and they concluded that the 'rates of postpartum hemorrhage were similar with both drugs, but oxytocin–ergometrine was associated with nausea, vomiting and hypertension' (McDonald *et al.*, 1993). Because of those side effects, and almost 180 years after its introduction to midwifery, ergot slowly became obsolete in the labor room and was replaced by synthetic oxytocin.

SPARTEINE

Sparteine sulfate, first isolated by Stenhouse in 1851, had been employed as a corrective for cardiac irregularities since 1873. Its atropine-like action was investigated by Tamba in 1921 and he deduced that it caused uterine contractions in experimental animals. Kleine of Germany introduced sparteine to obstetrics in 1939 and, although initial studies were disappointing, the drug became popular for the induction of labor (Moir, 1964; Clarke, 1975). Introduced to America in 1958, sparteine became widely used there until the mid-1960s when a number of adverse reports of its safety were published.

Embrey and Yates (1964) warned of the unpredictable uterine spasm caused by this ecbolic substance and, quoting the 'pulvis ad mortem' remark made by Hossack in relation to ergot in 1822, effectively rang the death knell for sparteine, which at one time was touted as the only 'safe' oxytocic drug.

QUININE AND THE OBE

Prior to the introduction of pituitary extract, there were a number of other drugs employed in the induction of labor. Included among them was quinine hydrochloride, given alone or in combination with the ubiquitous OBE – castor oil by mouth, a hot bath and a hot enema, and for which success rates of 25% to 80% were quoted. Castor oil contains ricinoleic acid which irritates the bowel, and in turn, the uterus. In cases of intrauterine death the synthetic estrogen, stilboestol, was administered to sensitize the uterus to subsequent quinine or oxytocin induction.

The action of quinine in the induction of labor was uncertain. It became apparent that quinine could cause fetal distress and intrauterine death and so the drug fell from favor (Clarke, 1975). Quinine is the principal alkaloid of cinchona and is obtained from the bark of the *Cinchona* or 'fever tree'. Cinchona first came to prominence in 1639 when it was introduced to Spain by Jesuits who were working in Peru. The bark, when powdered and administered as a potion, had the remarkable effect of reducing fevers and it also appeared to cure malaria. Cinchona, which is indigenous to certain parts of South America, was only one of a series of important new drugs imported to Europe from settlers in the New World.

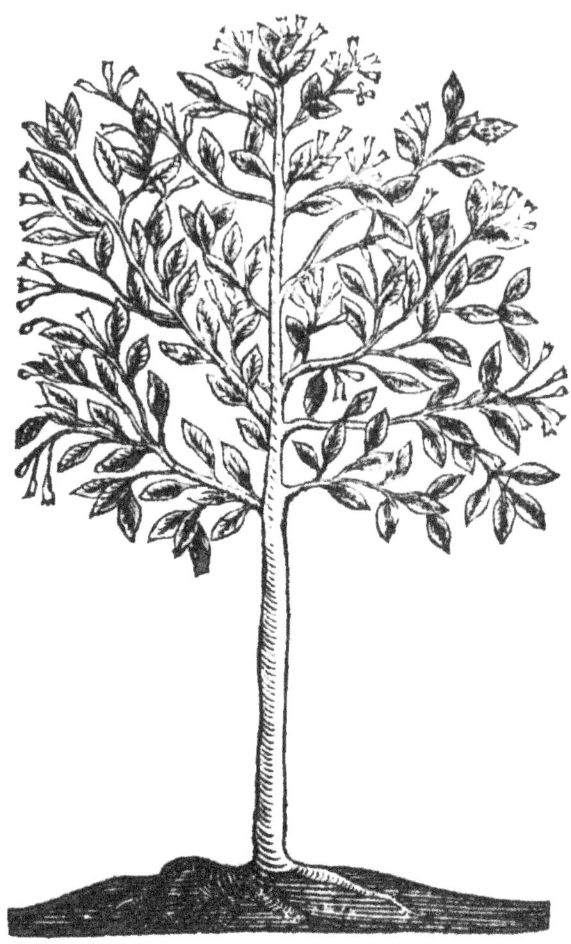

Figure 3 Cinchona plant, the source of quinine

PROSTAGLANDINS

Two American gynecologists, Kurzrok and Lieb, made a remarkable discovery in 1930 which was to have enormous implications for the world of biology, therapeutics and obstetrics. They found that strips of human uterus would contract or relax when exposed to human semen (Kurzrok and Lieb, 1930). A few years later, Goldblatt in England and von Euler in Sweden, reported the presence of a lipid-soluble smooth muscle contracting and vasopressor substance in the seminal fluid and accessory reproductive glands (Goldblatt, 1933; von Euler, 1934). Because of its site of identification, von Euler thought that the active factor was a secretion of the prostate gland and so in 1935 dubbed the substance 'prostaglandin' (PG).

The bioassays of the time were non-specific, so over 20 years were to elapse before technical advances permitted Bergstrom and his colleagues to isolate

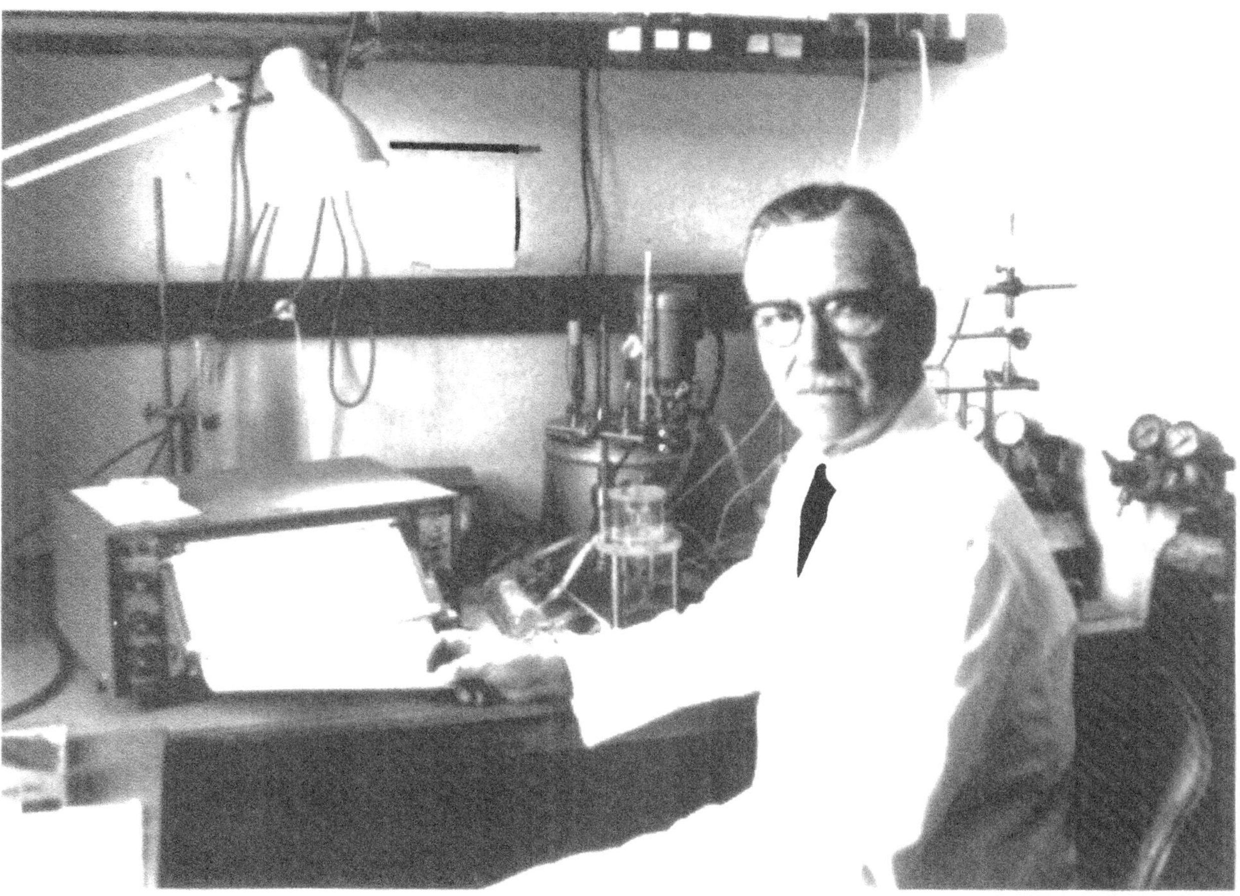

Figure 4 Ulf Svante von Euler (1905–1983)

prostaglandins E and F in crystalline form in 1960, and to elucidate their structure in the following year (Bergstrom *et al.*, 1962). PGs were found not to be stored in tissues but were biosynthesized when required. Arachadonic acid, itself derived from dietary linolenic acid, was found to be the most common precursor of PGs in humans. Prostaglandins participate in very many physiological processes, so inhibition of PG biosynthesis became an important study. A finding of great consequence was that salicylates, indomethacin and the non-steroidal anti-inflammatory drugs inhibit PG synthesis in a number of tissues.

From an obstetric point of view, Karim *et al.* (1968) and Bygdeman *et al.* (1968) underlined the value of PG in obstetrics. Karim, a London graduate who became professor and head of the Department of Pharmacology and Therapeutics in Makere, Uganda, studied the effects of continuous infusion of PGF2a in women at or near term. He and his colleagues found that PG stimulated uterine contractions, the patterns of which were similar to those in normal spontaneous labor, without a tendency to summation. The resting uterine tone did not increase and contractions were well spaced. Intravenous PG had unpleasant side effects so other methods of administration were researched.

Karim and Sharma (1971) used intravaginal PG to induce both labor and abortion. Meanwhile, Barr and Naismith (1972) experimented with PGE2 oral tablets for induction and found that 'The administration of PGE2a after amniotomy appears to be a satisfactory method of inducing labor at term. Maternal morbidity was rare ... uterine hypertonus was never recorded ... the infants were in satisfactory condition at birth'. As time went by, a large number of studies were carried out to determine the value and the correct role for PGs in obstetrics. The commonest usage was signaled by MacKenzie and Embrey (1977) who prescribed intravaginal PGE2 for ripening the cervix prior to induction of labor.

Mifepristone (RU 486)

The search for a 'medical' method of inducing early abortion led to the development of mifepristone (RU 486), an antiprogestogen. Etienne-Emile Baulieu, physician, biochemist and director of France's National Institute of Health and Medical Research, 'first conceived RU 486 as an aid to difficult births' (Sunday Times, 1995) but, by 1982, the drug was found to cause abortion of early human pregnancies. Subsequent trials revealed that a combination of mifepristone and prostaglandin analogue caused complete abortion in 95% of cases, with efficacy being linked to gestational age. Combined administration of mifepristone–prostaglandin became known as 'medical abortion' (Heard and Guillebaud, 1992). Frydman and colleagues of France suggested that, based on their experience, mifepristone could be used with safety to induce labor at term when the cervix was found to be unfavorable (Frydman *et al.*, 1991).

Misoprostol

The synthetic prostaglandin analogue, misoprostol, was found to have a 96% success rate in the medical treatment of incomplete miscarriage (Henshaw *et al.*, 1993) and, combined with methotrexate, was a 90–95% effective abortificient regimen up to 63 days after the last menstrual period (Crenin and Darney, 1993).

THE INDUCTION OF LABOR

This topic is dealt with in Chapter 21. There are interesting facts on various techniques in Fasbender (1906), Williams (1911), Beck (1942), Munro Kerr and Moir (1949), Clarke (1975), and O'Dowd and Philipp (1994), and good illustrations of hydrostatic bags and other methods for induction of labor in Williams and also in Beck.

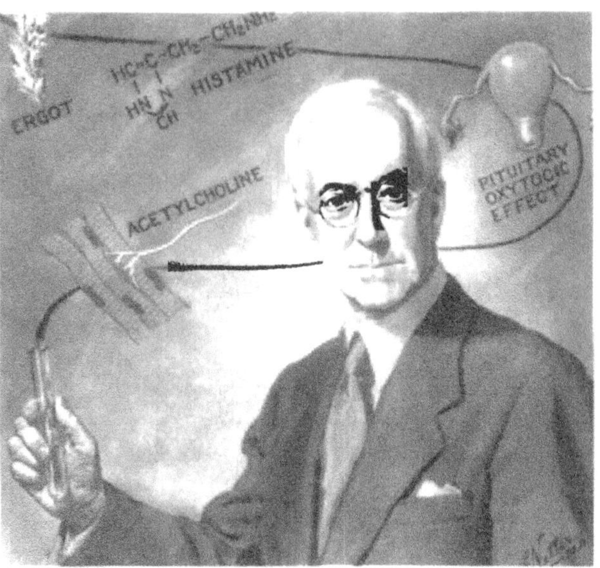

Figure 5 Sir Henry Hallett Dale (1875–1968)

BIOGRAPHIES

John Stearns (1770–1848)

John Stearns was born in Wilbraham, Massachusetts on 16 May 1770. He graduated from Yale University in 1789 and served his medical apprenticeship with Dr Erastus Sergeant of Stockbridge, Massachusetts. He gained distinction as a surgeon in the American Revolution and later studied in Philadelphia under Benjamin Rush, William Shippen Jr., and Caspar Wistar. Stearns then settled in Waterford, New York, where he practiced medicine. It was from there that he wrote his letter to a colleague with an account of the use of ergot in obstetrics. In 1817 he was elected President of the New York State Medical Society and was the first President of the New York Academy of Medicine. Having served as a Senator in New York State and Regent of the University, he moved to Albany. Stearns died on 18 March 1848 from an infection acquired during an autopsy (Findley, 1939).

Sir Henry Hallett Dale (1875–1968)

Born in 1875, Sir Henry Hallett Dale is famous for his outstanding contributions to physiology and pharmacology. A graduate of Trinity College Cambridge, he qualified as a doctor from St Bartholomew's Hospital

London in 1903. In the same year, Dale discovered the uterine stimulating effect of posterior pituitary gland extract. This eventually led to a dramatic change in the conduct of labor for countless women and their attendants. Dale was also involved in trials of crude ergot preparations. In 1936, he received the Nobel Prize for Physiology or Medicine (jointly with Otto Loewi) for his work on the transmission of nerve impulses, and in 1949 was bestowed with an Honorary Fellowship of the Royal College of Obstetricians and Gynaecologists (Peel, 1976). Shortly before Dale's death, during his 94th year in 1968, his old colleague and friend John Chassar Moir visited him in a Cambridge Nursing Home. After a happy but final encounter, Moir recounted that he left Dale's room with feelings of great sadness. When Dale died two weeks later the room was softly curtained 'for our little life is rounded with a sleep' (Moir, 1968).

References

Barr, W. and Naismith, W. C. M. K. (1972). Oral prostaglandins in the induction of labour. *BMJ*, **2**, 188–91

Beck, A. C. (1942). *Obstetrical Practice*, pp. 758–70. (Baltimore: Williams and Wilkins Co.)

Bell, W. B. (1909). The Pituitary body and the therapeutic value of the infundibular extract in shock, uterine atony and intestinal paresis. *BMJ*, **2**, 1609–13

Bergstrom, S., Ryhage, R., Samuelson, B. and Sjovall, J. (1962). The structure of prostaglandin E, F1 and F2. *Acta Chem. Scand.*, **16**, 501–02

Boissonas, R. A., Guttmann, S., Jacquenand, P. A. and Waller, T. P. (1955). A new synthesis of oxytocin. *Helvetica Chimica Acta*, **38**, 1491–95

Bygdeman, M., Kwon, S. U., Murkergee, T., and Wigvist, N. (1968). Effects of intravenous infusion of prostaglandin E1 and E2 on motility of the pregnant human uterus. *Am. J. Obstet. Gynecol.*, **106**, 567–72

Clarke, J. F. B. (1975). Medical Induction of Labour – A Review. In J. M. Beazley (ed.) The Active Management of Labour. *Clinics in Obstetr. Gynaecol.*, **2**(1), 49–79

Crenin, M. D. and Darney, P. D. (1993). Methotrexate and misoprostol for early abortion. *Contraception*, **48**, 339–48

Dale, H. H. (1906). On some physiological actions of ergot. *J. Physiol. (London)*, **34**, 163–206

Dale, H. H. (1909). The action of extracts of the pituitary body. *Biochem.* J., **4**, 427–47

Dale, H. H. (1953). *Adventures in Physiology with Excursions into Autopharmacology*. (London: Pergamon Press)

du Vigneaud, V. Ressler, C. Swan, J. M., Roberts, C. W., Katsoyannis, P. G. and Gordon, S. (1953). The synthesis of an octapeptide amide with the hormonal activity of oxytocin. *J. Am. Chem. Soc.*, **75**, 4879–80

Elbourne, D., Prendiville, W. and Chalmers, I. (1988). Choice of oxytocic preparation for routine use in the management of the third stage of labour: An overview of evidence from controlled trials. *Br. J. Obstet. Gynecol.*, **295**, 17–30

Embrey, M. P. and Yates, M. J. (1964). A tocographic study of the effects of sparteine sulphate on uterine contractility. *J. Obstet. Gynecol. Br. Common.*, **lxxi**.(1), 33–6

Eskes, T. K. A. B. and Longo, L. D. (1994). *Classics in Obstetrics and Gynecology*, p. 114. (London and New York: Parthenon Publishing)

Euler von, U. S. (1934). An adrenaline-like action in extracts from prostatic and related glands. *J. Physiol.* (London), **81**, 102–12

Fasbender, H. (1906). *Geschichte der Gerburtshilfe*, pp. 858–63. (Jena: Gustav Fischer)

Findley, P. (1939). *Priests of Lucina*, pp. 218–21. (Boston: Little Brown and Co.)

Frydman, R., Baton, C., Lelaidier, C., Vial, M., Bourget, Ph. and Fernandez, H. (1991). Mifepristone for induction of labour (letter) *The Lancet*, **337**, 488–9

Goldblatt, M. W. (1933). Depressor substance in seminal fluid. *J. Soc. Chem. Ind.*, **52**, 1056–57

Grieve, M. (1992). *A Modern Herbal*, pp. 338–9. (London: Tiger Books International)

Haggard, H. W. (1929). *Devils, Drugs and Doctors. The Story of the Science of Healing from Medicine-Man to Doctor*, pp. 216–19. (London: Heinemann)

Heard, M. and Guillebaud, J. (1992). Medical Abortion. *BMJ*, **304**, 195–6

Henshaw, R. C., Cooper, K., El-Refaey, H., Smith, N. C. and Templeton, A. A. (1993). Medical management of miscarriage: non-surgical uterine evacuation of incomplete and inevitable spontaneous abortion. *BMJ*, **306**, 894–5

Kamm, O., Aldrich, T. B., Grote, I. W., Rowe, L. W. and Bugbee, E. P. (1928). The active principles of the posterior lobe of the pituitary gland. *J. Am. Chem. Soc.*, **50**, 573–601

Karim, S. M. M. and Sharma, S. D. (1971). Therapeutic abortion and the induction of labour by the intravaginal administration of PGE2 and F2a. *J. Obstet. Gynecol. Br. Common.*, **78**, 294–300

Karim, S. M. M., Trussell, R. R., Hillier, K. and Patel, R. C. (1968). Induction of labour with prostaglandin F2 alpha. *BMJ*, **4**, 621–23

Kurzrok, R. and Lieb, C. C. (1930). Biochemical studies of human semen. 11. *Proc. Soc. Exp. Biol. (N. Y.)* **28**, 268–72

Leake, C. D. (1975). *An Historical Account of Pharmacology to the 20th Century*, p. 75. (Springfield, IL: Charles C. Thomas)

MacKenzie, I. Z. and Embrey, M. P. (1977). Cervical ripening with vaginal PGE2 gel. *BMJ*, **2**, 1381–84

McDonald, S. J. Prendiville, W. J. and Blair, E. (1993). Randomised controlled trial of oxytocin alone versus oxytocin and ergometrine in active management of third stage of labour. *BMJ*, 307, 1167–71

Moir, C. J. and Russell, C. S. (1943). An investigation of the effect of ergot alkaloids in promoting involution of the postpartum uterus. *J Obstet. Gynecol. Br. Emp.*, **50**, 94–104

Munro Kerr, J. M. and Moir, J. C. (1949). *Operative Obstetrics*, pp. 590–607. (London: Balliere, Tindall and Cox)

O'Dowd, M. J. and Philipp, E. E. (1994). *The History of Obstetrics and Gynaecology*, pp. 26–27, 267–68. (London and New York: Parthenon Publishing)

O'Driscoll, K. and Stronge, J. M. (1975). The Active Management of Labour. In J. M. Beazley (ed.) *Clinics Obstet. Gynecol.*, **2**(1), 3–16. (London: W. B. Saunders Co.)

Oliver, G. and Schaefer, E. A. (1895). On the physiological action of extracts of pituitary body and certain other glandular organs. *J. Physiol. (London)*, **18**, 277–9

Peel, Sir J. (1976). *The Lives of the Follows of the Royal College of Obstetricians and Gynaecologists 1929–1969*, pp. 9–11. (London: Heinemann Medical)

Rall, T. W. and Schleifer, L. S. (1985). Drugs Affecting Uterine Motility. In Goodman Gillman, L. S. Goodman, T. W. Rall and F. Murad (eds) *The Pharmacological Basis of Therapeutics*, pp. 926–45. (New York: Macmillan Co.)

Ringer, S. (1888). *A Handbook of Therapeutics*, p. 523. (London: H. K. Lewis)

Raynold, T. (1545). *The Byrth of Mankynde*. (London: Tho. Ray)

Sunday Times (1995). A life in the day of Etienne-Emile Baulieu. Color supplement, 10th September, p. 66.

Temkin, O. (1956). *Soranus' Gynecology*, Translation, pp. 175–86. (Baltimore: The Johns Hopkins Press)

Theobald, G. W. (1959). The choice between death from post-maturity or prolapsed cord and life from induction of labour. *The Lancet*, **1**, 59–65

Theobald, G. W., Graham, A., Gange, P. D. and Driscoll W. J. (1948). The use of posterior pituitary extract in physiological amounts in obstetrics. *BMJ*, **2**, 123–7

Theobald, G.W., Kelsey, H. A. and Muirhead, J. B. M. (1956). The Pitocin Drip. *J. Obstet. Gynecol. Br. Emp.*, **lxiii**, 641–62

Williams, J. W. (1911). *Obstetrics*, pp. 277–387. (New York: D. Appleton and Co.)

Section 5
Civilizations

25 The Orient

INTRODUCTION

China covers more than a fifth of Asia. It shares a large border with India, and both countries possess thousands of plants, many of which have medicinal properties. As they are so closely related, their respective materia medicae contain herbal medicines that are common to both countries. Drugs which entered the West from China and India include camphor (*Cinnamomum camphora*), cassia (*Cassia acutifolia*), ephedra (Ma-Huang, *Ephedra* sp.), ginseng (*Panax ginseng*), monkshood (*Aconitum napellus*), pomegranate (*Punica granatum*), rhubarb (*Rheum officinale*), star anise (*Illicium verum*) and the minerals arsenic, iron, mercury and sulfur. Some animal parts were also used in Chinese and Indian medicine but the vast majority of remedies were of plant origin.

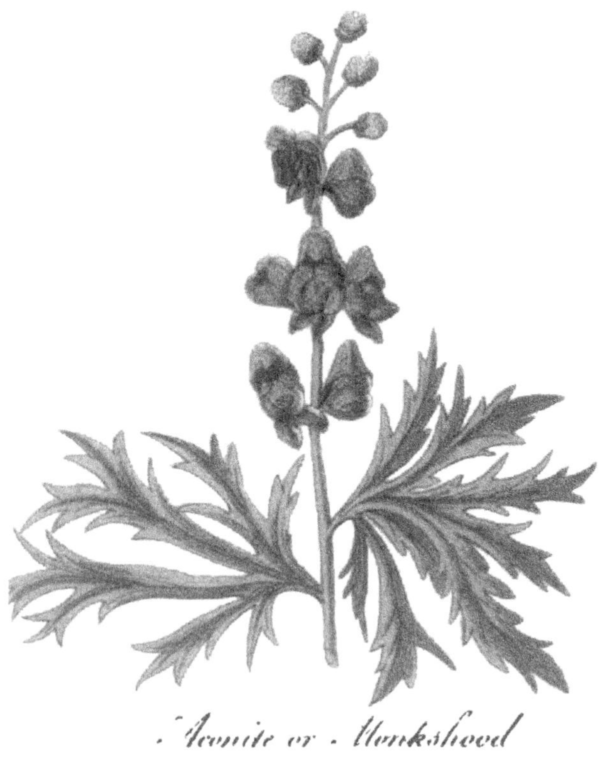

Figure 1 Monkshood (*Aconitum* sp.)

CHINA

Origins

China's history began over 7000 years ago in the fertile valleys of the Huang He, or Yellow River. The country was first united under Shih Huang Ti of the Ch'in dynasty (221–207 BC) from which the Western term 'China' developed. The Chinese call their country Ch'ung-Kuo, which means Middle Kingdom. They have a long and proud history and were the first to develop the compass, gunpowder, paper, porcelain, and silk cloth. Over the centuries, Japan, Korea, Vietnam and other Asian countries borrowed from Chinese art, language, literature, religion, technology and of course from it's rich medical heritage.

Mythology

According to Chinese mythology, the world came into existence with the death of Hun-Tun, the Emperor of the Center, whose name means Chaos. Many years later Chaos became an egg which gave birth to the earth, the sky, and a dwarf known as P'an-Ku. As the earth and sky expanded to their natural proportions poor P'an-Ku endeavored to fill the gap between. Inevitably he was torn apart and his body parts fell to earth and changed to various elements. P'an-Ku's semen became pearls, his marrow turned to jade, his sweat to rain and his body fleas became the human race. In another mythological version of creation the universe originated from the interaction of Yin and Yang, represented by the dwarf P'an-Ku and his wife. Yin was a cold, dark, moist, negative, and female form, while Yang was the active, dry, light, masculine, positive and warm principle. The two elements joined to form a balanced, perfect and totally interdependent entity.

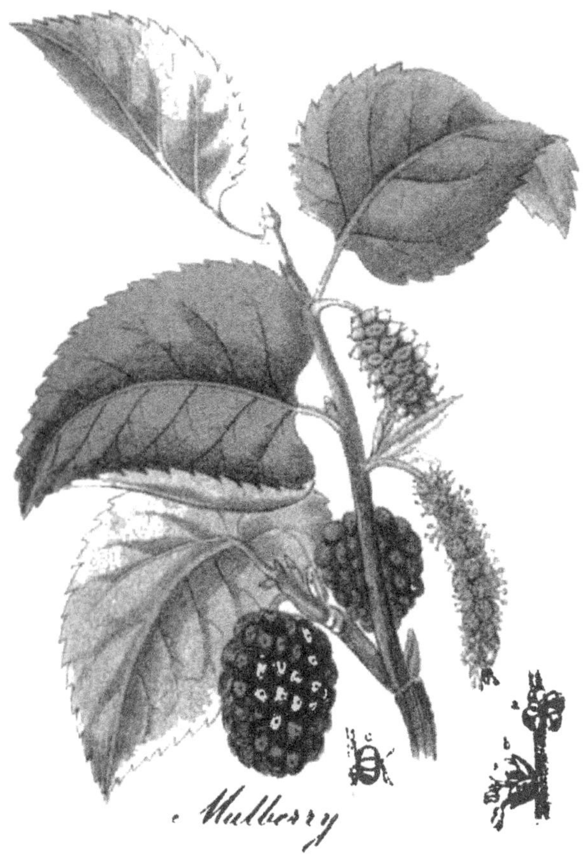

In an alternative story of the creation of the first humans, Nu-Kua, the creator goddess of ancient China, fashioned the first human beings. She modeled men and women from yellow clay but, becoming bored with her task, dipped a rope in the watery clay and trailed it behind her so that the formed figures and disparate blobs fell on the ground. The modeled figures became the noble and the rich while the blobs were the humble and poor. It was Nu-Kua who introduced the concept of marriage in mythological ancient China.

The semi-divine goddess Kuan-Yin (known in Tibet as Tara) was the most powerful being in the Chinese pantheon. Originally of mortal origin she was carried to heaven on a rainbow and transmuted into the divine world. Kuan-Yin was a feminine Avelokitesvara, a bodhisattva (Buddha to be), and as such was the embodiment of compassion. Dressed in flowing garments and bedecked with golden necklaces, she is the chief symbol of human clemency in the Orient. She was also the goddess of pregnancy and the ancient Chinese mother goddess, to whom infertile couples prayed. There was a popular belief that Kuan-Yin filled the ears of the rice plant with her own breast milk. She squeezed her breasts so strongly that her final drops of milk were tinged with blood and that was the origin of red rice.

Hsi-Wang-Mu was the Queen of the West and another powerful goddess of ancient China. She lived in a golden palace and every few thousand years threw a special birthday party for herself. On that special day the peach tree, p'an-t'ao, ripened and provided the fruit of immortality. She was the goddess of female energy, the essence of Yin and ruler of individual female beings. She dispensed peaches (*Prunus persica*) mixed with mulberry tree ashes (*Morus alba*) to help cure disease (Monaghan, 1990). The mythological Master of Healing was Yao-Shih, the Chinese name for Bhaishajyaguru Buddha, who ruled an Eastern paradise (Cavendish, 1991).

The Emperor Fu Hsi c. 2900 BC

The legendary ancient Emperor, Fu Hsi, introduced the 'pa-kua' symbol to represent the basic Yin–Yang elements and all their possible combinations. The outer core contained eight trigrams of combinations of the two. Each trigram was composed of broken lines for Yin and continuous lines for Yang. When arranged in pairs, the lines gave 64 possible Yin–Yang codes that were the key to the mysteries of the universe.

The Red Emperor, Shen Nung c. 2800 BC, and the *Pen-Ts'ao*

The Red Emperor, Shen Nung, is regarded as the father of Chinese pharmacy. He is said to have compiled the original Chinese materia medica which was handed down as an oral tradition until published in AD 1596/7 as the *Shen Nung Pen-Ts'ao*, The Materia Medica of Shen Nung. The Red Emperor also devised the first acupuncture charts. The herbal contained 365 drugs, all of which were personally tested by the Emperor. In later times the *Pen-Ts'ao* was enlarged, and in its final version contained approximately 2000 medications and many thousands of prescriptions. The *Pen-Ts'ao* remedies were administered as decoctions, mixtures, pills, plasters, powders, and suppositories. The definitive *Pen Ts'ao* comprised 52 volumes and its compilation was the work of Li Shih Chen, who had spent 30 years revising and updating the ancient Chinese materia medica. Each medicinal substance was described in detail with its locale, odor and taste, principal application, preparation, and use. The medications of the *Pen Ts'ao* were classified into 17 categories that included animals, birds, earth, fire, fruit, fish, grains, herbs, metals, insects, human body material, stones, water, and wood.

The Yellow Emperor, Huang Ti c. 2600 BC

The Yellow Emperor, Huang Ti, the legendary father of Chinese medicine, composed the *Nei Jing* (Canon of Medicine) a great compendium of Chinese medicine which was eventually committed to writing in the third century BC. The portion of the text that dealt with the prevention of diseases related a conversation between the Yellow Emperor and his Prime Minister. The *Nei Jing* laid out five treatment methods: apply acupuncture and moxibustion, cure the spirit, nourish the body, prescribe medications, and treat the entire body while restoring the patient to the right path of balance and harmony (the Tao). The *Nei Jing* dealt with many problems encountered by women. A modern translation is available (Veith, 1972). Another text entitled *The Discourses of the Yellow Emperor and the Plain Girl* dealt with Taoist beliefs regarding sexual matters.

The Yellow Emperor popularized the technique of acupuncture which drained off excess Yin or Yang and restored proper balance. The acupuncture technique that evolved meant piercing the skin with long needles. They could be inserted into any of the 365 points along the 12 meridians that course through the body to transmit its *Qi*, or active life-force. Each acupuncture point was related to a particular organ and, if properly used, it was thought that all illnesses could be corrected by the procedure. The acupuncture technique spread to Japan and Korea in the tenth century AD and to Europe by the seventeenth century. A similar approach to therapy, moxibustion, involved treatment with powdered plant substance, usually mugwort (*Artemisia vulgaris*). The moxa was burned over the patient's skin using the same meridians and points as acupuncture. The word 'moxa' is of Japanese origin and the technique of moxibustion may have originated in Egypt. The moxa was less energetic than acupuncture needles and better suited to children and old people or those weakened by disease.

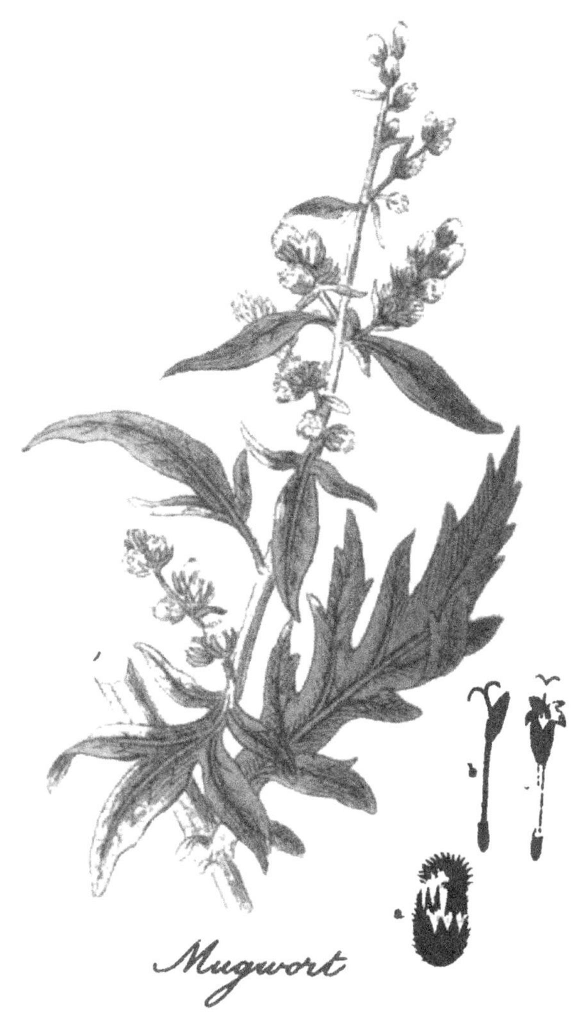

Figure 3 Mugwort (*Artemisia vulgaris*)

Zhou Dynasty (c. 1027–221 BC)

The duties and general organization of physicians was laid down during the Zhou dynasty and the compilation was known as the *Institutions of Zhou*. There were various categories of physicians including gynecologists, pediatricians and those who collected drugs.

Obstetrics was mainly carried out by midwives (Lyons and Petrucelli, 1987). The earliest known apothecaries were called Fang Shih. From the fifth century BC onwards prescriptions were painted on bamboo slats and contained information on drug quantity, dosage and use.

It was during the Zhou period that the theory of Chinese pulse lore was originated by Pien Ch'iao. Pulsology was further developed by Wang Shu-Hi (317–265 BC). The Chinese attached great diagnostic importance to the pulse, the varieties of which were sub-divided and investigated by touching different parts of the radial artery of either hand with the examining fingers, in the fashion of striking the keys of a piano. In this way, six sets of pulse data were elicited which were connected with the different organs and their diseases (Garrison, 1929). Europeans became aware of pulse lore when Michael Byom, a Jesuit missionary to China, first wrote on the subject in 1666.

Lao-Tzu and the Tao Way of Life, c. 600 BC

Lao-Tzu codified the Tao way of life of moderation, equanimity and morality as laid out in the *Tao-Te Ching*. Illness was caused by disregard of the Tao, and was also related to other forces such as the wind or conditions which led to inequality of the inner balance of Yin and Yang. Taoism and Chinese medicine focused on the prevention of illness as being the primary means of medical care but Taoist physicians also sought to influence health through medicinal drugs. The Yin–Yang of Chinese philosophy also extended to sexuality. Taoist physicians believed that one path to longevity lay in frequent and prolonged but non-ejaculatory sexual intercourse (Reid, 1993). A man's Yang could be strengthened by absorption of Yin released by his female partner during orgasm, but ejaculation of semen was detrimental as this would deplete Yang stores. If retained, the semen was recycled to nourish the brain.

Confucius 551–479 BC

Confucius was a Chinese philosopher and statesman who became a teacher after a long period of discontent and warring among the various groups who sought to gain control of China. Although he was China's greatest sage, little is known of his personal life. His name as we know it is a Latinized version of his Chinese name, K'ung Fu-Tzu. Confucianism became one of the principal religions of China, although it was a moral philosophy, or way of life, rather than a religion in the Western sense of the word. The Confucian doctrine was to achieve harmony through moral responsibility and great emphasis was placed on the five virtues of charity, justice, propriety, sincerity and wisdom. The medical philosophies of the era sought equilibrium, harmony and order through a delicate balance of Yin and Yang forces. Five literary classics of Confucian knowledge are extant and they contain a valuable insight into the condition of Chinese civilization of the time. Included in the texts are references to herbal medicines and physical therapy (Windridge, 1994). Dissection of the human body was not allowed during this era, so anatomical knowledge was only achieved through reasoning and observation of the animal kingdom. This situation continued in the nineteenth century, when anatomy was still taught by diagrammatic representation and artificial models rather than by dissection (Lyons and Petrucelli, 1987).

The Han Dynasty, 206 BC–AD 220

The first reference to anesthetics in Chinese medicine came during the lifetime of the great Han physician, Hua Tuo (AD 141–208). He used narcotic preparations which included Indian hemp (*Cannabis indica*, also known as bhang, hashish and marihuana, a psychotropic), monkshood (*Aconitum napellus*, contains aconite, an analgesic and sedative) and a variety of thorn apple (*Datura metel*, from the Hindi, *dhatura*, and containing atropine and other alkaloids). He also introduced the therapeutic Kung-Fu exercises which were based on the rhythmic movements of the bear, crane, deer, monkey and tiger. Towards the close of the Han dynasty, most of the elements which make up Chinese medicine were already firmly in place. These included dietary regulations, science, sexual code, spiritual beliefs, therapeutic exercises, and herbal pharmacopoeia. Angelica (*Angelica sinensis*), the second most important Chinese tonic after ginseng, was used at the time for menstrual disorders and is still prescribed for the same reasons in China and in

Western herbal medicine. Cinnamon (*Cinnamomum cassia*), ginger (*Zingiber officinale*), ginseng (*Panax ginseng*), pinellia (*Pinellia ternata*), and wormwood (*Artemisia* sp.) were also available for gynecological treatments. Those herbal remedies became popular in Europe and are still used.

Sun Szu-Miao, AD 581–682

Sun Szu-Miao summarized the medical knowledge to date and produced the *Ch'ien Chian Yao Fan* (A Thousand Golden Remedies). This text had three volumes devoted to gynecology and obstetrics, and offered hundreds of medications for women's diseases.

Li Shih-Chen, AD 1517–1593

Li Shih-Chen produced a famous herbal encyclopedia, *Pen Tshao Kang Mu*, in 1578 which took 27 years to complete. During that time, he traveled all over China in search of medicinal herbs. It is related that he consulted 360 medical treatises and 590 scientific works before he wrote his herbal. The text was contained in 52 book scrolls. It listed 1892 medicines and was highly illustrated. He classified herbs into 16 categories and also sub-divided individual remedies into plants, animals and minerals. Plants were further grouped into families based on the color of juice in their stalk and other characteristics. Nearly 12 000 prescriptions and formulae were described which had been collected over the course of his journeys all over the Empire. The herbal was widely distributed though China and neighboring countries and was also translated into European languages. It was about this time that the term 'Ben Cao' was introduced to describe the concept of herbal medicine. 'Ben' meant a plant stalk and 'Cao' was a grass-like plant. Ben Cao eventually included medicines derived from animal and mineral sources. In 1956 the People's Republic of China paid tribute to Li Shih-Chen when they issued a postage stamp bearing his likeness.

Chung Szi-Sung, c. AD 1700

Chung Szi-Sung in the *Secret Therapy for the Treatment of the Venereal Disease* reported using arsenic for the treatment of venereal disease. In the West, Paul Ehrlich reported the treatment of syphilis with the arsenic derivative Salvarsan (606) in 1910.

EARLY MEDICAL DEVELOPMENT

Traditional Chinese medicine originated in folk and religious practices and was contemporary with the growth of Ayurvedic medicine in India and the Hippocratic tradition in Greece. The term for medicine was 'Yao' while a doctor was called 'Yi'. Bian Que (407–310 BC) was said to be China's first true physician. He practiced acupuncture and medicine and introduced gynecological and pediatric treatments. The ancient medical books were written on white silk with a twig dipped in black varnish, or engraved on bamboo slats. After 200 BC they were written on mulberry-bark paper using a brush.

China's early development was influenced by contact with India and Tibet. Buddhism was introduced from India in the first century AD, as were some aspects of Ayurvedic medicine and Kung-Fu exercises related to Yoga. Contacts with the Arab world were also very important. In the second century BC the physician Chang Chien spent a decade in the study of the Arab drug treatments and medical concepts and introduced the new knowledge to Chinese medicine. The concept of humoral medicine also spread to China from Greece. The Medical Institution became organized by the end of the third century BC. The physicians were separated into groups which included alchemists, pharmacists, physicians, and veterinarians. By 165 BC, government examinations were introduced and an Imperial University was founded in 124 BC. During the period 200 BC–AD 200 the State medical service took control of all medical institutions and hospitals built by the Taoist and Buddhist communities. By the sixth century AD Chinese medicine had spread to Japan and Korea and by the tenth century, the full complement of Chinese medicine was accepted in Japan. In Southeast Asia, Arabic, Chinese and Indian medical systems developed concurrently. By the seventh century AD, an Imperial Medical College was established and there were medical colleges in the main provincial cities. In the eighth century AD the Chinese state authorities took responsibility for the development of pharmacopoeias and produced the *Guang Ji Fang* (General Formulary of Prescriptions). Centuries later European medicine again filtered into China during the era of Kublai Khan (1216–1294), founder of the Mongol Dynasty.

Throughout the dynasties to the seventeenth century AD, the principles and practice of Chinese medicine were consolidated, rather than moving into new fields of expertise, but the institutional structures for Chinese medicine declined after the weakening of the Empire, most especially after the seventeenth century (McGrew, 1985). Little was known about Chinese medicine in the West until the seventeenth century, when Jesuit missionaries were sent to Peking by Louis XIV. It was the Jesuits who coined the word 'acupuncture' from the Latin *acus*, needle, and *punctura*, pricking or puncture. The first European treatise on acupuncture was published in 1671 by Father Harvieu.

European medicine became popular in China and, by the turn of the twentieth century, Traditional Chinese Medicine (TCM) had fallen from favor. By 1911 only eight schools of TCM remained, and soon after the establishment of the Republic of China in 1912 the era of the traditional physicians appeared at an end. The situation was reversed after the Chinese Revolution and the formation of the People's Republic of China in 1949, under the leadership of Mao Ze-dong. Within a year it was established that there should be closer collaboration between doctors who practiced traditional medicine and those with modern training. China's administrators adopted a policy in favor of TCM, having for years suppressed it and replaced it with Western medicine. The China Academy of Traditional Chinese Medicine was established in 1955. In the following year medical colleges for TCM were established in Beijing, Shanghai, Chengdu and Guangzhou. Since then, TCM and Western medicine have become integrated in many parts of China.

Aspects of Chinese medicine

Physiology was dealt with as a humoral system, similar to that of Greco–Roman medicine, although the Chinese had five rather than four essential humors. The number five was very important to the ancient Chinese and carried mystical connotations. Most items could be divided in five, e.g. five solid organs, five drug types, five qualities, and so on. The physiological basis for body function was the interaction of Yin and Yang, the two principles which were believed to control all existence. Imbalance of Yin or Yang produced illness. The disease process was also related to meteorological influences, such as brightness of day, rain, twilight and the wind. Natural phenomena were classified into the five groups: earth, fire, metal, water and wood. The 'vital spirit' was known as Qi, and compared to the 'pneuma' or breath in Greek medicine. Qi suffused the body and its balance could be disturbed by any of six active disease-producing influences.

Chinese diagnostics included questioning the patient, observing the body, examination of the pulse, listening, smelling and tasting. Diagnostic statuettes were of particular importance for females. Modest upper-class ladies indicated the locations of their ailments, rather than being subjected to physical examination. Treatment was effected by acupuncture, diet or drug treatments, all of which adjusted the flow of Qi. Physical therapy was also important and various forms of massage and exercise were developed to keep the body fit. The Chinese also used dry cupping and massage. TCM stressed the importance of preventing illness rather than curing it.

Obstetrics and gynecology

Giovanni Maciocia (1998) in his *Obstetrics and Gynecology in Chinese Medicine* related the history of gynecology in China and offered an extensive bibliography of modern and historical books on the subject. It appears that the earliest records of gynecology date from the Shang dynasty 1500–1000 BC. Maciocia detailed the important obstetric and gynecological texts, or those medical texts which contained detailed tracts on the subjects over the subsequent centuries. Of importance from the historical point of view, Maciocia wrote that since the major colleges of TCM were established in 1956, the ancient books relating to obstetrics and gynecology have been reprinted, and many modern textbooks of TCM-style obstetrics and gynecology have been published. A short sample of Maciocia's detailed history follows.

Warring States Period (476–221 BC) *The Book of Mountains and Seas* contained herbal remedies for infertility. In this era, a gynecologist was a Dai Xia Yi which translates as one who treats diseases under the skirt belt.

Han Dynasty (206 BC–AD 220) The gynecologist was referred to as Ru Yi, a breast doctor, or Nu Yi a women's doctor. Books which dealt exclusively with gynecology before the Han dynasty have all been lost.

Wang Shu He in his Pulse Classic (*Mai Jing*, AD 280) discussed the qualities of the pulse in relation to various obstetric and gynecological abnormalities.

Sun Si Mio wrote the Thousand Golden Ducat Prescriptions (*Quian Jin Yao Fang*) in AD 652 and various forms of gynecological problems were mentioned.

The earliest book of obstetrics was written during the Tang dynasty (AD 618–960) and called the Treasure of Obstetrics (*Jing Xiao Chan Bao*).

Maciocia's historical essay is only a small part of his treatise on obstetrics and gynecology in Chinese medicine, the text of which runs close to 1000 pages. The book affords an intriguing view of a complex system, grounded in tradition, and quite unlike that of the West. Maciocia understands both approaches and explains the Chinese perception of diagnosis and treatment of various conditions while comparing the Oriental methods to those of the Occident.

From Maciocia's text we can also learn some Chinese terms of interest in obstetrics and gynecology. The uterus is known as the *Bao* or baby palace. Menstruation is *Jing*, and delayed periods translate as *Yue Jing Hou Qi*. Heavy periods are *Yue Jing Guo Duo*, while scanty menses are *Yue Jing Guo Shao*, and prolonged flow is *Jing Qi Yan Chang*. To regulate the period translates as *Tiao Jing*, and to warm the menses is *Wen Jing*. Pregnancy in Chinese terminology is *Zi* and the event was usually the cause of much joy, *Xi*.

Chinese medications

The Chinese believe that for every illness there is a corresponding natural remedy. Over the centuries they investigated many medicines which proved effective. Others were ineffective but may have had a magical or placebo effect. It is believed that drugs are animated with either harmful or helpful spirits and these affect a person's *Qi* (life force) and its balance. The word 'herb' as used in Chinese medicine includes some animal parts or minerals, although the vast majority of Chinese herbs were plants.

Medicines are classified according to their medicinal nature and taste. Their nature could be cold, hot, warm, cool or neutral. These attributes are known as the *Qi* of the medicine. The taste and smell of medicines subclassify them into the categories of sour, bitter, sweet, pungent, salty or tasteless (astringent). Notice is taken of drug compatibility, the volume used, and how it would be prescribed, either as an oral or external preparation.

Plant medications which entered the West from China include:

Camphor (*Cinnamomum camphora*), an analgesic, anti-inflammatory, antiparasitic, digestive and stimulant;
Cassia (*Cassia acutifolia*), a digestive, relieved vomiting and stimulated the circulatory system;
Ephedra (*Ephedra* sp.), the source of ephedrine, an anti-asthmatic and stimulant;
Ginseng (*Panax ginseng*), an 'all-heal' herb;
Monkshood (*Aconitum napellus*), the alkaloid isolated from it is aconitine, an analgesic, sedative and poison;
Pomegranate (*Punica granatum*), destroys intestinal parasites;
Rhubarb (*Rheum officinale*), laxative and uterine stimulant;
Star anise (*Illicium verum*), antibacterial and antifungal.

Other items of interest from the Chinese materia medica include:

Seaweed which contains iodine;
Siberian milkwort (*Polygala tenuifolia*) contains anti-spasmodics useful for menstrual pain;
Mulberry (*Morus alba*), is a source of rutin, an anti-hypertensive;
Willow (*Salix alba*) which yields the analgesic salicylic acid, first synthesized in 1838 and the basis for aspirin;
Opium poppy (*Papaver somniferum*) apparently did not enter into Chinese medicine until after 1000 BC. It was originally used for treating diarrhea but became

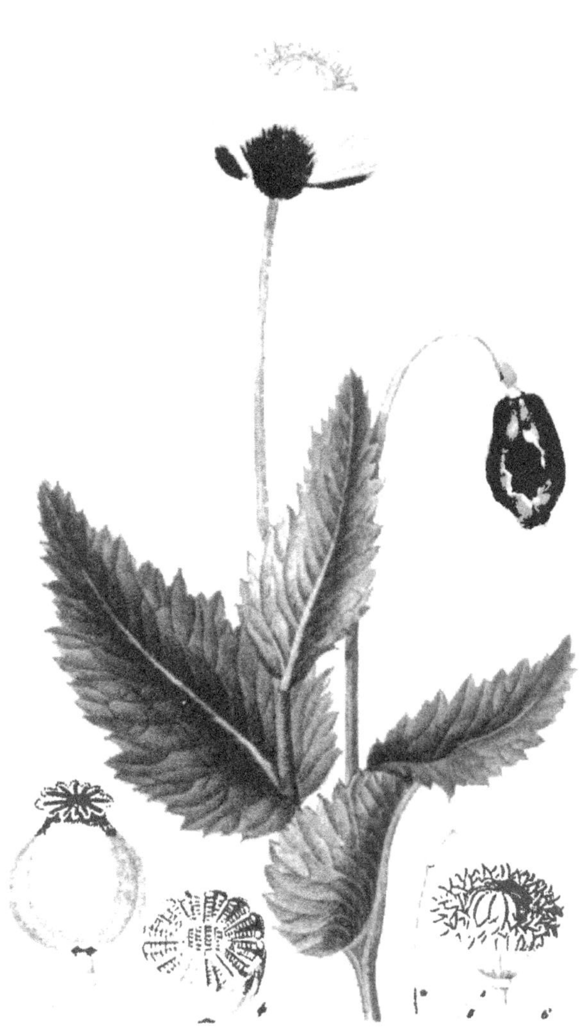

Figure 4 Opium poppy (*Papaver somnifera*)

a popular recreational drug in the sixteenth century, during the reign of the last emperor of the Ming dynasty, when alcohol was banned.

Dr Heny Lu (1994) tells the legends of some Chinese herbs in his *Chinese Herbal Cures*.

Animal parts such as Dragon teeth (powdered fossil bones), tiger hair, tips of antlers, toad skin or slime, rhinoceros horn, snake meat and sea mollusks, are all part of the Chinese materia medica which reached the West, but are little used here today. It has recently been proven that frog skin and scrapings from antlers have pharmacologically active compounds useful for therapeutics in humans.

Human organs and waste, such as young boys' urine for difficult childbirth, and a preparation of testicles and human sperm to treat impotence, are all used; while human placenta is advocated as an oxytocic. These therapies carry echoes of practice in the West where human products form a small but significant part of our materia medica. A recent addition to the repertoire is human foreskin. Discarded as redundant until recent times, except for witches' brews, it is reported that the human prepuce can be grown in culture to produce enough skin to cover a football field.

Minerals such as arsenic, iron, mercury (used as calomel for venereal disease), and sulfur have all found medicinal application in the West.

The Pharmacopoeia of the People's Republic of China

The People's Republic of China was founded on the 1st of October 1949. Soon afterwards, a meeting was called to discuss the creation of a National Pharmacopoeia. The first official Pharmacopoeia of the People's Republic of China (PPRC) was released in 1953 and contained 531 monographs of substances and articles. An addendum to the first edition was issued four years later on the basis of comments and suggestions by members of the Chinese Pharmaceutical Association. In that same year of 1957 it was decided that well-defined traditional Chinese medicines should be admitted to the Pharmacopoeia.

The second edition of the PPRC was released in 1963 and was enlarged to contain 446 monographs of traditional Chinese medications and 197 patent preparations in use by traditional Chinese physicians. The next edition of the Pharmacopoeia was in 1977 and the number of monographs devoted to Chinese herbal drugs was expanded. The fourth National PPRC was released in 1986. The first English version, based on that edition, was published in 1988, to encourage international exchange of information in the field of herbal medicine. The fifth edition of 1990 contained 1751 monographs of substances and articles. Of those, 509 were devoted to traditional Chinese medicaments, and 275 to Chinese patent preparations and single ingredient preparations. The English version (1992) contained 514 monographs of traditional Chinese medications, of which in excess of one third were used for women's disorders. Many of the compound Chinese patent medicines were also used for women's disorders. These latter medications can contain up to 25 or more ingredients in a single prescription.

Chinese materia medica for women

Maciocia (1998) listed 427 prescriptions for use in obstetrics and gynecology, with a further 70 patent medicines and 55 empiricals. Altogether, the prescriptions were based on 194 medicinal herbs, plus some animal and mineral parts. One such prescription, *Ren Shen Tang* (a ginseng decoction) contained 20 ingredients for the treatment of amenorrhea (*Bi Jing, Bi* meaning closed and *jing*, menstruation). A patent medicine known as *Quan Lu Wan* (whole deer pill) contained 25 ingredients and was used for the same indication.

The prescriptions have intriguing names, such as 'clearing the menses powder', 'arousing the uterus pill', or 'ovulation decoction'. Others carried names with less obvious objectives such as the 'female treasure decoction' and 'drain fire decoction'. Other prescriptions had cheerful-sounding titles such as the 'peaceful menopause' (*Geng Nian An*), or the 'happy menopause' (*Geng Nian Le*), while the remedy to promote lactation 'gushing spring powder' (*Xia Ru Yong Quan San*), and nostrums to 'calm the fetus' (*An Tai*), or to 'warm the menses' (*Wen Jing*) promised a happy outcome to treatment.

A SELECTION OF CHINESE MATERIA MEDICA

Ephedra

The Red Emperor described one of the plant substances especially associated with China, known as Ma-Huang (*Ephedra* sp.). *Ephedra* was used in ancient China as an anti-inflammatory or to induce perspiration and pyrexia (the former action is now ascribed to the oxazolidone content of the plant). The use of this medicinal plant found its way, via the trade routes, to Greece and from there to the rest of the known world. In 1887 Japanese investigators isolated an alkaloid which is one of the active principles of *Ephedra*

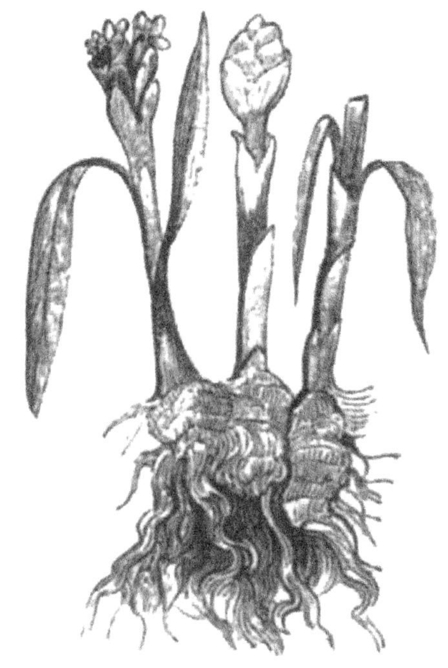

Figure 5 Ginger

and termed it ephedrine (pseudoephedrine was isolated from Ma-Huang at a later date). Ephedrine found application as a cerebral stimulant, mydriatic, vasoconstrictor, a potent monoamine oxidase inhibitor, and one of the most effective treatments for asthma. One form of *Ephedra* was called squaw tea and was used as an anti-syphilitic agent in North America. Ma Huang is currently advised in TCM for the 'night sweats' of the menopause (PPRC, 1992).

Ginger

Ginger, *Zingiber officinale* (Shen jiang, fresh, or Gan jiang, dried ginger) derives its name from the Greek, which in turn adopted the name from the East Indian Pali word, *singivera*. The ginger plant has been cultivated in India and China from earliest times. Its spicy taste, well known to the Greeks and Romans, was used to disguise the unpleasant odor of tainted fish and meat. Ginger had reached England by the eleventh century and was a common article of European commerce in the Middle Ages.

Ginger has a long history of medicinal use in China and India, and was used as an antiemetic to relieve nausea and vomiting. It is currently in vogue in the West as an anti-nauseant in early pregnancy and as an anti-spasmodic to relieve menstrual cramps. In China it is indicated to treat deficiency of Yang that can lead to abnormal uterine bleeding (PPRC, 1992). The ginger plant contains a large number of active constituents, and recent research reveals that it is an effective antiemetic with strong antibacterial and anti-fungal properties (Evans, 1996).

Ginseng

Ginseng is the dried root of the *Panax ginseng*, Ren shen in Chinese (the forked root of ginseng is similar to the Chinese written character for *ren*, which means man, while *shen* means essence). The term *Panax* derives from the Greek, *panakes*, a panacea, in allusion to the high value placed on it by the Chinese as an aphrodisiac and medication. In ancient China ginseng was especially prized as a treatment for wounds. Soldiers paid tribute to it's precious qualities by calling it *jin bu huan*, or 'gold-no-trade' (Reid, 1993).

Ginseng is prescribed to reinforce the vital energy, to increase longevity, and this 'man plant' is also used to treat frigidity and impotence (PPRC, 1992). *Panax* may also be used to treat heavy periods and problems in the puerperium (the Chinese term for the postnatal era is, *chan ru*, Maciocio, 1998). A number of ginseng preparations are available, including the cultivated and wild varieties, and the sun-dried and red ginseng types. The three main forms available in the West are Asiatic (*Panax ginseng*), American (*Panax quinquefolius*) and the Siberian (*Eleutherococcus senticosus*) and, although similar, they differ in their medicinal properties. Many substitutes and inferior specimens are being sold so the would-be purchaser should buy with caution.

Mulberry

The mulberry, *Morus alba*, was dispensed with the peach (*Prunus persica*) in the treatment of disease by the Queen of the West, Hsi-Wang-Mu. The leaves (sang ye), branches (sang zhi), root bark (sang bai pi), and the fruits (sang shen) are currently used in Western herbal medicine and are thought to have antibacterial properties. Mulberry leaves are the preferred food of the silkworm, *Bombyx mori*. Indian mulberry, *Morinda citrifolia*, and others of this genus, are astringents and purgatives. In TCM morinda root, *Morinda officinalis*, *Bajitian* in Chinese, is prescribed for infertility, impotence, menstrual disorders and seminal emission (PPRC, 1992).

Peach

The peach, *Prunus persica, Taoren* in Chinese, was originally called the malum persicum or Persian apple, reflecting the fact that the peach, a native of China, first became widely known in Europe when it had reached Persia on its westward journey (Ayto, 1994). In Chinese mythology, the peach was sacred to Hsi-Wang-Mu, The Queen of the West. Her mystic peach garden blossomed every 3000 years, and the gods' elixir of immortality was produced from its fruits. In Chinese mythology, the split peach represented the vulva and Shou-Lao, the god of longevity, was depicted seated on a deer (symbol of sexuality) within a split peach holding a coral scepter that represented the erect phallus. In Taoist terminology, a virgin was referred to as 'peach blossom'. A twig of the peach plant was used as a magic wand by ancient Chinese magicians. In Europe, the peach was the fruit of Venus and was sacred to the goddess Hymen.

The peach is an important part of the Chinese herbal pharmacopoeia and the semen persica, peach seed, is administered dry, blanched in boiling water, or stir-fried in the treatment of amenorrhea and dysmenorhoea (PPRC, 1992; Windridge, 1994). The seeds are also used in Western herbal medicine for menstrual disorders.

Placenta

The Pharmacopoeia of the People's Republic of China (PPRC, 1992) relates that the medication known as *Ziheche* or *Tai Pan* is the dried placenta of a healthy woman (placenta hominis). Preparation involves washing repeatedly until free from blood. The placenta is then steamed or boiled for a moment and dried. The dried placenta is broken in pieces and ground to a fine powder, and administered in a dose of up to 3 g. *Ziheche* is indicated for infertility and impotence, as a lactogenic, for seminal emissions, and for night sweats. A 'spoonful of sugar to make the medicine go down' is offered by Maciocia (1998) who writes that the 'sugar-coated placenta tablet', Tai Pan Tang Yi Pian, is available as a patent remedy, or combined with the herb Lu Jiao (*Cornus cervi*), to nourish the blood and the kidney essence in the treatment of infertility. Another source reveals that roasted placenta was prescribed as an oxytocic in China (Beau, 1972). Chen Ke-ji, Professor of Medicine at the China Academy of TCM, Xiyuan Hospital, advises powder of placenta, *Ziheche Fen*, for weakness after childbirth (Ke-ji, 1997).

In ancient times, the placenta was considered to be the unformed twin of the baby, and there were special rites performed during the disposal of the organ. In Egypt, the royal placenta bore the name of the moon god, Konshu, and was preserved for burial with the Pharaoh. For most people, the second birth was buried in a site of significance or disposed of by incineration. The placenta gained its Latinized name from Gabriel Falloppius (1523–1563) of Padua. He also coined the word 'vagina' and was the first to accurately describe the clitoris. In his *Observationes Anatomicae* of 1561, Falloppius detailed the anatomy of the oviducts which now bear his name, the Fallopian tubes. The word 'placenta' is Latin for cake and is borrowed from the Greek. Before the 'modern' term placenta became commonplace in the eighteenth century, the organ was variously known as the afterbirth, second birth, secondyne, secundine, hepar uterinum (uterine liver), placenta uterina (uterine cake) and other terms.

The placenta and cord (the navel string) have excited the interest of anatomists and obstetricians over the centuries. Among the many names associated with the organ is that of Thomas Wharton (1614–1673), who described the mucoid matrix of the umbilical cord now known as Wharton's jelly. In the nineteenth century, Bernhard Schultze (1827–1919) and J. Matthews Duncan (1826–1890) described the 'normal' presentation of the placenta at delivery as being the fetal or the maternal surface, respectively. Their contemporary, Carl Siegmund Crede (1819–1892), popularized abdominal expression of the placenta as a substitute for vaginal extraction, in an attempt to lessen the risk of 'flooding' during and after the third stage of labor. Placental studies revealed over 60 anatomical types and abnormalities. A full listing was included by William Hensyl in *Stedman's Medical Dictionary* (1990). This world-famous dictionary is called after Thomas Lathrop Stedman (1853–1938), who first introduced the text in 1911.

In his *History of Childbirth*, Jacques Gelis (1991) devoted a fascinating chapter to The Placenta: Double of the Child, which dealt with popular beliefs and superstitions related to the placenta. Placentogaphy, or the ingestion of cooked or raw placenta, was a custom among some 'primitive' and European societies until the eighteenth century. According to Gelis, placental opotherapy, or medication with placenta, has a long history. The remedy was used for a range of indications from freckles to inducing fertility. Thus, our predecessors hinted at an endocrine function of the placenta that was only scientifically highlighted by Josef Halban in 1904. The hormonal functions of the secondyne were of commercial interest to the pharmaceutical companies. Until the advent of acquired immune deficiency syndrome, many maternity units 'harvested' placentae which were sold on for production of cosmetics and hormones.

The umbilical cord was used in divination of the number of future children from the knots on the navel-string (Omphalomancy; Greek, *omphalos*, navel). The cord also provided blood vessels for grafting. Recent research has revealed that the blood that remains in the cord after it has been cut, provides a rich supply of stem cells, similar to those in bone marrow. If properly 'harvested', the cord blood can be transplanted later in life into the person from whom it was collected, with a guaranteed perfect match, to treat a number of life-threatening diseases. Placental products are proven treatment modalities but 'To eat, or not to eat?', therein lies the question.

Some traditional materia medica for women in the Pharmacopoeia of The People's Republic of China, 1992

Breast, for milk

Chuanmutong (armand clematis stem)
Guanmutong (Manchurian Dutchman's pipe stem)
Heizhongcaozi (fennel seed)
Jili (puncture vine caltrop fruit)
Lulutong (beautiful sweetgum fruit)
Tongcao (rice paper plant pith)

Xianmao (common *Curculigo* rhizome)
Zhongrushi (stalactite)
Ziheche (human placenta)

Breast, mastitis
Fengfang (honeycomb)
Gualou (snake gourd fruit)
Jigucao (Canton love pea vine)
Jili (puncture vine caltrop fruit)
Juhe (tangerine seed)
Lujiao (deerhorn (antler))
Mubiezi (cochinchina *Momordica* seed)
Qingpi (green tangerine peel)
Wangbuliuxing (cowherb seed)
Xiakucao (common selfheal spike)

Cervical cancer
Ezhu (zedoray rhizome)

Infertility
Aiye (argy wormwood leaf)
Bajitian (*Morinda* root)
Lurong (lurong (pilose antler))
Roucongrong (desert living cistanche)
Zishiyin (fluorite)

Labor, difficult
Jianghuang (turmeric)
Xiaoyelian (common *Sinopodophyllum* fruit)

Menopause, night sweats
Baishao (white peony root)
Baiziren (Chinese arbortivae kernel)
Guijia (tortoise shell)
Huangbai (amur cork tree)
Mahuanggen (*Ephedra* root)
Muli (oyster shell)
Wubeizi (Chinese gall)
Wuweizi (Chinese magnolia vine fruit)
Ziheche (human placenta)

Menstruation, amenorrhea
Chishao (red peony root)
Chuanxiong (Szechwan lovage rhizome)
Dahuang (rhubarb)
Danggui (Chinese angelica)
Daxueteng (sargent glory vine stem)
Guizhi (cassia twig)
Jianghuang (turmeric)

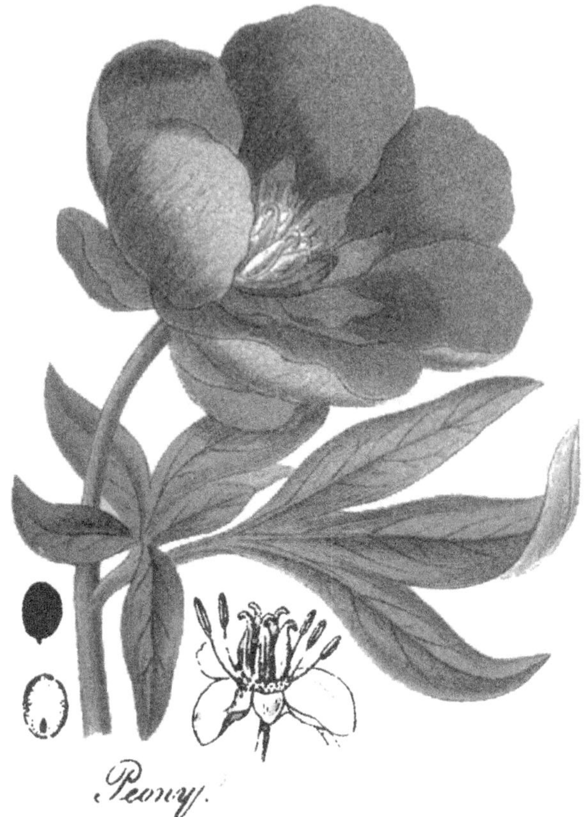

Figure 6 Red peony

Qiancao (India madder root)
Rougui (cassia bark)
Shuizhi (leech)
Taoren (peach seed)
Yimucao (motherwort herb)

Menstruation, for excess
Aiye (argy wormwood leaf)
Baifan (alum)
Cebaiye (Chinese arborvitae twig and leaf)
Duanxueliu (clinopodium herb)
Guijiajiao (glue of tortoise plastron)
Jiguanhua (cockcomb flower)
Lujiaojiao (deerhorn glue)
Luxiancao (pyrola herb)
Sangjishang (Chinese taxillus herb)
Xuduan (Himalayan teasel root)

Menstruation, painful
Chishao (red peony root)
Danggui (Chinese angelica)

Danshen (danshen root)
Mudanpi (tree peony bark)
Rougui (cassia bark)
Taoren (peach seed)
Wuyao (combined spicebrush root)
Xiaohuixiang (fennel)
Yimucao (motherwort herb)
Yuejihua (Chinese rose flower)

Placenta, retained
Chuanniuxi (medicinal cyathula root)
Jianghuang (turmeric)
Xiaoyelian (common *Sinopodophyllum* fruit)

Premature ejaculation
Longdon (Chinese gentian)
Shayuanzi (flatstem milkweed seed)

Puerperium, immoderate flowing of lochia
Yimucao (motherwort herb)

Puerperium, retention of lochia
Honghua (safflower)

Uterus, prolapse of
Chaihu (Chinese thorowax root)
Shengma (large trifoliolious bugbane rhizome)
Zhiqiao (orange fruit)
Zhishi (immature orange fruit)

Vagina, leukorrhea
Baiguo (*Ginkgo* seed)
Baitouweng (Chinese *Pulsatilla* root)
Chunpi (tree of heaven bark)
Guanmutong (Manchurian Dutchman's pipe stem)
Haipiaoxiao (cuttlebone)
Lianzi (lotus seed)
Shanyao (common yam rhizome)
Shanzhuyu (Asiatic cornelian cherry fruit)
Shiliupi (pomegranate rind)
Xianhecao (hairy vein agrimonia herb)

INDIA

India is the seventh largest country in the world and has the second largest population in Asia, after China. For hundreds of years India meant mystery and wealth. Early European explorers traveled to India for jewels, rugs, silks, and the spices for their condiments and medicines. It was this spice trade that led to the discovery of America by Christopher Columbus and to the colonization of India itself. India's most esteemed national song is *Vande Mataram* or 'I Bow To Thee, Mother'.

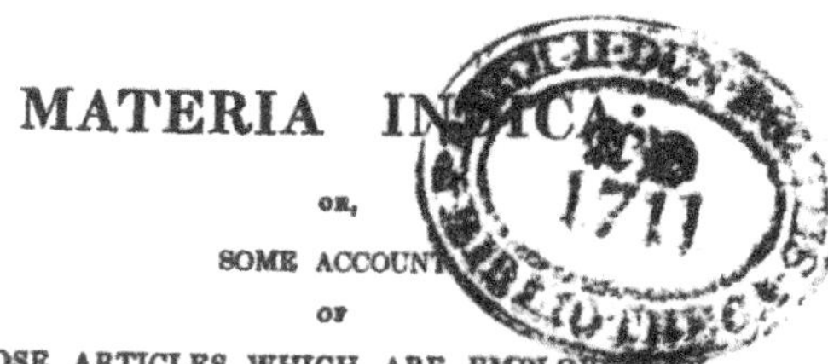

MATERIA INDICA;
OR,
SOME ACCOUNT
OF
THOSE ARTICLES WHICH ARE EMPLOYED BY
THE HINDOOS,
AND OTHER EASTERN NATIONS,
IN THEIR
MEDICINE, ARTS, AND AGRICULTURE;
COMPRISING ALSO
FORMULÆ,
WITH PRACTICAL OBSERVATIONS,
NAMES OF DISEASES IN VARIOUS EASTERN LANGUAGES,
AND A COPIOUS LIST OF ORIENTAL BOOKS IMMEDIATELY
CONNECTED WITH GENERAL SCIENCE,
&c. &c.

BY WHITELAW AINSLIE, M.D. M.R.A.S.
LATE OF THE MEDICAL STAFF OF SOUTHERN INDIA.

VOL. I.

LONDON:
PRINTED FOR
LONGMAN, REES, ORME, BROWN, AND GREEN,
PATERNOSTER-ROW.
1826.

Figure 7 Frontispiece from Ainslie's *Materia Indica* (1826)

Mythology

The goddess of married women and patroness of childbirth was Shashti the Sixth. She was worshipped on the sixth postnatal day, when the greatest danger of perinatal mortality was passed. Indian mythology is replete with other gods and goddesses of whom, Shiva and his partner Shakti, are examples. Shiva was the oldest god of the Vedic male trinity of Brahma–Vishnu–Shiva. As a sexual god, Shiva ensured the orgasmic ecstasy of his partner while absorbing the

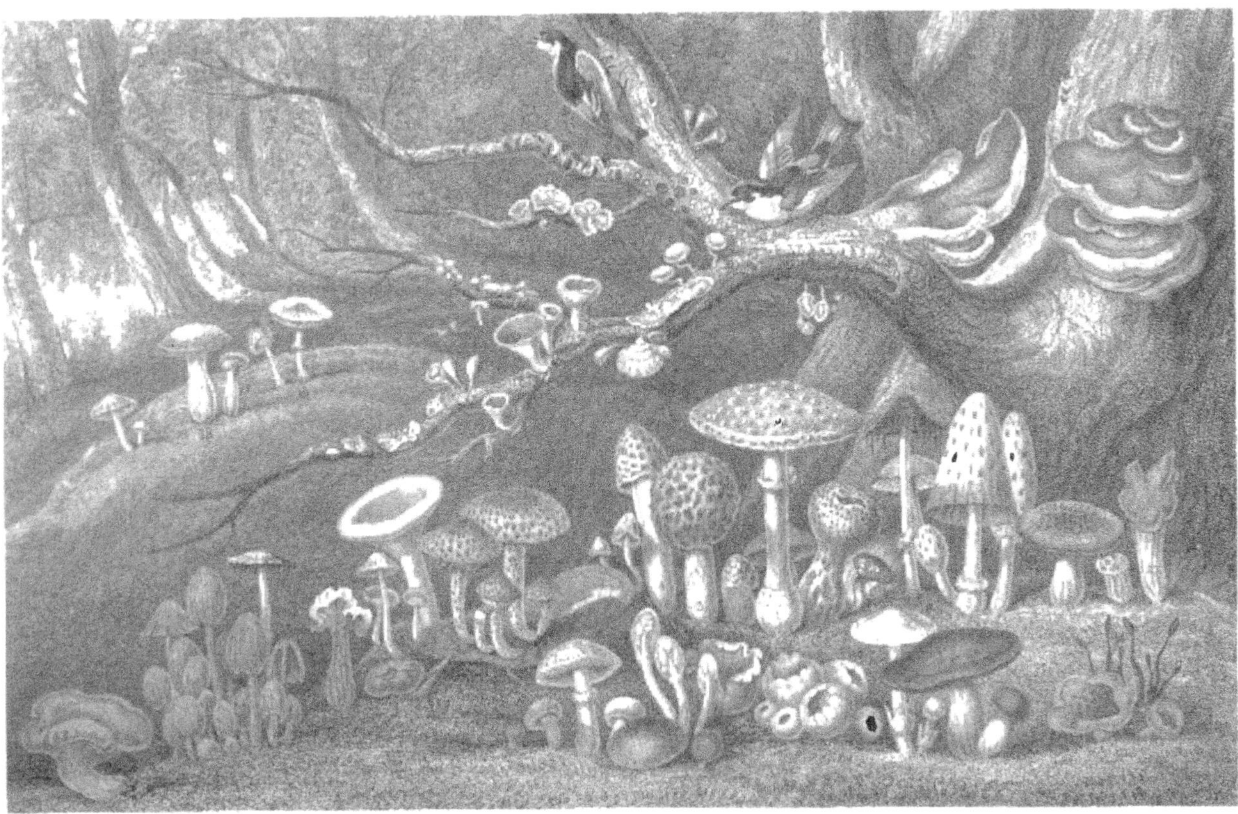

Figure 8 Fungi and their growth forms

sexual energy of her Yoni through his non-ejaculatory lingam. He advocated the female-superior position, maligned as a perversion by the Hindu priests. Every human orgasm reflected the perfect union of Shiva and Shakti, during which the *Bindu*, the seed of the universe, was produced. The food of the gods and goddesses was the *Soma*, possibly the fly agaric mushroom (*Amanita muscaria*) which, when dried, contains muscimol, a highly active psychedelic substance.

Shiva, often depicted with his much-adored lingam, was seldom shown alone as his power depended on his union with his goddess Shakti. The yoni or vulva was a Tantric object of worship and the goddess Kali was its personification. Kali was also known as Parvati, Shakti, Kunda or Cunti, the latter name giving rise to the commonly used slang word for the vulva. Shiva and Parvati argued as to which of them had in fact created the human race. Each decided to give birth separately to a new race of people without the aid of the other. Shiva, god of the lingam created the Lingajas, but they were dull and stupid. The goddess created the Yonijas, spirits of the yoni, who were well-shaped with fine sweet complexions. The two races waged war and the Yonijas won, but could not compare with humans (Walker, 1996). When it came to medicine, female dominance was not an issue, as it was well known that the male Divine Creator, Brahma, passed on the knowledge of medicinal plants to the original inhabitants of India thousands of years ago.

Development of medicine

The South Asian peninsula has been inhabited since the Stone Age, and agricultural communities appeared in the region about 10 000 years ago. From earliest times, there were contacts with the peoples of Mesopotamia and Central Asia. Inevitably, this led to exchange of ideas, information and trade. From the time of India's ancient Indus Valley civilization,

c. 2500–1500 BC, indigenous Indian plants found their way to other countries. Coriander seeds (*Coriander sativum*), which are native to India, were found in the tombs of Egyptian pharaohs, and it is also known that Indian plants were used in Mesopotamia for making dyes to color textiles. As time went by, Arab traders introduced Indian spices, as culinary and medicinal agents, to the peoples of the entire Mediterranean basin and thus to Northern Europe.

Little remains of the medical culture that flourished in ancient India. Archeological excavations at the ancient Indus cities of Harappa and Moheno-djaro, that flourished between 2500 and 1500 BC, reveal a sophisticated civilization with an advanced hygenic system of engineering that included bathing pools, drains and sanitary facilities. When the Indus civilization declined, Indo–European Aryan invaders overran the northwest area c. 1500 BC. Details of the Aryan culture, medicine and religion were committed to memory by hereditary priests, known locally as Brahmana, and were passed on in the Sanskrit language in a series of hymns collectively called the *Rig-Veda*. In his book *The Garden of Life* Naveen Patnaik of New Delhi quoted the complete text of a 'Hymn in Praise of Herbs' from the *Rig-Veda*, a sample of which reads ... 'You herbs, born at the birth of time, more ancient than the gods themselves ... let no malady destroy the lives within thy guardianship'. His bibliography is a good starting point for a study of books related to Indian plant medicines and contains a reference for a 1980 scientific synopsis of the *Charaka Samhita*, a famed medical treatise of ancient India – see below (Patnaik, 1993).

From the advent of the Aryans until the first century AD, medicine in India went through a number of stages. The first, or Aryan stage, later codified in the Sanskrit *Vedas* or texts, was introduced via Iran. It is related that the physician, Atreya Punavarsu, a founding member of the Ayurvedic (*Ayus*, longevity; *Veda*, knowledge) medical tradition, and his disciple, Agnivesh, collated the medical wisdom of the era and passed the information to subsequent generations of healers. The materia media of the Vedic period is contained in the *Ayurveda* which forms part of the Hindu repository of religious chants and poems known as the *Atharva Veda*. The *Ayurveda* itself has eight sections relating to health, one of which, the *Kaya Cikitsa*, deals with therapeutics. Its medicines were mainly of herbal origin. The Ayurvedic system of medicine emphasized the importance of preventive medicine, but also dealt with medications. The system was based on a doctrine of the three body humors – wind, bile and phlegm – and on the premise that the body must maintain a 'normal order'. Imbalance of it's five elementary substances – earth, fire, space, water and wind – would lead to disease.

The next stage of medical development was the introduction of the *Brahmanas* or commentaries on the *Vedas* (by Brahman priests) that were handed down as an oral tradition for almost 2000 years, until committed to text by the legendary physician, Caraka, probably in the first century AD. His treatise, *Caraka Samhita*, outlines 341 substances of plant origin, 177 of animal origin, and 64 mineral items that were use as medicines. A second medical text, by Susruta, (it also dealt with surgery) was the *Susruta Samhita*. With the *Caraka Samhita* these two tracts form the *Aryan Veda* (Van Alphen and Aris, 1995).

In southern India a separate system of medicine that was quite different to the Ayurvedic tradition evolved among the Tamil-speaking peoples. This was the *Tamil Cittar*, which became known as Siddah medicine. The method was believed to originate with the Lord Shiva and was passed by his wife Parvati to a number of medical teachers. The system was influenced by Tantrism and placed particular emphasis on the use of chemicals such as mercury, combined with magic, mysticism, religion, and Yoga (a *Yoga* is a standardized compound medication). The Tantric pharmacy contained over a 1000 biological products and was slowly assimilated into the Ayurvedic materia medica so that by the end of the fifteenth century the Ayurvedic pharmacopoeia had reached its final form (Cowen and Helfand, 1990; Jain, 1991).

Another stage of medical development was the appearance of Buddhist medicine, which entered India in the fifth century BC, and both Buddhism and Brahmanism flourished together until the end of the first millennium AD. Indian medicine was further influenced in the eleventh century AD by the spread of Islam, which introduced *Unani-Tibb* medicine, a system founded on that of Galen (AD 130–200) as interpreted by Avicenna (AD 980–1037) in his *Canon of Medicine*. *Unani-Tibb* medicine was popular in northern and central India.

In the fifteenth century, the European nations sought their own direct access to India, rather than having to trade with the Arabs who had a monopoly on Indian medicines and spices. The search for Ayurvedic medicines led Columbus to sail west to find a new access route to India, but he discovered America instead. The Portuguese sailed south and east on a similar mission and arrived at Goa. There, after years collecting the local plants, Garcia d'Orta wrote a commentary on the medical simples and drugs of India. When it was published in Goa in 1563, d'Orta's text was the first medical book printed in India. Vasco de Gama landed on the Malabar coast in 1498 and officials of the Dutch East India Company, of which he was a member, investigated the local plant life. Between 1686 and 1703 they produced a series of volumes on Indian medicine, illustrated by nearly 800 indigenous plants.

At the beginning of the seventeenth century the British arrived in India, in the form of the East India Company, and soon gained control of large parts of the country. European-based medical practices gradually prevailed, and in 1835 official support for Ayurvedic and Unani medicine was withdrawn. By 1858 the East India Company was dissolved and India was placed under direct British rule. In the same year, the British Pharmacopoeia was formalized and British physicians in India became increasingly critical of the indigenous drugs. Ayurvedic medicine declined after the mid-nineteenth century and retreated to a rural and mainly traditional family apprenticeship system. India gained it's independence in 1947, and since then interest in Ayurvedic medicine has flourished. Nowadays, orthodox medical practice is available, as are Ayurvedic, Unani, and other methods of healing (Van Alphen and Aris, 1995).

THE INDIAN MATERIA MEDICA

Whitlaw Ainslie (1826) 'Late of the Medical Staff of Southern India' wrote a valuable text in two volumes entitled *Materia Indica; or, Some Account of Those Articles Which Are Employed by The Hindoos, and other Eastern Nations, in their Medicine, Arts and Agriculture.* In his *Materia Indica* he listed diseases by their names in the various Eastern languages, a number of which referred to women's ailments. He detailed 191 rare books relating to medicine, pharmacy and science, from earliest times, that were available in Arabic, Ceylonese, Persian, Sanskrit, and 'Tamool' (Tamil). He also included a history of Ayurvedic medicine and discussed almost 900 Indian medications.

The entire first volume of *Review of the History of Medicine* by Thomas A. Wise (1867) was devoted to Asia. Wise, a Fellow of the Royal College of Physicians, Edinburgh, served in the Bengal Medical Service and dedicated his book to his esteemed friend, Sir James Young Simpson, Professor of Medicine and Midwifery of Edinburgh. Volume one contains chapters on The Profession in Ancient Hindostan; The Physiology and Structures of the Body; Hygiene and Surgery, and almost a 100 pages are devoted to Indian Materia Medica. Wise gave a detailed account of the 'simple medicines' derived from the animal, mineral and vegetable kingdoms and wrote about the classification, preparation and administration of the drugs and their weights and measures.

Oriental authors have interested themselves in aphrodisiacs and sexuality since earliest times, and an introduction to those arts may be found in *Kama Sutra of Vatsyayana*. This classic Sanskrit work of erotica was compiled by Vatsyayana at some time before the sixth century AD. Kama was the god of love in ancient Sanskrit literature, and *Sutra* simply means a book of aphorisms. Sir Richard Burton and F.F. Arbuthnot translated the text to English and that version of the *Kama Suta* was published in 1883. It is currently available in many English formats, and a complete translation of the original work is carried in a Wordsworth edition. The *Kama Sutra* deals with the emotional and physical aspects of sexuality, and contains a list of love potions with their ingredients, methods of preparation and manner of application. The translators include a lyrical description of the Padmini or Lotus woman, the perfect feminine essence whose ... 'Yoni resembles the opening lotus bud, and her love-seed (Kama salila) is perfumed like the lily that has newly burst' (Burton and Arbuthnot, 1995). In their concluding remarks, Burton and Arbuthnot wrote of the 'Anunga Runga' (stages of love), a Sanskrit text of the fifteenth century AD, that contained tracts on menstruation, fertility, miscarriage, labor, contraception, breast treatments, and love philters.

In recent times, Dr S.K. Jain (1991) in his *Medicinal Plants of India* updated the history of Indian books related to *Flora Medica*. He wrote that approximately 3000 species of Indian plants had therapeutic potential and, in his own work, he included the names of over 1800 medicinal herbs. The Indian Council of Medical Research has published a three-volume set devoted to Indian plant medicine, and each herbal monologue contained therein has details of published research relating to the pharmacological effects of Indian plant medicines (Satyvati, Ashok Gupta and Neeraj Tandon, 1987).

A SELECTION OF INDIAN MATERIA MEDICA

Cinnamon

Cinnamon species (Lauraceae family) provide two different commodities, camphor and cinnamon. The Ayurvedic physicians use the three aromatics, cardamom (*Elettaria cardamomum*), Indian cassia lignea (*Cinnamomum tamala* or bastard cinnamon) and Cinnamon cassia (*Tvak* in Sanskrit and *Dalchini* in Hindi) to disguise the taste of medicines. The Indian laburnum, *Cassia fistula*, *Aragvadha* in Sanskrit, *Amaltas* in Hindi, and the senna pods of *Cassia augustifolia*, were pulped and used as laxatives in pregnancy.

Cinnamon (*Cinnamomum loureirii*) is one of the oldest spices known to man and was recorded in China almost 5000 years ago. The Chinese 'five spices' are anise, cloves, fennel, star anise, and cinnamon. The inner bark (rougui), leafy twigs (gouzhi), fruits and oil of *Cinnamon loureirii* are all used as medication, as are the same parts of *Cinnamon zeylanicum* or Ceylon cinnamon also known as *Cinnamomum verum*. The search for, and determination of sea routes to, cinnamon-producing areas of the Orient, played a major role in colonial expansion (Bown, 1995).

In Greco–Roman obstetrics and gynecology, *Cassia* was employed to aid placental delivery and to treat inflammation of the uterus. In the seventeenth and eighteenth centuries *Cinnamon* was in vogue to induce menstruation, to prevent miscarriage, to avoid pregnancy sickness, induce labor, increase breast milk production, and as a medication for women's disorders in general. Cassia bark, cortex cinnamoni, or rougui, is currently indicated in TCM for amenorrhea, dysmenorrhea, frigidity and impotence, while the cassia twig, ramulus cassia, or guizhi, is also advocated for amenorrhea (PPRC, 1992).

Coriander

The popular culinary plant, coriander, *Coriandrum sativum*, *Dhanyaka* in Sanskrit, *Dhania* in Hindi, takes its name from the Greek *koris*, in allusion to the pungent odor of the unripe fruits. In ancient India, the leaves and seed were employed as an aromatic stimulant to aid virility. Coriander was introduced to Chinese medicine c. AD 600 and since then is known as *Hu*, foreign. Coriander seeds were found in the early Egyptian tombs, and the plant was a popular medication in classical Greece and Rome. Soranus (AD 98–117) noted its use to suppress lactation (Temkin, 1991). Coriander remains popular in TCM, where it is indicated as an aphrodisiac and emmenagogue. Coriander oil adds to the flavor of Chartreuse, gin and vermouth.

Cumin

Cumin, *Cuminum cyminum*, *Jiraka* in Sanskrit, *Jeera* in Hindi, takes its name from the Greek, *kyminon* and Latin, *cuminum*. It was among the earliest scented herbs used as a carminative and food seasoning. Several kinds of cumin are known, including the safed (white) and kala (black). The seeds are an ingredient of garam masal in India and a couscous seasoning in the Middle East. The cumin plant was especially important to Ayurvedic physicians as a treatment for early morning sickness, as a lactogenic for nursing mothers, and as a gripe-water preparation for infants. Cumin was replaced by dill (*Anethum graveolens*) or fennel (*Foeniculum vulgare*), to which was added alcohol and sugar to constitute Europe's answer for gripe-stricken infants. In Greco–Roman times, cumin was applied externally to dry up milk formation, and in pessary

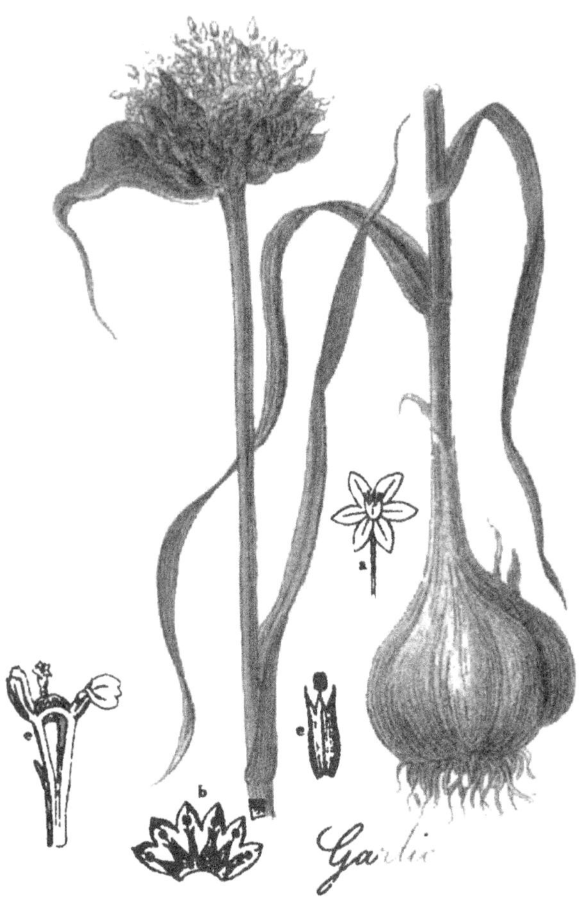

Figure 9 Garlic (*Allium sativum*)

form to treat amenorrhea and dysmenorrhea. In his *Materia Indica*, Whitelaw Ainslie (1826) related that ... 'French medical practitioners esteem these (cumin) seeds as "excitantes, carminatives et aperitifs", and formerly considered them as diuretic and emmenagogue'.

Garlic

The garlic, *Allium sativum*, *Rasona* in Sanskrit, *Lasan* in Hindi, takes its name from the Anglo-Saxon, *gar* (spear) and *lac* (a plant), and *Allium* is its Latin name. The specific and pervasive odor of the plant gave rise to the legend among Muslims that when Satan left the Garden of Eden after the fall of Adam and Eve, garlic sprang from his left footprint and onion from his right. Many other legends grew up around the plant, probably the best known relates that garlic keeps vampires at bay.

Garlic was treasured as a culinary and medicinal agent not only in ancient India and China but throughout the known world of the time. The Ayurvedic physicians prescribed garlic bulbs (*da suan*) for chest, heart and skeletal problems, while in reproductive medicine they prized it as an aphrodisiac and menstrual regulator. Allicin was isolated from garlic by Chester Cavallito in 1944 and the chemical was found to have broad-spectrum antibiotic effects. Garlic is said to have antithrombotic, hypolipidemic, hypoglycemic, hypotensive and other medicinal properties. John Heirman (1994) has written an entertaining and informative book entitled *The Healing Benefits of Garlic* which tells the story of the plant ... 'from Pharaohs to Pharmacists'.

Indian madder

The Indian madder, *Rubia cordifolia*, and other species in that family afford a red dye (rubia, *rubor*, Latin, red) that in ancient India symbolized blood, energy and the menstrual cycle. Its main pigment, alizarin, was synthesized by Graebe and Liebermann in 1868 and their discovery led to a decline in cultivation of the plant. In ancient India the plant was prescribed as a blood purifier and for menstrual irregularities or as a treatment for women after delivery (Patnaik, 1993).

Whitlaw Ainslie (1826) wrote of the 'Madder of Bengal', *Rubia manjista* (*Manjittie* in Sanskrit). He indicated that its qualities were similar to those of *Rubia tinctoria*, much used by European physicians as an emmenagogue, to treat chlorosis (iron deficiency anemia) and for difficult menstruation. In his *Flora Medica* (a worldwide survey of medicinal plants), John Lindley (1838), Professor of Botany in University College, London, cited the madder plant as an emmenagogue. Modern experts in plant medicine agree that madder is useful in menstrual disorders (Bown, 1995). Madder also has a long history in Chinese medicine; known as *Quiancao* it is currently used for amenorrhea and abnormal uterine bleeding (PPRC, 1992).

Lotus

The lotus, *Nelumbo nucifera*, is a beautiful water plant associated with divinity. Lotus is from the Greek, *lotos*, while *nelumbo* is the Sinhalese name for the Holy Lotus. In Asia the lotus is a symbol of the yoni and is associated with the goddess Padma (Shakti) from whom it gains its Sanskrit name (*Padma*). The god Brahma was styled 'Lotus-born', as he arose from the primal goddess's yoni. The Buddha first appeared floating on a lotus, with the soles of his feet resting on his thighs, a posture known in Yoga as the Lotus position. In China the custom of foot-binding evolved to produce artificially clubbed feet (known as golden lotuses). Maidens with golden lotus feet, a sign of great beauty, were deemed the most desirable for marriage.

In Greek mythology, Ulysses and his crew visited the sensual 'Land of the lotus-eaters' where those who ate the lotus fruit entered a state of blissful indolence. Pharmacological studies confirm that nuciferine, the major alkaloid isolated from the lotus, has divergent psychoactive effects, sufficient to explain torpor (Satyvati, Ashok Gupta, and Tandon, 1987). Barbara Walker (1996) opined that eating the lotus was a (sexual) custom of 'communion' with the feminine life principle. In traditional Indian medicine, the lotus was used for intestinal complaints, bleeding piles, and menorrhagia. The plant also found a place in TCM and is still advised for premature ejaculation, spermatorrhea and uterine hemorrhage (Windridge, 1994; PPRC, 1992). The indications for the use of this divine plant are similar in Western herbal medicine.

References

Ainslie, W. (1826). *Materia Indica; or, Some Account of Those Articles Which Are Employed by The Hindoos, and other Eastern Nation, in their Medicine, Arts and Agriculture*, pp. 100–1, 202–5. (London: Longman, Orme, Brown and Green)

Alphen, J. V. and Aris, A. (eds) (1995). *Oriental Medicine. An Illustrated Guide to the Asian Arts of Healing*, pp. 154–215, 19–146. (London: Serindia Publications)

Ayto, J. (1994). *Dictionary of Word Origins*, p. 387. (UK: Columbia)

Beau, G. (1972). *Chinese Medicine*, Translated by Lowell Bair, pp. 15–32, 141. (New York: Avon Books)

Bown, D. (1995). *The Royal Horticultural Society Encyclopedia of Herbs and their Uses*, pp. 261–2, 343. (London: Dorling Kindersley)

Burton, Sir R. and Arbuthnot, F. F. (1995). *The Kama Sutra of Vatsyayana*, Translation, pp. 11, 173. (Hertfordshire, UK: Wordsworth Editions)

Cavendish, R. (ed.) (1991). *Mythology. An Illustrated Encyclopaedia*, pp. 58–73. (London: Macdonald & Co.)

Cowen, D. L. and Helfand, W. H. (1990). *Pharmacy. An Illustrated History*, pp. 24–5, 25–6. (New York: Harry N. Abrams)

Evans, W. C. (1996). *Trease and Evans' Pharmacognosy*, pp. 281–4. (London: W. B. Saunders Company)

Garrison, F. H. (1929). *An Introduction to the History of Medicine*, pp. 73–7. (Philadelphia and London: W. B. Saunders Co.)

Gelis, J. (1991). *History of Childbirth. Fertility, Pregnancy and Birth in Early Modern Europe*, Translated by Rosemary Morris, pp. 165–72. (Oxford: Polity Press)

Heinerman, J. (1994). *The Healing Benefits of Garlic*. (Connecticut: Keats Publishing)

Hensyl, W. (ed.) (1990). *Stedman's Medical Dictionary*, pp. 1205–06. (Baltimore: Williams and Wilkins)

Jain, S. K. (1991). *Medicinal Plants of India*, pp. 63–7. (Michigan: Reference Publications Inc.)

Ke-ji, C. (ed.) (1997). *Chinese Patent Medicines*, p. 258. (Bejing: Hunan Science and Technology Press)

Lindley, J. (1838). *Flora Medica; A Botanical Account of all the more Important Plants Used In Medicine, in Different Parts of the World*, p. 446. (London: Longman, Orme, Brown & Green)

Lu, H. C. (1994). *Chinese Herbal Cures*, pp. 53–155. (New York: Sterling Publishing Co.)

Lyons, A. S. and Petrucelli, R. J. (1987). *Medicine. An Illustrated History*, pp. 121–53. (New York: Harry N. Abrams Inc.)

Maciocia, G. (1998). *Obstetrics and Gynecology in Chinese Medicine*, pp. 3–6, 579–83, 697, 707. (New York: Churchill Livingstone)

McGrew, R. E. (1985). *Encyclopaedia of Medical History*, pp. 56–9. (London: MacMillan Press)

Monaghan, P. (1990). *The Book of Goddesses and Heroines*, pp. 161–2. (Minnesota: Llewellyn)

Patnaik, N. (1993). *The Garden of Life. An Introduction to the Healing Plants of India*, pp. 1–14, 27. (London: Aquarian, Harper Collins)

Pharmacopoeia of the People's Republic of China (1992). English edition. Compiled by the Pharmacopoeia Commission of PRC, pp. 31, 187, 159–60, 281–4, 163, 308, 55, 179, 169, 229–30. (Beijing, China: Gaungdong Science and Technology Press)

Reid, D. P. (1993). *Chinese Herbal Medicine*, pp. 10–25. (Boston: Shambhala)

Satyvati, G. V., Ashok Gupta, K. and Tandon, N. (1987). *Medicinal Plants of India*, pp. 325–9. (New Delhi: Indian Council of Medical Research)

Temkin, O. (1991). *Soranus' Gynecology*, p. 221. (Baltimore: The Johns Hopkins University Press)

Van Alphen, J. and Aris, A. (eds) (1995). *Oriental Medicine. An Illustrated Guide to the Asian Arts of Healing*, pp. 19–99. (London: Serindia Publications)

Veith, I. (1972). *Huang Ti Nei Ching Su Wen, The Yellow Emperor's Classic of Internal Medicine.* (Berkeley: University of California Press)

Walker, B. G. (1996). *The Women's Encyclopedia of Myths and Secrets*, pp. 550, 935, 1097. (New Jersey: Castle Books)

Windridge, C. (1994). *The Fountain of Health. An A–Z of Traditional Chinese Medicine*, pp. 155–6, 337, 492–3. (Edinburgh and London: Mainstream Publishing)

Wise, T. A. (1867). *Review of the History of Medicine*, Vol. 1. (London: J. Churchill)

The Americas 26

INTRODUCTION

The plants and medicines of the Americas played a major role in the development of the materia medica for women's reproductive health. The stories of discoveries by the early settlers who gradually explored, through trial and error, the healing potential of local herbs, through to the laboratory synthesis of life-saving drugs in modern times, reflect similar tales from other continents. This chapter highlights some of the important steps along the way and further information may be gleaned from the chapters devoted to specific topics related to women's health.

THE NATIVE NORTH AMERICANS

The first settlers colonized the North American continent approximately 30 000 years ago, arriving in waves across the Beringia land-bridge that connected Siberia and Alaska during a former Ice Age. The Amerindians are thus descendants of an Asian stock related to the ancient Mongols. The Eskimos and the Aleuts of the Alaskan Islands arrived much later and are more closely related to present-day Eastern Asians.

The original Amerindians were big game hunters who had spread to most of North America by 9000 BC, but five thousand years later they had become reliant on foraging for smaller animals, fish and plant foods. Agriculture developed about AD 1000 and the city of Cahokia in Illinois had a population of many thousands and flourished and was occupied until 1550. When Christopher Columbus 'discovered' the Americas in 1492, there was already a population of up to six million Americans Indians, with hundreds of tribes and over 200 different languages. Each tribe had its own customs and way of life. The early settlers lived in close communion with their habitat, and their life-styles were remarkably green (Clairborne, 1973).

Indian medicine

The Indian medicine man played an important role in the tribal community and through a mixture of prayer and incantations, magical rattles and drums, and also the application of herbs or animal parts, helped to alleviate sickness. The medicine man had a collection of accouterments and carried medications in a bag, often fashioned from animal skin. Quite apart from the medicine men, the braves and squaws also learned herbal healing lore at the time of their initiation so that each member of a tribe had a basic understanding of plant medicine that was used to alleviate or even cure certain ailments.

The early European settlers were friendly with the native Americans and quickly delved into the native plant lore, thus enriching their own paltry stocks of medicines imported at great expense from Europe. The sharing of plant knowledge was a two-way process over several centuries, with inevitably some uncertainty about who introduced what medicine. Despite that, an analysis of Virgil Vogel's *American Indian Medicine* (1970) reveals that there are at least 80 drug remedies for women which can be directly attributed to information gained from the American Indians, while other sources indicate a much higher figure of over 350 such medications. Many of those remedies have achieved an international reputation and were included in a number of national pharmacopoeia until the mid-twentieth century. The following selection of plant medications illustrates the significance of native American Indian drugs.

Birthroot

Trillium erectum, bethroot, birthroot, Indian balm or squaw-flower, was used to treat vaginal discharge, heavy periods, and also to induce labor, to control postpartum hemorrhage, and as an application for sore nipples. It was listed in the *US National Formulary* from 1916 to 1947 (Vogel, 1970). The plant contains trillarin, a steroidal saponin, which has hormonal effects.

Blue cohosh

Caulophyllum thalictroides, or blue cohosh, is found in the rich moist woods of eastern North America. Its common name 'cohosh' is of Algonquin origin. Its alternative names of 'squaw root' and 'papoose root' illustrate its importance in native American Indian reproductive medicine (Bown, 1995). The plant was used to promote menstruation, to hasten childbirth, and also as a contraceptive, and was official in the *US Pharmacopoeia* from 1882 to 1905 (Weiner, 1980). It contains steroidal saponins, resins and the active alkaloids, caulophylline, laburnine and magnoflorine (Chevallier, 1996). Blue cohosh remains popular and is still used by herbalists and as an over-the-counter medicine for gynecological conditions.

Cramp bark

Viburnum opulus, cramp bark, or guelder rose, and the related *V. prunifolium*, contain scopoletin, a coumarin which has a sedative effect on the uterus. Useful for dysmenorrhea and threatened miscarriage, *Viburnum* was listed in all the major pharmacopoeias in the early part of this century (Squire, 1908) and remained in the *American National Formulary* until 1960. *V. prunifolium* contains salicin which also occurs in the willow, *Salix alba*, and from which salicylic acid was derived. Both salicin and salicylic acid are analgesic chemicals and were first synthetically prepared in 1852, but were found to cause marked gastric irritation. In 1899 the Bayer Company produced acetylsalicylic acid, known better by its proprietary name, aspirin (Griggs, 1997).

Squaw vine

Mitchella repens, or squaw vine, is an evergreen subshrub found in central and eastern North America. The plant was first used among women of the Cherokee and Penobscot tribes to ease labor, and hence gained its common name. It gained its official name from Dr John Mitchell (1711–1768) a physician and botanist from Urbana, Virginia. Squaw vine contains saponins, tannins and other chemicals. *Mitchella* was listed in the *US National Formulary* until 1947 and is still used as a uterine antispasmodic in herbal medicine (British Herbal Pharmacopoeia, 1991).

Squaw weed

Senecio aureus, golden ragwort or squaw weed, is a classic herbal 'female regulator' and was used by a number of North American tribes to ease childbirth and to treat female complaints. Until recently, it was grown in central Russia for the pharmaceutical industry. The appellation *Senecio* comes from the Latin, *senex*, old man, a reference to the white-haired seeds of the plant. Squaw weed contains toxic pyrrolizidine alkaloids. An extract is used in complementary medicine as an emmenagogue and for hot flushes. The closely related *S. triangularis*, found in Colorado, contains alkaloids that inhibit cancer growth in mice (Reynolds, 1982).

Sweetcorn

Zea mays, corn or sweetcorn, comes in five principal varieties and is an annual grass. Cultivated for nearly 6000 years in the Americas, it contains allantoin which stimulates growth and repair in tissues, and also a number of alkaloids. Corn smut, the fungus *Ustilago zeae*, contains the alkaloid ustilagine which has similar but lesser effects to ergot, and was used by the Zuni tribe in the southwest to induce labor. The fungus was listed in the *US Pharmacopoeia* from 1882 until 1894 (Vogel, 1970).

EUROPEAN DISCOVERY OF THE AMERICAS

In the second half of the fifteenth century, European sailors and navigators began to plan voyages that would take them beyond the limits of the 'known world'. This was partly the result of the new interest in exploration encouraged by the Renaissance, but the main reason was to set up new trading links with the spice and drug-producing countries of Asia, because direct land links between Europe and Asia had been completely severed as a result of the fall of the Byzantine Empire in 1453. The Portuguese sailed east and the Spanish sailed west. Christopher Columbus reached the West Indies in 1492, John Cabot discovered Newfoundland in 1497, and Amerigo Vespucci reached South America in 1499. For a time, Northern Europeans regarded America as a barrier on their way to the East but a major event in medical history would soon change that opinion.

Within a year of the discovery of the Americas, the first outbreak of epidemic venereal syphilis occurred in Europe. The initial epidemic of 1493 to 1494 was extremely malignant and proved fatal in its early stages. Treatment consisted of blood letting and the application of ungentum Saracenum, an ointment for common skin ailments which contained mercury and was named after the Saracen (Arab) physicians who introduced it to European medicine at the time of the Crusades in the twelfth to fourteenth centuries. High dosage mercury treatment was first used as a remedy for syphilis in 1496, by Georgio Sommeravia of Verona, and proved to be effective. Mercury remained the best treatment for syphilis until the introduction of bismuth by Felix Balzer in 1889, which in turn was displaced by the arsenic compound named 606 or Salvarsan (safe arsenic), developed by Paul Ehrlich (1854–1915) of Frankfurt in 1904. From 1914, Albert Keitel, of the Johns Hopkins, Department of Syphilis, and his successor, Joseph Earl Moore (1926) consolidated what became known as the 'continuous treatment' of syphilis with arsenicals.

Meanwhile, way back in the sixteenth century, mercury medication reigned supreme, giving rise to the well known saying 'A night with Venus means a lifetime with Mercury'. In mythology Mercury was a messenger of the gods, known to the Greeks as Hermes, and was the Roman god of merchandise, theft and eloquence. Treatment with mercury was severe and so the search for an alternative was imperative. That first alternative therapy came from the Americas and, long before the colonists became established in North America, a flourishing trade in drugs, particularly anti-syphilitic medicines, was established between South America and Spain in the years 1503–1508. The following nostrums appeared to be helpful and were exported to Europe where they were used extensively to treat the dreaded 'morbus gallicus'.

Guajacum

Guajacum or *Guajacum officinale* is a South American tree or evergreen shrub, of the bean–caper family, known by the Spanish name 'guayaco' (derived from a Taino Indian or Haitian word), and also known as guaiac, from which was extracted an aromatic medicinal resin. Spaniards living in the Caribbean discovered that the local Indians suffered from yaws, a condition which resembled European syphilis. The locals successfully treated yaws with a decoction of guajacum. The Spaniards began to treat syphilis in the same way as yaws and an apparent cure was effected after six weeks of therapy. By 1517, Emperor Charles V of Spain claimed that over 3000 Spanish syphilitics were cured by the use of guajacum alone (Griggs, 1981). The treatment was easier and apparently superior to mercury. A leading banking family, the Fuggers of Ausburg, became the main importers of guajacum to Europe and according to McGrew (1985) they made a fortune. As early as 1519, there was a famous woodcut showing a seller of guajac, in a book entitled *Morbus Gallicus* by Ulrich von Hutten, the German poet and reformer, who related his own battle with syphilis, and praised the effects of guajacum medication. Another famous illustration of the time was 'Guaiac and the Plague of Venus' by Jan van der Straet which dates from 1570, and shows the preparation and administration of medication derived from *Guajacum* (Wootton, 1910).

Treatment with guajacum caused pyrexia, and abatement of symptoms of syphilis. It is now know that it raises the body temperature in excess of 40 °C and can kill the spirochetes which cause syphilis. Pyrexial therapy was again used with success to treat syphilis in the 1930s but, despite treatment, the illness relapsed. Guajacum contains saponins and resin acids, and is an anti-inflammatory and diaphoretic agent. It was still listed in the British Pharmacopoeia this century as an anti-syphilitic agent and remains in the British Herbal Pharmacopoeia (1991) as a treatment for arthritis. The *Guajacum* flower is the national emblem of Jamaica.

Sassafras

Sassafras albidum, or sassafras, is an aromatic deciduous tree whose scent is said to have guided Christopher Columbus from the broad Atlantic to the eastern shores of America, but in reality the plant was discovered in Florida by the Spanish. Sassafras was another of the medicinal herbs to be exported to Europe and was used as an anti-syphilitic agent as early as 1560, but never achieved the notoriety and popularity of guajacum although it became 'official' and remained in all the major national pharmacopoeias until the early part of the twentieth century. The plant extract contains alkaloids and other active chemicals and is prescribed for arthritis by herbalists. The fragrant *Sassafras* has also been used as food flavoring and in root beer.

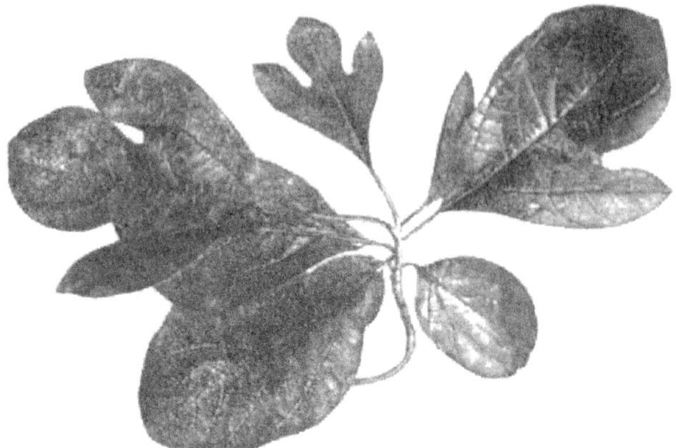

Figure 1 Sassafras

Smilax

The *Smilax* family contains about 200 species, and the form now known as smilax china, or china root, was imported to Spain from Mexico as a cure for syphilis in the late sixteenth century. The local Indians called the plant sarsa. From this and related plants was derived sarsaparilla, which also gained a reputation as an anti-syphilitic agent and was exported to Europe for centuries. The plant contains steroidal saponins, and a large number of pharmacologic agents, some of which have antibiotic properties. A plant extract was listed in many national pharmacopoeias until the twentieth century and is still used by herbalists as an anti-rheumatic agent and for various skin complaints (British Herbal Pharmacopoeia, 1991).

COLONIAL MEDICINE

As time went by it became obvious that the new lands were valuable in themselves, so potential settlers soon made their way across the broad Atlantic to a new life in America. The first successful English colony in North America was established at Jamestown, Virginia in 1607. In 1612 John Rolf introduced tobacco growing to the settlers. Tobacco was prescribed as a medication for chest complaints prior to its use as a recreational drug. The climate of Virginia suited the tobacco plant and the colonists soon began to export it. In 1620 the *Mayflower* arrived at Plymouth, near Cape Cod, and this settlement is considered the origin of the United States. The first of many 'Thanksgiving' days was held in November 1621 and the local Indian tribe joined in the festivities.

Throughout the Colonial period in America, from approximately 1600 to 1800, most routine medical care was based on folk or ethnic medicine. Medical treatment, where it existed, was similar to that practiced in Europe which was still laboring to break away from the archaic system set up by Galen (AD 130–200). Galenical theory held that the body was made up of four principal elements; earth, water, air and fire. These elements made up the four 'humors' of the body: blood, phlegm, yellow bile and black bile. Imbalance led to disease and could be treated by 'depletion', which involved blood letting, purging and sweating, or by 'restoration', which was accomplished by the use of diet or drugs.

In those first 200 years of the Colonial period the medical scene was heavily influenced by European healthcare practices and traditional European drugs were imported and accompanied by a variety of almanacs, herbals and textbooks such as *The Byrth of Mankynde*, the first textbook of consequence on midwifery in modern times. It was written by Eucharius Rosslin in 1513, with an English translation in 1552 by Raynold.

Another classic to reach the American colonies was translated by the renowned Nicholas Culpeper (1616–1654). Culpeper was an apothecary's apprentice

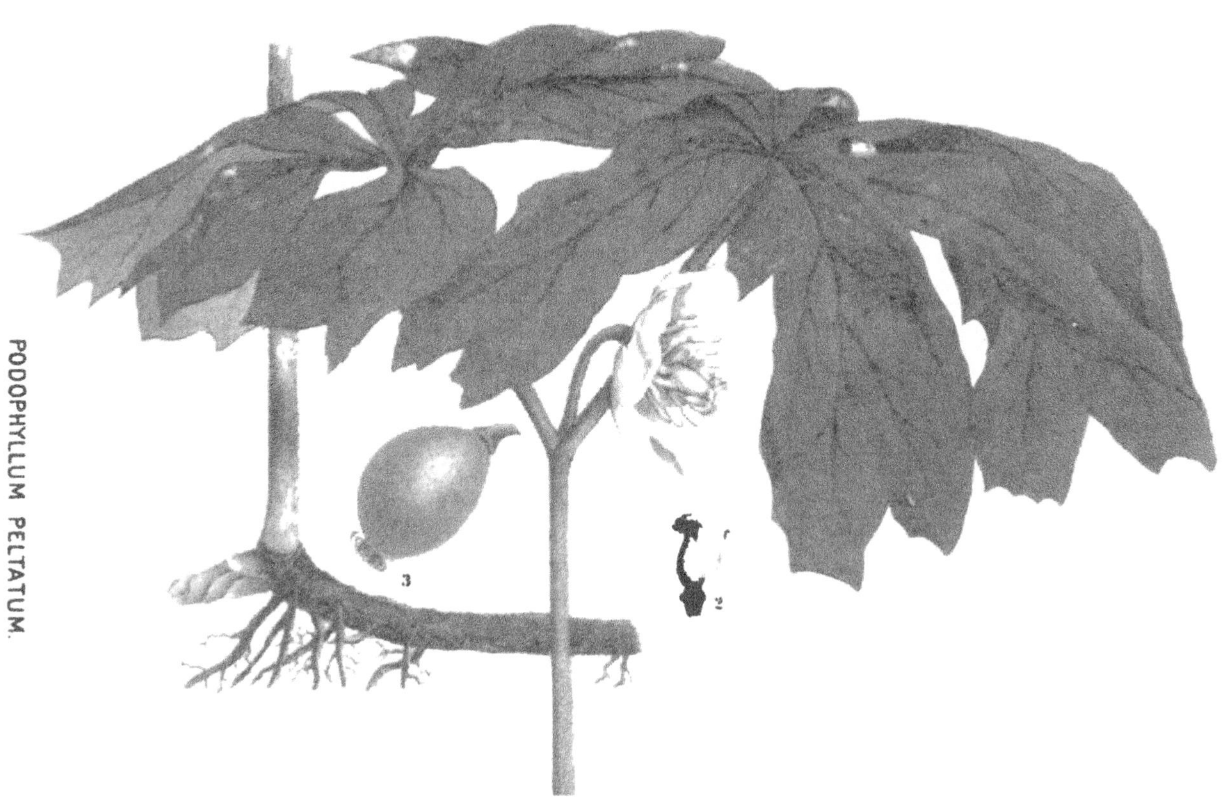

Figure 2 Sarsaparilla

who was destined to become a noted astrologer–physician in London. He was a prolific medical writer and his unauthorized translation of the London Pharmacopoeia of 1649 later became the first full-size medical book published in America, in Boston in 1720.

The early colonists were quick to investigate local resources and John Josslyn (1672) produced an early analysis of American medicinal plants. By the second half of the eighteenth century, Philadelphia had become the capital of medical botany in America. The dependency on Europe was severed and the new colony developed its own pharmaceutical industry. It is estimated that over 170 drugs used in colonial times became official in the *US Pharmacopoeia* or *National Formulary*, and remained so until the 1970s, a time when 50% of drugs still came from 'natural' sources.

Among the drugs imported by the colonists for general medical use were the purgatives, calomel (mercurous chloride), Glauber salts (sodium sulfate) and jalap (*Ipomea purga*). Other drugs used to cause 'depletion' were the emetics, tartar emetic (antimony potassium tartrate) and ipecac (*Cephaelis ipecacuanha*). Also important were lancets to deplete patients by bleeding. Pain was treated by the application of camphor (*Cinnamomum camphora*) as a counter irritant and by opium (*Papaver somniferum*) which was prescribed as a general purpose analgesic. Fevers were treated with cinchona bark (*Cinchona officinalis*, Peruvian or Jesuit's bark) that contains quinine. Skin ailments were medicated with mercury, the liquid metallic element also known as quicksilver or hydrargyrum. Then in the 1700s came European Patent Medicines. It is interesting when looking at this short list to note that some medications were exported to Europe from the Americas and then reimported by the early North American colonists. European imported drugs were dispersed throughout the colonies and,

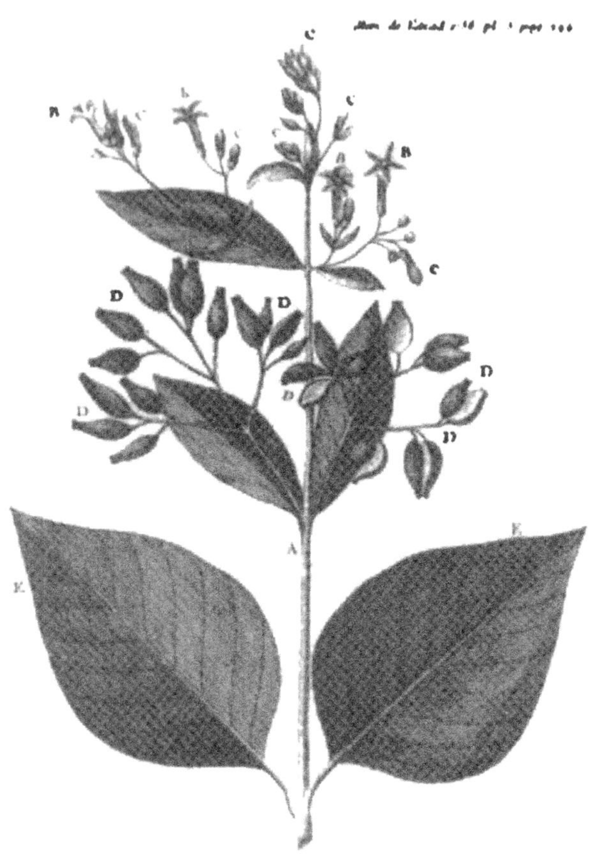

Figure 3 Cinchona, the source of quinine

when required, medications could be obtained from a variety of sources, including general drug dealers, midwives, ministers, plantation owners and surgeons (Der Marderosian and Yelvigi, 1976).

THE NINETEENTH CENTURY

During the early part of the nineteenth century the medical profession became well established in America. The story as it relates to women's medicine is detailed by Harold Speert (1980) in *Obstetrics and Gynecology in America. A History*. The formation of medical schools and the scientific approach to botanical medicine resulted in many advances, the most important of which, for our subject, were the application of ergot, the introduction of anesthesia and, of course, the use of antisepsis in surgery.

Ergot

John Stearns (1808), a doctor in Saratoga County, New York, gains the credit for introducing ergot to modern American obstetric practice. He wrote a letter at Waterford, New York, dated 25th of January 1807 to a Dr Samuel Akerly, physician to the New York City Dispensary in which he gave an account of the therapeutic use of ergot. This 'Account of the Pulvis Parturiens, a Remedy for quickening Childbirth' was published in the *Medical Repository of New York* in the following year.

Ergot is a fungus and is the winter resting stage of *Claviceps purpurea*, a parasite on rye, but sometimes also found on wheat and other grasses. The fungus grows from the infected plant to form a long black slightly curved body known as the sclerotium which stands out conspicuously from the ears of the rye. The word 'ergot' is derived from an old French word *argot*, a cock's spur, to which ergot has a marked similarity of form.

Midwives became aware that ergot could strengthen uterine contractions and there is evidence to show that ergot was in use by European midwives in the sixteenth century, but it was John Stearns who was responsible for the general introduction of the drug to 'official' midwifery care. His 'discovery' was investigated by Oliver Prescott, a Fellow of the Massachusetts Medical Society. Prescott (1813) read his *Dissertation on the Natural History and Medicinal Effects of the Secale Cornutum, or Ergot* at the annual meeting of the Society at Boston on 2nd June, and introduced ergot to a wider audience. His paper was translated into French and German and attracted the interest of European physicians to its medicinal use. Ergot was listed in the original edition of the United States Pharmacopoeia of 1820. (See also Chapter 3.)

Anesthesia

William Thomas Green Morton (1819–1868) introduced ether to clinical practice at the Massachusetts General Hospital on the 16th of October 1846. Oliver Wendell Holmes (1809–1894), anatomist and writer, at that time in practice in Boston, wrote to Morton and suggested that the state of etherization should be called 'anesthesia' and the term was quickly adopted. Ether salts are prepared by the action of sulfuric acid on that well-known plant derivative – alcohol. The year of 1997 was the 150th anniversary of the introduction of anesthesia to obstetrics by James Young Simpson (1811–1870) of Edinburgh, Scotland. He used ether anesthesia during a difficult delivery on the 17th January 1847 and later that year introduced chloroform. The champion of anesthesia in America was Walter Channing (1848) of Harvard, and his important book was entitled *A Treatise on Etherization in Childbirth*. Many more anesthetic discoveries were to follow during the nineteenth century. (See also Chapter 18.)

Coca

Erythroxylon coca, or coca, found in South America, contains a number of potent alkaloids, including cocaine which was first isolated from it in 1860 by Albert Niemann. His discovery was possible because of advances in plant chemistry earlier in the nineteenth century. Physicians and pharmacists depended on plant-derived drugs since antiquity but were unaware of the exact active plant constituents. In the 1770s to 1780s, Karl Wilhelm Scheele (1732–1786), a Swiss apothecary, isolated a number of organic acids from plants, but the main breakthrough came in 1803 to 1804 when the German pharmacist, Friedrich Wilhelm Serturner (1783–1841) isolated morphine, the active principle of opium (Serturner, 1806). He found the substance was alkaline and could form salts with acids. The term 'alkaloid' was introduced in 1818 to describe such complex organic nitrogenous substances by Karl Meissner, another German pharmacist, and through alkaloidal chemistry the active principles of many plants used in pharmacy were elucidated (Cowen and Helfand, 1990).

To return to the story of cocaine, the substance was tested in 1884 by Karl Köller, an ophthalmologist, and found to be an effective local anesthetic, and in a short time cocaine was introduced to obstetric care. William Stewart of Johns Hopkins Hospital in Baltimore experimented with the use of cocaine in conduction analgesia in 1885 (O'Dowd and Philipp, 1994). Advertising broadsheets for alkaloid products, including cocaine, in 1901 demonstrated not only the popular conception of the Indian medicine man as a healer but also pointed to the plant origin of the drug. Extract of the coca plant provided the basis for Coca-Cola until 1902 when cocaine was banned in the USA.

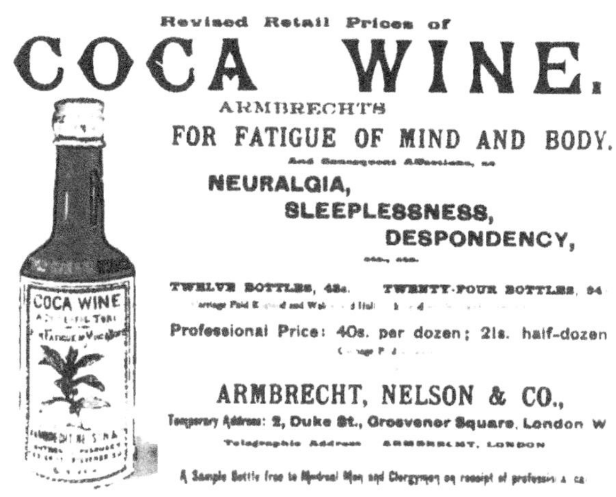

Revised Retail Prices of
COCA WINE.
ARMBRECHTS
FOR FATIGUE OF MIND AND BODY.
NEURALGIA,
SLEEPLESSNESS,
DESPONDENCY,
TWELVE BOTTLES, 42s.
TWENTY-FOUR BOTTLES, 84
Professional Price: 40s. per dozen; 21s. half-dozen
ARMBRECHT, NELSON & CO.,
Temporary Address: 2, Duke St., Grosvenor Square, London W
COCA WINE

Figure 4 Coca wine, a popular patent medicine

THE TWENTIETH CENTURY

What of more recent discoveries that visionaries could only dream of at the dawn of the new century? Who could have prophesied the enormous growth in the pharmaceutical industry which occurred after, and partially because of, World War Two, and that American drug firms would dominate the world market at the approach of the new millennium? The achievements of physicians, pharmacists and the drug firms were publicly honored by the US Postal Service which saw fit to release a stamp under the general umbrella of 'Pharmacy' in 1972. The following selection of highlights pays tribute to the innovators who led us from reliance on plant medicines to the stage where it became possible to standardize quality, eliminate impurities, make dosages more accurate and move towards a greater understanding of drugs' effects. This in turn led to the introduction of synthetic forms of medications which copied those available in nature and to the mass production of commonly used medications.

Prostaglandins

Two American gynecologists, Kurzrok and Lieb (1930), discovered that strips of human uterus relax or contract when exposed to human semen. In 1934 Ulf Svante von Euler (1905–1983) of Sweden identified the active principle as a lipid-soluble acid which he called prostaglandin (PGE). Research was inhibited by inadequate supplies of raw material until the discovery that the soft coral, *Plexaura homomalla*, was a rich source of inactive PGE, that was changed to an active form by scientists of the Upjohn Company. An alternative source of PGE was the red alga in lichens.

Curare

The well-known drug, tubocurarine, was isolated by Harold King (1935) from the plant, *Strychnos nux-vomica* and later from *Chondodendron tomentosum*. The introduction of tubocurarine, a skeletal muscle relaxant, was one of the most significant advances in clinical anesthesia. It heralded a new and safer era in obstetric anesthesia that would be responsible for a great reduction in maternal and perinatal mortality and morbidity. The origins of the story go back to the year of 1516, when an Italian 'gossip columnist' of his time, one Peter Martyr d'Anghera, wrote the first account of the use of arrow poisons by the South American Indians. He gave a detailed account of the preparation of the poison and how it was obtained from the sap of certain trees. In 1684 the word 'curare' was first used by Margavvius to describe the poison, and much was written about the drug, but it was not until 1935 that the active component, curare, was isolated.

Mexican yam

It is well known that estrogens can be obtained from plant sources including lignite, peat, petroleum, rape seed and pussy-willow (the common American willow, *Salix discolor*), and many other plants which contain phytoestrogens. There is, however, a fascinating tale about the yam plant, *Dioscorea mexicana*, and the synthesis of the female hormone, progesterone.

Yams are climbing vines with thick tubers, much like those of the sweet potato. More than 20 million tons of yams are grown for food each year in tropical countries. The plant was known in former times as 'colic root' and was used traditionally to ease menstrual cramps. In the 1940s the yam was found to contain steroidal saponins which yield diosgenin, the precursor of progesterone. The story of the rise to fame of the humble yam is due to one Russell Marker, an American research chemist at Pennsylvania State College, funded by the Park-Davis company (founded in 1867). He devoted much of his academic career in the late 1930s and early 1940s to work on steroids. Marker was aware that some plants had steroid precursors and became convinced that hormones could be produced more cheaply from plant sources. He investigated 400 plants and discovered that the Mexican yam (*Dioscorea mexicana*) contained steroidal saponins, including diosgenin, that could be chemically converted to progesterone and, in turn, the female hormone could be transformed to testosterone. Apart from the steroidal saponins, yam also contains alkaloids, tannins and starch. In 1944 Marker went on to found a new company named Syntex – from synthesis and Mexico. He left the company after two years but no patents had been taken out so his technique of producing progesterone was widely copied within a short time. Although not active orally, progesterone

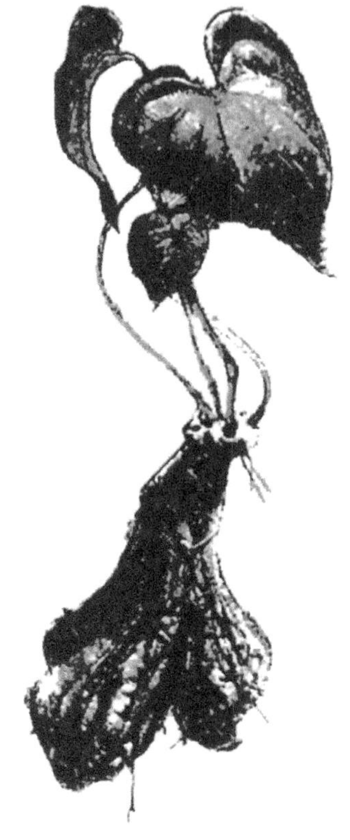

Figure 5 Mexican yam (*Dioscorea mexicana*)

was soon to be converted to a number of potent oral preparations, one of which was norethynodrel (Robertson, 1990).

Gregory Pincus, the father of the pill, worked as a biologist in Shrewsbury, Massachusetts. In 1953 he established the biological activity of norethynodrel in rabbits. He sought the clinical collaboration of John Rock of Harvard, and Celso Ramon Garcia, who at that time was working in San Juan City Hospital, Puerto Rico. Field trials were carried out there and the effectiveness of norethynodrel was confirmed. Ten mg of the compound with 0.15 mg ethinyl estradiol (mestranol) was marketed in 1957 as Enovid and prescribed for menstrual disturbances. The compound effectively blocked ovulation. In 1960 Enovid was approved for contraception in the USA and thus began the story of the oral contraceptive pill (Djerassi, 1992).

For almost 30 years the yam reigned supreme and, until 1970, the wild yam was the only source of diosgenin, but inevitably other sources were found, and the yam slid into relative obscurity. It blossomed again with a new life in complementary medicine, where it is one of the most popular sources of medication for female complaints.

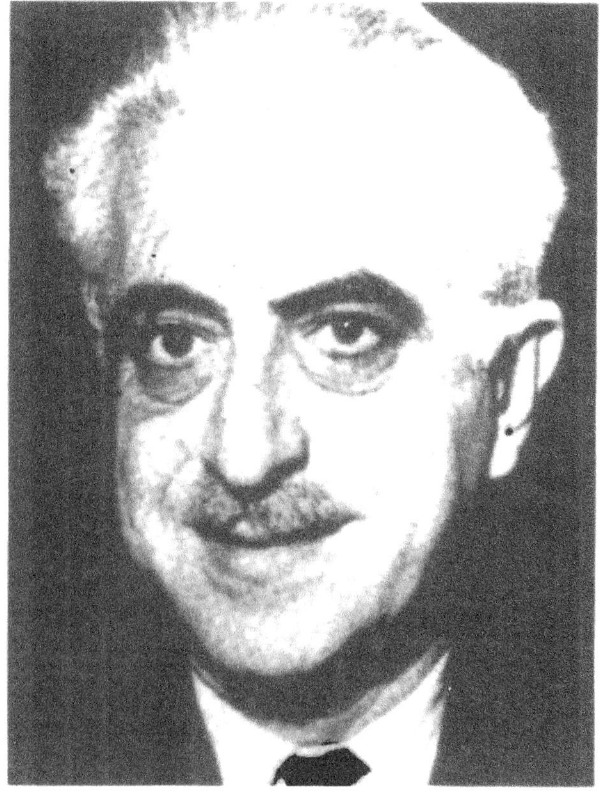

Figure 6 Gregory Pincus (1903–1967)

Antibiotics

In this era of cloning and chemical synthesis it is easy to forget that many antibiotic forms, including the aminoglycosides, cephalosporins, chloramphenicol, cytotoxic antibiotics, macrolides, penicillins, peptides and the tetracyclines, have been derived from fungi and soil micro-organisms. All antibiotics have had a major role to play in women's reproductive health and many were discovered or developed in America. A few of the agents are listed below. The first antibiotic was discovered in England but help was obtained from America to develop this wonderful new medical resource. (See also Chapter 19.)

Penicillin

Sir Alexander Fleming (1881–1955), a Scottish physician and bacteriologist at St Mary's Hospital, London, first noted the antibiotic effect of a mold, *Penicillium notatum*, in 1928 and isolated an active substance which he called penicillin (Fleming, 1929). At Oxford, England, a group of scientists, including Australian Howard Florey and German–British physician Ernst Boris Chain researched the clinical use of penicillin in laboratory animals from 1940 to 1941. Spurred on by favorable results, they sought to involve the British pharmaceutical industry but, due to the outbreak of World War Two, resources were scarce so Florey turned to America for help. The United States Department of Agriculture at Peoria, Illinois and, later, American pharmaceutical firms, produced massive quantities of the drug. In New York, John F. Mahony and associates (1943) showed that penicillin could cure syphilis, and the sulfonamides were no longer the first-line treatment for this centuries-old plague. Fleming, Chain and Florey were awarded the Nobel Prize in 1945.

Streptomycin

In 1944 Selman Waksman and his colleagues at the Agricultural College of Rutgers University discovered streptomycin. Waksman, a Russian-born American citizen, and his team tested over 10 000 cultures of *Streptomyces griseus* obtained from soil samples and eventually specimens taken from a chicken run were found to destroy bacteria, spirochetes and the tuberculosis bacterium, the active principle being streptomycin. Waksman was a Nobel Prize winner in 1952 (Lyons and Petrucelli, 1987).

Chloramphenicol

In 1949 Mildred C. Rebstock, of the Parke-Davis Company in Detroit, was the first to synthesize chloramphenicol (Duin and Sutcliffe, 1992). The antibiotic was isolated from soil samples containing *Streptomyces venezuelae*, an organism first found two years previously by Burkholder in soil samples collected in Venezuela.

Cancer therapy

Another area of great concern in this century is the topic of cancer. One of the first reliable anti-cancer drugs was isolated from the Madagascar periwinkle or Cayenne jasmine, *Catharanthus roseus*. The plant contains over 75 alkaloids, many of which are toxic, but from which were isolated vinblastine and vincristine, potent chemotherapeutic agents valuable in treating leukemia. Also known as *Vinca rosea*, Madagascar periwinkle contains reserpine (as found in *Rauwolfia serpentina*), a much used antihypertensive. The realization that plants contained such powerful chemicals has led to a search for other plant anti-cancer drugs (Evans, 1996).

Pacific yew

The biggest success story in plant medications of recent times concerns the Pacific yew, *Taxus brevifolia*. This evergreen coniferous tree is found in groves along the Pacific coast of North America and inland from British Columbia to Idaho. The Pacific yew has provided one of our latest wonder drugs, paclitaxel, or Taxol as we know it. It was described by Wani *et al.* (1971) and introduced much later to clinical practice. The bark of six trees is required to treat one patient with ovarian or breast cancer. Exploitation of *T. brevifolia* led to the Pacific Yew Act of 1992 which sought to conserve this wonderful medicinal asset. The closely related *T. baccata*, the common yew, provided the wood to make bows for archery many centuries ago. It was sacred to the ancient druids, and is to be found in churchyards, but unfortunately *T. baccata* contains only small amounts of active anti-cancer chemicals and, until recently, was only useful for research. The common yew is now used to produce paclitaxel.

Cotton

A more recent pharmaceutical is the New/Old plant wonder drug obtained from *Gossypium herbaceum*, cotton, or Levant cotton, which is now being touted for its hemostatic properties. Cotton is thought to have originated in India and was carried by traders to ancient Egypt c. 500 BC. Remains of the plant have also been found among archeological artifacts of ancient Peru c. 2000 BC. Apart from antibacterial and antiviral effects, its active constituent, gossypol, causes male infertility and stimulates the uterus. Cotton seed was used centuries ago by some North American Indian tribes to induce labor pains, and it was listed for its abortifacient properties in the USP from 1863 to 1950. It is still available as a herbal medication for treatment of amenorrhea (British Herbal Pharmacopoeia, 1991).

SELECTED AMERICAN INDIAN MEDICINES

Uses

Aphrodisiac
Joe Pye weed
Breast disease/inflammation
Fern, star grass, pine, pipsissewa, wintergreen
Breast engorgement/pain
Elder, red cedar, skullcap, spikenard, water
Breast, for milk
Corn, wild lettuce
Breast, sore nipples
Balsam fir, ipecacuanha, trillium
Contraception, oral
Indian turnip, milkweed
Diseases of urogenital organs
Blue cohosh, Joe Pye weed, juniper

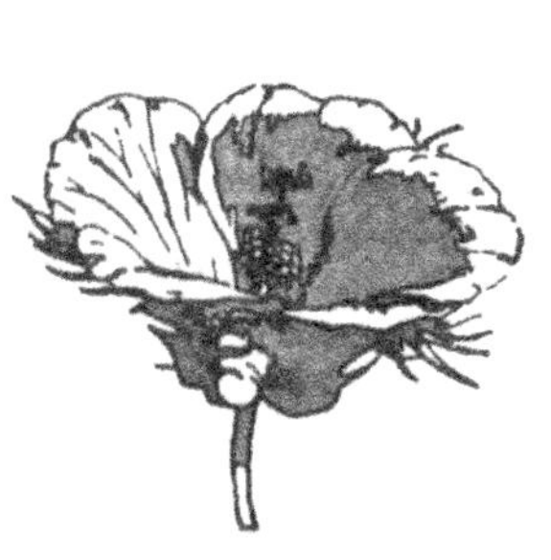

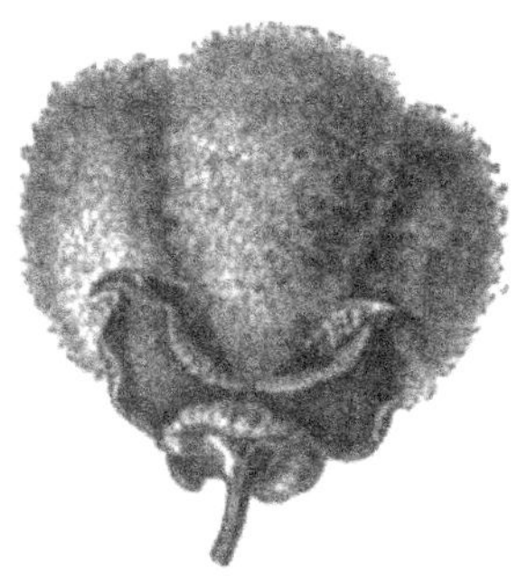

Figure 7 Cotton (*Gossypium* sp.)

Hemorrhage, unspecified
Butterfly weed, hawthorn, prickly ash, skunk cabbage, trillium

Labor, aid to
Blue cohosh, cedar, hardhack, lady's slipper, sumach, trillium

Labor, analgesia
Cotton, lady's slipper, partridge berry, squaw weed, wild cherry, wild yam

Labor, difficult
Blue cohosh, corn, elder or elderberry, slippery elm

Labor, oxytocic
Blue cohosh, corn, cotton, fleabane, squaw weed, tobacco, trillium

Labor, to cleanse after
Ash tree, Joe Pye weed, stillingia

Labor, unspecified
Burdock root, culver root, spikenard, squaw root, yellow root

Menstruation, for amenorrhea
Blue cohosh, pennyroyal, puccoon, red cedar, skunk cabbage, wintergreen

Menstruation, disorders of
Fleabane, hydrangea, Indian hemp, squaw root

Menstruation, for excess
Blue cohosh

Menstruation, painful
Fern, lady's slipper, pennyroyal, sumach

Menstruation, to cause
Arbor vitae, blue cohosh, buck bean, cotton, juniper, pulsatilla, saffron, skullcap, tansy, yarrow

Menstruation, to regulate
Stillingia, trillium, yellow dock

Menstruation, to stop
dogwood, golden seal

A

MANUAL

OF THE

MEDICAL BOTANY OF NORTH AMERICA

BY

LAURENCE JOHNSON, A.M., M.D.,

LECTURER ON MEDICAL BOTANY, MEDICAL DEPARTMENT OF THE UNIVERSITY OF THE CITY OF NEW YORK; FELLOW OF THE NEW YORK ACADEMY OF MEDICINE, AND OF THE NEW YORK ACADEMY OF SCIENCES; MEMBER OF THE COMMITTEE OF REVISION OF THE PHARMACOPOEIA OF THE UNITED STATES, MEMBER OF THE TORREY BOTANICAL CLUB, ETC.

NEW YORK
WILLIAM WOOD & COMPANY
56 & 58 LAFAYETTE PLACE
1884

Figure 8 Frontispiece from Johnson, *A Manual of the Medical Botany of North America* (1884)

Placenta, to deliver
Skullcap, slippery elm

Puerperium, postpartum hemorrhage
Corn, sumach

Uterus, disease of
Cranberry, wahoo

Venereal disease
Blue cohosh, butterfly weed, creosote bush, culver root, goldenseal, Joe Pye weed, puccoon, sassafras, slippery elm, wahoo, yerba santa

Vaginal discharge, leukorrhea, 'whites'
Blazing star, fleabane, hepatica, iron, lobelia, trillium, wild geranium, yarrow

Women's disorders (unspecified)

Bearberry, blue cohosh, hawthorn, Indian turnip, milkweed, partridge berry, pipsissewa, seneca, snake root, squaw weed, sumach

Remedies

Alder, anemone, angelica, arbor vitae, ash tree

Balsam fir, bayberry, bearberry, birch, blazing star, blue cohosh (papoose root; squaw root), buckbean, burdock, butterflyweed

Cedar (red), corn, corn smut, colic weed, cotton, cranberry (cramp bark), creosote bush, culver's root, wild carrot, wild cherry

Dogwood (American boxwood)

Elder, elm (slippery)

Fern, fleabane

Ginseng, goldenseal, grindelia, wild geranium, wild ginger

Hardhack, hawthorn, hepatica, hydrangea

Indian hemp, Indian turnip (American wake-Robin), ipecacuanha

Jimson weed, Joe Pye weed, juniper

Lady's slipper (American valerian; moccasin flower), lobelia, wild lettuce

Milkweed

Pennyroyal (squaw mint), partridge berry (squaw berry), pine, pipsissewa, poke root, prickly ash (angelica tree), puccoon (blood root)

Sarsaparilla, sassafras, skullcap, skunk cabbage, snakeroot, squaw flower, squaw root (black and blue cohosh), squaw weed, stargrass, stillingia (queen's delight), sumach

Tansy, tobacco, trillium (squaw flower)

Wahoo, water avens, wintergreen, witchhazel

Yarrow, yellow dock, yellow root, yerba santa, wild yam

NOTE

The American Indian medications listed are based on information culled from Vogel (1973). Other useful sources include: Bigelow (1817, 1818, 1820), Densmore (1974), Der Maderosian and Yelvigi (1976), Doane (1985), Hutchens (1973), Johnson (1884), Speert (1980), Stone (1962), and Weiner (1980).

References

Bigelow, J. (1817, 1818, 1820). *American Medical Botany*, Vols. 1, 2, 3. (Boston: Cummings and Hilliard)

Bown, D. (1995). *The Royal Horticultural Society Encyclopedia of Herbs*, p. 103. (London: Dorling Kindersley)

British Herbal Pharmacopoeia (1991). pp. 105–6, 107, 146, 197. (Bournemouth, UK: The British Herbal Medicine Association)

Channing, W. (1848). *A Treatise on Etherisation in Childbirth*. (Boston: Ticknor)

Chevallier, A. (1990). *The Encyclopedia of Medicinal Plants*, p. 73. (London: Dorling Kindersley)

Clairborne, R. (1973). *The First Americans. The Emergence of Man*, pp. 9–22. (New York: Time-Life Books)

Cowan, D. L. and Helfand, W. H. (1990). *Pharmacy. An Illustrated History*, p. 124. (New York: Harry N. Abrams)

Densmore, F. (1974). *How Indians Use Wild Plants for Food, Medicine and Crafts*. (New York: Dover Publications)

Der Maderosian, A. and Yelvigi, M. S. (1976). Medicine and Drugs in Colonial America. *Am. J. Pharmacy*, July–August, pp. 113–20

Djerassi, C. (1992). *The Pill, Pygmy Chimps and Degas' Horse*, pp. 49–65. (New York: Basic Books)

Doane, N. L. (1985). *Indian Doctor Book*. (North Carolina: Aerial Photography Services Inc.)

Duin, N. and Sutcliffe, J. (1992). *A History of Medicine*, p. 164. (London: Simon and Schuster)

Evans, W. C. (1996). *Trease and Evans Pharmacognosy*, pp. 420–2. (London: W. B. Saunders Co.)

Fleming, A. (1929). On the antibacterial action of cultures of a *Penicillium* with special reference to their use for the isolation of *B. influenzae*. *Brit. J. Exp. Path.*, **10**, 226–36

Griggs, B. (1997). *New Green Pharmacy. The Story of Western Herbal Medicine*, pp. 36, 211. (London: Vermillion)

Hutchens, A. R. (1973). *Indian Herbalogy of North America*. (Massachusetts: Shambhala Publications)

Johnson, L. (1884). *A Manual of the Medical Botany of North America*. (New York: William Woods and Co.)

King, H. (1935). Curare Alkaloids. Tubocurarine. *J. Chem. Soc.*, pp. 1381–9

Kurzrok, R. and Lieb, C. C. (1930). Biochemical studies of Human Semen. 2. *Proc. Soc. Exp. Biol. Med.*, 28, 268

Lyons, A. S. and Petrucelli, R. J. (1987). *Medicine. An Illustrated History*, p. 591. (New York: Harry N. Abrams Inc.)

Mahony, J. F., Arnold, R. C. and Harris, A. (1943). Penicillin treatment of early syphilis – A preliminary report. *Am. J. Publ. Health*, 33, 1387–91

McGrew, R. A. (1985). *Encyclopaedia of Medical History*, p. 329–34. (London: Macmillan)

Moore, J. E. and Keitel, A. (1926). The treatment of early syphilis. 1. A plan of treatment for routine use. *Bull. Johns Hopkins Hosp.*, 39, 1–15

Morton, T. G. (1846). Circular. *Morton's Leothon.* (Boston: Dutton and Wentworth)

O'Dowd, M. J. and Philipp, E. (1994). *The History of Obstetrics and Gynaecology*, p. 435–56. (London & New York: Parthenon Publishing)

Prescott, O. (1813). *A Dissertation on the Natural History and Medicinal Effects of the Secale Cornutum, or Ergot.* (Boston: Cummings and Holliard)

Reynolds, J. E. F. (ed.) (1982). *Martindale. The Extra Pharmacopoeia*, p. 1753. (London: The Pharmaceutical Press)

Robertson, W. H. (1990). *An Illustrated History of Contraception*, p. 121–138. (London & New York: Parthenon Publishing)

Serturner, F. W. (1806). Darstellung der reinen Mohnsaure (Opiumsaure) nebst einer chemischen untersuchung des opiums. *J. Pharm. für Aertze Apothexer*, 14, 47–93

Simpson, J. Y. (1847). Notes on the Employment of the Inhalation of Sulphuric Ether in the Practice of Midwifery. March. *Mon. J. Med. Sci.*, 9, 639–40

Speert, H. (1980). *Obstetrics and Gynecology in America: A History.* (Chicago: The American College of Obstetricians and Gynecologists)

Squire, P. W. (1908). *Squire's Companion to the latest edition of the British Pharmacopoeia*, p. 1233. (London: J. & A. Churchill)

Stearns, J. (1808). Account of Pulvis Parturiens, a Remedy for Quickening Child-birth. *The Medical Repository (New York).* Second Hexade, 5, 308–9

Stone, E. (1962). *Medicine Among The American Indians.* (New York: Hafner Publishing Company Inc.)

Vogel, V. (1970). *American Indian Medicine*, pp. 284–5, 293–4. (London: University of Oklahoma Press)

Wani, M. C., Taylor, H. L., Wall, M. E., Coggon, P. and McPhail, A. T. (1971). Plant antitumor agents. 5. The isolation and structure of taxol, A novel antileukemic and antitumor agent from *Taxus brevifolia. J. Am. Chem. Soc.*, 93, 2325–27

Weiner, M. A. (1980). *Earth Medicine – Earth Food*, p. 34, 42. (New York: Fawcett Columbine)

Wootton, A. C. (1910). *Chronicles of Pharmacy*, Vol. 2, pp. 111–3. (London: Macmillan and Co.)

Section 6
Appendices

Appendix I
Therapeutical classification of remedies

Alternatives
Medicines which gradually change and correct a morbid condition of the organs, so that abnormal conditions become normal and metabolism is increased.

Anesthetics
These are divided in **General** (by inhalation) and **Local** (by spray or other application to the part). General anesthetics abolish consciousness and reflex action, and so prevent the perception of painful and other stimuli in the sensory centers.

Analgesics or anodynes
Alleviate pain by lessening the excitability of nerves or nerve centers.

Anaphrodisian
Diminish sexual passion.

Anhidrotic
Check perspiration.

Antacid
Reduce the acidity of the gastric contents.

Anthelminty
Destroy intestinal worms (vermicides), or expel them from the alimentary canal (vermifuges).

Antidotes
Are mentioned under the several poisonous drugs.

Antilithic
Counteract lithiasis or lithemia i.e. a tendency to the deposit of uric acid or urates, or to the formation of the corresponding calculi.

Antiperiodic
Have the property of preventing the periodical attacks of certain fevers.

Antipyretic
Reduce and control the temperature in fever.

Antiseptic
Prevent decomposition by inhibiting the growth of micro-organisms.

Antispasmodic
Allay or prevent the recurrence of spasms.

Aperient
See cathartics.

Aphrodisiac
Increase sexual appetite.

Aromatic
See carminatives.

Astringent
Produce contraction of the tissues, diminution in the size of blood vessels and coagulation of the albuminous fluids; they improve digestion and check secretions, mucous discharges, and hemorrhages; or applied topically to stop bleeding and diminish discharges.

Carminative
Stimulate or aid the removal of flatus from the stomach and intestines, and relieve griping.

Cathartic
Promote intestinal evacuations.

Caustic
Destroy the vitality of the parts to which they are applied.

Cholagogue
Increase the amount of bile secreted.

Counterirritant
Stimulate and cause irritation or inflammation of the parts to which they are applied; they differ in their intensity of action and may be divided as follows:

Rubefacient – Agents which, when applied to the skin, produce local warmth and redness.

Vesicant or **Epispastic** – Those which raise a vesicle or blister.

Pustulant – Those which produce pustules.

Demulcent
Protect and thus allay irritation of the mucous membranes.

Deodorant
Destroy offensive odors and absorb foul gases.

Depilatory
Destroy living hair.

Desiccant
Check secretion and allay discharges from ulcers and wounds.

Diaphoretic
Increase the action of the skin and induce perspiration.

Disinfectant
Destroy the specific microbes or toxins of communicable diseases.

Diuretic
Promote the secretion of urine.

Ecbolic
Promote the contraction of the gravid uterus and facilitate the expulsion of the contents.

Emetic
Excite vomiting.

Emmenagogue
Maintain or restore a healthy condition of the menstrual discharge.

Emollient
Soften and relax the tissues, also protect sensitive surfaces; employed to allay irritation.

Epispastic
See Counterirritant.

Errhine
See Sternutatory.

Escharotic
See Caustic.

Expectorant
Promote the secretion of bronchial mucus or facilitate its expulsion.

Febrifuge
See Antipyretic.

Galactagogue
Increase the secretion of the mammary gland.

Hematinic
See Tonic, Blood.

Hemostatic
See Styptic.

Hypnotic
Induce sleep, and thus remove the consciousness of pain by lessening the excitability and functional activity of the brain cells.

Laxative
See Cathartic.

Mydriatic
Produce dilation of the pupil.

Myotic
Contract the pupil.

Narcotic
See Hypnotic.

Nutritive
Aid assimilation and improve the condition of the tissues.

Parasiticide
Destroy vegetable and animal parasites.

Purgative
See Cathartic.

Pustulant
See Counterirritant.

Refrigerant
Relieve febrile thirst and impart a feeling of coolness.

Rubefacient
See Counterirritant.

Sedative
Exert a soothing influence by diminishing pain, depressing vital activity, or tranquilizing abnormal

muscular movement (local, respiratory, nervine, gastric and cardiac).

Sialagogue
Increase the secretion of saliva.

Soporific
See Hypnotic.

Sternutatory
Cause sneezing and increase the nasal mucous secretion.

Stimulant
Increase the function of a part, or an organ (cerebral, nervine, stomachic, circulatory and local).

Stomachic
Directly promote the functions of the stomach and improve the appetite and digestion.

Styptic
Arrest bleeding.

Sudorific
See Diaphoretic. When diaphoretics act very powerfully, they are called sudorifics.

Tonic
Impart strength or tone to the functions of the body or its parts. (Acting through the blood and improving its qualities, nervine, stomachic and intestinal, cardiac, and mineral waters.)

Vasodilator
Causing dilation of the blood vessels.

Vermicide and vermifuge
See Anthelmintic.

Vesicant
See Counterirritant.

Abstracted from:

Squire, P. W. (1908) *Squire's Companion to the latest edition of the British Pharmacopoeia*, pp. 1333–41. (London: J. and A. Churchill)

Appendix II
Abbreviations commonly used in prescriptions

THE PRESCRIPTION

A medicinal formula. It has been divided into four constituent parts, suggested with a view to enabling the basis to operate, in the language of Aesclapius, 'Cito', 'Tuto', et 'Jucunde' – quickly, safely, and pleasantly.
These are:
Basis, or principal medicine.
Adjuvans: that which promotes its operation – 'Cito'.
Corrigens: that which corrects its operation – 'Tuto'.
Constituens: that which imparts an agreeable form – 'Jucunde'.

The 'Abbreviations commonly used in Prescriptions' were mainly taken from:
Hoblyn, R. D. (1878) *A Dictionary of Terms Used in Medicine*, pp. 518–22. (London: Whittaker & Co.)

Abbreviation	Latin (L) or Greek (G)	English
A, aa	ana (G)	of each
abdom.	abdomen (L)	the belly
abs. feb.	absente febre (L)	in the absence of fever
a.c.	ante cibos (cibum) (L)	before meals or food
add.	adde (L)	add
ad	ad (L)	to, up to
ad def. animi	ad defectionem animi	to fainting
ad grat. acid.	ad gratum aciditatem (L)	to an agreeable sourness
ad 2 vic.	ad duas vices (L)	at twice taking
ad lib.	ad libitum (L)	at pleasure
adst. febre	adstante febre (L)	when the fever is on
ad recid. praec.	ad recidivum praecavendum	to prevent a relapse
admov.	admove or admoveantur (L)	let there be applied
aeg.	aeger (L)	the patient
aeq	aequales (L)	equal
aggred. febre	aggrediente febre (L)	when the fever is coming on
Alt. dieb.	alternis diebus (L)	alternate days
Alt. hor.	alternis horis (L)	every other hour
aliquant	aliquantillum (L)	a very little
alt. noct.	alternis noctibus (L)	alternative nights
alvo adst.	alvo adstricta (L)	when the belly is bound

amb.	ambo (L)	both
amp.	amplus (L)	large
anodyn.	anodyne (G)	anodyne
apert.	apertus (L)	clear
applic.	applicetur (L)	let there be applied
aq.	aqua (L)	water
aq. bull.	aqua bulliens (L)	boiling water
aq. dest.	aqua destillata (L)	distilled water
aq. ferv.	aqua fervens (L)	boiling water
aq. frig.	aqua figida (L)	cold water
aq. font.	aqua fontana (L)	spring water
baln. tep.	balneum tepidum (L)	warm bath
BB. Bbds.	Barbadensis (L)	Barbados
b.d.	bis die (L)	twice a day
b.i.d.	bis in die (L)	twice a day
bis hor.	bis hora (L)	every half hour
bis ind.	bis in dies (L)	twice a day
Bull.	bulliat (L)	let it boil
C. or c.	cum (L)	with
C.C.	cucurbitula cruenta	cupping-glass
caerul	caeruleus (L)	blue
cap.	capiat (L)	let him take
cat.	catamplasma (L)	cataplasm
cath.	catharticus (L)	cathartic
cat. lin.	cataplasma lini (L)	poultice, linseed
cat. sinap.	cataplasms sinapis	poultice, mustard
cms	cras mane sumendus (L)	take tomorrow morning
CN	cras nocte (L)	tomorrow night
co.	compositus	compound
cochl.	cochleare (L)	spoonful
cochl. amp.	cochleara amplum (L)	heaped spoonful
cochl. infant	cochleare infantis (L)	child's spoonful
cochl. mag.	cochleare magnum (L)	tablespoonful
cochl. mod. (med.)	cochleare medium (L)	dessertspoonful
cochl. parv.	cochleare parvum (L)	teaspoonful
Col.	cola (L)	strain
Colat.	colatus (L)	strained
Colent.	colentur (L)	let them be strained
Collut.	collutorium (L)	mouth wash
Collyr.	collyrium (L)	eye wash
Comp.	compositus (L)	compound
conf.	confectio (L)	confection, sweetmeat
Cont. rem	continuentur remedium (L)	medicine to be continued

Cop.	copiosus	plenteous
Coq.	coque (L)	boil
Crast	crastinus (L)	for tomorrow
Cuj.	cujus	of which
Cujusl.	cujuslibet	of any
C.V.	cras vespere (L)	tomorrow evening
Cyath.	cyathus (L)	glassful
Deaur. pil	deaurentur pilulae	let the pills be gilt
Deb. spis.	debita spissitudine (L)	of proper consistency
Decub.	decubitus (L)	lying down
de d. in d.	de die in diem (L)	from day to day
Dej. alvi.	dejectiones alvi	stools
Det.	detur (L)	let it be given
Dext. lat	dextra lateralis	right side
Dieb. alt	diebus alternis (L)	on alternate days
Dieb. tert.	diebus tertiis	every third day
dil.	dilue (L)	dilute or dissolve
Diluc.	diluculo	at daybreak
dim.	dimidius (L)	one half
Dir. prop.	directione propria (L)	with a proper direction
Diuturn.	diuturnus	long-continued
Donec alv. bis dej.	donec alvus bis dejiciat (L)	until two stools have been obtained
dr	drachme (G)	dram
efferv.	effervescens (L)	effervescence, bubbling
Ejusd.	ejusdem (L)	of the same
Elect.	electuarium	electuary
Emp.	emplastrum	plaster
enem.	enemata (G)	clyster
Ex. aq.	ex aqua	in water
Ext. sup. Alut.	extende super alutam	spread upon leather
Ex. vel ext.	extractum	extract
Feb. dur.	febre durante (L)	while the fever lasts
Fem. intern.	femoribus internus (L)	to the inner thigh
F.h.	fiat haustus (L)	let a draught be made
fist. arm	fistula armata (L)	clyster-pipe and bladder fit for use
Fl.	fluidus (L)	liquid – by measure
fontic.	fonticulus (L)	an issue
fort.	fortis (L)	strong
Fot.	Fotus	fomentation
F.p.	fiat potio (L)	let a potion be made

F.pil. xij.	fiant pilulae duodecim (L)	make 12 pills
F.s.a.	fiat secundum artem (L)	let it be made skillfully
ft.	fiat (L)	let it be made
Ft. mist. or hst.	fiat mistura (haustus)	let a mixture (draught) be made
Ft. pulv.	fiat pulvis (L)	let a powder be made
F. vs.	fiat venaesectio (L)	let the patient be bled
Garg.	gargarisma (L)	gargle
Gel. quav	gelatina quavis (L)	in any kind of jelly
G.G.G.	gummi guttae gambiae (L)	gamboge
gr	granum (L)	grain
gutt. or gtt.	gutta (L)	drop
Gutt. quibusd.	guttis quibusdam (L)	with a few drops
Har. pil. sum. iij.	harum pilularum sumantur tres	let three pills be taken
H.d. or hor.decub	hora decubitus (L)	at bedtime
Hebdom.	hebdomada (L)	week
hestern.	hesternus	of yesterday
hirud.	hirudo (L)	leech
H.n.	hac nocte	tonight
Hor.decub.	hora decubitus (L)	at bedtime
Hor. un spatio.	horae unius spatio (L)	at the end of one hour
Hor.interm.	horis intermediis (L)	at the intermediate hours between what has been ordered at stated times
h.s.	hora somni (L)	at bedtime
i.c.	inter cibos (L)	between meals
Id.	idem (L)	the same
in d.	in dies (L)	daily
Inf.	infunde (L)	pour in
Inj. enem.	injicitur enema	let a clyster be given
inject.	injectio (L)	injection
In pulm.	in pulmento	in gruel
Lat. dol.	lateri dolenti (L)	to the painful side
lb	libra (L)	pound weight, or wine
linct.	linctus (L)	linctus
lin.	linimentum (L)	liniment
Liq.	liquor (L)	solution
Lot.	lotio (L)	lotion
M. or m.	misce (L)	mix
	mensura (L)	by measure

M. or m.	manipulus (L)	handful
mane pr. or M. prim.	mane primo (L)	early in the morning
Mediet.	medietas	half
Medioc.	mediocrim	middle-sized
min. or m.	minimum (L)	60th part of a fluid dram
mist. or M.	mistura (L)	mixture
Mitt.	mitte	send
Mitt. sang. ad 3xij. salt	mittatur sanguis ad uncias duodecim saltem	take away at least 12 ounces of blood
Mod. praes.	modo praescripto (L)	in the manner directed
Mor. sol.	more silto (L)	in the usual way
Narthec.	narthecium	gallipot
n.et m. (nmque)	nocte et mane (L)	night and morning
Nm.	nux moschata (L)	nutmeg
Noct.	nocte (L)	at night
O.	octarius (L)	pint
ol. lini s. i.	oleum lini sine igne	cold-drawn linseed-oil
o.m.	omni mane (L)	every morning
Omn. alt. hor	omnibus alternis horis (L)	every other hour
Omn. hor.	omni hora (L)	every hour
Omn. bid.	omni biduo (L)	every two days
Omn. bih	omni bihora (L)	every two hours
Omn. man	omni mane (L)	every morning
Omn. noct	omni nocte (L)	every night
Omn. quadr. hor.	omni quadrante horae (L)	every quarter of an hour
o.n.	omni nocte (L)	every evening
O.O.O.	oleum olivae optimum (L)	best olive oil
oz		ounce avoirdupois, or common weight, as distinguished from that prescribed by physicians in their orders.
P.	pulvis (L)	powder
	pondere (L)	by weight
	pilula (L)	pill
P.a.	parti affectae	to the affected part
p.a.	per anum (L)	by way of the anus
p. ae.	partes aequales (L)	equal parts
paracent. abd.	parakentesis abdominis (G)	tapping
Part. aeq.	partes aequales (L)	equal parts
Part. aff.	partem affectam (L)	the part affected

part.dolent.	partes dolentes (L)	the parts in pain
Part.vic.	partitis vicibus (L)	in divided doses
p.c.	post cibum (L)	after meals
P.D.	Pharmacopoeia Dublinensis	
P.E.	Pharmacopoeia Edinensis	
Per. op. emet.	peracta operatione emetici (L)	when the operation of the emetic is finished
per salt.	per saltum (L)	by leaps, without intermediary stages
Pil.	pilula (L)	a pill
P.L.	Pharmacopoeia Londinensis	
Plen.riv.	pleno rivo	in a full stream
Post sing. sed. liq.	post singulas sedes (L) liquidas (L)	after every loose stool
Ppt. vel prep.	praeparata (L)	prepared
P. rat. aet.	pro ratione aetatis (L)	in proportion to age
p.r.n.	pro re nata (L)	as occasion demands (repeated as required)
Pro pot.com.	pro potu communi (L)	a common drink
Prox. luc.	proxima luce	the day before
pug.	pugillus (L)	a grip between finger and thumb
pulv.	pulvis (L)	powder
P.U.S.	Pharmacopoeia of the United States	
q.	quaque (L)	each, every
q.d.	quaque die (L)	every day
q.i.d.	quater in die (L)	four times a day
q.l.	quantum libet (L)	as much as desired
q.p.	quantum placeat (L)	as much as desired
q.s.	quantum satis (L)	sufficient
q.q.h.	quaque quater hora (L)	every four hours
Qq.hor.	quaque hora (L)	every hour
q.suff.	quantum sufficit (L)	as much as suffices
quadrupl.	quadruplicato (L)	four times as much
Quamp	Quamprimum	immediately
quart. hor.	quater hora (L)	four-hourly
(4tis hor.	quater horis (L)	four-hourly
Quaq.	quaque (L)	every one
Quor.	quorum (L)	of which
quotid.	quotidie (L)	daily
q.v.	quantum vis (L)	as much as you please

Red. in pulv	reductus in pulverem (L)	powdered
Redig. in pulv	redigatur in pulverem (L)	let it be reduced to powder
Reg.hep.	regio hapatis	region of the liver
Reg.umb.	regio umbilici	region of the naval
Rep.	repetatur (L)	let it be repeated
R*x*	recipe (L)	take
S.A.	secundum artem (L)	according to art
scap.	scapula (L)	shoulderblade
scrob. cord.	scrobiculus cordis (L)	pit of the stomach
sed.	sedes (L)	a stool
semidr.	semidrachma (L)	half a dram
Semih.	semihora (L)	half an hour
Sept.	septem (L)	seven, a week
sesquih.	sesquihora (L)	an hour and a half
seq. luce.	sequenti luce (L)	the following day
Setac.	setaceum	a sieve
Sig.	signetur (L)	let it be labeled
Sign. n. pro.	signa nomine proprio (L)	label with proper name
sing.	singulorum (L)	of each
si n. val.	si non valeat (L)	if it is not enough
Si op. sit.	si opus sit (L)	if it is necessary
Si vir. perm.	si vires permittant (L)	if the strength will permit
Sol.	solution	solution
S.O.S.	si opus sit (L)	if it is necessary if there be occasion
Ss. or fs.	semis (L)	one half
s.s.s.	stratum super stratum (L)	layer upon layer
St.	stet (L)	let it stand
stat. or st.	statim (L)	immediately
Sub fin. coct.	sub finem coctionis (L)	when the boiling is nearly finished
sub-sulph.	sub-sulphas (L)	basic sulfate
Subtep.	subtepidus (L)	lukewarm
Suc.	succus (L)	juice
sum.	sumat (L)	let him take
sum. or s.	sumendum (L)	to be taken
sum. Tal.	sumat talem (L)	let the patient take one like this
Susunc.	sesuncia	an ounce and a half
S.V.	spiritus vinosus	ardent spirit of any strength
S.V.G.	spiritus vini gallici	brandy
S.V.R.	spiritus vinosus rectificatus	spirit of wine, alcohol

S.V.T.	spiritus vinosus tenuis	proof spirit or half and half spirit of wine and water
tab.	tabella (L)	tablet
t.d., t.i.d., t.d.s.	ter (in) die (summendum) (L)	take three times a day
temp. dext.	tempori dextro (L)	to the right temple
TO	tinctura opii (L)	tincture of opium Generally confounded with laudanum, which is, properly the wine of opium.
T.O.C.	tinctura opii camphorata	paregoric elixir
Tr. Vel tinct	tinctura	tincture
troch.	trochiscus (L)	lozenge
ult. praes.	ultimum praescriptus (L)	the last ordered
umb.	umbilicus (L)	navel
ung.	unguentum (L)	ointment
Usq. ut liq. anim	usque ut liquerit animus (L)	until fainting is produced
Ut dict.	ut dictum (L)	as directed
Utend.	utendus (L)	to be used
vap.	vapores (L)	inhalation
vent.	ventriculus (L)	stomach (belly)
Vom. Urg.	vomitione urgente	when vomiting begins
v.o.s.	vitello ovi solutus (L)	dissolved in egg yolk
V.S.	venaesectio (L)	bleeding
Zz	zingiber (L)	ginger

Appendix III
Sources of illustrations

Samuel Bard, *A Compendium of the Theory and Practice of Midwifery* (1808)

Benjamin, H. Barton & Thomas Castle, *The British Flora Medica*, Chatto & Windus (1877)

Victor Bonney, *A Textbook of Gynaecological Surgery*, Cassell & Co. Ltd. (1947)

Alan Brews, *Edens & Holland's Manual of Obstetrics* 11th ed., J. and A. Churchill Ltd. (1957)

O'Donel T. D. Browne, *The Rotunda Hospital 1745–1945*, E. & S. Livingstone Ltd. (1947)

O'Donel Browne, *A Manual of Practical Obstetrics*, John Wright & Sons Ltd. (1936)

Andrew M. Claye, *The Evolution of Obstetric Analgesia*, Oxford University Press (1939)

Nicholas Culpeper, *A Dictionary for Midwives* (1651)

Palmer Findley, *Priests of Lucina, The Story of Obstetrics*, Little, Brown & Co. (1939)

Margaret Goldsmith, *The Road to Penicillin*, Lindsay Drummond Ltd. (1946)

H. Laing Gordon, *Sir James Young Simpson and Chloroform (1811–1870)*, T. Fischer Unwin (1897)

Henry Jellett, *A Short Practice of Midwifery*, J. and A. Churchill (1930)

C. A. Johns, *Flowers of the Field*, George Routledge & Sons (1907)

Laurence Johnson, *A Manual of the Medical Botany of North America*, William Wood & Co. (1884)

J. M. Munro Kerr & J. Chassar Moir, *Operative Obstetrics*, Bailliére, Tindall and Cox (1949)

Thomas Keys, *The History of Surgical Anesthesia*, Schuman (1945)

Kunsthistorisches Museum, Schloss Ambras, Innsbruck, Austria

The Louvre, Dept of Antiquities, Paris, France

Clifford Lull & Robert Hingson, *Control of Pain in Childbirth*, William Heinemann (1945)

Aylmer Maude, *The Authorized Life of Marie C. Stopes*, Williams & Norgate Ltd. (1924)

François Mauriceau, *The Disease of Women with Child, and in Child-bed* (1668)

S. Maw, Son & Thompson, *Surgeons' Instruments*, Pardon & Sons (1891)

H. MacNaughton Jones, *A Practical Manual of Disease of Women and Uterine Therapeutics*, Bailliére, Tindall and Cox (1894)

H. MacNaughton Jones, *Practical Manual of Disease of Women*, Bailliére, Tindall, and Cox (1885)

Fielding Ould, *A Treatise of Midwifery in three Parts* (1742)

J. A. Paris. *Pharmacologia; comprehending The Art of Prescribing*, W. Phillips (1822)

Edith, L. Potter, *Rh...It's Relation to Congenital Hemolytic Disease & to Intragroup Transfusion*, The Year Book Publishers (1947)

Howard Riley Raper, *Man Against Pain*, Prentice Hall (1945)

William Rhind, *A History of the Vegetable Kingdom*, Blackie & Son (1870)

Sir Humphrey Rolleston & Alan Moncrieff (eds) *Essentials of Modern Chemotherapy*, Eyre & Spottiswoode (1941)

Eucharius Rösslin, *Der Schwangern Frauen und Hebammen Rosengarten*, M. Flkach, Jr. (1513)

Thomas Raynold, *The Byrth of Mankynde*, Tho. Ray (1545)

Jacob Rueff, *The Expert Midwife or An Excellent and most necessary Treatise on the generation and byrth of Man*, E. Griffin (1637)

William Smellie, *A Treatise on the Theory and Practice of Midwifery*, D. W. Wilson (1752)

Society of Gentlemen in Scotland, *Encyclopedia Britannica*, Vol. 1, Bell MacFarquhar (1771)

Marie Carmichael Stopes, *Contraception, It's Theory, History and Practice – A Manual for the Medical and Legal Professions*, John Bale, Sons & Danielsson, Ltd. (1924)

The Surgical Manufacturing Co. Ltd., *Catalogue of Surgical Instruments and Appliances, etc.*, The Surgical Manufacturing Co. Ltd. (1925)

Herbert Thomas, *Classical Contributions to Obstetrics and Gynecology*, Charles C. Thomas (1935)

Clifford White, Frank Cook & William Gilliat, *Midwifery*, Edward Arnold & Co. (1948)

J. Whitridge Williams, Obstetrics, *A Text-Book for the use of Students and Practitioners*, D. Appleton & Co. (1911)

Index

Printed and bound by CPI Group (UK) Ltd, Croydon, CR0 4YY
23/10/2024
01778254-0019